EMERGENCY CARE

EMERGENCY CARE

THE FIRST 24 HOURS

Catherine M. O'Boyle, R.N., M.A., C.E.N.
Associate Director, Emergency Services
Bellevue Hospital Medical Center
New York, New York

D. Karl Davis, R.N., Ed.D.
Associate Professor of Nursing
Hunter College–Bellevue School of Nursing
New York, New York

Barbara Ann Russo, R.N., M.Ed.
Associate Professor of Nursing
Hunter College–Bellevue School of Nursing
New York, New York

Terri J. Kraf, R.N., M.A., C.E.N.
Assistant Director, Emergency Services
Bellevue Hospital Medical Center
New York, New York

with a contribution by

Pamela D. Brick, M.S.
Assistant Research Scientist
Department of Immunology
    and Infectious Diseases
New York University
New York, New York

 APPLETON-CENTURY-CROFTS/Norwalk, Connecticut

Copyright © 1985 by Appleton-Century-Crofts
A Publishing Division of Prentice-Hall, Inc.

85 86 87 88 89 90/10 9 8 7 6 5 4 3 2

Prentice-Hall International, Inc., London
Prentice-Hall of Australia, Pty. Ltd., Sydney
Prentice-Hall Canada, Inc.
Prentice-Hall of India Private Limited, New Delhi
Prentice-Hall of Japan, Inc., Tokyo
Prentice-Hall of Southeast Asia (Pte.) Ltd., Singapore
Whitehall Books Ltd., Wellington, New Zealand
Editora Prentice-Hall do Brasil Ltda., Rio de Janeiro
Prentice-Hall Hispanoamericana, S.A., Mexico

Library of Congress Cataloging in Publication Data
Main entry under title:

Emergency care.

  Includes index.
  1. Emergency medicine.   I. O'Boyle, Catherine M.
[DNLM: 1. Critical Care.   2. Emergencies. WB 105 E5325]
RC86.7.E565   1985   616'.025   84-28441
ISBN 0-8385-2188-6

Design: Jean M. Sabato-Morley

PRINTED IN THE UNITED STATES OF AMERICA

This book is dedicated to
emergency care physicians and nurses everywhere,
to the ones who will follow them,
and in particular to those at Bellevue Hospital

CONTENTS

PREFACE

The purpose of this clinical text is to present succinct assessment parameters and suggested therapeutic modalities in the care of the emergency patient during the first 24 hours. Despite a diversity of settings and personnel, the requisite skills for acute emergency care are universal and quality emergency care is no longer limited to urban centers. We recognize that emergency department personnel are in a unique position to offer quality care that may significantly decrease morbidity and mortality. Furthermore, we believe that a collaborative team approach is the only effective way to provide this quality care, and therefore we have recognized the contributions of each team member—paramedic, nurse, and physician.

This text is intended to be a practical and theoretical book for emergency department personnel who are frequently confronted with the need to rapidly assess and manage acutely ill patients. The text is an attempt to assemble clinical information that will assist emergency personnel to better understand, recognize, and manage common emergency situations that are considered life-threatening. People differ in their opinion as to what is life-threatening. Some readers will find omissions whereas others will wonder why a topic is included. The authors have tried to include those emergencies considered life-threatening that are most frequently seen in an active urban emergency department.

Existing texts on emergency care nursing are primarily two dimensional, covering only signs and symptoms, and treatment. This text differs from others in that the format facilitates the identification of assessment parameters and therapeutic modalities with the option of retrospective review of pathophysiology underlying the assessment findings and the rationale supporting the therapeutic modalities. We assume that the reader has a basic understanding of anatomy, physiology, psychology, pharmacology, pathology, and physical assessment.

The uniqueness of this text is found also in its functional and conceptual approach. The text is divided into four sections. Section One serves as the foundation for the remainder of the book and provides an in-depth look at triage, assessment, and priority setting. In addition, because the clinical nurse is often working with an unknown, the use of algorithms is introduced to assist in establishing priorities and interventions in the emergency care of the acutely ill. Section Two presents both general and specific information related to shock syndromes and identifies differentiating assessment parameters and therapeutic modalities for treating those syndromes. The third section, the largest in the book, gives clear, concise, and complete presentations of a broad range of systemic emergencies including multisystem emergencies. The fourth section provides basic information related to administration and risk management and presents insights on such topics as medicolegal issues, communication, and documentation needs. Concluding the book are appendices rich in valuable information for all health care personnel.

We present this text in the hope that it will amplify present knowledge and understanding and increase clinical expertise in the most rewarding and challenging area—that of emergency care.

EMERGENCY CARE

SECTION ONE

TRIAGE

1. Triage Assessment Guide and Basic Triage

Recent trends indicate that there is an increased community reliance on the services of the emergency department. This has overburdened emergency department resources and has vastly compounded the difficulties of providing effective critical care to the emergency victim. In 1958, the nation's hospitals reported 18 million patient-visits to the emergency department; in 1968 the figure was 44 million and in 1977 it rose to 76 million. Health care has become an expensive commodity without concomitant improvement in health care. For the past 40 years, whereas the population of this country has increased by 53 million, the number of primary care physicians has remained static at about 120,000.

There is greater public sophistication and knowledge of health care practice and increasing confidence in and awareness of the hospital as an appropriate resource for primary as well as emergency health care. Many patients indicate a preference for using the emergency department because of its availability and convenience. Emergency services have become community health centers largely as a result of the decreased number of physicians practicing in the field of primary care, greater emphasis on specialization, and the unavailability of private practitioners during the evening hours and weekends, as well as the accessibility of the hospital around the clock, 7 days a week. Only the hospital is capable of providing the comprehensive sophisticated tools necessary to provide quality patient care.

With the increasing demand for emergency care, systems had to be developed to cope with the ever-burgeoning number of people presenting for emergency care. Triage, literally translated, sorting or selecting, was coined during the Napoleonic War (1812) because of the large numbers of casualties. Most contemporary emergency departments have instituted triage systems in order to rapidly assess and prioritize care in often congested waiting areas.

Currently, various triage systems utilize professional staff including nurses and physicians, paramedical staff such as physician assistants, and ancillary staff including clerks. Patient volume will determine which systems are most viable for a particular community. Effective triage implies that there must be viable alternatives within or near the emergency department to provide appropriate and expeditious treatment, particularly in high volume settings. It makes little sense to utilize a triage system if the only option available is that all patients, regardless of the severity of their illness, are treated in the emergency department. This can only lead to chaos, confusion, and interminable delays, not only for the acutely ill but also for those whose condition might be compromised without immediate medical attention. An outpatient department and/or a convenience clinic is essential and should emcompass some of the evening hours in order to meet the needs of the community. Effective triage is the cornerstone upon which an emergency department is built, and the portal of entry into the health care system.

The patients' initial experience in the emergency department can positively or negatively impact on their perception of the entire hospital. First impressions all too often are lasting impressions. The chaotic nature of the emergency department can be less frightening to the patient and his or her family when the triage nurse exhibits concern and interest. Privacy should be provided during the interview, examination, and treatment. Information regarding the process of care should be conveyed to the patient so that there is some reasonable expectation regarding the waiting time anticipated. A sign, prominently displayed, should inform the public that patients are seen relative to the acuteness of their illness or injury and not in a sequential fashion. The services rendered may also represent a necessary delay, and parameters for diagnostic testing and consultation should be explained.

It would be beneficial for some member of the staff to act as a liaison between the patient, the family, and the professional staff. Anxious family members are often overlooked in the haste of providing care to the acutely ill or injured patient. The few minutes necessary to reassure the family is an investment that will result in decreased anxiety as well as conveying a sense of caring.

TEN COMMANDMENTS OF EMERGENCY HEALTH CARE

1. Initial efforts should be directed toward airway, breathing, and circulation
2. All patients with head injury should be suspected of having concomitant spinal cord injury. The head and neck should be immobilized
3. Splint all suspected fractures
4. Critically ill appearing patients, regardless of the data, should receive priority in care
5. When in doubt, always up-triage
6. Attempt to identify the mechanism of injury
7. Apply ice to all strains and sprains to decrease swelling
8. Isolate all suspected infections or communicable diseases
9. All patients presenting for care must be seen by a physician and cared for in accord with the medical needs
10. Always be a patient advocate

TRIAGE ASSESSMENT GUIDE

If the patient arrives unconscious, use all available resources to elicit the nature of the emergency. Question friends, relatives, police, and ambulance personnel, in an effort to ascertain any history of prior illness, maintenance medications, allergies, or any emergency treatment rendered at the scene that may influence and modify management. As soon as the patient is correctly identified, affix an identification band to the patient's wrist. Proper identification will minimize the risk of error as patients frequently spend many hours in the emergency department before a disposition is made. This will not only facilitate patient flow, but will protect the patient and staff who are responsible for the care. It is also a legal and moral responsibility to protect all patient valuables, particularly for those patients who are unable to because of physical limitation of senility, confusion, disorientation, or intoxication. All valuables should be secured until the patient is either discharged or is able to assume responsibility for the property. Look for Medic-Alert tags which provide valuable information about the patient and any conditions or illnesses which might require immediate emergency intervention. If the patient is conscious, take a brief history including onset of, duration of, and associated symptoms. What precipitated the attack, what is the nature of the pain, does it radiate, and is it colicky, constant, localized to one area? The interviewer's appearance, attitude, and pattern of questioning will affect the patient's response. Allow the patient to express the problem, in his or her own words. Learn to develop an objective and nonjudgmental approach. Eye contact is a valuable method of controlling the interview situation. It establishes a sense of communication with the patient and conveys your interest. By watching the patient's response to questioning, the nurse can see if the patient understands what is being asked. Open-ended questions should be asked so that the patient will elaborate on various aspects of the illness or injury. Information not elicited with open-ended questioning must be obtained or refined through direct questioning. Try to focus on the immediate presenting problem and, should the patient wander too far afield, you may have to interrupt and redirect the line of questioning. The nurse should frame questions in understandable language and carefully weigh the value and reliability of the elicited responses.

At the conclusion of the interview, a rapid, and systematic assessment should be made. The purpose of this assessment is to record any deviations from the norm as they might provide helpful clues to the physician in determining diagnosis and treatment. This assessment will be performed at several different levels depending on the volume of patients being processed. When there is high volume utilization, basic triage will be performed which will encompass a rapid, systematic assessment in order to maximize the nurses' intervention skills. When there is low volume utilization, advanced triage utilizing clinical and diagnostic protocols will be used.

BASIC TRIAGE

The most valuable tool that the nurse possesses is his or her ability to accurately assess the patient's injury, and this involves the use of the senses of touch, sight, smell, and hearing.

- Sight: quality of respiration, unusual chest movements, obvious bleeding, color of skin and mucus membranes, cyanosis, and any disruption of the thoracic structure

- Touch: palpable disruption of bones, crepitus, localized area of pain, position of trachea, and carotid pulses
- Smell: odor of alcohol, urea, acetone, etc.
- Hearing: quality and volume of lung and heart sounds, gurgling, wheezing, and rasping sounds
- General: orientation, coordination, gross motor function, level of consciousness, and presence of other serious injuries

2. Systems Assessment

NEUROLOGIC ASSESSMENT

1. Conscious state which includes:
   a. Alertness
   b. Orientation
   c. Cognition (i.e., arithmetic computation)
   d. Memory
   e. Affect
   f. Perception
2. Respiratory pattern as judged by type and character of respirations
3. Pupils—size and reactivity
4. Extraocular movements (position at rest), voluntary movements, calorics
5. Motor activity which includes nonspecific findings, such as snout reflex, decorticate posturing, decerebrate posturing, hemiparesis, or seizure. Specific findings include tremor, asterixis
6. Vision—blurring, diplopia, and ocular pain should be noted
7. Headache—onset, localization, and intensity should be noted
8. Adequate cranial nerve function

Cranial Nerve	Patient Response
Olfactory (I)	Responds to pungent odors
Optic (II)	Can see to count fingers
Oculomotor (III)	No ptosis of eyelids; pupil equal and react to light
Trochlear, abducens (IV, VI)	Move eyes in all directions
Trigeminal (V)	Corneal reflex; feels tongue blade on oral mucosa
Facial (VII)	Smile and frown
Acoustic (VIII)	Can hear; answers questions
Glossopharyngeal (IX)	Gag reflex
Vagus (X)	Normal pulse rate
Spinal accessory (XI)	Shrugs shoulders
Hypoglossal (XII)	Sticks out and moves tongue

RESPIRATORY ASSESSMENT

1. Respiratory rate
   a. Apnea—absence or cessation of breathing
   b. Tachypnea—rapid breathing; respiratory rate of 20 or more per minute
   c. Bradypnea—slow breathing; respiratory rate of 10 or less per minute
2. Character of respirations
   a. Biot's or meningeal—total irregular and unpredictable respirations characterized by variations in depth of respirations, which are interrupted by pauses varying from 10 to 30 seconds
   b. Cheyne–Stokes—respiration in which there are rhythmic variations in intensity occurring in cycles (a cycle consisting of a period of increase in depth, then a decrease in depth, and then a period of apnea)
   c. Dyspnea—difficult, labored, or painful respirations
   d. Gurgling, rattling, or cracking sounds—caused by the passage of air through mucus or fluid in the large airways
   e. Hyperpnea—increased depth of respirations
   f. Pursed lip breathing—pathognomic of emphysema patients who purse their lips during exhalation to control the velocity of the expiratory effort
   g. Shallow—respirations in which the lungs are not fully expanded and with minimal movement of the chest cage; frequently indicative of physiologic splinting associated with pain
   h. Shortness of breath—rapid and shallow respiration
   i. Sighing—audible and prolonged inspirations followed by short expirations
   j. Stertorous—respirations which are noisy or snoring in character
   k. Stridor—harsh crowing sounds on inspiration, using accessory muscles producing a visible straining of the neck muscles
   l. Wheezing—whistling sounds heard either during inspiration or expiration
3. Changes in position or increased activity
   a. Can the patient lie flat in bed comfortably? How many pillows are used to sleep?
   b. Orthopnea—inability to breathe comfortably while supine
   c. Preferred position— preference for one side or the other may explain the localization of pathologic processes
   d. Dyspnea on exertion (DOE)—does the patient experience difficulty breathing with increased activity?
4. Persistent cough
   a. Onset
   b. Productive or nonproductive
   c. Presence of sputum—volume, color, odor, viscosity

CARDIOVASCULAR ASSESSMENT

1. Check neck veins for distention (i.e., congestive heart failure, cardiac tamponade)

2. Check temporal, carotid, brachial, radial, femoral, popliteal, dorsal pedal, and posterior tibial pulses for character and symmetry
3. Pulse Rate
   a. Bradycardia—pulse rate of 60 or less beats per minute
   b. Pulsus paradoxus—an exaggerated weakening of the pulse during normal inspiration; a cardinal sign of cardiac tamponade
   c. Running—a pulse rate so rapid that it is difficult or impossible to count
   d. Thready, weak, feeble—pulsations which have a decrease in volume and are very fine and scarcely perceptible
4. Regularity of pulse (dysrhythmias)
   a. Regular—separated by equal intervals of time
   b. Irregularly irregular—totally unequal time intervals between each beat (i.e., atrial fibrillation)
   c. Regularly irregular—a distinct pattern to the irregularity (i.e., atrial or ventricular trigeminy or bigeminy)
5. Pain (chest or referred pain, i.e., left arm, jaw, etc.)
   a. Location
   b. Description
   c. Precipitating factors
   d. Associated symptoms
6. Clubbing of digits—may be indicative of congenital heart disease, bacterial endocarditis, advanced cor pulmonale or inherited
7. Pitting edema—a common sign of congestive heart failure
8. Thrombophlebitis—pain, tenderness, erythema, and edema of the lower extremities
9. Acute arterial occlusion—agonizing pain in the affected extremity, which below the occlusion site is pale, cyanotic, and pulseless

GASTROINTESTINAL ASSESSMENT

1. If patient is vomiting, note the amount, color, and consistency of the material, i.e., coffee ground appearance of upper GI bleeding
2. Facial expression—note whether the patient appears relaxed, tense, or in pain
3. Abdomen—palpate for spasm, tenderness, guarding, rigidity, or distention
4. Nutritional state—outward signs of nutritional state may indirectly reflect GI function, i.e., starvation, alcoholism
5. Hydration—because serious fluid loss may accompany GI disease, the state of hydration is important
6. Skin—note jaundice, pallor, pigmentation
7. Bowel habits—check for constipation, diarrhea, form and color of stool, e.g., clay colored, tarry, fresh blood present
8. Mouth—check lips, oral mucosa, teeth, gingiva, and tongue
9. Pain
   a. Referred pain—upper abdominal or lower thoracic lesions producing irrita-

tion of the diaphragm often cause pain in the region of the distribution of the fourth cervical nerve

   b. Colicky pain—paroxysmal and excruciating pain exhibited by restlessness. The patient will frequently present with the knees drawn up to the chest

GENITOURINARY ASSESSMENT

1. Note the following on urination
    a. Frequency
    b. Urgency
    c. Dysuria
    d. Hematuria
    e. Incontinence
    f. Nocturia
    g. Pain
    h. Difficulty initiating stream
    i. History of previous UTIs, passing of stones, and venereal disease (history or active)

GYNECOLOGIC ASSESSMENT

1. Ascertain menstrual history—note any changes in cycle (increased or diminished blood flow)
2. Vaginal discharge—type, amount, and character
3. Venereal disease (history or active)
4. Method of birth control—oral or intrauterine devices
5. Bleeding—mild, moderate, severe (can usually be ascertained by noting how many sanitary napkins or tampons are needed to control flow)
    a. Menorrhagia—abnormally profuse menstruation
    b. Metrorrhagia—bleeding between periods
6. Pain—location, onset, duration (Mittelschmerz can be suspected by severe, recurrent pain in midcycle in women with regular menstrual cycle)

3. Initial Trauma Assessment

1. Complete and rapid assessment to establish a baseline to which signs and symptoms can be compared
    a. Evaluation regarding history of unconsciousness or posttraumatic amnesia.
    b. Check orientation to person, place, and time
    c. Palpate scalp for evidence of laceration, depression, or fracture

    d. Pupil size, symmetry, reaction, and accommodation to light. If the pupils are equal after the injury, then one pupil starts to dilate—there is evidence of a progressive lesion and immediate emergency intervention must take place. Systolic hypertension and/or bradycardia will be demonstrated

    e. Note response to painful stimuli and movement of extremities

    f. Observe for:
      Battle sign—ecchymosis behind the ears
      Raccoon eyes—orbital ecchymoses
      Rhinorrhea—spinal fluid from the nose
      Otorrhea—spinal fluid from the ear
      All of the above are signs of possible skull fracture

    g. Check for loose or maloccluded teeth which might be aspirated

    h. Examine the neck for pain, tenderness, muscle spasm, deformity, crepitus venous distention, or displacement of the trachea

    i. Check for splinting, asymmetry, or paradoxical respiration, which might lead to airway obstruction

    j. Blunt injuries to the thoracic wall (automobile steering wheel) may result in aortic rupture and may be suspected where there is a difference in pulse amplitude between the upper and lower extremities

    k. Palpate the ribs, noting crepitus, and identify the site of injury—rib fractures elicit pain on inspiration with a voluntary restriction of respiratory activity on the affected side

    l. Observe for traumatic flail chest which can be identified when the mobile portion of the chest wall moves paradoxically, being sucked in with inspiration and expanding outward with expiration

    m. Fracture of the sternum produces severe pain and the patient may be noted to breathe shallowly with the head and neck held forward rigidly. Inspection of the area may reveal evidence of depression and ecchymosis over the fracture site

    n. Gently palpate the spine for tenderness or muscle spasm

    o. Decreased sensation to touch or temperature, and an inability to move the extremities

    p. The spleen, liver, stomach, intestines, and pancreas are vulnerable to blunt injury. Frequent examination of the abdomen is essential to discover early signs of injury. Palpate the abdomen for spasm, tenderness, guarding, rigidity, and distention. Note facial expression. Is the patient relaxed, tense, or in pain? Early signs of splenic rupture might include tachycardia and abdominal tenderness

    q. Examine the pulses bilaterally in the neck and in the upper and lower extremities. Deviations of pulse, color, temperature, and sensory perception of opposite upper or lower extremities should be noted. The most accurate sign of major vessel damage is distal pulselessness

    r. A patient should be suspected of having a fracture when there is complaint of localized pain and loss of function, swelling, tenderness, deformity, muscle spasm, ecchymosis, or crepitation. It is important that an accurate account of the mechanism of injury be established. This information, coupled with a knowledge of patterns of damage commonly encountered, may be helpful in the diagnosis. All patients with suspected fractures should not be allowed food or fluids in the event that surgery is necessary

4. Advanced Triage

Emergency care can be facilitated if the triage nurse is permitted to initiate diagnostic testing. The use of clinical algorithms or operational protocols provides a logical system approach for the nurse to evaluate the ill or injured patient. These clinical assessment pathways are designed to lead the nurse through sequential decisions of appropriate diagnostic, therapeutic, and/or dispositional actions. Clinical algorithms have two primary advantages in the assessment process: (1) to identify and refer any patient with an acute problem for immediate medical intervention, and (2) to assist in the differential diagnosis and treatment of the patient. These operational protocols must be done under the supervision of a physician after approval by appropriate medical, nursing, and administrative personnel.

Because the triage nurse is most often dealing with an unknown etiology, the clinical algorithm will prove most helpful in determining a course of action. In the instance that the disease entity is well known and established, the disease-specific protocols will assist in the initial management.

5. Clinical Algorithms

For a definition of terms and abbreviations used in these algorithms, refer to pp. 67–68, following the clinical algorithms.

ABDOMINAL PAIN

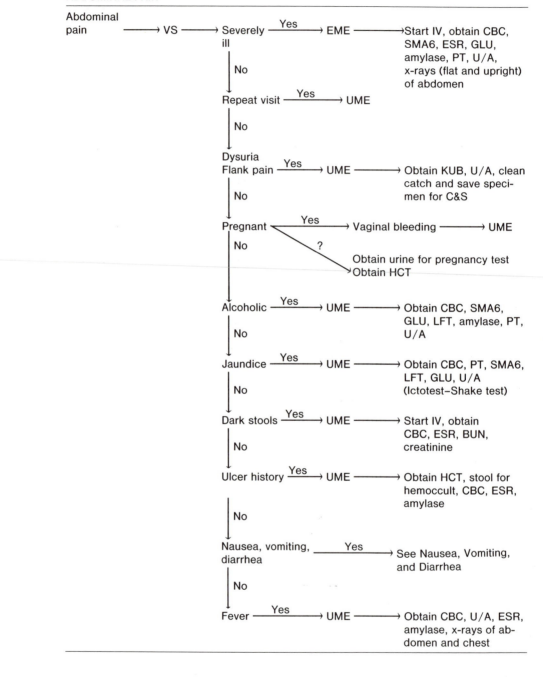

Abdominal pain ⟶ VS ⟶ Severely ill ——Yes——→ EME ⟶ Start IV, obtain CBC, SMA6, ESR, GLU, amylase, PT, U/A, x-rays (flat and upright) of abdomen

No ↓

Repeat visit ——Yes——→ UME

No ↓

Dysuria Flank pain ——Yes——→ UME ⟶ Obtain KUB, U/A, clean catch and save specimen for C&S

No ↓

Pregnant ——Yes——→ Vaginal bleeding ⟶ UME

No ↓   ?

Obtain urine for pregnancy test
Obtain HCT

Alcoholic ——Yes——→ UME ⟶ Obtain CBC, SMA6, GLU, LFT, amylase, PT, U/A

No ↓

Jaundice ——Yes——→ UME ⟶ Obtain CBC, PT, SMA6, LFT, GLU, U/A (Ictotest–Shake test)

No ↓

Dark stools ——Yes——→ UME ⟶ Start IV, obtain CBC, ESR, BUN, creatinine

No ↓

Ulcer history ——Yes——→ UME ⟶ Obtain HCT, stool for hemoccult, CBC, ESR, amylase

No ↓

Nausea, vomiting, diarrhea ——Yes——→ See Nausea, Vomiting, and Diarrhea

No ↓

Fever ——Yes——→ UME ⟶ Obtain CBC, U/A, ESR, amylase, x-rays of abdomen and chest

ABDOMINAL PAIN: PEDIATRIC

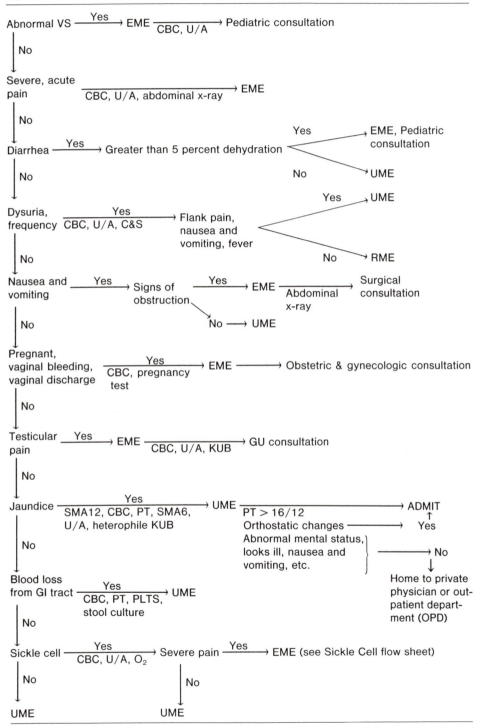

Abnormal VS ———Yes———→ EME $\overrightarrow{CBC, U/A}$ Pediatric consultation

No

Severe, acute
pain $\overrightarrow{CBC, U/A, abdominal x-ray}$ EME

No

Diarrhea ——Yes——→ Greater than 5 percent dehydration
                                  Yes → EME, Pediatric consultation
                                  No → UME

No

Dysuria,
frequency $\overrightarrow{CBC, U/A, C\&S}$ ——Yes——→ Flank pain, nausea and vomiting, fever
            Yes → UME
            No → RME

No

Nausea and
vomiting ——Yes——→ Signs of obstruction ——Yes——→ EME $\overrightarrow{Abdominal x-ray}$ Surgical consultation
                                No ——→ UME

No

Pregnant,
vaginal bleeding,
vaginal discharge $\overrightarrow{CBC, pregnancy test}$ ——Yes——→ EME ———→ Obstetric & gynecologic consultation

No

Testicular
pain ——Yes——→ EME $\overrightarrow{CBC, U/A, KUB}$ GU consultation

No

Jaundice $\overrightarrow{SMA12, CBC, PT, SMA6, U/A, heterophile KUB}$ ——Yes——→ UME

PT > 16/12 ————————————————→ ADMIT
Orthostatic changes ————————→ ↑ Yes
Abnormal mental status,
looks ill, nausea and } —————————→ No
vomiting, etc.
                                 ↓
                    Home to private physician or out-patient depart-ment (OPD)

No

Blood loss
from GI tract $\overrightarrow{CBC, PT, PLTS, stool culture}$ ——Yes——→ UME

No

Sickle cell $\overrightarrow{CBC, U/A, O_2}$ ——Yes——→ Severe pain ——Yes——→ EME (see Sickle Cell flow sheet)

No   No

UME   UME

THE ALCOHOLIC PATIENT

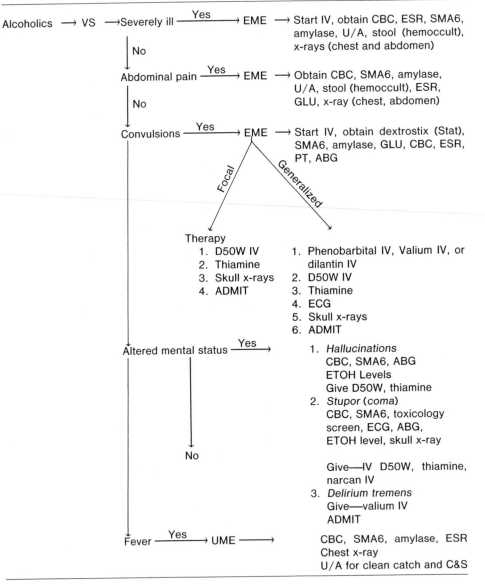

Alcoholics → VS → Severely ill ──Yes──→ EME → Start IV, obtain CBC, ESR, SMA6, amylase, U/A, stool (hemoccult), x-rays (chest and abdomen)

No

Abdominal pain ──Yes──→ EME → Obtain CBC, SMA6, amylase, U/A, stool (hemoccult), ESR, GLU, x-ray (chest, abdomen)

No

Convulsions ──Yes──→ EME → Start IV, obtain dextrostix (Stat), SMA6, amylase, GLU, CBC, ESR, PT, ABG

Focal / *Generalized*

Therapy
1. D50W IV
2. Thiamine
3. Skull x-rays
4. ADMIT

1. Phenobarbital IV, Valium IV, or dilantin IV
2. D50W IV
3. Thiamine
4. ECG
5. Skull x-rays
6. ADMIT

Altered mental status ──Yes──→

1. *Hallucinations*
   CBC, SMA6, ABG
   ETOH Levels
   Give D50W, thiamine
2. *Stupor (coma)*
   CBC, SMA6, toxicology screen, ECG, ABG, ETOH level, skull x-ray

   Give—IV D50W, thiamine, narcan IV
3. *Delirium tremens*
   Give—valium IV
   ADMIT

No

Fever ──Yes──→ UME ──→   CBC, SMA6, amylase, ESR
Chest x-ray
U/A for clean catch and C&S

ALTERED MENTAL STATUS

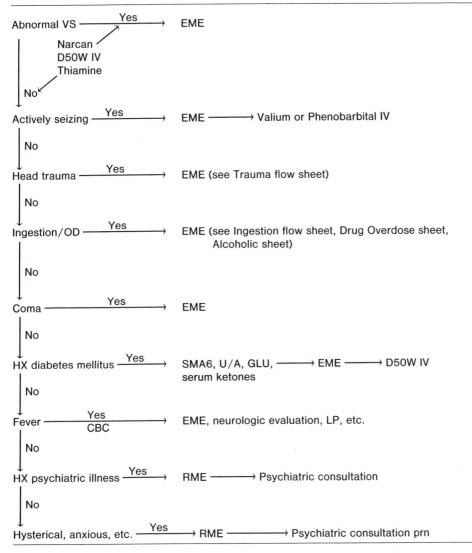

Abnormal VS ———Yes———→ EME

    Narcan
    D50W IV
    Thiamine

No

Actively seizing ———Yes———→ EME ———→ Valium or Phenobarbital IV

No

Head trauma ———Yes———→ EME (see Trauma flow sheet)

No

Ingestion/OD ———Yes———→ EME (see Ingestion flow sheet, Drug Overdose sheet, Alcoholic sheet)

No

Coma ———Yes———→ EME

No

HX diabetes mellitus ———Yes———→ SMA6, U/A, GLU, ———→ EME ———→ D50W IV
serum ketones

No

Fever ———Yes———→ EME, neurologic evaluation, LP, etc.
    CBC

No

HX psychiatric illness ———Yes———→ RME ———→ Psychiatric consultation

No

Hysterical, anxious, etc. ———Yes———→ RME ———→ Psychiatric consultation prn

PSYCHIATRIC ASSESSMENT

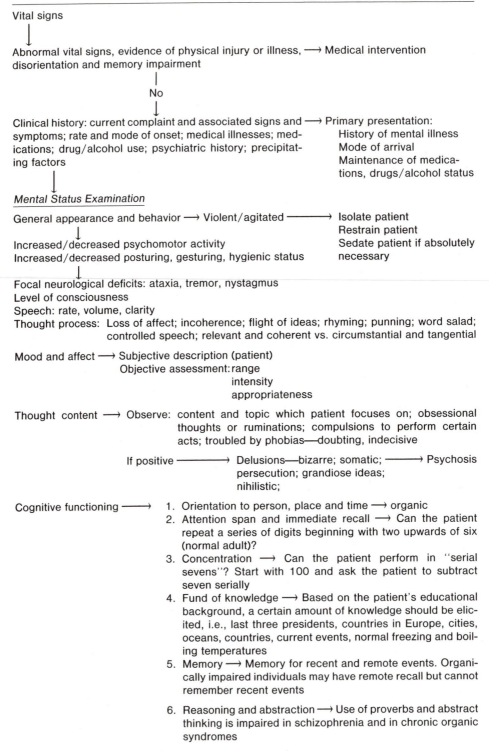

Vital signs

Abnormal vital signs, evidence of physical injury or illness, ⟶ Medical intervention
disorientation and memory impairment

No

Clinical history: current complaint and associated signs and ⟶ Primary presentation:
symptoms; rate and mode of onset; medical illnesses; med-
ications; drug/alcohol use; psychiatric history; precipitating factors

> History of mental illness
> Mode of arrival
> Maintenance of medica-
> tions, drugs/alcohol status

Mental Status Examination

General appearance and behavior ⟶ Violent/agitated ⟶ Isolate patient

Increased/decreased psychomotor activity
Increased/decreased posturing, gesturing, hygienic status

> Restrain patient
> Sedate patient if absolutely
> necessary

Focal neurological deficits: ataxia, tremor, nystagmus
Level of consciousness
Speech: rate, volume, clarity
Thought process: Loss of affect; incoherence; flight of ideas; rhyming; punning; word salad;
controlled speech; relevant and coherent vs. circumstantial and tangential

Mood and affect ⟶ Subjective description (patient)
Objective assessment: range
intensity
appropriateness

Thought content ⟶ Observe: content and topic which patient focuses on; obsessional
thoughts or ruminations; compulsions to perform certain
acts; troubled by phobias—doubting, indecisive

If positive ⟶ Delusions—bizarre; somatic; ⟶ Psychosis
persecution; grandiose ideas;
nihilistic;

Cognitive functioning ⟶
1. Orientation to person, place and time ⟶ organic
2. Attention span and immediate recall ⟶ Can the patient
   repeat a series of digits beginning with two upwards of six
   (normal adult)?
3. Concentration ⟶ Can the patient perform in "serial
   sevens"? Start with 100 and ask the patient to subtract
   seven serially
4. Fund of knowledge ⟶ Based on the patient's educational
   background, a certain amount of knowledge should be elicited, i.e., last three presidents, countries in Europe, cities,
   oceans, countries, current events, normal freezing and boil-
   ing temperatures
5. Memory ⟶ Memory for recent and remote events. Organi-
   cally impaired individuals may have remote recall but cannot
   remember recent events
6. Reasoning and abstraction ⟶ Use of proverbs and abstract
   thinking is impaired in schizophrenia and in chronic organic
   syndromes

Decreased level of
consciousness ⟶ History of alcohol, drug abuse, medical illness, medications
with psychiatric side effects

Abnormal physical findings—abnormal laboratory data, abnormal vital signs, tremor, rash, stiff neck, nystagmus, focal neurologic deficits, impaired cognitive functioning, hallucinations

Diagnosis ⟶ A. Organic

1. Drug/alcohol intoxication
2. Drug/alcohol withdrawal
3. Delirium
4. Dementia
5. Organic hallucinations
6. Organic affective syndrome
7. Organic delusional syndrome

B. Functional

Psychotic {
1. Schizophrenia—acute vs. chronic
2. Affective disorders—depressive
                              manic
                              bipolar
3. Paranoid disorders
4. Nonpsychotic disorders
      hysterical reactions—conversion symptoms, syncope, mutism
      grief reactions
      adjustment reactions
      character disorders
      anxiety disorders

Judgment ⟶ Assess patient's capacity for social judgment and decision
making

Insight ⟶ Patient's perceptions of his/her own limitations; patient's with
poor insight should be prime candidates for admission, as they
tend to be destructive and will not cooperate with plans for outpatient care

Differential diagnosis ⟶ 1. Acute vs. chronic schizophrenia
2. Neurologic impairment—cerebral lesion, seizure disorder
3. Acute drug toxicity (phencyclidine, amphetamines) vs. chronic phenothiazine therapy side effects
4. Medical emergencies—insulin shock, delirium tremens
5. Senile dementia, Alzheimer's disease
6. Mania
7. Depressive psychosis vs. neurosis

Admission criteria ⟶ Entire history, clinical picture, stress factors, degree of incapacitation, social support structure, and the benefits of hospitalization, should all be considered ⟶ No single symptom or diagnosis in and of itself justifies admission

1. *Acutely* psychotic—functional or organic
2. Actively suicidal or homicidal
3. Dangerous to self or others
4. Chronic illness decompensating
5. Moderate to severe impairment of functioning of recent onset

BACK PAIN

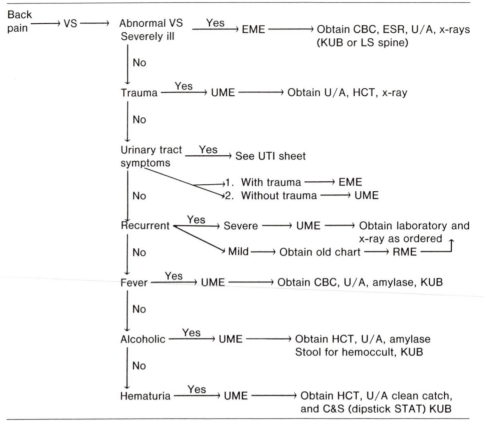

Back pain → VS → Abnormal VS Severely ill — Yes → EME → Obtain CBC, ESR, U/A, x-rays (KUB or LS spine)

No

Trauma — Yes → UME → Obtain U/A, HCT, x-ray

No

Urinary tract symptoms — Yes → See UTI sheet

No
1. With trauma → EME
2. Without trauma → UME

Recurrent — Yes → Severe → UME → Obtain laboratory and x-ray as ordered

No → Mild → Obtain old chart → RME

Fever — Yes → UME → Obtain CBC, U/A, amylase, KUB

No

Alcoholic — Yes → UME → Obtain HCT, U/A, amylase Stool for hemoccult, KUB

No

Hematuria — Yes → UME → Obtain HCT, U/A clean catch, and C&S (dipstick STAT) KUB

Therapy: IVs and/or analgesics as ordered while awaiting results of studies.

BURN

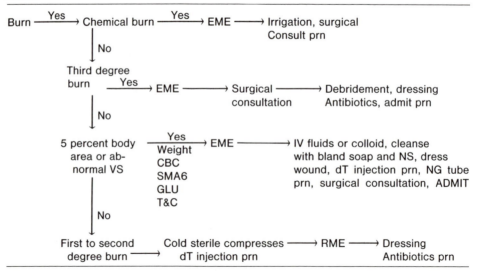

Burn — Yes → Chemical burn — Yes → EME → Irrigation, surgical Consult prn

No

Third degree burn — Yes → EME → Surgical consultation → Debridement, dressing Antibiotics, admit prn

No

5 percent body area or abnormal VS — Yes → EME → IV fluids or colloid, cleanse with bland soap and NS, dress wound, dT injection prn, NG tube prn, surgical consultation, ADMIT
Weight
CBC
SMA6
GLU
T&C

No

First to second degree burn → Cold sterile compresses dT injection prn → RME → Dressing Antibiotics prn

CHEST PAIN

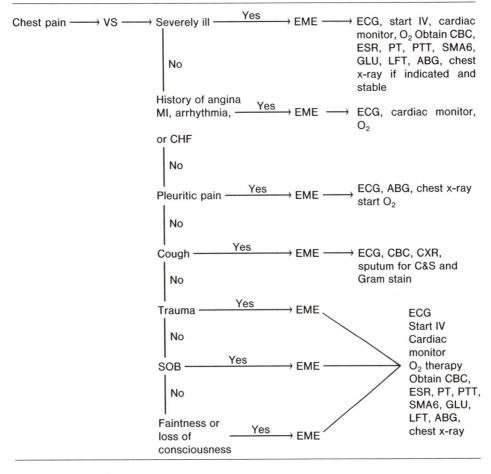

COMA

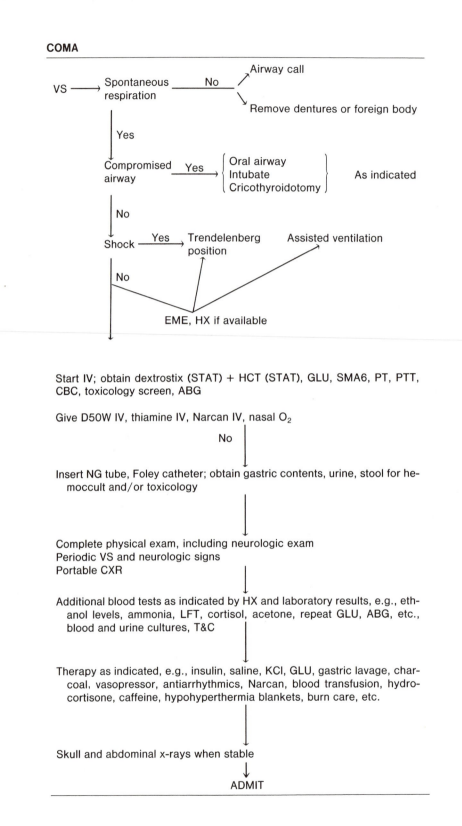

VS → Spontaneous respiration — No → Airway call

↘ Remove dentures or foreign body

↓ Yes

Compromised airway — Yes → { Oral airway / Intubate / Cricothyroidotomy } As indicated

↓ No

Shock — Yes → Trendelenberg position → Assisted ventilation

↓ No

EME, HX if available

Start IV; obtain dextrostix (STAT) + HCT (STAT), GLU, SMA6, PT, PTT, CBC, toxicology screen, ABG

Give D50W IV, thiamine IV, Narcan IV, nasal O_2

No

Insert NG tube, Foley catheter; obtain gastric contents, urine, stool for hemoccult and/or toxicology

Complete physical exam, including neurologic exam
Periodic VS and neurologic signs
Portable CXR

Additional blood tests as indicated by HX and laboratory results, e.g., ethanol levels, ammonia, LFT, cortisol, acetone, repeat GLU, ABG, etc., blood and urine cultures, T&C

Therapy as indicated, e.g., insulin, saline, KCl, GLU, gastric lavage, charcoal, vasopressor, antiarrhythmics, Narcan, blood transfusion, hydrocortisone, caffeine, hypohyperthermia blankets, burn care, etc.

Skull and abdominal x-rays when stable

↓

ADMIT

COMA: DIFFERENTIAL DIAGNOSIS

1. **With Focal Neurologic Deficit**
   Subdural hematoma, epidural hematoma
   Tumor
   Intracerebral bleed
   Abscess, cyst, hygroma
   Encephalitis
   Postictal
   Metabolic (increased or decreased glucose, hepatic encepha-
     lopathy, overdose, ingestion, carbon monoxide poisoning)

2. **Without Focal Neurologic Deficit**
   Subdural hematoma
   Subarachnoid hemorrhage
   Concussion
   Meningitis, encephalitis, CNS infections
   Postictal
   Metabolic (increased or decreased glucose, increased or de-
     creased sodium, uremia, hypoxia, acidosis, severe vitamin
     deficiency)
   Overdose, ingestion, carbon monoxide poisoning
   Hysteria
   Toxic encephalopathy (sepsis, typhoid, peritonitis, osteomyelitis,
     pneumonia, etc.)
   Arrhythmia
   Hypertensive encephalopathy

DIABETES MELLITUS

VS ⟶ abnormal VS —Yes→ EME ⟶ IV D25W
SMA6, GLU,   Pediatric consultation under age 15
U/A Urine
dipstick, | No
Dextrostix   ↓

Severely ill —Yes→ EME —Yes→ Comatose —Yes→ IV D50W → Further
ABG   abnormal   IV hydration   evaluation
CBC   affect,   Look for ke-
Weight   neurologic   toacidosis,
ECG   findings   hypoglyce-
Serum   mia, infec-
acetone | No   tion

| No
↓   Dehydrated —Yes→ IV hydration, further evalua-
                                                    tion

                              | No
                              ↓
                    Acidotic —Yes→ Follow ABG, lytes, serum, ace-
                                                    tone

                              | No
                              ↓
                    Febrile —Yes→ CBC, UA, CXR, urine C&S, etc.

Wants refill of medication —Yes→ Urine dipstick,
                                   prescription
| No
↓
Followed by private physician —Yes→ RME ⟶ Private physician
| No
↓
Family HX diabetes —Yes→ Polyuria, polydypsia, ⟶ RME
        mellitus   weight loss, recur-   Await
                          rent infections,   laboratory
                          enuresis, etc.   results

                              | No
                              ↓
                    Private physician or OPD

DIFFICULTY SWALLOWING

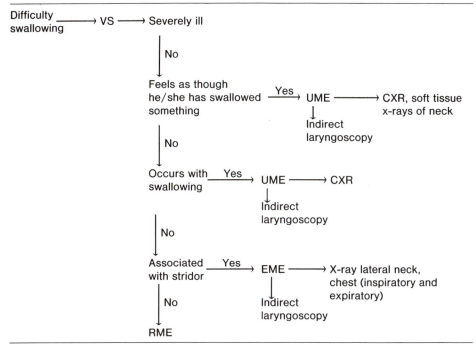

DRUG OVERDOSE

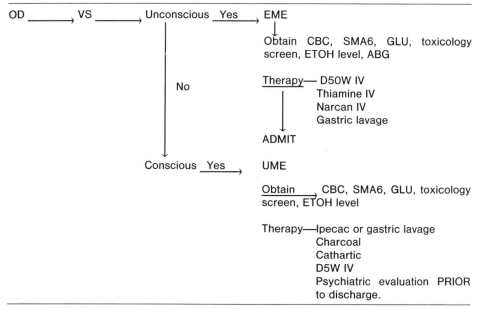

SHORTNESS OF BREATH

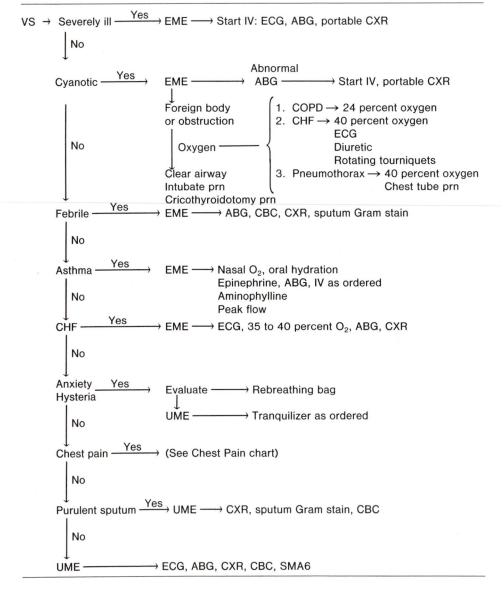

VS → Severely ill ——Yes——→ EME ——→ Start IV: ECG, ABG, portable CXR

│ No
↓

Cyanotic ——Yes——→ EME ——Abnormal——→ ABG ——→ Start IV, portable CXR

Foreign body
or obstruction

No   Oxygen ———

Clear airway
Intubate prn
Cricothyroidotomy prn

1. COPD → 24 percent oxygen
2. CHF → 40 percent oxygen
   ECG
   Diuretic
   Rotating tourniquets
3. Pneumothorax → 40 percent oxygen
   Chest tube prn

Febrile ——Yes——→ EME ——→ ABG, CBC, CXR, sputum Gram stain

│ No
↓

Asthma ——Yes——→ EME ——→ Nasal O_2, oral hydration
Epinephrine, ABG, IV as ordered
No   Aminophylline
Peak flow

CHF ——Yes——→ EME ——→ ECG, 35 to 40 percent O_2, ABG, CXR

│ No
↓

Anxiety ——Yes——→ Evaluate ——→ Rebreathing bag
Hysteria
            UME ——→ Tranquilizer as ordered
No

Chest pain ——Yes——→ (See Chest Pain chart)

│ No
↓

Purulent sputum ——Yes——→ UME ——→ CXR, sputum Gram stain, CBC

│ No
↓

UME ——————→ ECG, ABG, CXR, CBC, SMA6

RESPIRATORY DISTRESS: PEDIATRIC

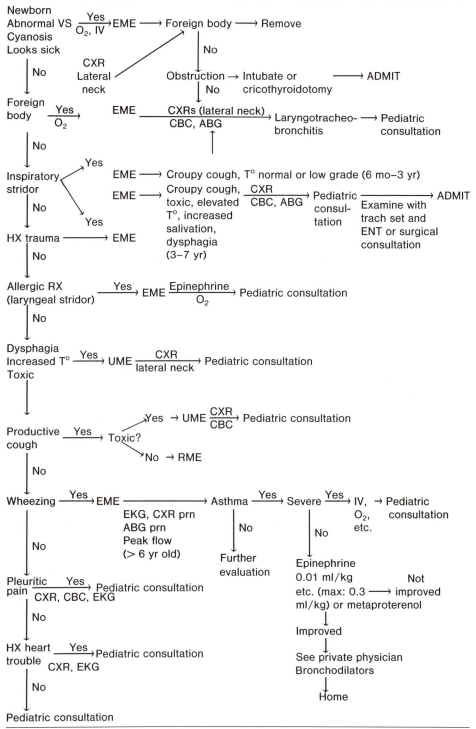

DIFFERENTIAL DIAGNOSIS: DYSPNEA

1. **Mechanical**
   Obstruction (foreign body, congenital malformations, inflammation, spasm)
   Elevation of diaphragm (e.g., ascites)
   Inadequacy of respiratory muscle (polio, myasthenia)
   Bony defects of thoracic cage
   Pleural effusion, pneumothorax, diaphragmatic hernia
   Pain in breathing (pleuritis, fractured ribs)
2. **Insufficient Oxygen Supply**
   Overexertion (including salicylate intoxication)
   Anemia
   High altitudes
   Cardiac failure
   Congenital heart disease
3. **Pulmonary Insufficiency**
   Distensibility (pulmonary congestion or fibrosis)
   Elasticity (e.g., emphysema)
   Pulmonary circulation
   Inflammation or infiltration of lungs
   Atelectasis
   Embolism
4. **Central Hyperventilation**
   Acidosis
   Drugs (e.g., ASA)
5. **Psychiatric**

DYSURIA, HEMATURIA, POLYURIA, NOCTURIA, ENURESIS, RETENTION

Abnormal VS $\xrightarrow{\text{Yes}}$ EME $\xrightarrow[\text{CBC, U/A}]{}$ Severe flank pain $\longrightarrow$ Analgesia
IV prn
KUB
Urology consultation

$\downarrow$ No

Febrile $\xrightarrow{\text{Yes}}$ Symptoms PN $\xrightarrow[\text{CBC, U/A}]{\text{Yes}}$ UME $\longrightarrow$ Compazine $\longrightarrow$?ADMIT
Severe nausea Urine C&S ASA
and vomiting SMA6, GLU KUB

$\downarrow$ No Toxic
Shaking chills

Hematuria $\xrightarrow[\text{U/A, BP, UME}]{\text{Yes}}$ HX trauma $\xrightarrow{\text{Yes}}$ KUB, IVP, Urology consultation
Weigh if child
HCT, CBC

$\downarrow$ No

Child with HX $\xrightarrow{\text{Yes}}$ Pediatric consultation
compatible with ADMIT
glomerulonephritis
high bp, edema

$\downarrow$ No No

Colicky pain $\xrightarrow{\text{Yes}}$ Analgesia $\longrightarrow$?IVP
KUB
$\downarrow$ No Urology consultation

Dysuria $\xrightarrow{\text{Yes}}$ U/A, Urine C&S

$\downarrow$ No

Frequency $\xrightarrow[\text{U/A}]{\text{Yes}}$ RME Clotting problem $\xrightarrow{\text{Yes}}$ PT, PTT, CBC
Dysuria

$\downarrow$ No

Polyuria or $\xrightarrow[\text{U/A}]{\text{Yes}}$ RME $\longrightarrow$ GLU in urine $\xrightarrow{\text{Yes}}$ Pediatric consultation or call private phy-
polydipsia, or blood sician or OPD
HX diabetes Blood
GLU

$\downarrow$ No $\downarrow$ No

Private physician for further W/U (SMA6, GTT, etc.)

Enuresis (evaluate for diabetes mellitus, $\longrightarrow$ Private physician referral (medical, pediat-
nocturnal seizures, UTI, DI) ric or urology)

$\downarrow$ No

Retention $\xrightarrow{\text{Yes}}$ EME, catheterize $\longrightarrow$ Urology consultation

$\downarrow$ No

Vaginal discharge $\xrightarrow{\text{Yes}}$ U/A clean catch or $\longrightarrow$ (See Vaginal Discharge sheet)
after perineal prep

DIFFERENTIAL DIAGNOSIS: HEMATURIA

Glomerulonephritis
Chronic nephritis
Vascular thrombosis
Renal tumor
Stones
Trauma
Foreign bodies
Cystitis
TB
SLE
Blood dyscrasias, sickle cell
Congenital abnormality

EYE

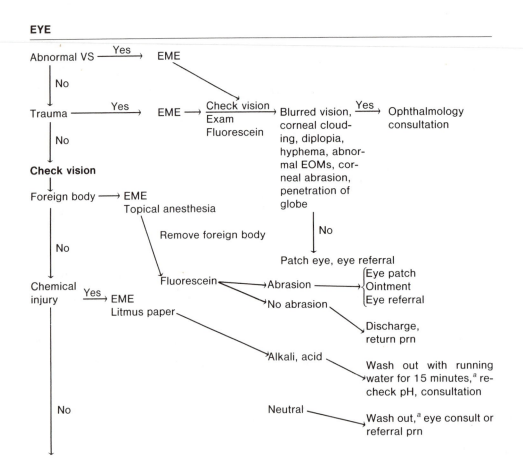

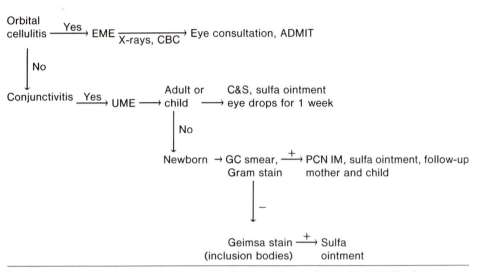

^a Wash out with running water for 15 minutes, then irrigate with normal saline for 30 to 60 minutes.

SIGNS OF INTRAOCULAR INJURY

Blood in anterior chamber (hyphema)
Distortion, dilatation, or paralysis of pupil
Shallow anterior chamber compared to
  other eye
Black fundal reflex
Gray shadows in fundus

28

EAR

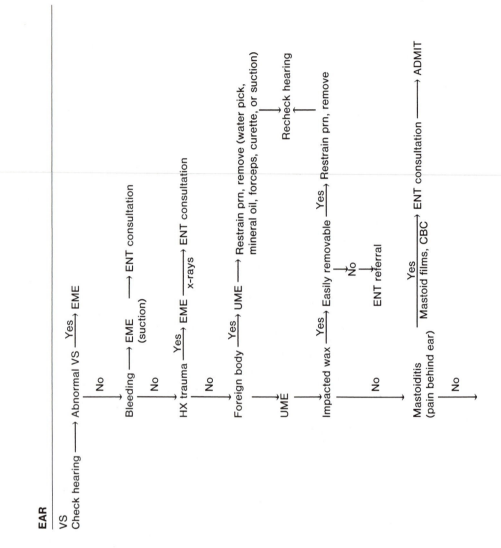

VS
Check hearing $\longrightarrow$ Abnormal VS $\xrightarrow{\text{Yes}}$ EME

$\downarrow$ No

Bleeding $\longrightarrow$ EME $\longrightarrow$ ENT consultation
(suction)

$\downarrow$ No

HX trauma $\xrightarrow{\text{Yes}}$ EME $\longrightarrow$ ENT consultation
x-rays

$\downarrow$ No

Foreign body $\xrightarrow{\text{Yes}}$ UME $\longrightarrow$ Restrain prn, remove (water pick, mineral oil, forceps, curette, or suction)

$\downarrow$ UME $\longrightarrow$ Recheck hearing

Impacted wax $\xrightarrow{\text{Yes}}$ Easily removable $\xrightarrow{\text{Yes}}$ Restrain prn, remove

$\downarrow$ No $\quad\quad\quad\quad$ $\downarrow$ No

$\quad\quad\quad\quad\quad\quad\quad$ ENT referral

$\downarrow$ No

Mastoiditis $\xrightarrow{\text{Yes}}$ Mastoid films, CBC $\longrightarrow$ ENT consultation $\longrightarrow$ ADMIT
(pain behind ear)

$\downarrow$ No

29

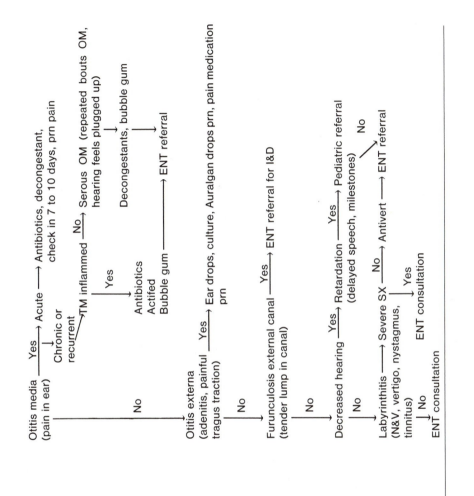

30

NOSE

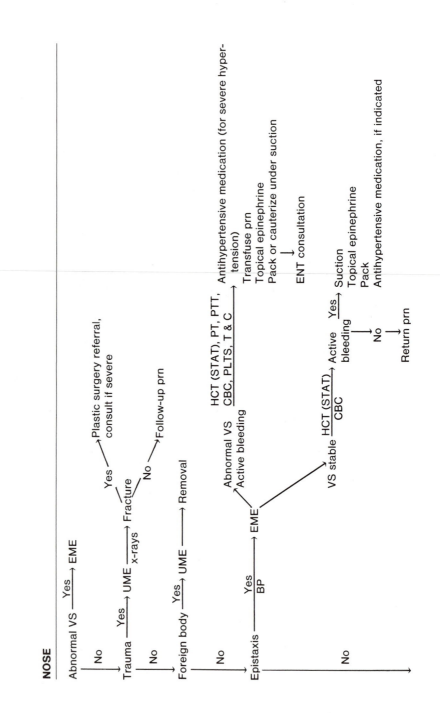

Abnormal VS — Yes → EME

No ↓

Trauma — Yes → UME — x-rays → Fracture — Yes → Plastic surgery referral, consult if severe
— No → Follow-up prn

No ↓

Foreign body — Yes → UME → Removal

No ↓

Epistaxis — Yes → EME

  BP

  → Abnormal VS / Active bleeding → HCT (STAT), PT, PTT, CBC, PLTS, T & C → Antihypertensive medication (for severe hyper-tension)
  Transfuse prn
  Topical epinephrine
  Pack or cauterize under suction
  → ENT consultation

  → VS stable → HCT (STAT) / CBC → Active bleeding — Yes → Suction
  Topical epinephrine
  Pack
  Antihypertensive medication, if indicated
  — No → Return prn

No →

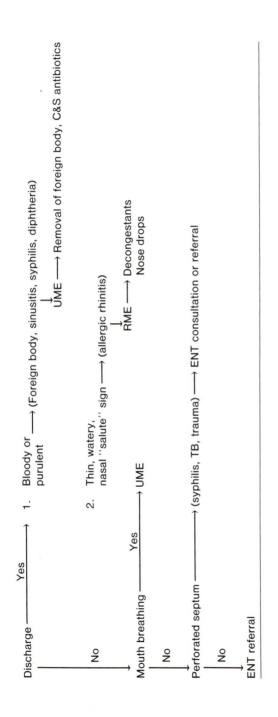

Discharge ——Yes——→ 1. Bloody or ——→ (Foreign body, sinusitis, syphilis, diphtheria)
                         purulent
                                    ↓
                                   UME ——→ Removal of foreign body, C&S antibiotics

                      2. Thin, watery,
                         nasal "salute" sign ——→ (allergic rhinitis)
                                                        ↓
                                                       RME ——→ Decongestants
                                                               Nose drops

         ——No——→ Mouth breathing ——Yes——→ UME

                              ——No——→ Perforated septum ——→ (syphilis, TB, trauma) ——→ ENT consultation or referral

                                                ——No——→ ENT referral

CAUSES OF EPISTAXIS

Adenoidal hypertrophy
Trauma
Allergic rhinitis
Sinusitis
Polyps
Infections—ARF, scarlet fever, measles,
  varicella, syphilis, diphtheria, typhoid
  fever
Telangiectasis
Blood dyscrasias
Hypertension

CAUSES OF MOUTH BREATHING

Adenoidal hypertrophy
Cystic fibrosis
Leukemia
Hypothyroidism
Deviated nasal septum
Polyps
Choanal atresia
Foreign body
URI
Bronchial asthma

THROAT

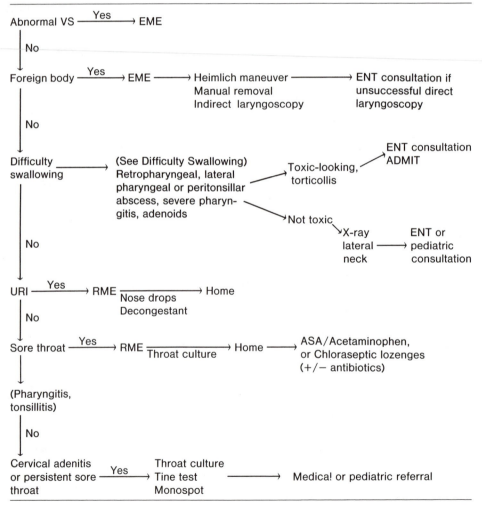

COUGH: ADULT

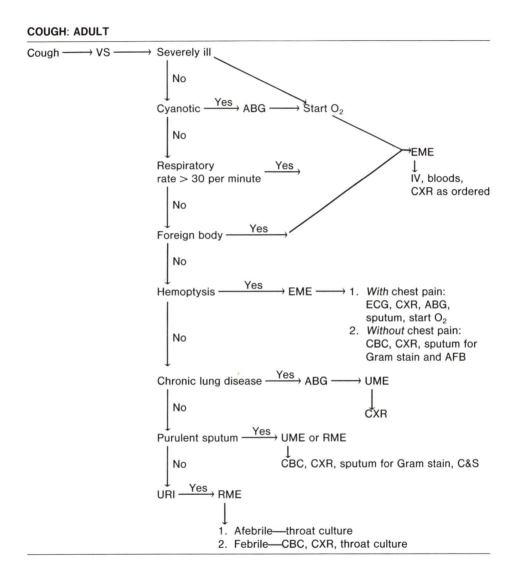

COUGH: PEDIATRIC

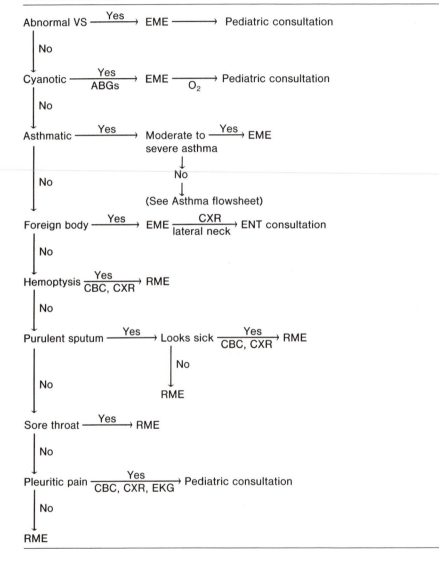

HEADACHE

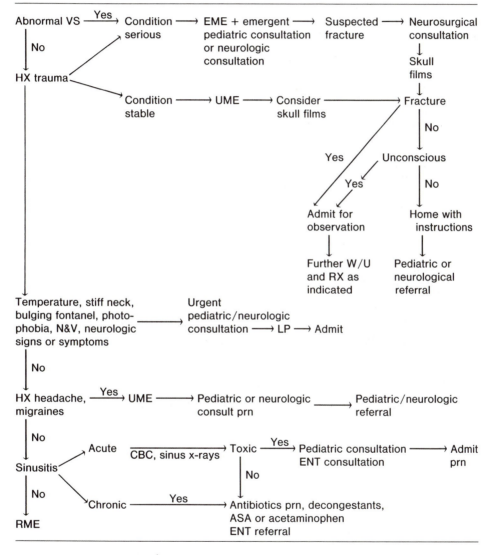

DIFFERENTIAL DIAGNOSIS: HEADACHE

I. Functional (tension)
II. Organic
   A. Vascular
      1. Hypertension
      2. Angioma, AV malformation
      3. Subarachnoid hemorrhage
   B. Mass lesion
      1. Tumors
      2. Brain abscess, cyst
      3. Subdural hematoma
   C. Infections
      1. Meningitis
      2. Encephalitis
      3. Sinusitis
      4. Other (e.g., tonsillitis, other febrile illnesses)
      5. Post LP
   D. Ocular
   E. Musculoskeletal
      1. Whiplash
      2. Head trauma
      3. Tension

Indications for Lumbar Puncture
1. Meningeal signs—nuchal rigidity, Kernig and Brudzinski signs
2. Full fontanel
3. Paradoxical irritability, e.g., infant who is irritable when picked up and quiet when on table
4. First seizure with or without fever
5. Infant less than 2 months with unexplained temperature or lethargy

HEART: PEDIATRIC

Abnormal VS $\xrightarrow{\text{Yes}}$ EME $\xrightarrow[\text{CXR}]{\text{ABG, ECG, IV,}}$ Pediatric consultation

    ↓ No

HX of ARF or $\xrightarrow{\text{Yes}}$ Fever $\xrightarrow[\text{ASO, CXR}]{\text{CBC, ECG, ESR,}}$ EME $\longrightarrow$ Pediatric consultation
congenital lesion   blood culture, TC,

                      ↓ No

  ↓ No   EME

Arthritis nodules $\xrightarrow[\text{TC, ECG, ESR}]{\text{Yes}}$ EME $\longrightarrow$ Pediatric consultation
Erythema marginatum

  ↓ No

Irregular pulse $\xrightarrow[\text{ECG,}]{\text{Yes}}$ EME $\longrightarrow$ Pediatric consultation
           Cardiac monitor

  ↓ No

CHF (wheezing, dyspnea, edema) $\xrightarrow[\text{ECG, ABG, CXR}]{\text{Yes}}$ EME $\longrightarrow$ Pediatric consultation

  ↓ No

(Infants can present with failure to thrive, poor feeding, vomiting, etc.)

Pleuritic pain $\xrightarrow[\text{ECG, CXR, CBC, ESR}]{}$ EME $\longrightarrow$ Pediatric consultation

  ↓ No

UME

HYPERTENSIVE EMERGENCIES

Assessment parameters ⟶ Differential diagnosis

1. Acute hypertensive encephalopathy
2. Acute (L) ventricular failure
3. Acute coronary insufficiency
4. Intracranial hemorrhage
5. Acute dissecting aortic aneurysm
6. Malignant and accelerated hypertension
7. HTN with excessive cathecholamines

Therapeutic Interventions
1. Diuretics
     furosemide (Lasix) and
     ethacrynic acid (Edecrine)

   Antihypertensives
   a. Adrenergic blockers
      alphamethyl dopa (Aldomet)
      clonidine (Catapres)
      prazocin (Minipres)

   b. β-blockers
      Propranolol and others

   c. Peripheral adrenergic
        blockers
      reserpine
      guanethidine monosulfate (Ismelin)

   d. Vasodilators
      hydralazine (Apresoline)
      sodium nitroprusside (Nipride)
      diazoxide (Hyperstat)

GENERAL PRINCIPLES IN TRIAGE OF INGESTIONS

1. Try as best you can to identify the ingested material, e.g., send someone back home to retrieve it, if necessary, or, in the case of a prescription drug, call pharmacy that dispensed the medicine. Use Poisindex to identify toxic ingredients.
2. The initial history should include the time of the ingestion and the quantity ingested (a swallow for a 3-year-old child is approximately 4 to 5 ml).
3. Save all vomitus and urine for later identification if substance ingested has not been identified.
4. Inquire as to history of previous ingestions or pica. All children under 6 years of age should have blood lead level drawn.
5. Counsel parents regarding safety precautions to follow at home in the future.

INGESTIONS

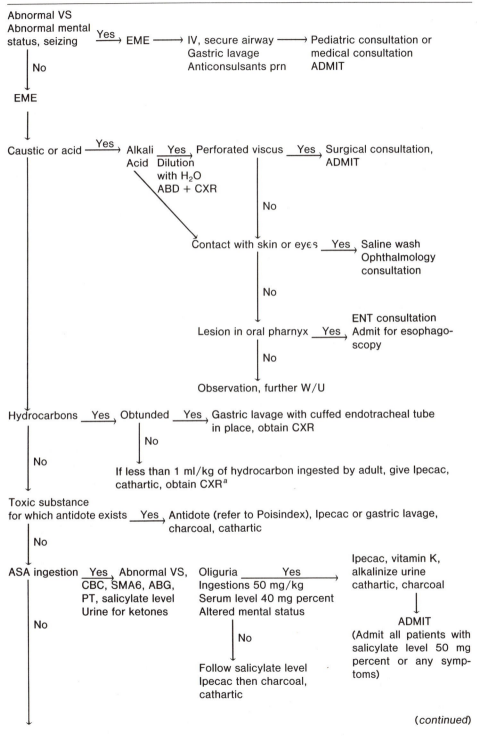

(continued)

INGESTIONS (Continued)

Lead ingestion → Yes, KUB, CBC, U/A → Symptomatic (irritable, clumsy, lethargic, hyperactive) or shows signs of advanced intoxication (ataxia, convulsions, coma, HT, bradycardia) → Yes, ADMIT

No ↓

Unknown substance

Yes ↓

Ipecac followed by charcoal and further W/U (salicylate level, FeCl$_3$ test, barbiturate level, etc.) treatment as indicated

No ↓

Follow-up by private physician

[a] 1. If more than 1 ml/kg of hydrocarbon is ingested by an adult, vomiting should be induced. Vomiting should *not* be induced in children.

2. If pesticide, heavy metal, benzine, or toluenem is ingested, vomiting should be induced both in children and adults.

COMMON INGESTIONS

The ingredients of all the following substances should be known and checked carefully in the Poisindex before deciding on a treatment plan.

No Treatment Usually Required	Removal Necessary If Large Amounts Ingested
Ballpoint inks	Aftershave lotion
Bar soap	Body conditioners
Battery (dry cell)	Colognes
Bubble bath soap	Deodorants
Candles	Fabric softners
Chalk	Hair sprays
Clay (modeling)	Hair tonic
Crayons with A.P., C.P. or C.S. 130–46 designation	Indelible markers
Dehumidifying packets	Matches (more than 20 wooden matches or 2 books of paper matches)
Detergents (anionic)	No Doz
Eye makeup	Oral contraceptives
Fishbowl additives	Perfumes
Hand lotion and cream	Suntan preparations
Ink (blue, black, red)	Toilet water
Lipstick	
Newspaper	
Pencils (lead and coloring)	
Putty and Silly Putty	
Sachets	
Shaving cream and shaving lotions	
Nonliquid shoe polish (occasionally, aniline dyes are present)	
Striking surface materials of matchboxes	
Sweetening agents (saccharin, cyclamate)	
Thermometers	
Toothpaste	

HYDROCARBON INGESTIONS

1. Induce emesis regardless of amount if hydrocarbon contains
   Heavy metals
   Pesticides
   Camphor
   Halogenated solvents
   Benzene
   Petroleum ether or benzine or other toxic substances
2. Emesis indicated if > 1 ml/kg ingested hydrocarbons, such as gasoline, kerosene, turpentine, and naphthas, in adult; do not vomit in child

DRUGS ABSORBED BY ACTIVATED CHARCOAL

Acetaminophen	Muscarine
Amphetamines	Nicotine
Antipyrine	Opium
Aspirin	Oxalates
Atropine	Parathion
Barbiturates	Penicillin
Cantharides	Phenol
Chalorpheniramine	Phenolphthalein
Cocaine	Propoxyphene
Colchicine	Primaquine
Digitalis	Quinine
Diphenylhydantoin	Salicylates
Glutethimide	Sulfonamides
Iodine	Stramonium
Ipecac	Strychnine
Methylene blue	Theophylline
Morphine	

RECOMMENDED STOCK LIST OF ANTIDOTES TO RELATED TOXINS

Antidote[a]	Medication (Toxin)
Activated charcoal	General
Ammonium chloride	Phencyclidine, amphetamines, strychnine
Antivenin (crotalidae), Polyvalent (Wyeth)	Crotalid snake bites
Antivenin (lactrodectus mactans), (MSD)	Black widow spider bites
Atropine	Cholinesterase inhibitors
Bentonite (7%) (Fuller's Earth)	Paraquat (herbicide)
Botulinus antitoxin (ABE-Trivalent)	Available from local health department (or Center for Disease Control)
Calcium chloride	Oxalates, fluoride, ethylene glycol
Chlorpromazine (Thorazine)	General, amphetamines
Corn starch	Iodine
Cyanide kit (amyl nitrite, sodium nitrite, sodium thiosulfate	Cyanide
Deferoxamine mesylate (Desferal)	Iron
Dextrose in water (50%)	Hypoglycemic agents
Diazepam (Valium)	General
Dimercaprol (BAL, British anti-Lewisite)	Arsenic, mercury, gold
Diphenhydramine (Benadryl)	Phenothiazines
Dopamine HCl	Hypotension
Edrophonium chloride (Tensilon)	Anticholinergic agents
Ethylenediaminetetraacetic acid, Ca (Calcium EDTA)	Lead, zinc, and other heavy metal
Ethyl alcohol (100%)	Methyl alcohol, ethylene glycol
Haloperidol (Haldol)	General
Ipecac, syrup of	General
Magnesium sulfate (Epsom salts)	General
Methylene blue (1% solution)	Methemoglobinemia
N-acetylcysteine (Mucomyst)	Acetaminophen
Naloxone hydrochloride (Narcan)	Opium alkaloids, pentazocine, propoxyphene
Nitroprusside	Hypertensive management
Oxygen	Carbon monoxide, cyanide
d-Penicillamine	Copper, lead, mercury, arsenic
Phenobarbital	General
Phospho-Soda (Fleet's)	General
Physostigmine salicylate (Antilirium)	Anticholinergic agents: antihistamines, atropine, tricyclic antidepressants
Pralidoxime chloride (2-PAM chloride)	Cholinesterase inhibitors
Protamine sulfate	Heparin
Pyridoxine hydrochloride	Ethylene glycol, isoniazid, monomethyl-hydrazine-containing mushrooms
Sodium bicarbonate (5% solution)	Iron, general
Thiamine hydrochloride	Thiamine deficiency
Vitamin K_1 (Aquamephyton)	Oral anticoagulants

[a] Each emergency department should have all of the above readily available to its staff. Some of these antidotes may be stored in the pharmacy, others may be available from the Center for Disease Control, but the precise mechanism for locating each one *must* be known by each staff member. These antidotes will be discussed in the management of the case studies covered in this text.
(*From* Goldfrank, L. R. *Toxicologic Emergencies* (2nd ed.). New York: Appleton-Century-Crofts, 1982, p. 15.)

THE FERRIC CHLORIDE REACTION

1. Principle

Many compounds react with Fe^{+++} to form colored derivatives. To interpret results, remember the following

a. It is a relatively sensitive test requiring relatively high concentrations of the reacting metabolite (salicylate is an exception).

b. Phosphate ions yield cloudy precipitates which may mask positive result.

c. Many compounds yield only a transient color.

d. Best done on fresh urine.

2. Reagent

The standard reagent is 10 percent $FeCl_3$. Modified reagents used in specialized laboratories are not considered here.

3. Procedure

Add 2 drops of reagent to 1 ml of urine. Mix and observe color immediately and on standing.

4. Interpretation (see chart, following)

A negative result does not rule out disease.

INTERPRETATION OF FERRIC CHLORIDE REACTION

Clinical Condition	Reacting Compound	Color Produced	
		10 Percent FeCl₃	*Phenistix*
Normal	Phosphates	Brown to white precipitate which can obscure positive test	
Phenylketonuria	Phenylpyruvic acid	Green, stable for few hours	Grey-Green
Maple syrup urine disease	Branch chain keto acids	Grey-green to green, stable	
Histidinemia	Imidazole pyruvic acid	Dark green, stable	
Tyrosinemia	P-hydroxphenyl pyruvic acid	Green, fades in seconds	Green
Alkaptonuria	Homogentistic acid	Blue-green, fades in seconds	
Oast house disease	Hydroxy butyric acid	Purple fading to red-brown	
Ketosis	Acetoacetic acid	Purple-red, fades in minutes	
Direct bilirubinemia	Bilirubin	Green, stable	
Melanoma	Melanin	Grey precipitate, turning black	
Carcinoid	5-hydroxyin-dolacetic acid	Blue-green	
Salicylate ingestion	Salicylates	Purple, stable	Purple
PAS ingestion	P-amino salicylic acid	Red-brown	Red-brown
Phenothiazine ingestion	Phenothiazine derivatives	Blue-purple	Purple
Lyson ingestion	Lysol	Green	
Antipyrine and acetophenetidine ingestion	Antipyrine acetophenetidine derivatives	Cherry red	
L-Dopa ingestion	L-Dopa metabolites	Green	

JAUNDICE

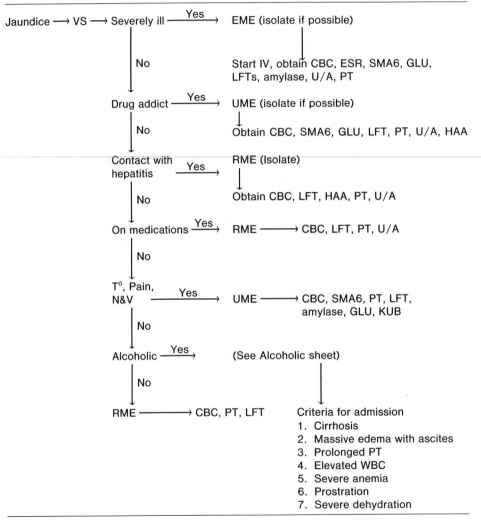

Jaundice → VS → Severely ill ——Yes——→ EME (isolate if possible)

│ No

Start IV, obtain CBC, ESR, SMA6, GLU, LFTs, amylase, U/A, PT

Drug addict ——Yes——→ UME (isolate if possible)

│ No

Obtain CBC, SMA6, GLU, LFT, PT, U/A, HAA

Contact with hepatitis ——Yes——→ RME (Isolate)

│ No

Obtain CBC, LFT, HAA, PT, U/A

On medications ——Yes——→ RME ——→ CBC, LFT, PT, U/A

│ No

T°, Pain, N&V ——Yes——→ UME ——→ CBC, SMA6, PT, LFT, amylase, GLU, KUB

│ No

Alcoholic ——Yes——→ (See Alcoholic sheet)

│ No

RME ——→ CBC, PT, LFT

Criteria for admission
1. Cirrhosis
2. Massive edema with ascites
3. Prolonged PT
4. Elevated WBC
5. Severe anemia
6. Prostration
7. Severe dehydration

JOINT PROBLEM

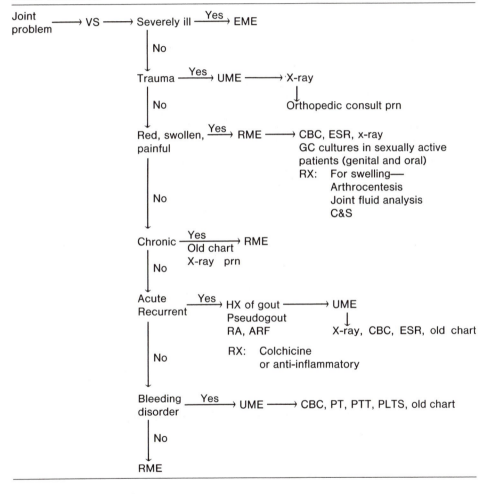

Joint problem $\longrightarrow$ VS $\longrightarrow$ Severely ill $\xrightarrow{\text{Yes}}$ EME

No

Trauma $\xrightarrow{\text{Yes}}$ UME $\longrightarrow$ X-ray

Orthopedic consult prn

No

Red, swollen, painful $\xrightarrow{\text{Yes}}$ RME $\longrightarrow$ CBC, ESR, x-ray
GC cultures in sexually active patients (genital and oral)
RX: For swelling—
Arthrocentesis
Joint fluid analysis
C&S

No

Chronic $\xrightarrow[\text{Old chart}]{\text{Yes}}$ RME
X-ray   prn

No

Acute Recurrent $\xrightarrow{\text{Yes}}$ HX of gout $\longrightarrow$ UME
Pseudogout
RA, ARF

X-ray, CBC, ESR, old chart

RX: Colchicine
or anti-inflammatory

No

Bleeding disorder $\xrightarrow{\text{Yes}}$ UME $\longrightarrow$ CBC, PT, PTT, PLTS, old chart

No

RME

NAUSEA, VOMITING, DIARRHEA

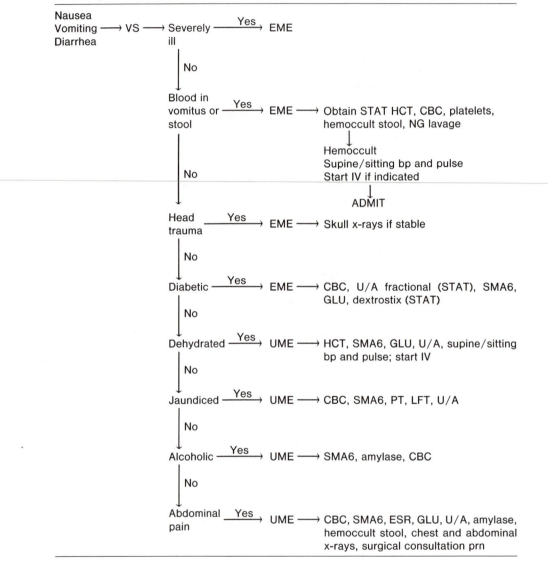

Nausea
Vomiting ⟶ VS ⟶ Severely ——Yes——→ EME
Diarrhea   ill

                      ↓ No

                   Blood in
                   vomitus or ——Yes——→ EME ⟶ Obtain STAT HCT, CBC, platelets,
                   stool   hemoccult stool, NG lavage

                                                          ↓

                                                   Hemoccult
                                                   Supine/sitting bp and pulse
                      ↓ No   Start IV if indicated

                                                          ↓
                                                       ADMIT

                   Head ——Yes——→ EME ⟶ Skull x-rays if stable
                   trauma

                      ↓ No

                   Diabetic ——Yes——→ EME ⟶ CBC, U/A fractional (STAT), SMA6,
                                                   GLU, dextrostix (STAT)
                      ↓ No

                   Dehydrated ——Yes——→ UME ⟶ HCT, SMA6, GLU, U/A, supine/sitting
                                                   bp and pulse; start IV
                      ↓ No

                   Jaundiced ——Yes——→ UME ⟶ CBC, SMA6, PT, LFT, U/A

                      ↓ No

                   Alcoholic ——Yes——→ UME ⟶ SMA6, amylase, CBC

                      ↓ No

                   Abdominal ——Yes——→ UME ⟶ CBC, SMA6, ESR, GLU, U/A, amylase,
                   pain   hemoccult stool, chest and abdominal
                                                     x-rays, surgical consultation prn

DIFFERENTIAL DIAGNOSIS: DIARRHEA

Infection
  Non-GI: OM, UTI, pneumonia
  GI: Staph, *Shigella*[a], *Salmonella,*[a] *E. coli,* viral, amoebiasis,[a] parasites[a]

Toxins
  Staph, *E. coli, Clostridia,* cholera

Allergy

Disaccharidase deficiency
  Primary or acquired after diarrheal illness

Inflammatory
  Enterocolitis, ulcerative colitis

Nervous excitement

Antibiotic Rx

Obstruction
  Intussusception, volvulus, appendicitis, foreign body ingestion, tumor

Miscellaneous
  Hyperthyroid, uremia, megacolon

Malabsorption

Tumors (e.g., neuroblastoma)

Ingestions

N.B. Bleeding with diarrhea: enterocolitis, ulcerative colitis, amoebiasis, parasites, intussusception, megacolon, iron ingestion, and many other medications.

[a] Stools can contain blood.

DIARRHEA: PEDIATRIC

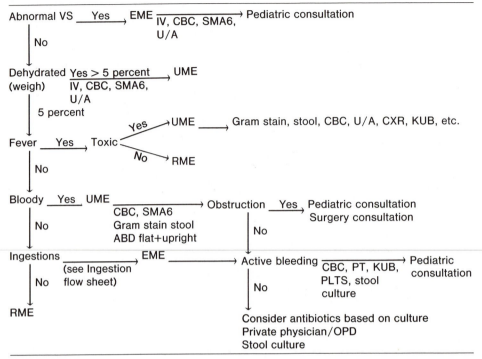

Abnormal VS —Yes→ EME $\overline{IV, CBC, SMA6,}$ → Pediatric consultation
U/A

No ↓

Dehydrated —Yes > 5 percent→ UME
(weigh) $\overline{IV, CBC, SMA6,}$
U/A

5 percent ↓

Fever —Yes→ Toxic —Yes→ UME ——→ Gram stain, stool, CBC, U/A, CXR, KUB, etc.
—No→ RME

No ↓

Bloody —Yes— UME $\overline{CBC, SMA6}$ → Obstruction —Yes→ Pediatric consultation
Gram stain stool   Surgery consultation
ABD flat+upright   No ↓

No ↓

Ingestions ——————→ EME ————→ Active bleeding $\overline{CBC, PT, KUB,}$ → Pediatric
(see Ingestion   PLTS, stool   consultation
No flow sheet)   No ↓   culture

RME   Consider antibiotics based on culture
Private physician/OPD
Stool culture

EVALUATION OF DEHYDRATION IN INFANTS

	0–5 percent	5	5–10 percent	10–20 percent
Dry membranes	+	+	+	+
↓ skin turgor, sunken eye grounds		+	+	+
↓ intraocular pressure			+	+
depressed fontanel			+	+
↓ bp, ↑ HR				

VOMITING: PEDIATRIC

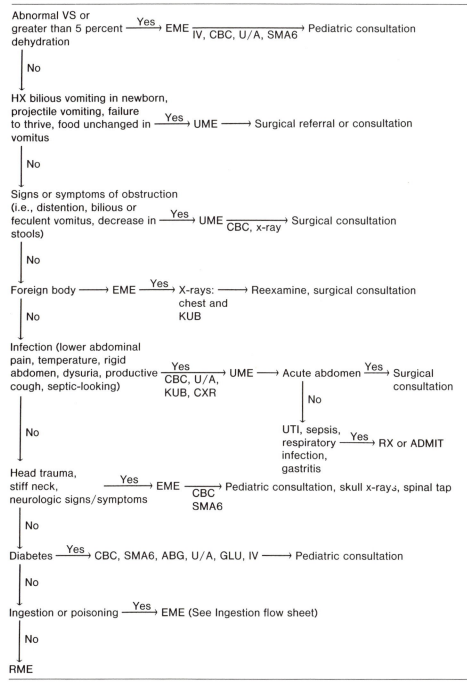

Abnormal VS or
greater than 5 percent ——Yes——→ EME ——IV, CBC, U/A, SMA6——→ Pediatric consultation
dehydration

| No

HX bilious vomiting in newborn,
projectile vomiting, failure
to thrive, food unchanged in ——Yes——→ UME ——→ Surgical referral or consultation
vomitus

| No

Signs or symptoms of obstruction
(i.e., distention, bilious or
feculent vomitus, decrease in ——Yes——→ UME ——CBC, x-ray——→ Surgical consultation
stools)

| No

Foreign body ——→ EME ——Yes——→ X-rays: ——→ Reexamine, surgical consultation
| chest and
| No   KUB

Infection (lower abdominal
pain, temperature, rigid
abdomen, dysuria, productive ——Yes——CBC, U/A, KUB, CXR——→ UME ——→ Acute abdomen ——Yes——→ Surgical
cough, septic-looking)   consultation
| | No
|
| No   UTI, sepsis,
| respiratory ——Yes——→ RX or ADMIT
| infection,
| gastritis

Head trauma,
stiff neck, ——Yes——→ EME ——CBC SMA6——→ Pediatric consultation, skull x-rays, spinal tap
neurologic signs/symptoms

| No

Diabetes ——Yes——→ CBC, SMA6, ABG, U/A, GLU, IV ——→ Pediatric consultation

| No

Ingestion or poisoning ——Yes——→ EME (See Ingestion flow sheet)

| No

RME

OBSTETRICS–GYNECOLOGY

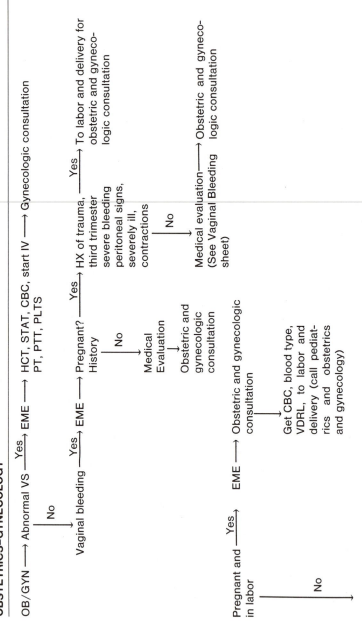

OB/GYN ——→ Abnormal VS ——Yes——→ EME ——→ HCT, STAT, CBC, start IV ——→ Gynecologic consultation
PT, PTT, PLTS

No

Vaginal bleeding ——Yes——→ EME ——→ Pregnant? ——Yes——→ HX of trauma, ——Yes——→ To labor and delivery for
History   third trimester   obstetric and gyneco-
                                     severe bleeding   logic consultation
No   peritoneal signs,
                                     severely ill,
Medical   contractions
Evaluation
↓   No
Obstetric and
gynecologic   Medical evaluation ——→ Obstetric and gyneco-
consultation   (See Vaginal Bleeding   logic consultation
                                     sheet)

Pregnant and ——Yes——→ EME ——→ Obstetric and gynecologic
in labor   consultation
                                 ↓
                                 Get CBC, blood type,
No   VDRL, to labor and
                                 delivery (call pediat-
                                 rics and obstetrics
                                 and gynecology)

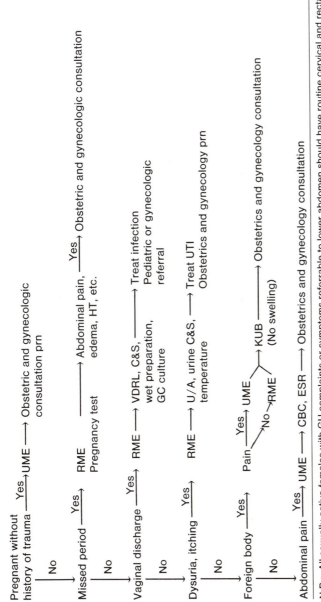
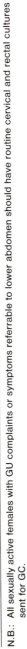

Pregnant without history of trauma — Yes → UME → Obstetric and gynecologic consultation prn

↓ No

Missed period — Yes → RME Pregnancy test → Abdominal pain, edema, HT, etc. — Yes → Obstetric and gynecologic consultation

↓ No

Vaginal discharge — Yes → RME → VDRL, C&S, wet preparation, GC culture → Treat infection / Pediatric or gynecologic referral

↓ No

Dysuria, itching — Yes → RME → U/A, urine C&S, temperature → Treat UTI / Obstetrics and gynecology prn

↓ No

Foreign body — Yes → Pain — Yes → UME → KUB (No swelling) → Obstetrics and gynecology consultation
Pain — No → RME

↓ No

Abdominal pain — Yes → UME → CBC, ESR → Obstetrics and gynecology consultation

N.B.: All sexually active females with GU complaints or symptoms referrable to lower abdomen should have routine cervical and rectal cultures sent for GC.

VAGINAL BLEEDING

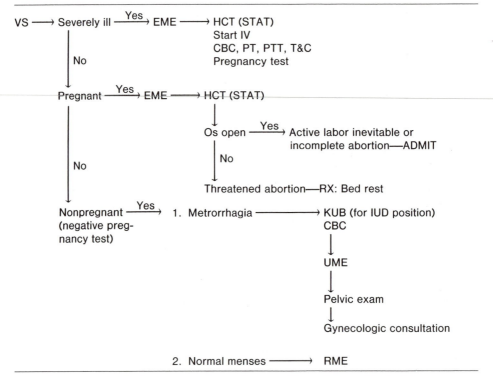

TRIAGE OF ORTHOPEDIC TRAUMA—GUIDELINES FOR ORDERING X-RAYS

A. Vital Signs
Recording of vital signs is the first step in the triage of all patients. Patients who present with trauma should have vital signs performed. If their vital signs are compromised, they should be immediately triaged and if necessary, the surgical team should be called.

B. Examination
The patient should be examined carefully before x-rays are ordered.
1. The injured area should be assessed.
   Is a fracture present? Is there swelling, tenderness, decreased range of motion, or deformity? Is an x-ray necessary? Is the fracture open or closed? Is the nerve supply (motor and sensory) intact? Is the blood supply intact? Is bleeding present?
2. Particular care must be taken to exclude reciprocal injuries at distant sites.
   Does the patient who has fallen and fractured his or her heel have a compression fracture of the spine? Does the patient with a forearm fracture have a dislocation at the elbow or wrist (usually two joints proximal, i.e., heel–knee–hip–LS)? Does the patient with diastasis (disruption) of the tibiofibular joint at the ankle have an associated fracture of the fibula at the knee?
3. The triage nurse must be aware that pain in one area may be referred from somewhere else. For example, hip problems can often present with pain in the knee, back to legs, wrist or elbow, etc.
4. Finally, the patient must be stabilized before he or she is sent to x-ray. Vital signs must be stable, bleeding controlled, wounds properly dressed, etc. Patients with spine injuries must be adequately immobilized and great care must be exercised when transporting these patients.
5. Patients who are seriously ill or who have sustained serious trauma to the head, face, or spine should be assessed by a physician before x-rays are ordered and should be accompanied by a staff member if sent to the x-ray department.
6. Patients with painful fractures should be splinted and medicated before being sent to x-ray. Patients with open fractures should receive a DT booster, if indicated, the Hypertet if history is unclear. If medication is given, the patient should be observed for a reasonable time before being sent to x-ray. Consent for surgery should be obtained, if necessary, before medication.

C. How to Order X-Rays
It is most important when ordering x-rays to give the radiologist enough information to interpret the films. The following information should be included on the request form.
1. Age of injury
2. How the injury occurred (mechanism of injury), if relevant, e.g., eversion injury to left ankle
3. Description of the findings (gross deformity, soft tissue swelling, point tenderness, decreased range of motion)

Instructions for Specific Sites
1. Hand
   a. Digit—Ask for AP, lateral, and oblique of specific digits involved. DO NOT ask for "hand views."
   b. Carpal and metacarpal bones—AP, lateral, and oblique of hand. If patient is tender in anatomical snuff box, order special scaphoid (navicular) view.
   c. Wrist—AP, lateral, and oblique of wrist.
2. Forearm—AP and lateral views.
3. Elbow—AP, lateral, and oblique views.
4. Upper arm—AP and lateral of humerus.
5. Shoulder—Internal and external rotation and axillary views. Orthopedics may want a transthoracic view as well for a shoulder dislocation. If shoulder separation (acromioclavicular ligament tear) is suspected, order weight-bearing views.

(continued)

TRIAGE OF ORTHOPEDIC TRAUMA (Continued)

6. Clavicle—AP and apical lordotic views.
7. Sternum—AP, lateral, and oblique views.
8. Ribs—AP and oblique views. State which side and also estimate which rib(s) is/are involved. Always get CXR with rib series to rule out pneumothorax or hemothorax. However, a chest x-ray is adequate to rule out a rib fracture.
9. Pelvis—AP view only.
10. Hips—AP and lateral views. Always order pelvis with hip film to rule out fracture of the other hip. Order frog leg lateral in children if slipped femoral epiphysis or ischemic necrosis of femoral head is suspected.
11. Femur—AP and lateral views. With suspected fracture of the femur, order x-ray of hip on same side to rule out a dislocation of the hip.
12. Knee—AP, lateral, and oblique views. If patella injury is suspected, ask for knee views and a tangential (skyline) view.
13. Tibia/fibula—AP and lateral views.
14. Ankle—AP, lateral, and oblique views. With persistent pain following a sprained ankle, one can order stress films to rule out ligamentous injury.
15. Foot—AP, lateral, and oblique views.
16. Toes—Ask for AP, lateral and oblique views. DO NOT ask for "foot views."
17. Skull—AP, both laterals, and Townes view (skull series).
18. Facial bones—Order Waters view and lateral view of face. This does not include orbits, nasal bone, zygomatic arches, temporomandibular joints, or mandible. All of these must be ordered separately.
19. Spine
    a. Cervical—AP, lateral, and odontoid (open mouth) views. If spondylosis is suspected, order an oblique view.
    b. Dorsal—AP and lateral
    c. Lumbar—AP, lateral, and coned-down views of L5–S1. If spondylolisthesis or spondylosis is suspected, order an oblique view.
    d. Sacrum and coccyx—AP and lateral

D. Comparison Views
Comparison views are important to order in young children who are still in a growth phase (e.g., right and left knees).

E. Pregnancy
Any female who is of child bearing age should be assessed for possible pregnancy before x-rays are ordered.

F. Radiation
Female and male patients who require x-rays other than the pelvis should be told to request shielding.

G. Child Abuse
Any child who presents repeatedly with orthopedic trauma or who has suspicious injuries should be assessed for possible child abuse.

RASH

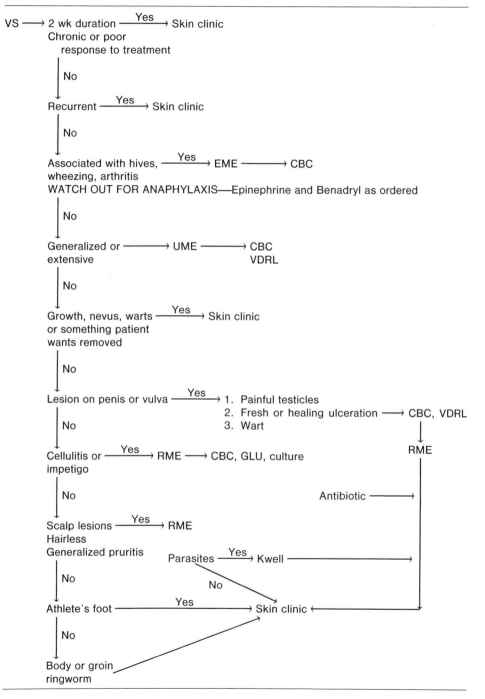

RASH: PEDIATRIC

Abnormal VS ——Yes——→ UME

⏐ No
↓

Petechiae below ————————————————→ EME ——→ Rule out meningococcemia, ASA
neck or purpura   ingestion, and sepsis

＼
CBC, platelet count, PT, PTT,
⏐ No   Rumple Leede, Gram stain
            of petechiae
↓

Ecchymoses or ————————————————→ UME ——→ Rule out bleeding disorders,
hematoma   CBC, platelet count,   leukemia
              Rumple Leede, PT, PTT
⏐ No
↓

Urticaria ——Yes——→ Dyspnea, wheezing ——Yes——→ EME (RX for anaphylaxis), epinephrine,
                                                      Benadryl, O_2, IV prn
⏐ No
↓

Infectious disease ————————→ RME, isolation precautions
(measles, rubella,
chicken pox)

⏐ No
↓

Lesions around vulva, ——VDRL——→ RME ——→ Darkfield GC cultures and Gram stain
rectum, or penis   Social services consultation

⏐ No
↓

Orbital cellulitis ——Yes——→ UME ————————————→ Pediatric consultation, ADMIT
or peri-orbital   CBC, blood cultures,
                             sinus x-rays
⏐ No
↓

Herpes (face/eyes) ——Yes——→ Pediatric consultation, ophthalmology consultation

⏐ No
↓

Abscess, boil ——Yes——→ RME ——→ I&D if fluctuant ————→ Private physician/OPD

⏐ No
↓

RME ————→ Private physician/OPD

RECTAL PAIN: BLEEDING

Abnormal VS ──Yes──→ EME ──→ HCT (STAT), CBC ──────→ Sigmoidoscopy
PT, PTT, PLTS, T&C   Admit prn
stool hemoccult,
IV, NG tube

│ No
↓

Swallowed blood ──Yes──→ RME
(HX epistaxis, etc.) CBC

│ No
↓

Medication/ingestion ──Yes──→ EME (See Ingestion flow sheet)
(aspirin, steroids,
iron poisoning)

│ No
↓

Trauma/Foreign body ──Yes──→ EME X-ray (chest + KUB)──→ Surgical consultation
               CBC

│ No
↓

Fissure, local
Drainage, abscess ──────→ RME ──────→ Surgical consultation prn

│ No
↓

Diarrhea ──Yes──→ (See Diarrhea flow sheet) Abnormal VS ──Yes──→ EME
                            or 5 percent
│ No   dehydration
↓

Nocturnal itching ──────→ RME ──────→ Treat if positive
(parasites) Scotch tape   Private physician/OPD
          test

│ No
↓

Purpura ──────────────→ UME ──────→ Hematology or
                     CBC, PLTS, pediatric consultation
                     PT, PTT

│ No
↓

RME ──→ Stool hemoccult,
      CBC, PT, PTT

SEIZURES

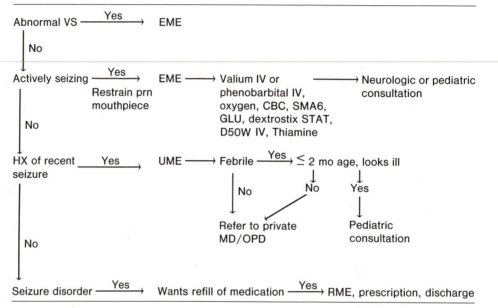

SHOCK

Abnormal
  VS
   ↓
  EME ——————→ IV, general support
               (Foley, CVP, etc.)
               ABG, CBC, EKG
                     ↓

Hemorrhage T&C, HCT, (STAT), CBC ——→ volume expansion,
                                        blood

                             HCT (STAT)
Intravascular volume ___Yes___ Trauma ___T&C___ volume expansion,
                                    X-ray for   surgical consultation
                                    fracture

                                Fluid loss

                                    Burn ——→ Cleanse+cover
                                               Tetanus prophylaxis,[a]
                No
                                               PCN, IV

                                  Gastroenteritis ——————————→ plasma
                                  (HCO_3^-, N+V, and diarrhea) expander

                                  DM/DI ——→ Plasma expander
                                  insulin prn, HCO_3^-, ABG, U/A, etc.

Cardiogenic/obstructive blood flow ——→ EKG, CXR, etc. vasopressors
                                           antiarrhythmic
  ↓ No

Infection ___Yes___ Blood cultures, antibiotics, steroids, IV
  ↓ No

Anaphylaxis ___Yes___ EPI, O_2, benadryl, steriods, vasopressor, aminophylline
  ↓ No

Neurogenic ___Yes___ Head injury ___Yes___ Stabilize ——→ Skull films, neurosurgery
                                ↓ No
  No
                      Spine injury ___Yes___ Stabilize ———→ X-rays
                                  ↓ No

                      OD ———→ Stabilize ———→ Lavage, charcoal
                                             etc.
Endocrine ___Yes___ IV, SMA6, GLU, CBC

---

[a] Tetanus immunization: < 6 yrs DPT; > 6 yrs DT; > 13 yrs dT

DIFFERENTIAL DIAGNOSIS: SHOCK

1. **Hemorrhage**
   Trauma to abdominal organs—liver, spleen
   Thrombocytopenia
   DIC

2. **Fluid Loss**
   Gastroenteritis
   Severe burn
   Diabetes mellitus, diabetes insipidus

3. **Sepis**
   Gm-negative infection, meningococcemia, immunologic deficiency

4. **Cardiogenic, Obstructive**
   Myocarditis, RHD, pulmonary embolus, tension pneumothorax
   Tamponade

5. **Neurogenic**
   Spinal cord transection, head injury (epidural)
   Intracranial pressure

6. **Anaphylaxis**
   Food or drug allergy, insect sting

7. **Endocrine**
   Adrenogenital syndrome, pituitary insufficiency

DEFINITION OF SHOCK IN CHILDREN

1. Blood pressure low and/or unobtainable
2. Urine output < 10 ml/kg/24 hours or < 0.5 ml/kg/hr
3. Alternation in mental status
   a. Infants: weak or absent cry, apathetic
   b. Children: disoriented and stuporus, apathetic
4. Associated findings
   Mottled or pale skin, sunken eye grounds
   Cool extremities
   Poor capillary filling
   Shallow respirations (acidosis)
   Rapid, weak pulse

Blood Pressure

1. Newborn: flush method (supine position, 5 cm cuffs applied to wrist or ankle)
   First week of life: mean flush bp: 41 ± 8 mm Hg
   1 to 12 months: mean flush bp: 72 ± 10 mm Hg
2. Older child: (cuff width should cover two thirds of upper arm)

Average Blood Pressure				Heart Rate (at rest)		
Age (yr)	Systemic	Diastolic		Age	Average	Range
1				Newborn	120	(70–170)
2				1–11 months	120	(80–160)
3				2 years	110	(80–130)
4	85	60		4	100	(80–120)
5	87	60		6	100	(75–115)
6	90	60		8	90	(70–110)
7	92	62		10	90	(70–110)
8	95	62		12[a]	90	(70–110)
9	98	64		14[a]	85	(65–105)
10	100	65		16[a]	80	(60–110)
11	105	65		18[a]	75	(55–95)
12	108	67				
13	110	67				
14	112	70				
15	115	72				
16	118	75				

[a] Values for girls (boys tend to have a heart rate 5 beats/minute slower than girls).

SICKLE CELL ANEMIA

Sickle cell ——→ abnormal VS ——Yes→ EME ——————→ O₂, IV fluids, analgesia
anemia   CBC   CBC,
        with   reticulocytes
        reticulocytes   count, U/A
        count | No

Fever ————Yes————→ UME ——→ Pediatric ———→ Admit if febrile or
      CXR, bone films   consultation   patient looks ill
      (if indicated, urine   if indicated
      and blood culture,
  | No U/A, IV hydration, O₂)

Thrombotic crisis ————Yes————→ EME CXR, Severe pain ——Yes→ IV
          Look for precipi-   Abdominal   analgesia
          tating cause   x-ray U/A,   O₂   ADMIT
          (infection,   SMA6,   No ——→
          dehydration,   Amylase
          acidosis,   Hydration
  | No   hypoxia)   analgesia ——→ Reevaluation
                                     O₂

Aplastic crisis (severe anemia, low ——Yes→ ADMIT
                 or absent reticulocytes,   O₂
  | No   CHF etc.)

Sequestration crisis (shock, severe anemia or ————Yes————→ ADMIT
                    enlarged spleen)   IV saline, O₂
  | No   T&C

Hemolytic crisis ——Yes→ (look for G6 PD def, Coombs and autoim-
                   mune hemolysis, falling HCT, infection, ——————→ ADMIT
  | No   etc., pink serum)   IV saline, O₂
                                                 T&C

Miscellaneous problems (folate def, gallstones, ——Yes→ UME ———→ Consult
                          hepatitis)   pediatrics,
  | No   hematology,
                                               surgery prn

Mild pain ——Yes→ UME ———→ Analgesia, O₂
  | No

  ↓
RME

SINUSITIS

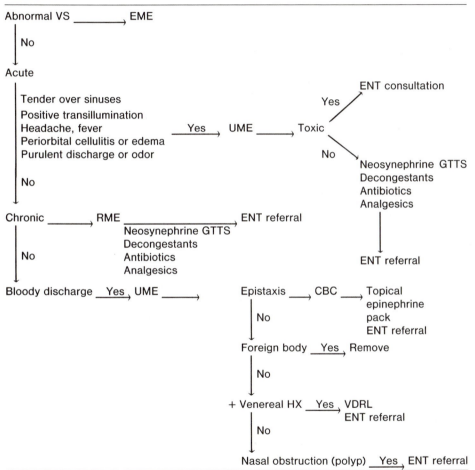

SMOKE INHALATION

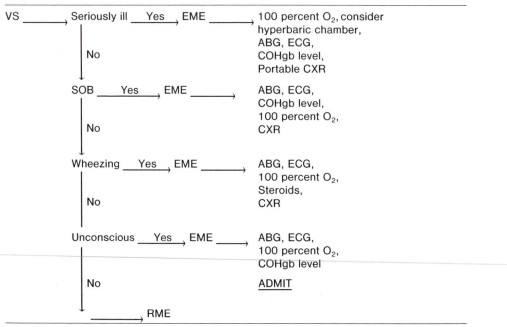

VS ⟶ Seriously ill ─── Yes ⟶ EME ⟶ 100 percent O_2, consider
hyperbaric chamber,
ABG, ECG,
COHgb level,
Portable CXR

No

SOB ─── Yes ⟶ EME ⟶ ABG, ECG,
COHgb level,
100 percent O_2,
CXR

No

Wheezing ─── Yes ⟶ EME ⟶ ABG, ECG,
100 percent O_2,
Steroids,
CXR

No

Unconscious ─── Yes ⟶ EME ⟶ ABG, ECG,
100 percent O_2,
COHgb level

No   ADMIT

⟶ RME

TRAUMA

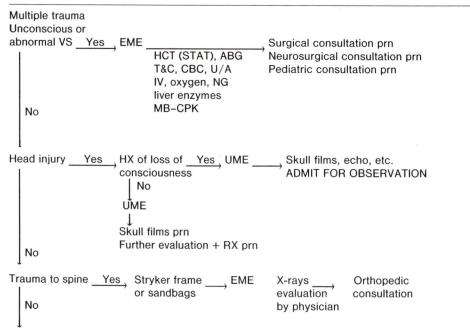

Multiple trauma
Unconscious or
abnormal VS ─── Yes ⟶ EME ⟶ Surgical consultation prn
HCT (STAT), ABG   Neurosurgical consultation prn
T&C, CBC, U/A   Pediatric consultation prn
IV, oxygen, NG
liver enzymes
No   MB–CPK

Head injury ─── Yes ⟶ HX of loss of ─── Yes ⟶ UME ⟶ Skull films, echo, etc.
consciousness   ADMIT FOR OBSERVATION
No
UME

Skull films prn
Further evaluation + RX prn
No

Trauma to spine ─── Yes ⟶ Stryker frame ⟶ EME   X-rays ⟶ Orthopedic
or sandbags   evaluation   consultation
No   by physician

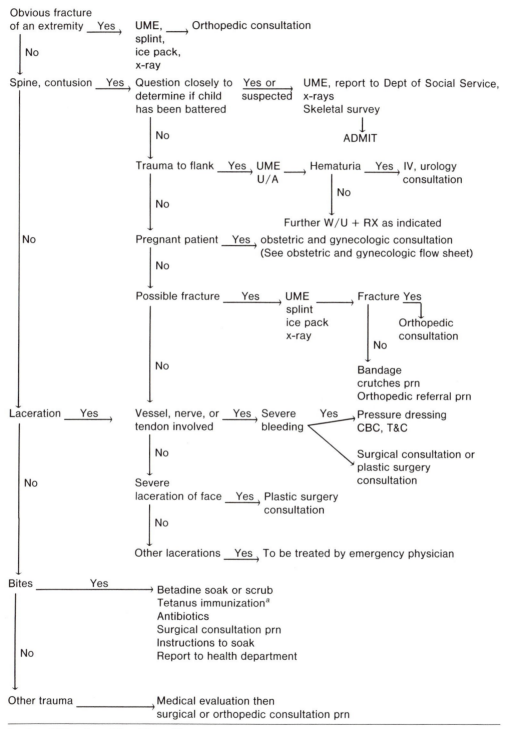

Obvious fracture
of an extremity ___Yes__→ UME, ___→ Orthopedic consultation
splint,
│No
ice pack,
↓
x-ray

Spine, contusion ___Yes__→ Question closely to ___Yes or__→ UME, report to Dept of Social Service,
determine if child   suspected x-rays
has been battered   Skeletal survey
│No   ↓
↓   ADMIT

Trauma to flank __Yes_→ UME ___→ Hematuria __Yes_→ IV, urology
U/A   consultation
│No   │No
↓   ↓
Further W/U + RX as indicated

│No   Pregnant patient __Yes_→ obstetric and gynecologic consultation
(See obstetric and gynecologic flow sheet)
│No
↓

Possible fracture ___Yes___→ UME ___→ Fracture Yes
splint   ┐
ice pack   Orthopedic
x-ray   │No   consultation
│No   ↓
↓   Bandage
crutches prn
Orthopedic referral prn

Laceration __Yes__→ Vessel, nerve, or _Yes_→ Severe __Yes_→ Pressure dressing
tendon involved   bleeding   CBC, T&C
│No   ╲ Surgical consultation or
↓   plastic surgery
│No   Severe   consultation
laceration of face _Yes_→ Plastic surgery
consultation
│No
↓
Other lacerations __Yes_→ To be treated by emergency physician

Bites _____Yes_____→ Betadine soak or scrub
Tetanus immunization[a]
│   Antibiotics
Surgical consultation prn
Instructions to soak
│No   Report to health department
↓

Other trauma _____→ Medical evaluation then
surgical or orthopedic consultation prn

[a] < 6 yrs DPT; > 6 yrs DT; > 13 yrs dT.

URETHRAL DISCHARGE

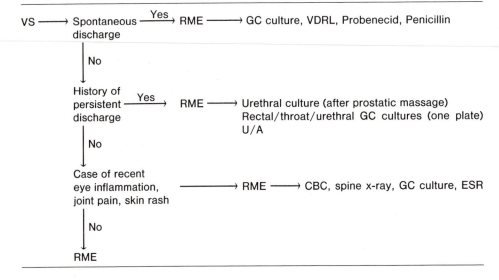

DEFINITION OF TERMS AND ABBREVIATIONS

ABG	arterial blood gases	GTTS	drops
ACH	acetylcholine	HAA	hepatitis associated antigen
ACTH	adenocorticotropic hormone	HCO_3	bicarbonate
ADH	antidiuretic hormone	H_2CO_3	carbonic acid
AFB	acid fast bacillus	HCT	hematocrit
ARF	acute rheumatic fever	Hg	mercury
ASO	acute streptozyme O test	Hgb	hemoglobin
AV	atrioventricular	HTN	hypertension
AVM	arteriovenous malformation	Hx	history
BAL	British antilewisite	I&D	incision and drainage
bid	2 times a day	IgA, etc.	immunoglobulin A, etc.
BMR	basal metabolic rate	IM	intramuscular(ly)
bp	blood pressure	I&Os	inputs and outputs
BUN	blood urea nitrogen	IPPB	intermittent positive pressure
C&S	cuture and sensitivity		breathing
CAT	computerized axial tomography	IU	international unit(s)
CBC	complete blood count	IV	intravenous(ly)
cc	cubic centimeter(s)	IVP	intravenous pyelogram
CHF	congestive heart failure	kg	kilogram(s)
CO_2	carbon dioxide	K/O	keep open
COPD	chronic obstructive pulmo-nary disease	KUB	kidney, ureter, and bladder x-ray
CPK	creatine phosphokinase	L&D	labor and delivery
cu mm	cubic millimeter(s)	lb	pound(s)
CVP	central venous pressure	LDH	lactic dehydrogenase
CXR	chest x-ray	LFT	liver function test; direct bili,
D5W	5 percent dextrose in water		total bilirubin, alkaline phos-
D50W	50 percent dextrose in water		phatase, LDH, SGOT
dc	direct current	LOC	loss of consciousness
DI	diabetes insipidus	LP	lumbar puncture
DIC	disseminated intravascular coagulopathy	LS	lumbosacral
DPT	diphtheria, pertussis, tetanus	LVEDP	left ventricular end-diastolic pressure
DT	diphtheria, tetanus	mEq	milliequivalent(s)
ECG	electrocardiogram	mg	milligram(s)
EEG	electroencephalogram	MI	myocardial infarction
EME	emergent medical exam	mIU	mili-international unit(s)
EMT	emergency medical techni-cians	ml	milliliter(s)
ENT	ear, nose, and throat	mm	millimeter(s)
EOM	extraocular movements	mOsm	milliosmole(s)
EPI	epinephrine	N & V	nausea and vomiting
ER	emergency room	neb	nebulized
ESR	erythrocyte sedimentation rate	ng	nanogram (= millimicrogram)
ETOH	ethanol	NG	nasogastric
FIO_2	forced inspiratory oxygen	nm	nanometer (= millimicron)
GC	gonococcus	nmole	nanomole
GI	gastrointestinal	non-urgent	RME; routine medical exam
GLU	glucose	npo	nothing by mouth
g	gram(s)	NS	normal saline
GTT	glucose tolerance test	NVD	nausea, vomiting, diarrhea
		OD	overdose
		OM	otitis media

(continued)

DEFINITION OF TERMS AND ABBREVIATIONS (Continued)

O&P	ova and parasites	SGOT	serum glutamic oxaloacetic transaminase
OPD	outpatient department		
P_{CO_2}	carbon dioxide pressure	SGPT	serum glutamic pyruvic transaminase
P_{O_2}	oxygen pressure (or tension)		
Pa_{CO_2}	arterial carbon dioxide pressure	SL	sublingual
		SLE	systemic lupus erythematosus
PA_{O_2}	alveolar oxygen pressure		
PBI	protein-bound iodine	SMA6	Na, K, Cl, CO_2, BUN, creatinine
PCN	penicillin		
PE	physical exam	SOB	shortness of breath
PEEP	positive end-expiratory pressure	SQ	subcutaneously
		stat	at once
pH	hydrogen-ion concentration	SX	signs
PLTS	platelets	TB	tuberculosus
PN	pneumonia	T&C	type and crossmatch
po	orally	TC	throat culture
PPD	purified protein derivative	tid	3 times a day
prn	as needed	TM	tympanic membrane
Ps_{O_2}	arterial oxygen pressure	TPR	temperature, pulse, respirations
PT	prothrombin time		
PTT	partial prothrombin time	u	unit(s)
q 4 hours, etc.	every 4 hours, etc.	U/A	urinalysis
		UME	urgent medical exam
qd	every day	URI	upper respiratory infection
qid	4 times a day	UTI	urinary tract infection
RA	rheumatoid arthritis	VDRL	venereal disease research lab
RAIU	radioactive iodine uptake	VS	vital signs
RHD	rheumatic heart disease	WBC	white blood cell
RME	routine medical exam	wt	weight
R/O	rule out	W/U	workup
RX	treatment	/	per
SBE	subacute bacterial endocarditis	<	less than
		>	more than
SC	subcutaneously		

ACKNOWLEDGMENTS

These algorithms were initially prepared in 1973 by Lewis Goldfrank, M.D., and Jerome Ernst, M.D., at the Morrisania City Hospital. They were subsequently adapted by the emergency department nursing staff at the hospital, which was then closed in 1976. In 1976, the algorithms were extensively adapted by Harold Osborn, M.D., at the North Central Bronx Hospital. They were further modified by the emergency department nursing staffs at the North Central Bronx and Montefiore Hospital and Medical Center. In 1979, the algorithms were expanded by Clark Haber, M.D., and Alan Kulberg, M.D. to meet the needs of the Bellevue Hospital Center and New York University Medical Center.

Although the impact of many nursing staff will be seen throughout these algorithms, True Samms, R.N., who was the Emergency Department Nursing Supervisor at Morrisania, the North Central Bronx, and New York University, was most influential in their evolution. In addition, the imprint of Harold Osborn, M.D., Director of Residency Training in Emergency Medicine at the Lincoln Hospital Center in the Bronx, Alan Kulberg, M.D., Assistant Director of Emergency Services at Bellevue and the Director of Pediatric Emergency Services, Clark Haber, M.D., Attending Physician at University Hospital Emergency Services, and Lewis Goldfrank, M.D., Director of Emergency Services at Bellevue and University Hospitals is seen throughout. In offering these credits I apologize in advance to anyone of the hundreds of physicians and nurses who contributed to the formation of these algorithms and was not given adequate credit for the efforts that made them so functional.

Triage References

Christensen-Szalanski, J. J., Diehr, P. H., Wood, R. W., Tompkins, R. K. Phased trial of a proven algorithm at a new primary care clinic. *American Journal Public Health*, 1982, **72**(1), 16–21.

Flomenbaum, N., & Goldfrank, L. Diagnostic testing in the emergency department. *Topics in Emergency Medicine*, 1983, 1–8.

George, J. E. The emergency room: Entry to the health-care system. *Hospital Topics*, 1969, **47**(10), 69–74.

Goldfrank, L., Weisman, R., & Flomenbaum N., Teaching the recognition of odors. *Annals of Emergency Medicine*, 1982, **11**(12), 684–686.

Hospital statistics. Chicago: American Hospital Association, 1977.

Komaroff, A. L., & Winickoff, R. *Common acute illness*. Boston: Little Brown, 1977.

Lanros, N. *Assessment and intervention in emergency nursing*. Bowie, Md.: Robert J. Brady Co., 1978.

Larsen, K. T., et al. Triage: A logical algorithm alternative to a non-system. *Journal of American Coll. Emergency Physician*, 1973, **2**(3), 183–187.

Prior, J. A., & Silverstein, J. S. *Physical diagnosis*. St. Louis: C.V. Mosby, 1977.

Priorities of treatment. In *Emergency war surgery* (United States issue of NATO handbook prepared for use by the medical services of NATO nations). Washington, D.C.: U.S. Government Printing Office, 1975, p. 158.

Rada, R. T. The violent patient: Rapid assessment and management. *Psychosomatics*, 1981, **2**(2), 101–109.

Rund, D. A. *Essentials of emergency medicine*. New York: Appleton-Century-Crofts, 1982.

Rund, D. A., & Rausch, T. S. *Triage*. St. Louis: C.V. Mosby, 1981.

Russo, R. M., Gurruraj, V. J., & Allen, J. Ambulatory care triage. *American Family Physician*, 1974, **9**, 125–130.

Turner, S. R., Golden rules for accurate triage. *Journal Emergency Nursing*, 1981, **7**(4), 153–155.

Vickery, D. M. *Triage*. Bowie, Md.: Robert J. Brady Co., 1975

White, H. H. When you're faced with an unconscious patient. *Medical Times*, 1980.

SECTION TWO

SHOCK

1. Shock Syndromes

- Hypovolemic
    - Hemorrhage
    - Burns
    - Intestinal obstruction
    - Dehydration
- Cardiogenic
    - Myocardial infarction
    - Cardiac tamponade
    - Arrhythmias
    - Direct trauma to heart
    - Pulmonary emboli
- Neurogenic
    - Spinal anesthesia
    - Vasomotor center trauma
    - Spinal cord injury
    - Uninterrupted severe pain
    - CNS depressant drugs
    - Brain and brainstem damage
- Septic
    - Bacteremia
    - Septicemia

2. Assessment Parameters

Refer to Table 1 on the following pages.

TABLE 1. SHOCK SYNDROMES: ASSESSMENT PARAMETERS

	Hypovolemic	Cardiogenic	Neurogenic	Septic Hyperdynamic	Septic Hypodynamic
Cardiac function	Increased	Severely diminished	Diminished	Increased	Decreased
Cardiac output	Decreased	Decreased	Decreased	Increased	Increased
Pulmonary wedge pressure	Decreased	Increased	Decreased	Low to normal	High to increased
Central venous pressure	Decreased	Increased	Decreased	Low to normal	Increased
Pulse and heart rate	Rapid and possibly irregular	Increased	Decreased	Increased	Decreased
Arterial pressure	Decreased	Decreased	Decreased	Decreased	Decreased
Blood pressure	Normal to decreased	Decreased	Decreased	Normal to decreased	Normal to decreased
Venous reserve	Severely decreased	Increased	Decreased	Increased	Increased

Arteriolar resistance	Increased	Increased	Decreased	Severely decreased	Severely decreased
Respirations	Rapid and deep initially then decreased	Rapid and possibly irregular then decreased	Decreased	Rapid and deep then decreasing	Rapid and deep then decreasing
Arterial P_{CO_2}	Decreased	Decreased	Decreased	Decreased	Decreased
Arterial pH	Decreased leading to metabolic acidosis	Decreased leading to metabolic acidosis	Decreased leading to metabolic acidosis	Decreased leading to metabolic acidosis	Decreased leading to metabolic acidosis
Skin	Cold, pale, moist	Cold, pale, moist	Cold, pale, moist	Warm, dry, flushed	Cold, pale, moist
Temperature	Normal to decreased	Normal to decreased	Decreased	Elevated	Subnormal
Urinary output	Decreasing	Decreasing	Decreasing	Decreasing	Decreasing
Mental status	Anxious to lethargy to coma	Impaired to lethargy to coma	Impaired	Impaired to coma	Impaired to coma
Musculoskeletal response	Weakness and fatigue	Weakness and fatigue	Weakness and fatigue	Weakness and fatigue	Weakness and fatigue

See Figure 1 for monitoring checklist.

3. Pathophysiology for Assessment Validation

HYPOVOLEMIC SHOCK

Shock is a clinical syndrome characterized by signs and symptoms which arise when the cardiac output is insufficient to fill the aterial tree with blood for adequate perfusion of organs and tissues. Basically, there are three contributors to shock: a reduction in the amount of blood volume; dysfunction in the pumping status of the heart; and an alteration in the distribution of circulating blood volume. Despite its etiology, shock creates severe changes systematically as well as metabolically and homeostatically. The state of shock is usually viewed in two stages: early shock and late shock (Figs. 1 and 2).

Hyperventilation is usually the first sign of early shock, especially in hypovolemic shock. This hyperventilation causes a drop in the $Paco_2$. A sympathetic nervous system compensatory mechanism is triggered that in turn stimulates both α- and β- adrenergic receptors in the sympathetic nervous system. Stimulation of the α-receptors causes arterial vasoconstriction depriving tissues such as skin, bowel, kidney, liver, and muscle of adequate blood supply, and diverting it to the heart and the brain. In addition to arteriolar vasoconstriction, there is a severely reduced vascular capacity. These changes are responsible for the cold moist skin, and the relative normalcy in blood pressure in early stage shock. Stimulation of the β-receptors results in increased heart rate and myocardial contraction. Excessive stimulation of β-receptors may cause the development of arrhythmias, especially in those patients suspected as septic, or with a pulmonary embolism.

A hypovolemic or hypotensive state causes a fluid shift from the interstitial space into the vascular compartment. This fluid shift occurs because of a reduced blood pressure in the capillary bed and a disturbance in the factors related to fluid exchange across the capillary membrane. As a result of the fluid and plasma exchange, there is an engorgement of the capillaries from the aggregation of white blood cells, red blood cells, and platelets. This phenomenon causes a sludging of the microvasculature and the possibility of emboli formation, and possibly respiratory complications. Urinary output is compromised because of the reduced arterial pressure and the vasoconstriction of the renal arterioles. Reduced pressure in the renal afferent arterioles activates the renin-angiotensin system which leads to sodium retention by the kidneys. Stimulation of this system activates ADH production which causes water retention.

If the shock state is not self-limiting or corrected the continual sympathetic stimulation will be devastating to the body. A continuous cycle of decreased cardiac output and decreased tissue perfusion inevitably ends in death. Decreased blood flow through the microvasculature causes ischemic hypoxia of surrounding tissues which in turn produces drastic effects on energy availability. Cellular metabolism is altered and becomes anaerobic. The pyruvic acid and hydrogen ions produced as the first step in glycolysis cannot enter the Krebs cycle without oxygen. As a result

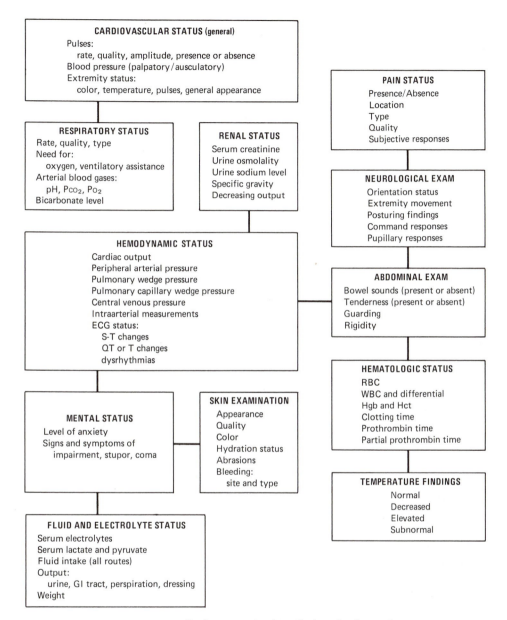

Figure 1. Physiologic profile for assessing/monitoring shock events.

the pyruvic acid and hydrogen ions combine and form lactic acid which induces metabolic acidosis. The shift from aerobic to anaerobic glycolysis depresses protein synthesis, causes severe electrolyte and acid–base disturbances, and depletes the body of glycogen stores. As cellular hypoxia continues, the cells are damaged which

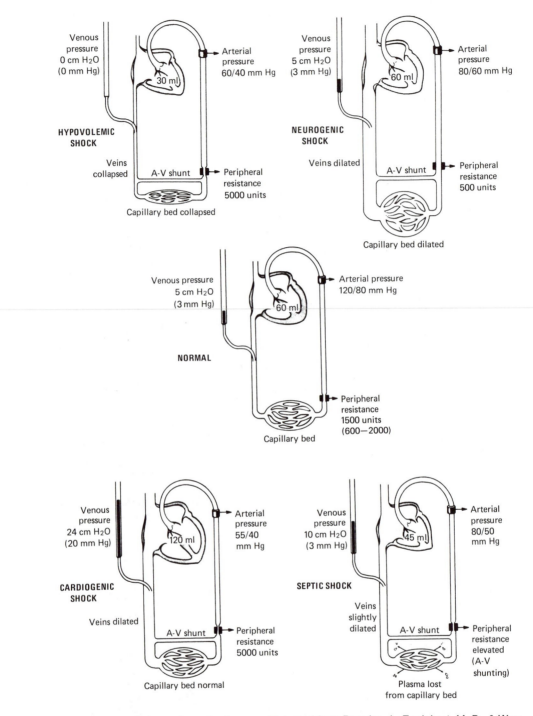

Figure 2. Shock: hemodynamic changes. (*Adapted from Dunphy, J., Englebert, M. D., & Way, L. W. Current Surgical Diagnosis and Treatment. Los Altos, Calif.: Lange Medical, 1973, p. 213.*)

disrupts their lysosomes, thus freeing their enzymes. These enzymes assist in the continual destruction of cells, and in addition, combine with inactive kininogens to form active kinins. The best known of these are bradykinin, histamine, and serotonin, which cause severe vasodilation, and may reduce cardiac output by depressing the heart.

Shock is a multisystem insult, and with decreased metabolism, comes deterioration of organ and system function. Ischemic or damaged intestine may spill bacteria and/or bacterial products across or through the mucosal barrier, allowing endotoxins to enter the bloodstream, which contribute to additional vasoconstriction and cardiac depression. Interstitial edema and atelectasis may develop as a result of damaged pulmonary capillary endothelium. Decreasing creatinine clearance tests are indicative of renal damage even though urinary output is fairly well maintained. Ischemic changes in the gastric mucosa causes erosions and stress bleeding. It is theorized that ischemic changes in the pancreas cause the release of proteolytic enzymes, which either stimulate the myocardial toxic factor (MTF) or alter plasma proteins to form toxic factors. This MTF factor interferes with the function of calcium ions in the myocardium by reducing its contractility. Continued hypoxia and inadequate perfusion to the brain causes deterioration in mentation, and is seen early in septic shock.

In the final stages of shock there is another fluid shift. This shift is generally opposite to that in the early stages of shock and produces a severe hypovolemia regardless of the etiologic factors or the kind of shock. Failure of the sodium pump to maintain a low sodium concentration allows sodium and water to enter the cell, producing intracellular edema, and further aggravating the ever increasing hypovolemia. With the continuation of this late shock state, the capillary endothelial cells swell, leaving enlarging intercellular capillary spaces which allow the leakage of protein molecules and the entry of red blood cells into the interstitial fluid space. This leak, combined with the increasing intracellular edema results in fluid leaving the circulation. This capillary leak is seen early in septic shock.

The increasing amounts of vasoactive substances accumulating in the capillaries and the fluid shift to the interstitial space produces a progressive decrease and slowing of effective circulation. The sludging within the capillaries, as well as chemical changes, cause stagnation and aggregation of red blood cells and intravascular clotting.

CARDIOGENIC SHOCK

Serious impairment of the pumping ability of the heart is the primary etiologic factor in the development of cardiogenic shock. A result of this impairment is a drastic reduction in arterial pressure and cardiac output. The most frequent cause of cardiogenic shock is myocardial infarction; however, cardiac tamponade, arrhythmias, or direct trauma to the heart may also produce cardiac shock (Fig. 2).

When ventricular dysfunction is present, stroke volume falls because of inadequate ventricular pressure to eject its capacitance of blood. This reduced ejection pressure causes an increase in the left ventricular end-diastolic pressure. Compensatory sympathetic response initiates an increase in venous flow by increasing vasoconstriction, and enhances contractility of the undamaged portion of the myocardium. As a result, diastolic inflow remains at a relatively normal level and end-diastolic volume remains high. As myocardial damage progresses, or additional demands are made on the heart, cardiac output and stroke volume are dramatically reduced and the compensatory mechanisms are unable to quell the progression of cardiac shock.

Pressures within the left atrium and left ventricle become elevated as a result of increased end-diastolic and end-systolic pressures. As a result of these elevated pressures there is a rise in the pulmonary circulation and a concomitant elevation in the pulmonary wedge pressure, and a possible increase in the central venous pressure.

Cardiogenic shock, like hypovolemic shock, commands the same biochemical, sympathetic, and hormonal responses producing essentially the same assessment findings with the exception of elevation of pulmonary wedge pressure, possible elevation of central venous pressure, and the possibility of irregularities in the pulse.

NEUROGENIC SHOCK

Neurogenic shock develops when there is a reduction in or a loss of vasomotor tone. Etiologic factors include spinal anesthesia, direct damage or trauma to the vasomotor center in the medulla, spinal cord injury, uninterrupted severe pain, central nervous system depressant drugs, metabolic effects on the vasomotor center such as decreased levels of blood sugar, and brain and brainstem damage (Fig. 2).

Loss of vasomotor tone results in decreased peripheral resistance and in decreased arterial pressure. As the vascular capacity increases, the dilated blood vessels retain a larger volume of blood. As a result, a normal amount of blood is unable to sufficiently fill the general circulatory system. This inadequate filling causes a drop in the main systemic pressure and a decreased return of venous blood to the heart. Cardiac output and arterial pressure declines as venous return is diminished. If uncorrected, neurogenic shock will activate the same compensatory responses as in hypovolemic shock, and will generally follow the same pathophysiologic course.

SEPTIC SHOCK

Septic shock is a condition caused by a systemic infection in which microorganisms and/or their products are found in the blood. It is indicative of invasive infection and carries a very poor prognosis. Gram-negative organisms are the most common cause of septic shock, although some forms of gram-positive cocci may be responsible (Fig. 2).

Two theories exist as to the etiology of septic shock. One implicates the bacteria themselves and the other cites the toxins released by the bacteria. In any case, it is most apparent that there is a primary defect in cellular uptake of oxygen or a defect in cellular utilization of oxygen.

Septic shock may present as a hyperdynamic state with a normal to high cardiac output, a normal or low central venous pressure, a low total peripheral resistance, and an increasing anaerobic metabolism. This hyperdynamic state is considered a high output–low resistance type of shock, and the patient's skin appears warm, dry, and flushed. Liberation of exotoxins stimulate the release of vasoactive kinins which initiate vasodilatory effects on small arteries and veins. This vasodilation causes a decrease in peripheral arteriolar resistance as well as a decrease in venular resistance. As a result of this decreased resistance, there is a pooling of blood in the capillaries which further reduces the effectiveness of the blood volume.

In contrast, there is a hypovolemic aspect to septic shock because of the movement of fluid into the inflamed areas. The combination of hypovolemia and decreased myocardial failure produces a hypodynamic state of septic shock. In this low output–high resistance form, just as in hypovolemic shock, there is a reduced cardiac output, a fall in systemic arterial pressure, a low central venous pressure, and a normal to increased peripheral resistance. With this form of septic shock, the patient presents with a pale, moist, and cool appearance.

As the pathophysiologic state continues, the same sympathetic, biochemical, and hormonal mechanisms are ushered into action providing essentially the same assessment parameters as exist in hypovolemic and cardiogenic shock.

Basically, the abnormality in septic shock is inadequate tissue perfusion resulting from stagnation and shunting of circulation secondary to endotoxin release as seen by vasoconstriction, reduction in cardiac output, hypotension, and renal failure.

4. Management Modalities

I. Identify and alleviate primary etiologic factors
  A. Control bleeding
  B. Drain abscesses
  C. Emergency surgery for abdominal complications
  D. Pericardiocentesis (cardiac tamponade)
II. Provide oxygen therapy to promote optimal ventilation and relief of hypoxia
  A. Ventilator mask
  B. Endotracheal intubation
III. Institute measures to support management modalities by establishing the following:
  A. Catheters
    1. CVP line
    2. venous line

    3. intraarterial line
    4. PCWP line
    5. Foley catheter
    6. nasogastric tube
  B. Laboratory tests
    1. CBC
    2. type and crossmatch
    3. serum electrolytes
    4. arterial blood gases
    5. lactate levels
    6. blood cultures
IV. Monitor continuously for trends and response to management modalities
  A. Temperature
  B. Pulse
  C. Respirations
  D. bp
  E. CVP
  F. Pulmonary wedge pressure
  G. Level of consciousness
  H. Skin quality and appearance
  I. Arterial pH
  J. Bicarbonate levels
  K. Hemoglobin levels
  L. Serum electrolytes
  M. Urinary output
  N. Urine sodium levels
  O. Urine osmolarity
  P. Subjective responses
V. Promote and institute measures aimed at restoring acid–base, electrolyte, and fluid balance
  A. Correct respiratory alkalosis
  B. Correct metabolic acidosis
  C. Administer sodium bicarbonate
    1. maintain arterial pH of 7.35 to 7.50
    2. maintain Pa_{CO_2} between 30 and 40 mm Hg
    3. maintain HCO_3 between 20 and 26 mEq/L
  D. Fluids
    1. to maintain CVP between 12 and 15 cm H_2O
    2. to maintain PWP not less than 15 and not more than 20 mm Hg
  E. Types of fluid
    1. crystalloid solutions
      a. Ringer's lactate
      b. buffered electrolyte solution without lactate
    2. colloid solutions
      a. albumin (5 percent)

        b. plasma

        c. plasmanates

     3. blood (to maintain hemoglobin between 12.5 and 14 g percent)

  F. Fluid challenge (especially in hypovolemic and cardiogenic)

VI. Restore, maintain, and support cardiac function and output

  A. Digoxin (rapid and multiple small doses, IV; loading dose—0.5 mg; 0.25 mg q 1 hour until optimal effect achieved)

     1. assess for digitalis toxicity

     2. assess for arrhythmias

  B. Dopamine (low dose of 2 to 15 μg/kg/minute)

  C. Epinephrine (1 to 5 μg/minute) (assess for arrhythmias)

  D. Isoproterenol (1 to 4 μg/minute)

     1. contraindicated in myocardial infarct, pulmonary embolism, and septic shock

     2. assess for

        a. tachyarrhythmias

        b. angina

        c. ST–T changes

     3. manage with

        a. norepinephrine

        b. high dose dopamine

  E. Calcium chloride (1 g per 2 to 4 units of blood)

     1. assess for digitalis toxicity

     2. assess for arrhythmias

VII. Restore and maintain hemodynamics and metabolism

  A. Steroids (specifically in septic and hypovolemic shock)

     1. hydrocortisone (75 to 200 mg q 6 hours, IV bolus)

     2. Solu–Medrol (50 mg/kg slow infusion over 20 to 30 minutes)

        a. assess for hyperglycemia and manage with insulin

        b. assess for urine sodium retention and correct imbalance

        c. assess for potassium loss in urine and correct imbalance

        d. assess for steroid induced ulcer and manage with antacids and cimetadine

  B. Vasopressors (not in hypovolemia)

     1. dopamine

     2. metaraminol

     3. norepinephrine

     4. isoproterenol

     5. phenylephrine

     6. methoxamine

     7. dobutamine

  C. Vasodilators (not in hypovolemia and septic shock)

     1. chlorpromazines (1 to 2 mg q 3 to 5 minutes until effect achieved)

        a. assess for drowsiness and lethargy

        b. assess for CNS changes

      2. nitroprusside IV, especially in cardiogenic shock

      3. nitroglycerine IV, especially in cardiogenic shock

  D. Diuretics

      1. furosemide

      2. mannitol

      3. ethacrynic acid

      4. thiazides

  E. Antiarrhythmics

      1. lidocaine

      2. procainamide

      3. quinidine

  F. Anticoagulants

      1. heparin (especially in septic shock)

VIII. Promote measures designed to combat infection or counteract reduced resistance to infection

  A. Prophylactic antibiotic therapy

  B. Specific antibiotic therapy for identified organism(s)

  IX. Institute mechanical modalities for continual support of vascular system

      1. Shock trousers (shunts blood from legs and abdomen to vital organs)

      2. Intraaortic balloon pump (controls amount of blood in aorta)

5. Rationale Underlying Management Modalities

Initial effort must be directed toward establishing the etiologic factor(s) while appropriate emergency measures are being instituted. Any bleeding must be controlled either by tourniquet or by direct pressure to the site. Administration of oxygen ensures that the patient is adequately ventilated, so that the blood reaching the tissues is optimally oxygenated and that the arterial Po_2 is maintained to at least 80 mm Hg. Measures to support management modalities, such as catheters and laboratory tests cited, establish baseline values and initial diagnostic data.

    Evaluation of the baseline data help determine the types and amounts of fluids to be used to restore maximum stroke volume. Particular factors to be evaluated are pulse rate, blood pressure, central venous pressure and pulmonary wedge pressure, urinary output, skin perfusion, and metabolic states. If ordered, a fluid challenge should be administered to assess the hemodynamic response to an increased circulatory volume. Despite the fluids administered, the circulatory blood volume must be appropriate to sustain a central venous pressure between 12 and 15 mm Hg and a capillary wedge pressure between 15 and 20 mm Hg. The exception to this would be in those individuals who had previously high cardiac pressures. Ringer's lactate is usually the emergency solution of choice, but is contraindicated in cirrhotic states, advanced septic shock, and in any shock state accompanied by metabolic alkalosis. In these instances, a buffered electrolyte solution is preferred. A poor response to the initial fluid protocol might indicate the need for administering plasma, 5 percent salt-poor albumin or plasmanates. Utilization of these colloidal solutions helps to maintain the blood's colloidal osmotic pressure at a relatively normal level. If blood is used either to treat hemorrhage or to maintain the hemoglobin at a normal level for better intravascular volume, it must be accompanied by calcium chloride administration. Citrate in the whole blood causes ionized calcium deficiencies, which in turn interferes with the heart's contractility. Whatever fluid protocol is established, it is grossly important to scrupulously monitor the vascular pressure trends and the intake and output to assess for signs and symptoms of fluid overload or fluid depletion.

Acid–base disturbances, such as metabolic acidosis, that do not respond to ventilatory support and fluid administration, can be corrected by the intravenous use of sodium bicarbonate to counteract the rising lactate levels. Arterial blood gas levels determine the need for, and the amount to be given.

Restoration, maintenance, and support of cardiac function is of major significance in this critically ill patient. Digitalis and digitalis preparations in small doses may be used to improve myocardial function. The use of such drugs may predispose the patient to increased incidence of arrhythmias because of the increased myocardial oxygen demands, and therefore, must be monitored closely. If arrhythmias develop, antiarrhythmic drugs are administered. Vasoactive pharmacologic agents are also used to alter peripheral vascular resistance and improve cardiac output. Adrenergic vasopressors often help to keep blood flowing to the heart, brain, and other organs in adequate amounts to ward off irreversible shock. The choice of vasopressor oftentimes depends on whether the shock state stems mainly from cardiac failure, impaired peripheral vessel function, or a combination of both. Dopamine is currently the agent of choice in attempting to increase cardiac and urinary output. Dopamine is a valuable choice in all types of shock because it selectively constricts certain blood vessels, while at the same time dilates those vessels innervating the heart, brain, mesentery, and kidneys. This latter action counteracts its α-adrenergic vasoconstricting activity with only a slight increase in heart rate. Dopamine also activates dopaminergic receptors in the kidney which increases urinary output. Another frequently used β-stimulator is isoproterenol. A contraindication to this drug is the development of tachycardia, which if left uncorrected will decrease diastolic filling time. Patients receiving β-stimulating drugs must be closely monitored for signs and symptoms of excessive β-stimulation. These signs include angina, tachyarrhythmias, premature beats, and ST–T changes on electrocardiographic readings. β-stimulators are contraindicated in states of low peripheral resistance (e.g., septic shock), severe tachycardia or in myocardial irritability. In such cases an α-adrenergic agent may be used such as high dose dopamine or another α-stimulator such as norepinephrine (Levophed).

The use of vasodilators is only indicated in those individuals with an expanded blood volume, and who still show evidence of continual vasoconstriction and poor tissue perfusion. Therefore, their use is contraindicated in hypovolemic and septic shock. A variety of vasodilators, such as chlorpromazine, nitroprusside, and nitroglycerin may be used to correct this vasoconstriction. Nitroprusside and nitroglycerin are especially valuable in treating cardiogenic shock. A positive assessment parameter is improvement in skin perfusion and urinary output.

Diuretic therapy is recommended only after extracellular volume has been restored, and when all therapies have failed to increase urinary output. Electrolyte imbalance from diuretic therapy must be frequently assessed and corrected immediately.

The use of steroids remains controversial; however, their administration appears valuable. The rationale for their use includes suppressing the systemic reaction to endotoxins, increasing cardiac output, decreasing peripheral arterial resistance, controlling fever and toxicity, minimizing cellular damage by stabilization of lysosomes, and in supporting adequate cortisone levels in the face of cortisone deficiencies brought on by prolonged stress. Hyperglycemia, gastric bleeding and ulceration, sodium retention, and potassium loss are problems that may result from steroid therapy. Hyperglycemia can be managed by using insulin; gastric ulceration may be managed with antacids and/or cimetidine, and electrolyte imbalances corrected appropriately.

Measures to combat infection or counteract reduced resistance to infection are instituted by the prophylactic use or antibiotic–antiinfective therapy or by specific antibiotic–antiinfective therapy for identified organism(s).

In persistent shock, especially in septic shock, intravascular coagulopathy may be present. If laboratory data demonstrate a severe decrease in the platelet count and concentrations of prothrombin, fibrinogen, and Factors V and VIII, heparin therapy may be instituted to antagonize thrombin formation.

Mechanical modalities may be necessary for the continual support of the vascular system. One of these is the pneumatic antishock trousers which can be used to control intraabdominal, lower extremity and pelvic bleeding, as well as a means of shunting blood from the abdomen and the legs to other vital organs of the body. Another mechanical support is the intraaortic balloon. This device can be introduced into the descending thoracic aorta for the purpose of reducing the work load of the left ventricle by lowering left ventricular systolic pressure. In so doing, there is an increase in coronary artery blood flow, an increase in peripheral tissue perfusion, and a decrease in the systolic afterload work of the heart.

Shock References

Cohen, S. Nursing care of the patient in shock. Part 2: Fluids, oxygen and the intra-aortic balloon pump. *American Journal of Nursing*, 1982, **82** (9), 1401–1422.

Concannon, J. E. Antishock trousers. *Journal of Family Practice*, 1982, **15** (2), 349–352.

Ellenbogen, C. Treatment priorities for septic shock. *American Family Physician*, 1982, **25** (2), 163–167.

Gaffney, F. A. Hemodynamic effects of medical anti-shock trousers (MAST garment). *Journal of Trauma*, 1981, **21** (11), 931–937.

Goldfarb, R. D. Cardiac dynamics following shock: Role of circulating cardiopressant substances. *Circulatory Shock*, 1982, **9** (3), 317–334.

Goldman, D. A., Mala, D. G., & Rhaney, F. S. Guidelines for infection control in intravenous therapy. *Annals of Internal Medicine*, 1973, **79**, 848.

Maher, A. B. A systems approach to nursing the patient with multiple system failure. *Heart Lung*, 1981, **10** (5), 866–867.

Marx, J. A. Objective approach to the management of shock. *Annals of Emergency Medicine*, 1982, **11** (3), 167–168.

McCaffree, R. D. Shock: How to recognize its early stages and what to do about it. *Medical Times*, 1979, **107** (9), 25.

Mohr, J. A., & Coussons, T. Septic shock. *Medical Times*, 1979, **107** (9), 39.

Moylan, J. A. Emergency medicine: Shock—do's and don'ts of the trade. *Proceedings of the Annual Meeting of the Medical Section of the American Council of Life Insurance*, 1981, **6**, 153–164.

Pepine, C. J., Nichols, W. W., & Alexander, I. A. Guidelines to evaluation and management of shock. *Hospital Medicine*, 1979, **15** (3) 88–119.

Poole, G. V. Comparison of colloids and crystalloids in resuscitation from hemorrhage shock. *Surgery of Gynecology and Obstetrics*, 1982, **154** (4), 577–586.

Pure, V. K. The pathophysiology of septic shock. *Internal Medicine*, 1982, **67** (1), 5–8.

Snow, N. Intra-aortic balloon counterpulsation for cardiogenic shock from cardiac contusion. *Journal of Trauma*, 1982, **22** (5), 426–429.

Symposium on new concepts in shock therapy. *Advances in Shock Research*, 1980, **3**, 1–296.

Whitmen, G. Intra-aortic balloon pumping and cardiac mechanisms: A programmed lesson. *Heart Lung*, 1978, **6**, 1034.

Whitsett, T. L. Medical management of shock: Drugs of choice and their choice. *Medical Times*, 1979, **107** (9), 59.

Wilson, R. F. The diagnosis and management of severe sepsis and septic shock. *Heart Lung*, 1976, **5** (3), 422.

Zamova, B. Management of hemorrhagic shock. *Hospital Medicine*, 1979, **15** (7), 6.

SECTION THREE

SYSTEMIC EMERGENCIES

A. NEUROMUSCULAR EMERGENCIES

1. Cerebrovascular Accident

ASSESSMENT

Refer to Tables 2 and 3 on the following pages.

PATHOPHYSIOLOGY

Cerebrovascular accident (CVA) is one of the most common neurologic disorders seen today. The vascular problems usually arise in the conducting arteries which form an extensive network over the hemispheres and communicate with penetrating arteries which nourish the brain. The cerebral circulatory route is usually symmetrical, but variations commonly exist which can confuse the clinical picture. Specific areas of the brain are fed by more than one artery and extensive anastomoses exist in the cerebral cortex which extend across the corpus callosum. There also exists great variability in the collateral blood flow of the circle of Willis. In addition, the presence of concomitant metabolic factors affect the clinical picture of a CVA.

A cerebrovascular accident may be classified by its pattern of clinical progression or by its vascular problem. A transient ischemic attack (TIA) produces deficits that develop suddenly and then disappear, however, one third of these patients will eventually develop a cerebral infarct. A stroke-in-evolution is one in which the deficits appear over time with a series of sudden events. In a completed stroke, deficits are maximal at the onset with little improvement seen later.

Cerebral *thrombosis* is the most frequent cause of a CVA and has its greatest incidence during the middle or later years of life. The commonest cause is arterio-atherosclerotic vessel changes which predispose to clot propagation, edema, anaerobic glycolysis, and alterations in cerebral functions.

Lipid atherosclerotic plaques gradually build up in an irregular pattern on the intima of arteries. Some plaques remain soft and necrotic whereas others become

TABLE 2. CEREBROVASCULAR ACCIDENT: ASSESSMENT FINDINGS ASSOCIATED WITH DIFFERENT VASCULAR PROBLEMS

Parameter	Cerebral Thrombosis	Cerebral Embolism	Cerebral Hemorrhage	Cerebral Aneurysm–AVM
Mode of onset				
Time	Usually occurs at rest; Takes minutes to hours	Occurs at any time; Within seconds to minutes	Occurs at any time; Very sudden	Occurs at any time; Very sudden
Activity; Prodrome; Headache	Unrelated to activity; TIAs common; Suboccipital; mild or none	Unrelated to activity; No warning; Localized: fleeting, and/or moderate	During activity or stress; No warning; Severe	Unrelated to activity; No warning; Severe: migraine type
Preexisting disease	Atherosclerosis: Evidence of risk factors (smoking, oral contraceptives, hyperlipidemia, hypertension, diabetes mellitus), inflammatory processes (vasculitis, meningitis, encephalitis, periarteritis, temporal arteritis) Infections of face, sinus, or middle ear Trauma or mechanical obstruction by masses Polycythemia Dehydration in elderly	Sequelae of cardiac disease: (mural thrombus from atrial fibrillation, MI, prosthetic valves, septic emboli in SBE) Atheromatous plaques off carotids or aortic arch Air or fat embolism Inflammatory diseases (TB, syphilis, fungus)	Hypertension Ruptured aneurysm or sclerotic vessel Secondary to anticoagulation Blood dyscrasias (acute leukemia, hemophilia, polycythemia, thrombocytopenia) Trauma Systemic disease (lupus erythematosus, hepatic disease)	Hypertension May follow infections and/or arteriosclerotic processes Associated with polycystic kidneys and coarctation of the aorta AVM are developmental defects
Common findings				
LOC	Mostly confusion	Transient or prolonged loss	Rapid progression to coma	Transient or lasting loss
Blood pressure	Hypertensive	Normotensive	Hypertensive	Hypertensive

	Thrombosis	Embolism	Hemorrhage	Aneurysm / AV malformation
Meningeal irritation	None	None	Nuchal rigidity	Nuchal rigidity + Kernig and Brudinski signs
Bruit	Heard over involved artery or opposite carotid artery, subclavian or back of neck	Not usual	Not usual	Heard in neck carotids, mastoid process and eyes
Seizures	May occur with venous thrombosis; otherwise not usual	Not usual	Focal seizures possible	Seen prior to AV malformation rupture
Diagnostic tests CSF	Clear: No change in pressure unless swelling is great	Clear: No change in pressure ↑ WBC, lymphs if sepsis. ↑ protein	Grossly bloody: Pressure elevated if bleed great. ↑ protein	Grossly bloody: Pressure elevated if bleed great. WBC and RBC rise proportionately
CAT scan	If early, necrotic tissue seen: Later, cavitation	If early, hemorrhage can be seen in the infarct: Otherwise negative	Identifies size and location of bleed	Detects area of intracerebral bleed
Angiography	Arteries of circle of Willis or their branches will show narrowing or obstruction	(Same as for thrombosis)	Hemorrhagic area seen as an avascular zone surrounded by stretched and displaced arteries and veins	Typical aneurysm pattern Characteristic pattern of AV malformation
Brain scan	May show marked uptake in affected area	(Same as for thrombosis)	Normal	Increase in uptake in area of AV malformation
Skull x-rays	Calcification of carotids Pineal shift to opposite side may be seen	Very little shift of pineal	Shift of pineal to opposite side	Partial calcification of walls of aneurysm

Focal neurologic findings: Involvement of specific cerebral arteries produces the specific deficits seen in the patient with a cerebrovascular accident whether it be due to thrombosis, embolism, hemorrhage, aneurysm, or arteriovenous malformation. (See next pages.)

TABLE 3. ORIGIN OF FOCAL NEUROLOGIC DEFICITS IN A CEREBROVASCULAR ACCIDENT

	Internal Carotid	Vertebral Artery	Basilar Artery	Middle Cerebral Artery	Anterior Cerebral	Posterior Cerebral
Motor deficits	Contralateral upper extremity weakness may progress to face and tongue	Ipsilateral paralysis of palate, vocal cords; decreased gag reflex; dysphagia; hoarseness Ipsilateral ataxia of limbs with falling or toppling to affected side	Contralateral or bilateral hemiparesis in one or four limbs Dysphagia Ataxia which may be severe Upper extremity static tremor	Contralateral flaccid hemiplegia or hemiparesis or monoparesis Dysmetria, if nondominant side	Contralateral hemiplegia greater in foot and leg but may involve proximal arm Contralateral grasp reflex Gegenhalten rigidity Gait apraxia Paraplegia possible	Mild contralateral hemiparesis Contralateral ataxic tremor Hemiballismus or hemichoreoathetosis Ataxia
Sensory deficits	Contralateral paresthesias in arm, face, and tongue	Ipsilateral decreased facial response to pain Contralateral decrease in pain and temperature sense Loss of taste	Contralateral or bilateral loss of sensation including the face	Contralateral hemianesthesia Loss of proprioception, fine touch and localization	Mild sensory losses in contralateral lower extremity	Contralateral hemisensory losses May have thalamic pain Depression and/or distortion of taste
Speech deficits	If dominant side, expressive aphasia	None	Dysarthria with slurring	If dominant side, global aphasia	Laconic spoken responses, akinetic mutism—if bilateral involvement; speaks in whispers Perseveration	If dominant side, receptive (sensory) aphasia

Visual deficits	Ipsilateral transient loss of vision (amaurosis fugax)	Ipsilateral Horner syndrome (miosis, ptosis, decreased sweating) Nystagmus Diplopia	Ipsilateran Horner syndrome Some degree of blindness Nystagmus Diplopia Ipsilateral horizontal gaze palsy Oscillopsia	Contralateral homonymous hemianopsia or impairment of conjugate gaze opposite to site of lesion	None	Incomplete or contralateral homonymous hemianopsia Alexia, dyslexia without dysgraphia Anomia for color and faces Ipsilateral third nerve palsy with contralateral palsy Topographic disorientation for surroundings
Other neurologic deficits	None	Vertigo Nausea, vomiting Hiccups	Vertigo Nausea, vomiting Memory disturbances Partial deafness, tinnitus Stupor, coma	Opposite side neglect Variations in alertness; stupor and coma possible	Mental confusion Amnesia Easily distracted No will power or initiative (abulia) Urinary incontinence	Recent memory loss Stupor, coma

hard and calcified. These degenerative changes in the plaques eventually involve both the intima and media coats of arteries. A plaque may ulcerate, lead to stenosis of a vessel, and/or cause an acute occlusion of an artery.

Atherosclerotic plaques propagate clot formation. Platelets are attracted to the roughened lining of the vessel and become injured. Injured platelets release thromboplastin which in combination with other clotting factors, acts on circulating prothrombin, converting it to thrombin. Enzymatically, thrombin converts fibrinogen to fibrin which forms a meshwork of tiny strands that entangle blood cells to form a clot. This clot may remain stationary (thrombus) or it may break off (embolus).

Thrombotic stenosis and/or occlusion of an artery leads to ischemia or infarction of the brain tissue that artery supplies. The ischemic portion involved undergoes necrosis. A pale infarct occurs when the necrotic brain tissue is liquefied and removed by the normal body processes leaving behind scar tissue or small cysts filled with clear fluid. A red infarct is believed to be due to red blood cells leaving the damaged artery wall and invading the necrotic brain tissue.

Because the brain is so dependent upon an adequate supply of oxygen, ischemia resulting in hypoxia of brain tissue can produce devastating effects. Without oxygen, cellular metabolism switches to anaerobic glycolysis for energy. This type of metabolism is inefficient and results in an increase in lactate production, carbon dioxide retention and failure of the sodium–potassium pump. These events lead to acidosis, brain swelling, and the possibility of increased intracranial pressure.

The focal signs of a CVA usually correlate with the artery occluded. However, the effects of the occlusion may vary for a number of reasons. The degree of deficits depends upon the size of the artery occluded, the function of the now ischemic tissue, and the presence of adequate collateral circulation. In addition, because of the variable arterial anastomoses, brain tissue distal to the thrombus may be affected leading to a decrease in cerebral blood flow and metabolism in that part of the brain.

A second type of ischemic CVA is due to the occlusion of an artery by material from outside of the brain. *Embolism* is the second leading cause of a CVA. The onset of this type is sudden, not related to time or activity and can affect all age groups.

Embolic material may arise from a number of sources. Whereas cardiac pathology is the most common source, embolic material can be composed of a small fragment of a blood clot, atheromatous plaque, or tumor. Emboli may originate with thrombotic or suppurative processes elsewhere in the vascular tree and body. In adults and the aged, a fragment of a mural thrombosis that occurs in association with atrial fibrillation or myocardial infarction may break off and embolize to the brain. In children and young adults, cerebral emboli are associated with rheumatic heart disease and endocarditis. Fat embolism to the brain can occur after a long bone fracture and an air emboli can result from lung trauma. Most emboli are sterile but could be septic.

The occlusive nature of embolic material causes ischemia and infarction of cerebral tissue that artery serves. Like thrombus formation, clot formation with resolution usually occurs. Red infarcts result mainly from embolic phenomena. Because the occlusion is so rapid, greater amounts of tissue death are seen with embolism as there is little time for collateral or anastomotic vessels to dilate and compensate for the decrease in perfusion. Septic emboli may lead to encephalitis, abscess formation or a mycotic aneurysm which may later rupture. Embolic events are usually multiple in nature and it is wise to look for infarcts in other organs.

The degree of deficits seen with cerebral embolism depends upon the size of the embolus and the artery involved. In sequential order, these arteries are most commonly affected: middle cerebral, vertebral, basilar, and inferior cerebellar. An embolus may disintegrate into smaller emboli and travel causing a confusing clinical picture.

Intracerebral hemorrhage is the third leading cause of a CVA. This type of stroke affects all age groups and both sexes. If coma is an early presenting sign, the prognosis is poor.

Hypertension is frequently associated with intracerebral hemorrhages. With time, it initiates a series of events that damage arterial walls. The smaller arteries which branch off the large caliber arteries are subject to the greatest strain. Their walls eventually weaken and dilate to form saccular aneurysms. Under the right conditions, these microaneurysms will rupture and bleed into brain tissue. For some unexplained reason, the lenticulostriate vessels seem to be the most vulnerable to this series of events.

A small or lacunar intracerebral hemorrhage may remain circumscribed and local. Phagocytic mechanisms remove the sanguinous material leaving behind a cystic cavity filled with brown hemosiderin stained borders. In approximately 6 months, only a cleft may remain. Brain tissue adjacent to the cyst may appear edematous and show other changes. However, if the bleeding is minimal, survival is possible with function returning slowly. Rebleeding at the same site is uncommon.

Massive intracerebral hemorrhages are commonly fatal. This bleeding tends to pass along cerebral tissue planes and may extend to the adjacent ventricle or rupture into the subarachnoid space. Larger hemorrhages may obliterate the putamen, thalamus, pons, and cerebellum. Hemorrhages secondary to anticoagulation therapy, bleeding diathesis, and trauma tend to involve other areas of the brain such as the frontal, temporal, or occipital lobes and can be distinguished from hypertensive hemorrhage.

The prognosis is extremely poor with a massive intracerebral hemorrhage. The accumulation of blood, an irritant to brain tissue, leads to cerebral swelling, compression, and displacement of cerebral tissue and increased intracranial pressure. The deficits are related to the size of the bleed and the areas of the brain involved. Putaminal hemorrhage often produces a clinical picture similar to middle cerebral artery occlusion but there is a greater change in the level of consciousness. Thalamic hemorrhage tends to produce greater sensory than motor losses and unusual eye signs. Pontine hemorrhage results in early coma, pin point pupils that react to light and decerebrate posturing. Cerebellar hemorrhage presents with sudden dizziness, vomiting, and truncal ataxia. Intracerebral hemorrhage may lead to signs of herniation and death very rapidly. Cerebellar hemorrhage has the best prognosis, if the hematoma can be evacuated rapidly.

Rupture of a cerebral aneurysm or vascular malformation may produce a combination of intracerebral and/or subarachnoid hemorrhage. This type of hemorrhage accounts for the fourth leading cause of CVA. Aneurysm rupture tends to occur in the middle to later years of life whereas vascular malformation hemorrhage is most likely to present in childhood or during young adult years.

Aneurysms vary in their size, shape, and location. They range from 1 to 10 centimeters in diameter and change over time. Fusiform aneurysms appear as rather uniform dilatations of the entire circumference of a blood vessel whereas saccular (berry) aneurysms, the most commonly seen in adults, appear as a pouch with a small neck protruding from a vessel. Aneurysms can occur anywhere but have a propensity at sites of arterial bifurcations and branching. Cerebral aneurysms are seen most frequently in the vessels of the circle of Willis and near the basilar surface of the skull.

Aneurysms are usually asymptomatic, but can cause clinical symptoms because of their propensity to grow. Symptoms result from rupture, pressure on surrounding structures, and thrombosis. Larger aneurysms can erode the bones of the skull and sella turcica plus compress adjacent cerebral tissue and nerves. Rupture tends to be related to extreme physical or emotional stress and is accompanied by an unusually severe headache. The patient may loose consciousness or be drowsy and confused. Signs of meningeal irritation such as nucchal rigidity are common as is a low grade fever. If unconsciousness persists, the prognosis is poor. In many cases the neurologic deficits clear as the effects of vasospasm are reduced. However, there is a strong tendency for aneurysms to rebleed in 6 to 8 weeks. If the bleeding blocks the flow of cerebrospinal fluid, hydrocephalus may develop.

Vascular malformations represent a developmental tissue defect. There appears to be no distinction between an artery, vein, or capillary because the layers of these vessels is missing. To compensate, adjacent arteries try to nourish the abnormal vessels and their surrounding tissue. Soon these vessels become enlarged, engorged, and tortuous, resulting in a poorly organized mass of arteries and veins which convey blood under very high pressure.

Vascular malformations usually come to clinical attention because of seizures or rupture producing hemorrhage. A chronic headache is a common complaint prior to rupture. Bruit over the eyeball, carotid artery, or mastoid also suggests this type of malformation. The progression and course of a rupture is the same as for a ruptured aneurysm.

From the foregoing material it should be apparent that not only must a distinction be made between ischemia and hemorrhage as the basis for the presenting clinical picture, but also that other processes that could lead to the same deficits be ruled out.

The triage nurse plays a major role in obtaining the history of the patient while others care for the patient's immediate resuscitative needs. Questioning should focus upon the immediate prodromal events of the situation as well as the patient's life style, concomitant medical–surgical problems, recent or past injuries or surgery and medications (prescribed and over-the-counter) the patient has taken. The history of a sudden, rapid onset of neurologic deficits helps to rule out other neurologic problems that may produce a similar clinical picture.

The physical examination of the patient usually gives a fairly accurate clinical hypothesis but this must be validated with laboratory and other diagnostic studies. The usual blood and urine screening studies are performed as for any acutely ill patient. If it is possible, the first special study done should be a CAT scan. This remarkable machine, in a noninvasive manner, is capable of diagnosing intracranial hemorrhage and differentiating it from an ischemic process in the majority of cases.

When a CAT scan is not available, lumbar puncture (LP) is done to examine the cerebrospinal fluid (CSF). Blood in the CSF is usually found in all cases where subarachnoid hemorrhage has occurred, in some cases of intracerebral hemorrhage, and rarely found in patients with an ischemic origin to their CVA. Cerebral edema results in a rise in CSF pressure in some types of CVA patients.

There are certain risks in performing a LP when intracranial pressure is already elevated. Withdrawal of CSF could disrupt this pressure to such an extent that herniation of cerebral tissue downward through the tentorial notch or foramen magnum occurs. If the patient is at high risk of this occurrence, a hyperosmolar agent may be infused prior to the LP. If signs of deterioration occur during the LP, the procedure is stopped and a hyperosmolar solution administered along with high doses of a steroid.

Examination of the arterial vessels (angiography) can be performed to obtain a clearer picture of the pattern of the arterial supply and drainage in the brain. It is most helpful in the ischemic type of CVA and when confusion exists as to the basis of hemorrhagic CVA (e.g., ruptured aneurysm, AV malformation, or hypertensive intracerebral hemorrhage). This can be a very stressful test and at times is delayed in the patient with a hemorrhage problem, if severe hypertension already exists.

Radioactive technetium is the most commonly used substance for brain scanning. The area of infarction in an ischemic CVA shows an increase in uptake of this substance. However, it may not become positive for 4 to 5 days and thus, may not be done as part of the emergency room workup.

Skull x-rays are still considered useful tools in assessing patients with a presumed CVA. Typically, they show evidence of the effects of a mass in the brain which causes the pineal structure to shift. These films also depict calcifications of the arteries and are helpful in ruling out fractures that could have led to intracranial bleeding.

MANAGEMENT

I. Detect and correct airway obstruction
   A. Assess respiratory rate, depth, and pattern. Auscultate breath sounds. Report any rales, adventitious sounds or areas of consolidation
   B. Test swallowing and gag reflexes and ability to handle secretions
   C. Position on side to promote drainage of secretions

    D. Obtain stat chest x-ray; monitor the blood gases

    E. If airway is obstructed

        1. remove dentures; provide for their safe keeping

        2. suction gently, but frequently, using aseptic technique

        3. insert an oropharyngeal airway and secure it

    F. If ventilation is unsatisfactory, insert a cuffed endotracheal tube and assist ventilation mechanically. Suction tube frequently

    G. Administer oxygen as prescribed with humidification

    H. Carefully observe that patient does not hyper- or hypoventilate

  II. Evaluate and maintain adequate circulation to the tissues

    A. Take and record the bp q 15 to 30 minutes; report hypo- or hypertension

    B. Examine the peripheral pulses. Note their strength, quality, symmetry, and the presence of bruit

    C. Obtain a stat ECG: Continuous cardiac monitoring may be prescribed to detect myocardial or valvular disease that may be the source of emboli

    D. Monitor the serum electrolytes, osmolarity, BUN, glucose, and bleeding profile

    E. Insert a nasogastric tube and attach it to low suctioning

    F. Insert an indwelling urinary catheter; send samples to laboratory for urinalysis, electrolytes, and osmolarity

    G. Obtain rectal temperature; if elevated, monitor q 2 to 4 hours

    H. Establish an IV line for fluid and drug administration

        1. initial fluids should not be hypotonic (e.g., 5 percent D/W)

        2. start 0.45 percent in 2.5 percent D/W (or its equivalent)

        3. run in slowly or as prescribed

    I. Administer thiamine chloride 100 mg IV, if prescribed

    J. Keep accurate intake and output records

 III. Detect changes in neurologic status

    A. Prepare patient and assist with evaluative studies as ordered (e.g., CAT scan, brain scan, lumbar puncture, skull x-rays, etc.)

    B. Record the neurologic vital signs q 15 to 30 minutes

        1. level of consciousness and orientation

        2. pupillary responses: size, position, roundness, reaction to light, and accommodation; test extraocular eye movement in all directions; perform oculocephalic test or oculovestibular tests

        3. vision: note presence of visual field defects; papilledema

        4. motor responses: assess strength of hand grasp. Note spontaneous movements (e.g., myoclonic jerks, seizures), absence of movement and body posture or position assumed by patient; or best motor response on the Glasgow Coma Scale

        5. reflex activity: evaluate gag, swallow, blink, Babinski, Kernig reflexes

        6. sensory responses: note areas of anesthesia, hyperasthesia

    C. Describe communicating ability of patient (e.g., dysarthria, aphasia)

    D. Describe respiratory pattern: examples: Cheyne–Stokes, central neurogenic hyperventilation, apneustic breathing, ataxic breathing, depressed breathing, apnea

E. Report signs of increased ICP: decreasing LOC, pupillary changes, decrease in motor and sensory responses, increased blood pressure, slow pulse (Cushing reflex), papilledema

IV. Reduce intracranial pressure

A. Monitor ICP device, put in place after CAT scan. Normal pressure equals 4 to 14 mm Hg (50 to 200 mm H_2O)

B. Hyperventilate to a P_{CO_2} 20 to 25 mm Hg

C. Administer dexamethazone (Decadron)

   1. dosage: bolus of 10 mg IV followed by 4 mg IV q 4 to 6 hours as prescribed
   2. monitor the blood glucose, stool guaiac, urine for sugar and acetone, serum electrolytes; look for opportunistic infections

D. Administer mannitol or glycerol, as prescribed

   1. selection of drug depends upon physician
   2. dose of mannitol is 250 ml 20 percent solution given IV over 10 to 20 minutes
   3. dose of glycerol is 1 to 5 mg/kg/day in divided doses po
   4. with mannitol, observe for a rapid diuresis
   5. with both drugs, monitor serum osmolarity, blood glucose levels

V. Control seizure activity

A. Institute seizure precautions on all CVA patients

B. Observe seizuring activity. Record onset, spread, limbs involved, and postictal state. Protect patient from injury

C. Administer anticonvulsant medication as prescribed (e.g., Dilantin)

D. Drugs may be used prophylactically in CVA patients whose problem is due to ruptured aneurysm. For other types of CVA drugs not usually prescribed until seizures occur

VI. Reduce the incidence of further emboli or thrombotic insult

A. Administer anticoagulant or antiplatelet drugs as prescribed

   1. Heparin 5 to 10,000 U IV followed by a continuous infusion or repeated bolus of large dose, depending on clotting time *or* low dose heparin therapy at 5,000 U sc, q 8 hours

      a. maintain clotting time at double the control using Lee–White whole blood clotting time or PTT
      b. monitor for hemorrhagic side effects: skin purpura, hematuria, bleeding gums, blood in the stool
      c. have antidote ready: Protamine sulfate 2 mg/ml solution (mix 5 ml of a 1 percent solution in 20 ml of saline). Inject slowly, no more than 50 mg/10 minutes
      d. protect the patient from injury while receiving this drug

   2. Coumarin agents: Coumadin or Warfarin

      a. dose: Coumadin 75 mg/day; Warfarin 2 to 15 mg/day
      b. maintain prothrombin time between 17 and 19 seconds
      c. monitor for hemorrhagic side effects as above
      d. have antidote ready: vitamin K 50 mg IV or IM
      e. protect patient from injury while receiving this drug

3. Platelet antiaggregants
   a. drug and dose: aspirin 300 mg/day or every other day
      Dipyridamole—50 mg tid
      Sulfinpyrazone—200 mg tid
   b. observe for side effects: gastric irritation, aggravation of peptic ulcer disease, headache, dizziness, flushing, rash

VII. Maintain blood pressure within normal limits in hemorrhagic CVA
   A. Monitor bp q 15 to 30 minutes; rapid lowering is avoided
   B. Keep patient on complete bedrest, assist in all activities. Avoid straining or coughing. Provide a nonstimulating environment
   C. If diastolic pressure is consistently above 120 mm Hg, antihypertensive medication and/or diuretics may be prescribed

VIII. Detect and prevent recurrent hemorrhage from aneurysm or AV malformation
   A. Observe for signs of a rebleed: retro-orbital headache, confusion, decreased LOC, nucchal rigidity, sudden frontal headache, positive Kernig and Brudzinski sign
   B. Obtain baseline plasma fibrin levels. Administer antifibrinolytic agent
      1. drug: E-aminocaproic acid (Amicar) 30 to 36 g/day IV mix 30 to 36 g in 1 liter 2½ percent dextrose 0.45 percent saline solution
      2. infuse over 24 hours, using a microdrip and run slowly. Rapid infusion will lead to bradycardia, arrhythmias, marked hypotension
      3. observe for side effects: nausea, cramps, diarrhea

IX. Provide physical and emotional support to patient and family
   A. Keep patient and relatives informed of the rationale for acute care activities
   B. Explain to relatives the need for surgery, if indicated
   C. Allow patient (if possible) and family to ask questions and express fears
   D. Recognize that a communication disorder exists. Reassure the patient that the condition is known to staff
   E. Explain all activities by speaking slowly and softly
   F. Anticipate needs as much as possible
   G. Nurse must see that the patient is flat with head only slightly elevated
   H. Apply antiembolic stockings to both legs
   I. Place feet up against a board; elevate paralyzed arm
   J. Place body in correct alignment
   K. Offer skin, oral, and eye care as required
   L. Keep linens clean and wrinkle free

RATIONALE

The goals of emergency care for the patient with a CVA are to identify the type of CVA, prevent further neurologic damage and to treat life-threatening crisis situations. The general supportive modalities are similar for most CVA patients and the topic has been approached in this manner.

The immediate priority is to assure adequate oxygenation of the body's tissues and to prevent aspiration and/or hypercapnea. A good airway must be established, especially if the patient has a decreased level of consciousness. Placing the patient in the lateral decubitus position with the face turned toward the mattress promotes the drainage of oral secretions. The oropharynx should be suctioned frequently and gently to avoid raising intracranial pressure (ICP). A nasogastric tube will decompress the stomach, prevent aspiration of vomitus or secretions, and allows for easier ventilation. Serial blood gases are performed to monitor ventilatory efforts. Hypoventilating is to be avoided because it produces hypercapnea and respiratory acidosis which in turn increases cerebral blood flow and adds to the problem of increasing ICP.

Acutely ill patients require frequent monitoring of their physiologic status to detect trends and to evaluate their status. In the early stages, a patient with a CVA is frequently in a very unstable condition. Therefore, vital signs are taken every 15 to 30 minutes, cardiac performance is monitored, peripheral pulses assessed, and blood studies done to detect the physiologic status of this patient.

An inadequate circulation to the body's tissues leads to ischemia and tissue hypoxia which can produce pathologic changes in themselves and delay the identification of the underlying problem. An intravenous line is set in place and is used for fluid and drug administration. Hypotonic solutions are avoided with CVA patients, because they add to cerebral edema. Most patients only need enough fluids to keep them in fluid and electrolyte balance.

Another important indicator of physiologic functioning besides the sensorium and blood pressure is the urinary output. Urinary output is a reflection of renal blood flow which is dependent on cardiac output. Accurate measurement of input and output (I&O) is very necessary and will warrant the insertion of an indwelling urinary catheter.

The repeated neurologic assessments serve many functions. They establish a baseline of information for future reference, they provide information relating to the stabilization or deterioration of the patient's condition and they help define and/or locate the disease process. The complications of CVA include: increased ICP, additional emboli formation, expanding clot formation, and/or rebleeding. The medical and nursing staff must be alert to the signs of these catastrophic events.

Cerebral edema is a possible complication of all types of CVA. It is probably due to low arterial perfusion through ischemic or infarcted areas resulting in hypoxia, plus venous obstruction which causes the extravasation of cellular fluid into the interstitial fluid spaces of the brain. As the brain volume increases and eventually reaches cranial limits, the brain is pushed through weak points of the meninges, giving rise to herniation and displacement of structures. The nurse is always on the alert for signs of increasing ICP.

Clinical findings of increased ICP include rapid deterioration of LOC, progressive enlargement of one pupil. It is possible in some emergency centers to monitor ICP with special monitoring devices. A subarachnoid bolt, an intraventricular cannula, or an epidural probe may be used. The normal intracranial pressure ranges from 4 to 14 mm Hg. Any elevations are reported. The monitor can detect ICP before clinical signs are evident.

Immediate and prompt measures are taken to reduce the pressure to avoid further brain damage. Steroids are given intravenously. The exact mechanism by which these drugs reduce cerebral edema is not known at this time. Some researchers believe that they are capable of stabilizing capillary endothelium and reducing vascular permeability.

The hyperosmolar agent used to reduce cerebral edema related to a CVA may be glycerol because the rebound effect of mannitol increases cerebral pressure. Regardless of the physician's choice, the nurse must be certain that all urine is accurately measured and vital signs monitored when these agents are used.

Anoxic areas of the brain, collection of blood in the subarachnoid space and hypertensive encephalopathy are some of the possible causes of seizures in the CVA patient. They do not occur with regularity and therefore, treatment is withheld until there is evidence of this complication. Anticonvulsants are used prophylactically in CVA patients whose basic problem is a ruptured aneurysm. The nurse takes the usual seizure precautions; notes seizure activity and administers the prescribed medication.

The medical management of cerebral ischemia is fraught with controversy. Once the CVA is completed, little can be accomplished with medication or surgery. However, patients with transient ischemic attacks, strokes-in-evolution and completed strokes associated with minor deficits (where the risk of a more serious stroke is great) might respond favorably to aggressive anticoagulation therapy. The decision to use anticoagulation depends upon the patient's condition and the past medical history (e.g., gastric ulcers, bleeding problems, liver disease, renal disease, etc.).

One aim of anticoagulation is to inhibit the thrombin system. Heparin quickly neutralizes thrombin by combining with circulating cofactors and antithrombin III. Coumarin agents are taken orally and their effects take longer to observe. These agents alter the synthesis of vitamin K-dependent clotting factors (e.g., Factors III, VII, IX, X). The nurse administers these drugs and closely observes for the clinical and laboratory evidence of bleeding. The nurse must be familiar with the appropriate antidotes and have them readily available for emergency use.

Antiplatelet agents (e.g., aspirin) are used for patients in whom the coumarin drugs and heparin are contraindicated. The goal of this therapy is to interfere with platelet functioning and thus delay clotting. Bleeding is also a problem with antiplatelet agents because the dosage is high. The antidote is a platelet transfusion or fresh frozen plasma. Whereas it is true that to date there is no clinical proof that any of these drugs will prevent a clot from forming, many physicians feel that they are beneficial.

The danger of recurrent hemorrhage, vasospasm, and hydrocephalus exists in patients who have a CVA resulting from hemorrhage. It is believed that rebleeding occurs from lysis of the blood clot covering the original bleeding point in the brain. The drug, E-aminocaproic acid inhibits antifibrinolysin action, thereby retarding clot breakdown. This drug is usually administered intravenously and the nurse would observe for its side effects. The complications of vasospasm and hydrocephalus usually occur later in the hemorrhage process, thus their treatment shall not be discussed for it would not fall into the realm of the emergency department.

The CVA patient's degree of recovery depends heavily upon the type of emergency care received. Nurses play a vital role in identifying trends in the patient's condition and instituting acute care activities to maintain proper organ functioning. The nurse must also consider the relatives and the role they play in the decision making process. She or he can begin the rehabilitative process, which may be quite long, by proper positioning, ROM, relieving pressure, and keeping the patient free from iatrogenic infection. Most patients with a CVA are admitted to hospital for further observation, care, and possible surgical procedures.

2. Craniocerebral Trauma

ASSESSMENT

   I. Presenting clinical picture
      A. Acutely ill patient
      B. Most likely unresponsive or with vacillating LOC
      C. Bleeding, if scalp lacerated
      D. Respirations may be rapid and noisy; pulse may be slow or rapid.
      E. Bp usually elevated; pulse pressure may be wide
      F. Look for Battle sign; raccoon eyes, epistaxis
      G. Note any otorrhea or rhinorrhea
      H. Temperature may or may not be elevated
  II. Precipitating and/or contributing factors
      A. Primary brain injury or distress (see Table 4 for an overview of common brain injuries)
         1. Trauma (blunt or missile)
            a. concussion, contusion, laceration
            b. fractures
            c. epidural hematoma
            d. subdural hematoma
         2. Vascular lesions (see CVA)
         3. Infections (see Meningitis)
         4. Neoplasms
         5. Status epilepticus (see text on Status Epilepticus)
      B. Secondary causes (these must be ruled out)
         1. Metabolic encephalopathies (e.g., DKA, HHNK, uremia, etc.)
         2. Hypoxic encephalopathies (e.g., severe CHF, COPD, anemia, etc.)
         3. Toxicity (e.g., heavy metals, CO, drugs, alcohol)
         4. Physical causes (e.g., heat stroke, hypothermia)
         5. Deficiency states (e.g., Wernicke's encephalopathy)

TABLE 4. AN OVERVIEW OF COMMON BRAIN INJURIES

Basilar Skull Fracture

a. Fracture of cribiform plate, basisphenoid sinus and paranasal sinus as evidenced by a mucosal tear; rhinorrhea, otorrhea, CSF leaks increase likelihood of infection

b. Injury to blood vessels (e.g., carotids, venous sinuses) leads to hemorrhage, AV fistulas, or thrombosis. Battle sign, raccoon eyes occur. Cranial nerve injury common (e.g., I, II, VII, VIII)

c. Admit for observation. Complications may require surgery

Vault Fracture

a. Fracture could be linear, comminuted, depressed,or stellate. May also be simple or compound fracture

b. Linear fractures commonly associated epidural hematoma

c. Admit for observation; simple analgesia for pain. Surgical intervention required for depressed comminuted or compound fracture

Contusion/Laceration

a. Acceleration–deceleration. Direct bruising of brain at site of impact (coup). Indirect bruising at pole opposite impact (contrecoup)

b. Cortex and white matter of brain are bruised and necrotic. Many petechial hemorrhages. Cerebral edema common. Complications: subarachnoid bleeding, focal neurologic deficits, and seizures

c. Admit for observation and general supportive care. Surgery may be required to remove necrotic tissue and control bleeding

Epidural Hematoma

a. Collection of blood between the skull and the dura. Direct low speed blunt head injury associated with linear fracture which injures meningeal artery or vein

b. Initially unconscious; then lucid interval; then progressive decrease in LOC and hemiparesis. Seizures may be seen. Herniation may occur rapidly

c. Intubate, hyperventilate, start steroids, and hyperosmolar agent. Prepare OR or perform exploratory burr holes in the emergency room

Subdural Hematoma

a. Collection of blood usually venous beneath the dura and the underlying arachnoid. Acute type follows high speed impacts resulting in massive bleeding from torn dural sinuses. Severe brain damage and unremitting coma are common. Chronic type follows trivial trauma. There is a gradual drift into coma. Headache, confusion, LOC fluctuates

b. Active bleeding carries a high mortality

c. Admit for observation and diagnostic studies. If patient deteriorating, rapid surgical intervention is needed

Intercerebral Hematoma

a. Hemorrhagic area larger than 5 mm located within brain substance. Predisposition to frontal and temporal lobes

b. Stupor, progressively worsening headache, and progressing contralateral hemiparesis

c. Admit for observation and supportive care. Surgery indicated if lesion is accessible

C. Collect all available data such as

1. Time of occurrence. Mechanisms of injury (blunt, missile)
2. Was coma immediate? Was there a lucid period? If so, how long?
3. Did anyone observe a period of apnea or cyanosis?
4. Was much blood lost?

D. Identify the existence of other injuries and past medical conditions

III. Evaluate the degree of neurologic injury
- A. Assess the LOC (using 1 or 2, below, or both)
  1. Using these descriptions
     - a. clouding of consciousness: inattentiveness
     - b. delirium: disoriented, fearful, irritable, sensory distortions
     - c. stupor: incomplete arousal to painful stimuli
     - d. coma: unarousable and unresponsive to stimuli
  2. Using the system of the Glasgow Coma Scale, determine a score for
     - a. Best motor response (in either arm)
       6 points—obeys simple commands
       5 points—localizes noxious stimuli*
       4 points—flexion withdrawal from stimuli
       3 points—abnormal flexion (decorticate rigidity) to stimuli
       2 points—abnormal extension (decerebrate rigidity) to stimuli
       1 point—no motor response to stimuli
     - b. Best verbal response (after arousal)
       5 points—oriented, able to converse, knows person, place, time
       4 points—confused, not fully oriented
       3 points—verbalizes, may use expletives, nonsensical speech
       2 points—vocalizes, moans or groans that are not recognizable words
       1 point—no vocalization, no sound or response to noxious stimuli
     - c. Eye opening (determine minimum stimulus that evokes opening of one or both eyes)
       4 points—eyes open spontaneously
       3 points—eyes open to speech, in response to a command or name
       2 points—eyes open to noxious stimuli
       1 point—no eye opening in response to noxious stimuli
     - d. Findings of scores of 7 or less qualifies as coma
- B. Assess pupillary responses
  1. Describe the roundness and size of both pupils. Normal is 2 to 3 mm in diameter and symmetrical
  2. Describe equality of each pupil in reaction to light. Terms used are brisk, sluggish, nonreactive (fixed). Brisk reactive pupils indicates midbrain is intact. In the presence of decreased LOC, decreased EOM with corneal reflexes, reactive pupils suggest metabolic abnormality or drug ingestion
  3. Test and describe consensual light reflex. Normal is when one eye is stimulated with light, the other responds
  4. Chart and report abnormal findings. Some common examples are:
     - a. unilateral dilated and unreactive pupils may mean ipsilateral cranial nerve III compression and impending uncal herniation. Seen in epidural hematoma and other deteriorating conditions
     - b. small, pinpoint reactive pupils suggest localized involvement of the

---

*Noxious stimuli include external or supraorbital compression and/or calf and nipple pressure.

pons or effects of drugs or medications. Could also suggest central or cerebellar herniation syndromes

  c. midposition fixed pupils (3 to 5 mm diameter) suggests midbrain dysfunction. Unequal midposition, fixed pupils is seen with gluthethimide (Doriden) overdose

  d. fully dilated, unreactive pupils indicate the end result of cranial nerve III compression, toxicity from atropine or scopolomine, anoxia, or ischemia

  e. bilateral unreactive pupils suggest intracranial mass lesion

  f. a defective direct light reflex, but an intact consensual reflex (Marcus–Gunn pupil) suggests unilateral optic nerve damage

C. Assess corneal (blink) reflex and motility of the face
  1. this tests cranial nerves V and VII (trigeminal and facial)
  2. it is one of the last activities to disappear

D. Perform fundoscopy
  1. observe for papilledema which suggests increased ICP
  2. observe for subhyaloid hemorrhage which suggests ruptured aneurysm

E. Assess extraocular movements (EOM) as defined by 1 or 2, below
  1. Test the oculocephalic response (doll's head maneuver—DHM)
    a. do not perform, if patient has a potential cervical cord injury
    b. move patient's head from one side to another vigorously, noting eye movements
    c. normal is positive and means eye movement lags behind head movement
    d. negative is when the eyes remain fixed in midline
    e. negative findings suggest brainstem injury
  2. Test the oculovestibular reflexes (caloric testing with ice water)
    a. do not perform if CSF or blood is leaking from ear
    b. normal alert response: eyes move away from irrigated side
    c. normal unconscious response: deviation of eyes to the irrigated side

F. Assess the status of the lower pons and medulla
  1. test functioning of cranial nerves IX and X; check the gag reflexes. This is another reflex that is among the last to disappear
  2. observe and describe spontaneous respirations:
    a. Cheyne–Stokes—suggests thalamic lesion, metabolic problem
    b. central neurogenic hyperventilation—suggests midbrain and upper pons lesion but could also be due to metabolic acidosis and hypoxia
    c. apneustic breathing—suggests lower pontine damage. Usually accompanied by cluster breathing
    d. ataxic breathing and gasping respirations (Biot)—suggests damage to medulla
    e. depressed breathing—suggests medullary depression of drug induced nature
    f. hyperventilation—suggests metabolic acidosis or respiratory alkalosis

G. Assess motor responses (in addition to Glasgow Coma Scale)
  1. observe for spontaneous movements
     a. seizuring activity—especially focal but usually generalized
     b. myoclonic jerks—suggest metabolic encephalopathies
     c. absence of movements on one side or asymmetry suggests hemiparesis
  2. Observe for responses to induced movements
     a. In addition to Glasgow Coma Scale, test integrity of corticospinal tract by tickling nose. Normal response is to scratch nose. If movement is poorly organized and unilateral, damage evident
  3. test reflex movements: check for absence or presence of tendon reflexes
     a. test the biceps, triceps, Achilles, patellar
     b. elicit Babinski sign
     c. test the corneal and gag
  4. describe motor tone and posture
     a. grasp reflex and forced grasping. Stroking or stimulating the palms causes patient to grasp and hold on against resistance. Suggests massive bilateral cerebral dysfunction. May occur unilaterally with frontal lobe tension
     b. paratonia (gegenhalten, counter holding) is a constant, semivoluntary, plasticlike increase in muscle resistance when moved passively (e.g., legs, arms, trunk, neck). Suggests diffuse forebrain disruption. First sign of progressive rostural–caudal deterioration. Also seen in diffuse hemisphere dysfunction
     c. decorticate rigidity appears as flexion of the wrists, arms, and digits. Upper extremities adducted and flexed at the shoulder. Hands internally rotated. Legs are extended and inwardly rotated with plantar flexion. Could be bilateral or unilateral. Unilateral suggests spastic hemiplegia. Bilateral suggests lesion in the pons and involves internal capsule, basal ganglia, and thalamus
     d. decerebrate rigidity appears as extension, adduction and hyperpronation of upper extremities plus extension and plantar flexion of lower extremities. Could include opisthotonus with clenched teeth and jaws and erect head. Suggests lesion at the lower midbrain, upper pons area
     e. flaccidity is the absence of muscle tone or weak flexor responses. Suggests rostural–caudal brainstem compression of or across the pons at the level of cranial nerve V
IV. Conduct diagnostic studies to establish a definitive diagnosis
  A. Collect blood and urine samples for RBC, Hgb, Hct, bleeding profile, WBC and differential, electrolytes, glucose, BUN, creatinine, liver profile, enzyme studies, serum osmolarity, toxic screen, arterial blood gases
  B. Obtain a CAT scan; visualizes most focal pathology. Should be first test done
  C. Obtain plain skull films (if CAT scan not available). However, may be done

to detect depressed skull fracture, CSF leaks, and when bullet wounds are cause of injury
D. Obtain cervical spine x-rays (if indicated)
E. Prepare for cerebral arteriography (if CAT scan not available) as ordered
F. Prepare for a nuclear brain scan (if CAT scan not available) as ordered
G. Prepare for echoencephalogram (if prescribed), not commonly done in emergency situation
H. Measure ICP (may be done immediately following resuscitative measures). A subarachnoid bolt or ventricular cannula may be inserted (some hospitals defer this until ICU transfer)
I. EEG evoked potential (not usually done in emergency department)
J. BER (brainstem evoked response), not usually performed in emergency department)

PATHOPHYSIOLOGY

In the human adult, the delicate cerebral structures were practically sealed off from the remainder of the body. The brain is surrounded by a bony strong box, wrapped tightly by membranes, nourished by a generous blood supply, and further protected by a blood–brain barrier and CSF. The design is well-conceived. However, the lifestyle of modern man places him at risk for disrupting this design and disturbing the delicate tissues and equilibrium of cerebral structures. Close to 4 percent of the total population in the United States in 1975 sustained some type of head injury. Today, that figure has most likely risen. Head injuries are most commonly caused by automobile accidents, but also occur as a result of industrial accidents, sport injuries, falls, or assaults from a variety of sources.

The pathophysiologic changes associated with primary traumatic injuries are described in this section of the text. The reader is referred to different parts of the text where other primary and/or secondary causes of cerebral insults are discussed.

The biologic responses of the brain to trauma are both physical and cellular. It is obvious that physical events such as blunt blows or missile types of head trauma directly injure cranial bones and blood vessels. Many neurologists call this the primary injury. In an effort to explain some of the biomechanical effects of the primary injury, principles relating to the effects of force and motion have been borrowed from the physical sciences. The laws of motion are replete with concepts such as acceleration, deceleration, velocity, recoil, gravity, and shearing which the neuropathologists have used to explain the diffuse effects of head trauma on cerebral tissue.

Once the primary effects are initiated, cerebral equilibrium is disrupted and further insult is added to the brain. Secondary insults such as hypotension, hypoxemia, hypercarbia, increased intracranial pressure, and infection increase the brain's vulnerability. These secondary effects of head trauma are the real causes of the high morbidity and mortality of head injuries.

Mechanical force to the head could lead to a concussion. This clinical syndrome is characterized by immediate and yet temporary impairment of neural functioning. Rotational and/or linear acceleration–deceleration forces result in the derangement of the reticular activating system (RAS) leading to a loss of consciousness, shearing of axons, intercerebral pressure changes in addition to other widespread microscopic damage. The patient has impaired memory for events preceding the injury (retrograde amnesia) and those following the injury (anterograde amnesia). Recovery usually involves periods of restlessness, agitation, confusion with gradual increasing periods of rational behavior until normality returns. Depending upon the severity, patients may be admitted for observation. Children with a concussion, as well as some adults, are sent home with precise instructions concerning the observations the family must make for the next 24 to 48 hours.

Skull fractures are commonly produced by blunt injury to the skull. They may be closed (simple) or open (compound). Basilar skull fractures are usually associated with severe trauma and commonly injure the cribiform plate of the ethmoid bone, the basisphenoid sinus, and the paranasal sinus. Dural tears frequently accompany these fractures. If the fracture occurs at the anterior fossa, it may cause conjunctival hemorrhage, periorbital ecchymosis (raccoon eyes), loss of smell, and epistaxis. A fracture at the middle fossae near the temporal bone will probably lead to otorrhea, tinnitus, possible deafness, and facial paralysis. Posterior fossa basilar fractures result in pharyngeal bleeding and ecchymosis in the neck and behind the mastoid (Battle sign). Basilar fractures are quite serious because of the potential infection from CSF leaks and injury to large blood vessels and to cranial nerves.

Vault fractures are less serious and yet demand attention. They usually involve a scalp tear which requires copious irrigation and repair. Linear vault fractures are recognized by the inward bending of the skull at the site of the blow and the outward bending of the bones around this indentation. These fractures may be depressed or compound. They require surgical intervention for repair.

Whereas blunt injuries may not always produce a skull fracture, they result in injury to brain tissue at the site of impact and at sites remote from the impact. When there is contusion or laceration of the crests of cerebral tissue at the point of impact, the lesion is called a coup lesion. If there is a lesion opposite the site of impact, it is called a contrecoup lesion. Contrecoup occurs because the brain tissue lags behind the acceleration–deceleration of the skull and thus hits other parts of the skull. Therefore, the signs and symptoms of contrecoup lesions are not reflective of the original site of impact. Patients must be observed closely for the effects of both events.

The contusions caused by a coup or contrecoup injury can be severe and are associated with focal neurologic signs. These types of injuries produce a bruised necrotic cortex and white matter with varying amounts of petechial hemorrhages and edema. In addition, subarachnoid bleeding frequently occurs. The most common areas involved are the orbital surface of the frontal lobes and the frontotemporal connection of the hemisphere because of the irregularities of the bones in these regions (e.g., orbital roof or sphenoid wing). Contusions may result in cerebral edema and seizure activity. Surgery is required in many cases.

Missile injuries to the skull are those produced by penetration and/or perforation. Missiles come in all sizes, shapes, types and the extent of the damage produced is reflective of these factors in addition to velocity and direction of entry and exit. Bullet wounds are the most serious example. They may have an explosive effect; they may ricochet or may displace multiple bone and bullet fragments throughout the cerebral tissue. Missile type injuries cause lacerations, destruction of tissue, bleeding, edema, and many other microscopic changes.

Low speed, blunt head injuries (e.g., falls, impacts with objects) occur most often in the area of the middle meningeal artery or vein and could result in an accumulation of blood above the dura and beneath the skull. This is an epidural hematoma (EDH) and for the most part is not very common. It is readily correctible by surgery, if it is not associated with other lesions. An EDH may be contrecoup to the original injury.

The classical picture of EDH in 33 percent of the cases is one of a loss of consciousness at the time of injury. This is followed by a variable period of consciousness, called the lucid interval, which may range from 6 to 18 hours. Then the patient experiences headaches which become more severe, decreasing LOC, dilatation of the ipsilateral pupil, decerebrate posturing, and hemiplegia of the contralateral limb.

The lucid interval is significant for it represents the lapse of time between the original loss of consciousness and the beginning of the signs of deterioration and displacement of tissue through the tentorial notch. A short lucid period suggests brisk, probably arterial, bleeding.

The classical picture of EDH gives the examiner localizing signs. In 80 percent of the cases, the side of the dilated pupil is the location of the mass. However, the dilated pupil is also the first sign of uncal herniation. In 50 percent of the cases, the side of the initial hemiplegia is contralateral to the clot because of the pressure of expanding mass on the origins of the corticospinal tract. However, the absence of the classical signs does not rule out the diagnosis because one third of the patients with EDH never lose consciousness and another third never have a lucid interval and remain unconscious.

In most cases the lesion is readily diagnosed and treated. The CAT scan and skull films will usually depict a linear skull fracture across the middle meningeal groove. Because the physical effect of this hematoma leads to rapidly increasing ICP, it must be identified and treated fairly quickly. The hematoma is frequently localized to the area under the point of blunt impact. For this reason, some neurosurgeons operate without the aid of diagnostic tests, especially if the patient's condition is rapidly deteriorating. In more stable patients, the CAT scan or angiography and skull films locate the lesion. At times, however, burr holes may need to be done in the emergency room.

A subdural hematoma (SDH) by definition is a collection of blood between the dura mater and the arachnoid mater. It occurs more frequently than EDH and is classified as acute (occurring within 24 hours), subacute (within 1 to 15 days) and chronic (taking over 15 days). This division depends upon the interval between the time of injury and the onset of the symptoms. However, clinically the distinction is less clear because the patients present with some disturbance in their LOC.

Subdural hematomas can be found anywhere within the cranium, but most frequently are located over the cerebral convexities. Although 50 percent of acute SDH are associated with skull fractures, blunt trauma and bleeding diathesis could lead to it. In most cases it is the high speed of the impact which disrupts the cortical veins draining the dura or dural sinuses which leads to massive bleeding. This type of hematoma may or may not be associated with underlying cerebral contusion or laceration. When it is associated with these events, some physicians refer to it as a complicated acute SDH. The mortality rate for complicated SDH is extremely high, especially if the lesions are bilateral.

The symptoms occur at the outset of the injury. The patient appears in the emergency room unconscious and most likely with signs of deterioration. The lesions of acute SDH cause a shift in the midline structures of the brain which can be picked up by CAT scan or angiography. Only immediate diagnosis plus medical and surgical intervention can prevent mortality. In many cases the damage is so profuse that surgery may only temporarily relieve the condition and the patient succumbs from the secondary effects of the damage.

Subacute SDH resembles acute SDH in most aspects. However the history is one of increasing somnolence and stupor followed by a deterioration in the LOC. It still, however, carries a high mortality rate.

Chronic SDH is less fatal, more subtle, and tends to occur in older persons. In the elderly, brain atrophy prolongs the trajectory of cortical veins as they enter the superior sagittal sinus, thus making them more vulnerable to rupture by even minor rotational acceleration. This hematoma evolves slowly. The original traumatic event may have been so inconsequential that it went unnoticed by patient and family.

As the hematoma evolves in chronic SDH, it becomes encased in a fibrous capsule which is lined with vascular tissue. In time, the enclosed blood clot becomes osmotically active and draws fluid into its interior. The expanding lesion displaces cerebral structures and eventually cerebral cellular functioning. However, many patients survive with small chronic SDH which resolve spontaneously.

The expanding lesion of a chronic SDH gives rise to the confusing yet deteriorating clinical picture. Behavioral changes are commonly the initial signs. However, these changes are misdiagnosed as senile dementia, psychosis, or drug toxicity, and the chronic SDH goes undetected. The patient who abuses alcohol is at high risk of such misdiagnosis because falls and disorientation are components of the alcoholic state. The triage nurse needs a high index of suspicion to recognize this problem. A period of observation and diagnostic studies clears up the confusion. If severe progressive deficits surface (e.g., increasing ICP, pupil changes, or decreasing LOC), surgical intervention may be required.

Cerebral edema habitually accompanies craniocerebral trauma. In the case of expanding lesions, the edema is probably due to obstruction of venous outflow resulting in the escape of fluid into the extravascular space. If the amount of this extravasation is small, it can be absorbed by the surrounding vessels and enter the subarachnoid space thus keeping the volume equilibrium stable. If the amount is large, it increases the pressure inside the brain.

It is widely believed that other cerebral injuries evoke mechanisms that primarily affect the capitance vessels and lead not only to venuous stasis, but also a decrease in cerebral blood flow (CBF). Any decrease in CBF to an area will lead to hypoxia of the cells in that area. Hypoxic tissues switch to anaerobic metabolic pathways to obtain needed energy in the form of ATP. When this system fails, fluid imbalance and acidosis of cerebral tissue result. Without energy, the sodium–potassium pump cannot function. This results in an accumulation of sodium and water inside the glial cells. Lactate production increases with anaerobic glycolysis resulting in depressed nerve cell activity and dilated blood vessels which only add to the increasing pressure. As the tissues swell they cause more pressure, more anoxia, and more pressure. A vicious cycle is started that must be interrupted.

Regardless of the underlying mechanisms producing the edema, the swollen tissues have nowhere to expand, forcing the intracranial pressure to rise. As the limits of the cranium are reached, the brain is pushed through folds of the dura. Herniation is usually rostrocaudal with uncal herniation through the tentorial notch the most common. Once this occurs, the midbrain is compressed as well as the third cranial nerve which gives rise to the typical pupillary dilatation, fixation, and other changes. Central herniation syndrome produces herniation transtentorially disturbing the diencephalon, midbrain, pons, and medulla. Sequentially, the first sign is decreasing alertness and Cheyne–Stokes respiration with small reactive pupils. Masses in and around the cerebellum herniate through the cerebellar tonsils and force tissue down through the foramen magnum. Expanding lesions in the frontal lobe could herniate under the rigid falx cerebri. The latter two types of herniation are not common.

In summary, craniocerebral injuries produce their effects by primary and secondary mechanisms that lead to brain swelling. Edema cannot be handled easily in this enclosed area and its damaging effects are spread throughout the brain. When the intracranial pressure reaches its limits, cerebral tissue herniates through select areas of the dura. This only leads to life threatening damage to the vital structures of the brainstem. Death will quickly follow unless these cascading events are halted.

Assessment of the patient with craniocerebral injuries must be done accurately and rapidly, especially if the patient is unconscious. A neurologic checksheet should be started and the patient sequentially tested every 15 minutes. The first testing establishes a baseline to which later findings are compared and can be used to estimate the eventual outcomes for this patient. Most centers are now combining the Glasgow Coma Scale scoring along with the usual neurologic assessment parameters. These assessment devices complement each other and should be used with this in mind.

The triage nurse makes a rapid system survey and tries to obtain as much of a history as possible from those who accompany the patient to the hospital. Obvious craniocerebral injuries are not difficult to detect, however, the more subtle epidural and/or subdural hematomas require a high index of suspicion. The importance of adequate record keeping cannot be overemphasized. All observations must be documented, if they are to be of any help to the entire team.

Because other injuries frequently accompany head trauma, a careful search must be made for them. The nurse should assume a cervical cord injury until proven otherwise. For this reason, the oculovestibular method of testing extraocular eye movements is preferred to the oculocephalic method. Another assumption is that the patient has an increase in the intracranial pressure and thus, all efforts are made to prevent straining or performing activities (e.g., coughing) that increase intracranial pressure.

MANAGEMENT

I. Establish and maintain a patent airway
   A. Clear the airway without flexing or turning the head
   B. Insert an oropharyngeal airway
   C. Assist ventilations with a bag and mask; preferably with oxygen 50 percent to maintain Po_2 at 30 torr
   D. Avoid gastric dilatation by not exerting excessive pressure on the bag
   E. Insert a nasogastric tube if stomach appears distended
   F. Obtain x-rays of the neck to rule out cervical neck injury
   G. Draw baseline blood studies; auscultate the lung fields
   H. Initiate an IV line for fluid and drug administration
   I. Under these controlled conditions and with the possible use of muscle relaxants or thiopental, an endotracheal tube may be inserted
   J. Continue controlled hyperventilation
   K. Obtain a CAT scan or other studies as prescribed
   L. Keep head of bed elevated 15 to 30 degrees; limit suctioning to 15 seconds
II. Ensure an adequate circulation to the body's system
   A. Obtain and monitor the bp, pulse, and respirations q 15 minutes
   B. Provide for continuous cardiac monitoring
   C. Insert a urinary catheter and monitor urine output
   D. Monitor serum electrolytes, glucose, BUN, and osmolarity
   E. Start IV fluids; saline with glucose solution preferred
   F. A central venous pressure line may be requested
   G. If shock is present, search for its cause while treating it
II. Detect the direction of changes in the neurologic status
   A. Evaluate the following q 15 minutes. Report all changes from baseline data
     1. LOC as determined by the Best Motor Response on the Glasgow Coma Scale
     2. pupillary size, roundness, and reaction to light
     3. the presence of corneal and gag reflexes
     4. extraocular eye movements as defined by oculovestibular and/or oculocephalic responses
   B. Report any unilateral dysfunctions, change in body posture and/or seizure activity
IV. Detect and treat increased intracranial pressure
   A. Report immediately clinical signs (e.g., decreases in LOC and in motor responses, pupillary dilatation) of increased ICP

B. Assist with the insertion of an ICP monitoring device (e.g., subarachnoid screw or ventricular cannula). Observe the monitor for intermittent waves of increased pressure which would be over 20 torr
C. Hyperventilate to P_{CO_2} levels prescribed. May be moderate, P_{CO_2} of 30 to 35 torr; and high, P_{CO_2} of 25 to 30 torr
D. Administer steroids as prescribed. Usually prednisolone (Decadron)
E. Administer hyperosmolar diuretic agents
 1. initial therapy may be high dose bolus of mannitol (Osmitrol) 1 to 2 g/kg injected over 5 to 10 minutes (or 250 ml of a 20 percent solution) Maintenance therapy: smaller boluses mannitol 0.15 to 0.3 g/kg q 1 to 2 hours
 Continuous therapy: mannitol 0.05 to 0.15 g/kg/hour
 2. monitor serum osmolarity: report all readings near or above 315 to 320 mOsm/L
 3. monitor urine output, cardiac functioning, serum glucose, electrolytes
F. Administer furosemide and/or ethacrynic acid as prescribed
G. Be prepared to institute barbiturate therapy
 1. pentobarbital (Nembutal) most commonly prescribed
 2. doses: IV loading dose based upon body weight; followed by hourly doses
 3. criterion: EEG has equal lengths of burst suppression pattern. Blood barbiturate levels not a good indicator
 4. neurologic activity now monitored by brainstem evoked responses (BER)
 5. respirations must be mechanically controlled
H. Be prepared to assist with cranial trephination (burr holes) if indicated
V. Control of posttraumatic seizures
A. Treatment may be initiated in the presence of prolonged unconsciousness, skull fracture, neurologic deficits, and substantiated hematoma
B. Administer phenytoin (Dilatin) as prescribed
 1. doses: loading 1000 mg (adults) over first 24 hours
 maintenance—300 to 400 mg daily
C. Observe the onset, progression, and postictal states of the patient who seizures. Record all observations systemically. (See Chapter on Status Epilepticus.)

RATIONALE

One of the major goals in the emergency management of craniocerebral injuries is to provide adequate cerebral oxygenation. The cumulative effects of the primary and secondary pathologic processes in the brain result in hypoxia. As an organ, the brain is extremely sensitive to oxygen deprivation and without oxygen cerebral cells die. Cerebral oxygenation problems are treated by increasing the oxygen carrying capacity of the blood and assuring its delivery to the brain. The adequacy of this approach is assessed by serially examining the arterial blood gases and cardiovascular parameters.

Once the nose and mouth are clear, an oropharyngeal airway is inserted. Ventilations should be assisted with a bag, mask, and oxygen. It has been shown that once the airway is patent, patients spontaneously hyperventilate. However, cerebral hypoxia still exists and supplemental oxygen up to 50 percent may be prescribed. Intubation is deferred until later because it is frequently accompanied by coughing and straining which adds to the problem of increased ICP. In some centers, intubation is performed only under anesthesia and with the use of muscle relaxants.

Gastric dilatation can be caused by excessive external pressure on the ventilatory bag. When the stomach is distended, diaphragmatic excursions are compromised. A nasogastric tube attached to low suctioning relieves this problem as well as avoids any aspiration of secretions.

The possibility of hemorrhagic shock should be suspected in all patients who have suffered trauma. Hypotension can result from the decreased volume and the ensuing hypoxic acidemia. The decreased volume and hypoxia allow fluid to escape from the capillaries and the venous pooling that follows can impair cardiac functioning. Management consists of correcting the hypoxia and replacing the volume. A central venous pressure line would be inserted to monitor the functioning of the right heart once fluid replacement is started. Solutions are infused rapidly until the CVP reaches 2 to 6 cm of water. The fluid in this situation cannot be hypotonic (e.g., 5 percent D/W) because it lowers serum osmolarity thus adding to the cerebral edema. An isotonic solution of saline and glucose is preferred. Vital signs are monitored closely. Urine output is the crucial indicator of organ perfusion, thus an indwelling urinary catheter is inserted. Serially monitor the serum electrolytes, osmolarity, glucose, and BUN to assess the effectiveness of therapy.

The neurologic assessment continues throughout the management phase to rapidly detect any deterioration that is taking place so that appropriate intervention strategies may be taken. The most important parts of the neurologic assessment parameters are the LOC (as defined by the Best Motor Response on the Glasgow Coma Scale), pupillary size, reaction to light, corneal and gag reflexes, and extraocular eye movements. The assessment is done systematically to identify rostural–caudal changes in the patient's condition.

Another major goal in the emergency management of patients with craniocerebral injuries is to detect and treat increased intracranial pressure (ICP). An increase in ICP is assumed present when the patient is first seen in the emergency room until proven otherwise. This is the reason all precautions are taken to avoid activities which could induce additional increases in pressure (e.g., intubation).

The detection of increased ICP demands alert and frequent neurologic testing. Clinical signs of this event include a rapidly deteriorating LOC with or without progressive enlargement of one pupil. In some settings it is now possible to directly measure ICP. Normal pressure is defined as below 15 torr and pressure readings over 20 torr are indicative of intracranial hypertension. A device such as a subarachnoid screw can be attached to a portable monitoring device for emergency use.

The advantages of continuous ICP monitoring are numerous. The intermittent waves of increased pressure, which occur in many cases before the clinical signs appear, indicate an increase in ICP thus allowing prompt treatment and possibly titration of treatment to correct the problem before significant neurologic deterioration has taken place. If muscle paralysis or barbiturates are used, ICP monitoring is the only tool (other than brainstem evoked potentials) available to follow the neurologic status of the patient.

Hyperventilating the patient relieves increased ICP in most cases. Hyperventilation leads to hypocarbia which is followed by vasoconstriction. Vasoconstriction lowers ICP by lowering intravascular blood volume. Despite widespread cerebral injury, the cerebral blood vessels retain their reactivity to low carbon dioxide levels. Falls in ICP are seen soon after this therapy is initiated. However, with prolonged use, the ICP may rise. There does not appear to be detrimental effects on the body when the P_{CO_2} is at 20 torr. The cerebral blood flow is lowered but this does not appear to cause problems except in those cases where cerebral blood flow is already lowered. The nurse must be certain as to the level of P_{CO_2} the physician wishes to maintain and frequently check the blood gases to be certain that this level is reached.

There is conflicting evidence for the use of corticosteroids in managing cerebral hypertension. Some studies report no statistical differences in outcomes between those patients treated and those not treated, whereas other studies report a dramatic reduction in mortality rates of those treated with steroids. Most likely steroids will be prescribed although substantiating data concerning their mechanism of action is not available at this time. The commonly used preparation is dexamethasone (Decadron). It may initially be given in high or low doses. Once begun, it continues over a period of days and then is tapered. The nurse monitors the serum glucose and electrolytes as a measure of the patient's response. Antacids may be prescribed to control the drug-induced hyperacidity; urines for sugar and acetone should be checked to detect an imbalance in carbohydrate metabolism; and the patient should be monitored for opportunistic infection. Whereas the side effects of steroid therapy do not occur during the patient's stay in the emergency department, it is worthwhile to review them.

Cerebral hypertension can be reduced by administering hyperosmolar diuretic agents. Hyperosmolar agents induce an osmotic gradient between the brain and the intravascular compartment thus promoting the movement of water out of the brain cells into the intravascular compartment. A 20 to 25 percent solution of mannitol (Osmitrol) is preferred over urea osmotic agents because of mannitol's reduced rebound effects. In some cases mannitol may not be used if the cerebral blood flow is high because it may further increase it and worsen a condition of hyperemia.

Mannitol may be administered as a bolus or by continuous infusion. A high dose bolus is usually required for the initial emergency control of ICP in patients showing evidence of rapid deterioration. Maintenance therapy can be carried out with smaller boluses every 1 to 2 hours. Continuous infusion may be needed for the first 48 hours. Close monitoring of the serum osmolarity is vital. It should not rise above 320 mOsm/L because irreversible cardiopulmonary and renal complications can occur. In addition, because hyperglycemic hyperosmolar nonketotic syndrome can occur in diabetic patients or in those who are receiving high doses of steroid, the serum glucose must be monitored.

Other diuretics used to treat intercranial hypertension are furosemide (Lasix) and ethacrynic acid (Edecrin). These are very potent, rapid acting, "loop" diuretic agents which can be given intravenously. When given in conjunction with mannitol, the hyperosmolar action appears to be enhanced. With both the hyperosmolar agents and diuretic agents, the nurse must accurately monitor the intake and output as well as the serum electrolytes. Imbalances created by these diuretic agents must be treated.

In 60 minutes, if all other strategies have been used to lower cerebral hypertension and if the patient's ICP remains above 20 torr and the serum osmolarity above 320 mOsm/L, barbiturate therapy may be initiated. Initially, this treatment was used empirically to lower body metabolism and thus rest and protect the brain. Recently, encouraging results have been reported on the ability of barbiturates to lower ICP, in situations where all else has failed. The exact mechanism for this action awaits elucidation.

The newness of this therapy is manifest by the wide variety of drug doses being prescribed. Short-acting pentobarbital (Nembutal) is the drug most commonly prescribed. A loading dose is given based upon body weight which is followed by hourly doses. Because barbiturate blood levels vary widely in these patients, the EEG is used as a criterion measure. The aim is equal lengths of the burst–suppression pattern. The intravenous preparation of this drug is highly alkaline and necrosis can occur if the drug extravasates into the tissues.

Barbiturates in the doses prescribed for these patients suppresses all neurologic activity except brainstem evoked responses. Constant vigilant attention must be provided. Respirations are mechanically controlled because spontaneous respirations are abolished. In addition, cardiac toxicity and hypotension due to barbiturate ingestion must be guarded against. Once begun, the average length of time required for this therapy has been under 5 days.

Interventions aimed at reducing cerebral hypertension give the surgeon valuable time to stabilize the patient prior to operative intervention. However, if the patient's condition deteriorates rapidly, cranial trephination (burr holes) may need to be done in the emergency department. If surgical intervention is not a viable option for this patient, the need for continuous surveillance necessitates transfer to an intensive care unit.

3. Cervical Cord Injury

ASSESSMENT

I. Presenting clinical picture
   A. Usually a young person with spine immobilized on stabilization board.
   B. LOC: may be alert, have decreased LOC, or be unresponsive.
   C. May complain of acute pain in neck; have limited motion in neck; or neck

is tender to touch. Pain behind the ears or occipital headache suggests injury to the odontoid process of C-2
    D. Open neck wound will be seen if gunshot or stabbing has occurred
  II. Obtain historical data to elicit clues as to mechanism of injury
    A. Search for bruising or abrasions on the chin, forehead, occiput, tip of shoulder, and scapular region
    B. Question patient as to the pattern of injury
       1. hyperextension of the neck:
          a. indirect force: (e.g., rear-end auto collision). This type of injury is associated with muscle, ligament, and soft tissue trauma, commonly called a whiplash
          b. direct force: e.g., falling forward and striking face or forehead. This type of injury associated with paralysis without injury or dislocation of vertebrae
       2. hyperflexion of the neck or flexion–rotation of the neck (e.g., body in forward motion and head strikes an immovable object). This type of injury occurs in head-on type of auto collisions or could occur when a person falls backwards and violently hits the back of the head. It usually is a deceleration type of injury associated with dislocation
       3. vertical compression injury (e.g., diving into a shallow body of water) This type of injury usually compresses the vertebral bodies and causes comminuted fractures with cord displacement
       4. penetrating injury (e.g., bullet or knife wounds). This injury varies in symptoms depending upon point of entry, angle of entry, structures involved, and exit of bullet
 III. Alterations in respiratory system functioning
    A. Chest excursions minimal to none; diaphragmatic breathing (abdomen protrudes on inspiration); muscles of nose, mouth, and neck may be attempting to carry on process of respiration
    B. Breath sounds are diminished; cough is ineffective
    C. Trachea may be deviated, if only half of diaphragm is involved
    D. Vital capacity and tidal volume are diminished
    E. Increased P_{CO_2} levels on blood gas analysis; oxygen levels may be satisfactory early in injury
    F. Obtain a chest x-ray
    G. May have compounding existing problems (e.g., fractured ribs, lung contusions, history of smoking or lung disease, paralytic ileus)
 IV. Alterations in the cardiovascular system functioning
    A. Hypotensive (bp near 100/60)
    B. Bradycardia (pulse around 50 to 60/minute)
    C. May be evidence of poor venous circulation: cold, cyanotic limbs
    D. Central venous pressure probably low
    E. ECG indicates sinus bradycardia
    F. Fluctuation in body temperature
    G. Hypovolemic shock only if:

      1. bp falls below 70 mm Hg, pulse rate increases

      2. decreases seen in LOC

      3. urinary output falls below 30 ml/hour

      4. CVP decreases below baseline

V. Alteration in neuromuscular system functioning

  A. Palpation of spine may show areas of tenderness, gaps between spinous process

  B. LOC: Usually alert but must be monitored

  C. Pupillary functioning: usually normal but must be monitored

  D. Sensory impairment as defined by testing dermal segments of the spinal nerves. All dermatomes must be examined frequently to determine ascending or transverse progression. Examples of areas supplied by cord segments. Losses in these segments suggests the level of the lesion:

      1. C-2—2 inches behind the ear

      2. C-3—anterior portion of neck

      3. C-4—top of shoulder

      4. C-5—anterior lateral shoulder

      5. C-6—thumb

      6. C-7—ring and middle finger

      7. C-8—little finger

      8. T-1—median aspect of arm

      9. T-4—nipple line

     10. T-10—umbilicus

     11. T-12—pubis

     12. L-1—below iliac crest

     13. L-4—median ankle, great toe

     14. S-1—top of fifth toe

     15. L-5—dorsum of the foot

     16. S-3,4,5—perianal area

  E. Motor impariment as defined by testing myotome reference. Muscle tone is usually flaccid immediately after injury. Muscle responses must be tested frequently to determine ascending or transverse progression of lesion. Some examples of cord lesions and their loses are:

      1. C-1 to C-4—total quadriplegia with loss of respiratory functioning

      2. C-4 to C-6—quadriplegia with some sparing of elbow and wrist movement and diaphragm, diaphragmatic breathing

      3. C-6 to C-7—quadriplegia with elbow flexors intact; wrist extensors may be intact, diaphragmatic breathing

      4. C-7 to C-8—quadriplegia, good elbow movements, fair wrist movements, no hand movements, diaphragmatic breathing

      5. T-1 to T-12—paraplegia with varying degrees of intercostal and abdominal muscle losses

      6. Below L-2—mixed picture of motor losses and dysfunctions in elimination

  F. Reflexes: usually areflexic below level of the lesion. Baseline data on all superficial and deep tendon reflexes must be obtained because of possible progressing ascending or transverse deterioration. Examples of select reflexes and their controlling center are:

1. superficial reflexes
   a. nasal (sneeze)—brainstem and upper cord
   b. upper abdominals—T-7,8,9,10
   c. lower abdominals—T-10,11,12
   d. cremasteric—L-1
   e. plantar—S-1,2
   f. anal—S-4,5
2. deep tendon reflexes
   a. biceps—C-5,6
   b. triceps—C-6,7
   c. periosteoradial—C-6,7,8
   d. wrist (flexion)—C-6,7,8
   e. wrist (extension)—C-7,8
   f. patellar—L-2,3,4
   g. achilles—S-1,2
3. visceral reflexes
   a. ciliospinal—T-1,2
   b. bulbocavernosus—S-2,3,4
   c. bladder and rectal—S-2,3,4

VI. Alterations in GI system functioning
   A. Abdomen appears distended; bowel sounds not audible
   B. Paralytic ileus a common occurrence; vomiting with or without aspiration could occur
   C. If abdominal or dorsolumbar trauma also exists, hemorrhage into the abdominal or retroperitoneal space could occur. A four quadrant paracentesis may be done to assess this situation
   D. Stress gastric ulcers and bleeding may develop

VII. Alterations in genitourinary functioning
   A. Bladder areflexive leading to retention of urine and possible reflux

VIII. Alterations in the metabolic and integumentary systems
   A. Hypoperfusion of tissues leading to metabolic acidosis
   B. Respiratory insufficiency leading to respiratory acidosis
   C. Skin may show areas of blotching, discoloration, or lack of color
   D. Skin temperature may vary in different parts of the body
   E. Diaphoresis may be seen above the level of the lesion whereas anhidrosis is observed below the level of the lesion

IX. Detect the extent of the injury and for concomitant problems
   A. Draw bloods for RBC, Hgb, Hct, WBC, and differential, glucose, BUN, creatinine, electrolytes. Blood gases. Type and crossmatch
   B. X-rays of spine: usually oblique views in addition to anterioposterior views
   C. Routine views of the pelvis and spine below the level of the lesion will alert examiner to hidden fractures in anesthetized areas

D. In some cases tomograms, epidurogram, or myelogram may be ordered
E. A four quadrant abdominal paracentesis may be done to rule out hemorrhage in the abdominal peritoneal space
F. Sample of urine sent for routine analysis

PATHOPHYSIOLOGY

Spinal injuries are among the most devastating of injuries. They often affect vigorous young people and are a result of sport, vehicular and/or industrial accidents, falls, or missile types of trauma. The sequelae of spinal trauma can leave an individual paralyzed and helpless for the remainder of his or her life.

The vertebral column which extends from the base of the skull to the coccyx is constructed as a somewhat movable, rodlike structure that provides the body axial support and protection for the spinal cord. The vertebrae are essentially bony rings that weakly articulate with each other posteriorly and are separated anteriorly by fibrocartilagenous discs. These intervertebral articulations are weak points and are easily injured by flexion, extension, or rotational stress. Fractures and dislocations occur most commonly at points where a relatively mobile portion of the column meets a relatively fixed segment of the column (e.g., between lower cervical area and upper thoracic segment). Thus, most cord lesions are between C-4-7, T-1 and the thorocolumbar junction, T-11-12, L-1.

The lesions capable of producing spinal injury are multiple. Biomechanical injuries to the spinal column can be caused by compression, flexion–rotation, hyperextension, and hyperflexion types of stress. They may result in fractures, fracture–dislocations, tears of ligaments and discs, and other soft tissue trauma. Any one of these lesions may be unilateral or bilateral or they may be partial or complete. Thus, the clinical picture of a patient with spinal trauma varies widely. It is only with frequent neurologic testing and good x-ray studies that a fairly accurate picture of the injury can be ascertained. The history of the injury gives the examiner valuable clues.

Spinal cord concussion occurs when there is a transient loss of cord function. It occurs most frequently when the neck is hyperextended suddenly by an indirect force. This is seen in rear-end auto collisions and results in the so-called whiplash injury. The sudden acceleration of the struck vehicle throws the head backward. The head recoils, hyperflexes, and finally returns to a neutral position. If the backward hyperextension of the head is unimpeded by a headrest, structures such as the neck muscles, esophagus, larynx, and mandibular ligaments are stretched. In 12 to 24 hours after the injury, the patient experiences dysphagia, hoarseness, pain on chewing, limited mouth opening, neck stiffness, and pain. The spinal cord recovers completely, but the patient may be left with residual discomfort.

Whereas the exact mechanisms leading to spinal cord destruction are still under study, discernible changes take place in the injured cord. Early pathologic changes include petecchial hemorrhages in the gray matter resulting from decreased blood supply and hypoxia. Edema and hypoxia probably contribute to the release of catecholamines which lead to further hemorrhage, inflammatory responses and necrosis. In many spinal centers, neurosurgeons attempt to delay these changes by cooling the injured cord segment, blocking the effects of norepinephrine, and administering large doses of steroids.

Thus, the degree of neurologic losses may not be static. In fact, pathologic changes may extend above or below the damaged segment and lesions at C-7–T-1 may be missed because it is difficult to view them on x-ray. It is most important that precautions be taken during the rescue and emergency care of this patient to avoid extending the amount of tissue damaged. Late deficits that appear are related to intramedullary cyst formation or syringomyelic cavities.

Complete functional cord transection is followed by three devastating events. First, loss of all voluntary motor activity in the body parts innervated by the spinal segments reflective as a flaccid paralysis. Second, loss of all sensation below the level of the lesion because of the interruption of the spinal pathways. Third, loss of most reflexes below the level of the injury. The loss of reflexes greatly reduces the excitability of descending axons for a variable period of time resulting in a condition called spinal shock, which can be life-threatening.

Spinal shock is a temporary condition usually lasting 3 to 6 weeks. It has profound effects on the autonomic nervous system. With lesions above T-6, the sympathetic nervous system is compromised because sympathetic outflow occurs between T-1 and L-2. Interruption or lack of sympathetic tone leads to disruptions in blood pressure, heart rate, thermal regulation, bladder, bowel, and sexual dysfunction.

In the early stages of injury before adaptation occurs, the cardiovascular effects of a lack of sympathetic tone are hypotension and bradycardia. Hypotension is reflective of the inability of the capitance vessels to reflexly contract, especially in response to postural changes. Vasodilation occurs resulting in a decreased venous return to the heart. If the hypotension is not accompanied by other pathology (e.g., hypovolemia), it stabilizes at approximately 100/60 mm Hg which is sufficient to perfuse the vital organs. However, pooling of blood in the extremities with resultant clot formation is a constant threat to these patients.

Bradycardia is reflective of unopposed vagal tone on the sinoatrial node. In previously healthy people, the bradycardia poses no problem. However, if the rate falls below 48 beats/minute, the physician might consider anticholinergic drugs such as atropine which block the action of the vagus nerve, if given in large doses, or adrenergic drugs such as norepinephrine which stimulate cardiac activity might be considered. There may be occasions when it is best to insert a temporary transvenous pacemaker until the cardiovascular system has accommodated. Bradycardia is worsened by states of hypothermia and/or hypoxia.

The other autonomic manifestations of spinal shock arise from different mechanisms. Thermal regulation is interrupted because the sympathetic spinal neurons innervating skin effector organs concerned with body temperature are severed from the descending influences of the hypothalamic thermoregulatory center. There is a loss of sweating below the level of the lesion, if the lesion is above T-9–T-10. If the lesion is above C-8, all thermoregulation is lost and the patients tend to assume the temperature of the environment they are in, thus producing hypo- or hyperthermia.

A loss of central control on the gastrointestinal tract leads to temporary gastric distention and paralytic ileus. If there are associated abdominal injuries, peristalsis could immediately cease. If not, peristalsis ceases within 24 hours and persists for the next 3 to 4 days or longer. The combination of hypotension, decreased or absent bowel sounds, and a decreased hematocrit might lead the examiner to suspect an acute abdomen. However, unless the pulse is increased, there is no need for a four quadrant paracentesis. It is the tachycardia that signals the onset of other pathology (e.g., hypovolemia, infection).

After a spinal cord injury, the urinary bladder loses its ability to contract. It becomes atonic. In some cases even the peristaltic waves in the ureters cease. This areflexive state may last many weeks. An indwelling urinary catheter avoids over-distending the bladder and limits the amount of urine that remains in the bladder which could give rise to an infection.

The respiratory complications of spinal cord injury can develop at any time and are most commonly seen in patients with cervical cord injuries during the acute stage. The lesion produces paralysis of the intercostal muscles and varying degrees of impairment of the diaphragm. In addition to other possible chest problems that must be ruled out, this patient has an impaired cough mechanism, which allows secretions to accumulate. Diaphragmatic breathing can lead to an increased physiologic arteriovenous shunting or ventilation–perfusion mismatching. A distended abdomen can interfere with diaphragmatic breathing thus reducing the vital capacity. The danger of vomiting and aspiration of abdominal contents with the resultant chemical pneumonia and bronchospasms is a real threat to these patients.

Incomplete spinal cord transection gives rise to varying clinical pictures. In central cord syndrome, the injury usually results from a direct force (e.g., fall and striking of forehead or chin on a hard surface) which causes the neck to hyperextend. The elderly are quite prone to this type of injury. Forced hyperextension in the presence of cervical spondylosis further narrows the spinal canal. The cord is pinched or crushed between the osteophytes and the thickened posterior ligament. Tissue swelling impairs venous circulation and results in progressive central hemorrhaging. In young people, torn fragments of the annulus or cartilage plates of the discs could be thrust into the spinal canal and give rise to central hemorrhage. This central damage affects the medial and parts of the lateral pyramidal tracts as well as the anterior horn cells. Clinically, the patient has a greater motor deficit in the arms than the legs. Sensory losses are variable and there may be a loss of pain and temperature sensation but preservation of touch. However, rapidly developing quadriplegia could follow this injury. Immediate recognition and surgical intervention cures this paralysis.

The anterior cord syndrome could be called the anterior spinal artery syndrome. In this situation, the anterior spinal artery is compressed by bone or cartilage spicules resulting in all but the dorsal columns of the cord being damaged. Motor function, temperature, and pain sensation are lost bilaterally below the injured segment. However, there is some preservation of touch, vibration, and position sense.

When only half of the spinal cord is damaged, the resulting syndrome is referred to as the Brown–Sequard syndrome. This type injury results in ipsilateral loss of motor functioning as well as loss of vibratory sense below the level of the lesion. In addition, there will be a contralateral loss of pain and temperature sensation.

The detailed neurologic assessment and other studies establish the degree of impairment and approximates the level of the injury. A precise assessment of all motor and sensory activities is performed not only to ascertain if any activities are preserved below the level of the lesion, but also to serve as a baseline of data to compare later assessments. It is not uncommon for the dysfunctions to ascend or transverse during the first 24 to 48 hours after the injury. A loss of function higher than two segments or the appearance of a second level of cord dysfunction usually indicates that the cord had been injured in more than one place. Following the clinical assessments, radiographic examinations are performed to validate the clinical impression, rule out associated injuries, and serve to aid the neurosurgeon in making management decisions.

MANAGEMENT

   I. Prevent further damage to the spinal cord
      A. Keep the neck and spine immobilized continuously
      B. Do not remove stabilization board or cervical collar
      C. Do not release skull traction that has already been put in place
      D. Obtain assistance when x-rays and special tests are requested
      E. Use log-rolling technique when moving patient
  II. Maintain a patent airway and adequate ventilations
      A. Monitor respiratory effort, vital capacity, and tidal volume q 15 to 30 minutes
      B. Pass a nasogastric tube and attach to low suctioning
      C. Monitor serial blood gases
      D. If an oral airway is in place, suction only the mouth. Avoid tracheal suctioning to reduce vagal stimulation which could lead to cardiac arrest
      E. If tracheal suctioning is required, precede it by oxygenation and possibly by administering atropine. Monitor heart rate closely during tracheal suctioning
      F. If pneumothorax or hemothorax is present, be prepared to assist with chest drainage
      G. When vital capacity falls below 1000 liters, and/or P_{CO_2} nears 50 and P_{O_2} is below 60, prepare for mechanically assisted ventilations
      H. A nasotracheal intubation tube attached to a mechanical volume respirator with oxygen may be required
      I. Continue to monitor tidal volume and blood gases
 III. Maintain an adequate circulation to all body tissues
      A. Monitor bp and pulse q 5 to 10 minutes until stable (anticipate a low bp and slow pulse)
      B. Initiate an IV line for drug and fluid administration. Do not allow fluids to flow fast. Limit IV fluids to 600 to 1000 ml/24 hours

C. Insert an indwelling urinary catheter. Measure all output
D. Assess peripheral pulses for rate, rhythm, and quality
E. Continuously monitor cardiac functioning. Sinus bradycardia is to be expected
F. If bradycardia falls to a rate between 44 and 48 beats/minute:
1. anticholingeric drugs (e.g., atropine) or adrenergic drugs (e.g., noradrenaline) may be prescribed
2. a transvenous pacemaker may be inserted
G. Apply thromboembolic stockings to lower limbs to support venous return
IV. Detect and correct signs of hypovolemia and electrolyte imbalances
A. Hypovolemic shock symptoms include
1. bp below 70 mm Hg systolic
2. rise in pulse rate
3. decreased LOC
4. decreased urine output, CVP, and hematocrit
B. Restore fluid volume
1. colloids or crystalloid solutions may be prescribed
2. monitor bp, pulse, and CVP during fluid replacement
3. record urinary output frequently
4. auscultate the chest for rales because pulmonary edema is a frequent hazard
C. Search for the cause of hypovolemia
D. Monitor serum electrolytes and blood gases to assess adequacy of treatment
V. Monitor neurologic status to detect changes in status
A. Keep an accurate flow sheet of all observations
B. Perform motor testing as described in assessment
C. Perform sensory testing as described in assessment
D. Compare current findings with baseline data. Validate findings with another observer. Report all deviations to physician
E. Administer steroids as prescribed
VI. Detect and treat problems in elimination
A. Observe for the development of hypokalemia and alkalosis caused by loss of gastric fluid
B. Monitor the characteristics of the gastric fluid plus the amount
C. Measure the abdominal girth and record
D. Because stress ulcers are common, cimetidine (Tagamet) may be prescribed to decrease gastric acid secretion
E. Keep patient npo until bowel sounds return
VII. Correct the deformity and stabilize the spine
A. Assist with the insertion of devices to apply skull traction
1. secure the Gardner–Wells device, cervical traction pulley, and adjustable arm clamp
2. prepare the skin above the ears below temporal ridge
3. have a local skin anesthetic ready for injection

   4. the points are advanced according to directions and seated
   5. indicator protrusion should be at 1 mm
   6. apply weights as prescribed (principle is 5 lb/disc space) the usual transporting weight is 10 to 15 lb; 25 to 40 lb may be required for lower cervical cord injuries
   7. repeat lateral views of cervical spine in 20 minutes
   8. keep head in extension to prevent redislocation
B. Prepare patient for surgery

RATIONALE

Recovery from spinal cord injury depends to a large extent on the prevention of further injury during the rescue and emergency treatment period plus the prevention of secondary complications (e.g., hypoxia) that compromise functional neural tissue.

The patient is assessed and cared for in the emergency room with the spine stabilized on a board or in some acceptable manner. All efforts are aimed at preventing active or passive movements of the patient's spine. Clothing is cut away along the seams. Nothing is pulled over the head. If emesis occurs, the patient attached to the board is turned sideways to avoid aspiration or may be log-rolled with sufficient number of people. A nasogastric tube should be inserted immediately in the event of emesis to avoid aspiration.

At the scene of the accident and in the emergency room, the top priority is the maintenance of adequate airway and ventilation. Usually the patient breathes diaphragmatically. Blood gas analysis indicates whether this is sufficient. In the early stages, it commonly is not sufficient and respiratory failure occurs. Nasotracheal intubation is preferred to oral intubation because it avoids neck movements. In some centers, a tracheostomy is performed if there are no facial or mandibular injuries.

A volume respirator plus oxygen is necessary to assist with adequate ventilations. Oxygen delivery is assessed by serially measuring the Po_2 levels. The oxygen tension of the spinal cord falls quickly below minimal requirements and is very sensitive to hypoxia. To prevent hypoxic damage to the nerves, the Po_2 is maintained at 80 mm Hg or above.

Whereas suctioning is necessary to keep the airway clear, it is not without hazard. Incorrect suctioning could stimulate the vagus nerve endings in the oropharynx and carina resulting in further slowing of the heart rate. The nurse should watch the cardiac monitor for just such an event and be prepared to administer medications (e.g., atropine, norepinephrine) to combat the problem. Offering increased oxygen before suctioning and, in some cases, medications forestalls this event.

An important distinction must be made between the signs of neurogenic (spinal) shock and hemorrhagic or hypovolemic shock (see Section Two, Shock Syndromes). The patient with a cervical cord injury is in neurogenic shock but there may be coexisting hypovolemia and hemorrhage. A careful search must be made for conditions such as a myocardial infarct, lung contusion, abdominal bleeding if the situation is warranted. The signs of these shock syndromes in the cervical cord injured patient are a further lowering of the blood pressure, a low CVP, a decrease in LOC, a decrease in urine output, and a slight increase in pulse.

Hypovolemia when diagnosed must be treated. However, the rapid infusion of intravenous fluids in this patient frequently leads to pulmonary edema. The blood pressure, CVP, pulse, and urinary output must be carefully monitored during fluid administration that is intended to make up losses. Blood tests such a serum osmolarity, electrolytes, blood gases, and hematocrit determine the type of fluid to be replaced.

Once the respiratory and circulatory systems are fairly stable, a detailed neurologic survey as well as all other systems are assessed. The neurologic assessment must include motor and sensory functioning in the sacral area. Even with complete paralysis, sacral sparing may be found. This is an encouraging sign for it signals the potential for partial or complete functional return. Conversely, the lack of spinal sparing may be the single clue that the cord has been damaged. The neurologic assessments are repeated often because progression of the lesion can and does occur. Thus, the need for good record keeping.

Steroid therapy is commonly initiated during the emergency care of this patient. High doses of dexamethasone (Decadron) are used as loading doses and then administered every 4 to 6 hours. Steroids in some manner reduce the edema by promoting sodium and water excretion. Dexamethasone prevents the loss of potassium which may be decreased in the injured tissues of the cord.

Because gastrointestinal peristalsis ceases during spinal shock, a nasogastric tube is passed and attached to low suctioning. The nurse must observe for hypokalemia and metabolic alkalosis if an excessive amount of fluid is withdrawn. In addition, a sample of gastric fluid should be tested for blood, because stress ulcers and bleeding could occur. The nurse will frequently auscultate for bowel sounds. The patient remains npo until bowel sounds return.

An indwelling urinary catheter is inserted because the bladder is atonic and the sphincter tone is increased. The bladder becomes easily overdistended, especially if intravenous fluids are given. The catheter allows for accurate output recording and this is a valuable clue to assessing the perfusion of a vital organ. It might also prove beneficial in detecting bladder injuries. The nurse must use strict aseptic technique during the catheter's insertion as well as in maintaining a closed collection system.

There is much discussion over the role of conservative management of cord injuries versus aggressive surgical management. In large emergency centers, the treatment plan is usually a team decision in consultation with the patient and family. There are occasions where a closed reduction of a spinal dislocation necessitates the insertion of skull traction while the patient is in the emergency department. The newer Gardner–Wells apparatus is relatively easy to use. Muscle relaxants may be prescribed before this therapy is begun.

During the stay in the emergency department, the patient must be protected from extremes in temperature. Special care must begin for correct positioning and avoidance of pressure. The nurse, as well as all others, should explain in calm un-hurried tones what is occurring and why it is necessary. The patient is not uncon-scious and most likely fear will quickly turn to panic if the staff appears unable to meet his or her needs.

After the patient is stabilized and the neurosurgical consultants have conferred, the patient may be taken to surgery, a neurosurgical intensive care unit, or a spinal cord center for further treatment and care.

4. Meningitis

ASSESSMENT

I. Presenting clinical picture
  A. General findings and behavior
    1. moderate to acutely ill patient with a history of URI
    2. mental status: confused, disoriented, restless, delirious, might be halluci-nating or experiencing seizures
    3. complains of violent headache, malaise, stiff neck, backache
    4. TPR and bp: usually elevated temperature, bp may be normal, low, or high
  B. Neurologic findings
    1. LOC: depressed; patient could be comatose
    2. cranial nerve findings (depends on which nerves involved)
      a. optic nerve: visual losses, photophobia
      b. oculomotor, abducens, trochlear: if involved, altered pupillary re-sponses, altered eye movements, strabismus, diplopia
      c. acoustic: tinnitus, nystagmus, vertigo, hearing loss
      d. glossopharyngeal: dysphagia
    3. Motor findings (suggestive of meningeal irritation)
      a. body position: rigid spine, head could be retracted
      b. nucchal rigidity upon neck flexion
      c. positive Kernig sign
      d. positive Brudzinski sign
      e. seizure activity
      f. paresis possible
    4. sensory findings
      a. hypersensitivity in most cases
      b. hyperalgesia also possible
  C. Respiratory system alteration (suggests brainstem involvement)
    1. respiratory difficulty
    2. alteration in the rate, pattern, and depth of respirations
    3. secretions might collect in oropharynx, if swallowing is interfered with

    D. Cardiovascular system alteration
       1. weak, rapid pulse
       2. could be dehydrated if in septic shock
       3. could be normovolemic if SIADH exists
    E. Alterations in other body systems
       1. gastrointestinal: vomiting common; some nausea
       2. skin: petechial–purpuric rash, if meninococcus

II. Precipitating and/or contributing events
    A. Head trauma
       1. closed head injury with fracture or defect of cribiform plate (suspect pneumococcus)
       2. open head injury (wide variety of oganisms)
       3. if rhinorrhea present (suspect pneumococcus)
    B. Parameningeal infections
       1. sinusitis, chronic otitis, chronic mastoiditis (usually pneumococcal but could be *H. influenzae* in the very young)
       2. osteomyelitis (skull), brain abscess
    C. Anatomic defects
       1. meningomyelocele, midline pilonidal sinus tract, invading tumors of the head and neck (a wide variety of organisms)
    D. Systemic sepsis
       1. *Staphylococcus* septicemia
       2. pneumonia (pneumococcus)
       3. skin lesions (meningococcus)
    E. Underlying systemic illnesses
       1. splenectomy and sickle cell anemia (pneumococcus and meningococcus)
       2. Systemic malignancy (wide variety of organisms)
       3. Immunosuppressed patients and those in renal failure or on dialysis (fungal infections, gram-negative enteric rods and hospital-acquired pathogens)
       4. cancer patients (cryptococcus, pneumococcus, *Listeria*, gram-negative rods)
    F. Community factors
       1. presence of an epidemic or increase in number of cases in the hospital or community
    G. Age factor (when underlying focus is not found)
       1. children and adolescents
          a. after 2 months: *H. influenzae, N. meningitidis*
          b. after 4 years: meningococcus (*H. influenzae* rare)
       2. adults
          a. after 20 years: pneumococcus (meningococcus rare)

III. Alteration in laboratory and/or other diagnostic tests
    A. Hematologic studies: Bloods are drawn for RBC, Hgb, Hct, and examination of a peripheral smear. A WBC and differential is drawn. Leukocytosis is a common finding

B. Chemistries and metabolic studies: Bloods are drawn for electrolytes, BUN, creatinine, glucose, arterial blood gases, and serum osmolarity
C. Blood coagulation studies: Findings depend upon the severity of the patient's condition
D. Lumbar puncture for CSF analysis
   a. opening pressure usually high; increased cell count and protein; decreased glucose content. Fluid appears purulent
   b. microscopic examination should include Gram stain, AFB to r/o tuberculosis; india ink preparation to r/o cryptococcus and wet smear to r/o fungi and amoebae
   c. bacteriologic studies include culture and specimens for AFB, fungi, amoebae
   d. Other studies: Counterimmunoelectrophoresis to r/o meningococcus, *H. influenzae*. Serologic tests to r/o syphilis, cryptococcal, coccidioidal antigen, or antibody
E. Skull films: r/o basilar fracture, parameningeal foci
F. CAT scan and radionucleotide scan to locate brain abscess and detect hydrocephalic condition
G. Chest x-ray to r/o pneumonia or respiratory mass
H. ECG
I. Cultures of the nose, throat, blood, and urine
J. Urine studies: routine analysis, electrolyte and osmolarity if SIADH is suspected

PATHOPHYSIOLOGY

Meningitis is an inflammatory process involving the membranes of the central nervous system. When referred to as leptomeningitis, the pia and arachnoid mater are involved. If all the meninges are involved, the term used is pachymeningitis. In the event that the process spreads to the cerebral parenchymal tissues, it is called meningoencephalitis.

The number of offending organisms that could lead to meningitis is large. They include bacteria, viruses, spirochetes, parasites, and fungi. There appears to be a typical age distribution for select bacterial meningitis. From 2 months to 4 years of age, the *Hemophilus influenza* and the *Neisseria meningitidis* are the most common offenders. From ages 4 through 20, meningococcus is the common agent whereas from 20 years through adulthood, diplococcus pneumonia gains prominence.

The chronologic history of the progression of bacterial meningitis frequently discloses a prior upper respiratory illness. A sore throat, cough, or earache usually existed from one to several weeks before the onset of other symptoms. The presence of a sore throat frequently precedes neisserial infections; a cough could be the forerunner of meningococcal or pneumococcal infection; and an earache could be the precursor to *Hemophilus influenzae* infection. However, there are a number of cases who have no prior history of a respiratory disease. These particular patients have a rapid onset of the disease process and appear in the emergency department in an unconscious state. A petechial or purpuric rash precedes and accompanies meningococcal meningitis.

Another large group of people at risk to develop meningitis are those with reduced or altered defense mechanisms. The very young and the very old are considered high risk groups. Patients who have a history of malignancy, diabetes mellitus, renal failure, and those who abuse alcohol are at greater risk because of their reduced nutritional reserves and metabolic imbalances. Treatments that place a patient at risk for meningitis include radiotherapy, dialysis, organ transplant, and cancer chemotherapy. These treatments frequently depress the host's immune system and ability to fight off infection. Whereas sporadic meningococcal infections occur in 5- to 10-year cycles and are usually confined to circumscribed areas (e.g., army camps, residential schools), bacterial meningitis more commonly occurs in a setting of some associated disease(s) or condition. The origin of the bacterial meningitis must be sought, if the correct therapy is to be prescribed.

It is hypothesized that the pathophysiologic cascade of events start with a metastatic foci of infection becoming established in the choroid of the lateral ventricles leading to a choroiditis and an ependymitis. This inflammatory process pours organisms into the ventricles and CSF. Thus, the organisms are carried to all parts of the CNS by the CSF. As the organisms proliferate, they produce the toxic effects of infection plus a purulent exudate. On gross examination of the brain and cord, the cortical and basal surfaces of the brain are covered with this exudate as is the spinal cord. The meningeal vessels appear greatly dilated. There is evidence of hemorrhage, vascular congestion, and thrombosis of the cortical veins. The ventricles appear moderately dilated, somewhat hyperemic and their lining roughened. Microscopically, the subarachnoid space is filled with a purulent polymorphonuclear exudate which at times is seen to penetrate the perivascular sheath. The pressure in the subarachnoid space is greatly elevated.

Inflammation of the meninges results in meningeal irritation and accounts for a number of symptoms seen with meningitis. Irritated meninges at the posterior basilar cranial area leads to a stiff neck, nuchal rigidity on testing, and retraction of the neck. Low back pain is due to the spinal meningeal irritation and pulling which produces muscle spasms. Positive Kernig and Brudzinski signs are indicative of meningeal irritation. When the meninges of the neck and the lumbar area are very taut, the patient may manifest an opisthotonus body position. The severe headache is also reflective of meningeal irritation.

Increased intracranial pressure (ICP) is a consequence of three mechanisms in meningitis. First, the toxic effects of the inflammatory process produce a local cellular swelling and outpouring of CSF. Second, focal circulatory changes of a venous and/or an arterial nature contribute to this rise. The venous thrombosis or venous obstruction which occur decrease fluid drainage of cerebral cells resulting in fluid collection in the cerebral tissues. Arteritis leads to brain ischemia and infarct which produce a local swelling of surrounding tissues. Third, an obstructive communicating hydrocephalus can lead to an increase in ICP. This type of hydrocephalus results from an obstruction to the flow of CSF and is believed to be due to a thickening fibrotic change in the meninges at the base of the brain.

Cranial nerve involvement in meningitis is reflective of two pathophysiologic processes. First, disturbances in functioning could result from direct extension of the infectious process into the area where the cranial nerves extrude from the brainstem. For example, if pressure surrounds the optic nerve, the retinal vessels dilate. The patient experiences blurring of vision, diplopia, and photophobia. On examination, the optic disc appears choked (papilledema).

A rise in ICP is the second mechanism by which cranial nerves become involved in meningitis. When the cerebral pressure above the tentorial notch is sufficiently increased, the uncal lobe of a hemisphere herniates through this notch and pushes up against the structures of the brainstem. The pathways of the cranial nerves lie alongside the brainstem and if they are stretched or displaced, characteristic signs are observed. Disturbances in cranial nerves III, IV, and VI result in changes in pupillary responses and eye movements. Interference with cranial nerves IX, X, and XI leads to dysphagia and dysarthria. Tinnitus, ataxia, and hearing loss suggest cranial nerve VIII involvement. Vomiting could result from a lesion in the vestibular nuclei or involvement of cranial nerves V, VII, IX, X, and XII. Facial weakness occurs because of cranial nerve VII involvement.

Because the midbrain, pons, and medulla are the structures that comprise the brainstem, pressure or displacement of these structures can have grave consequences. The reticular activating system runs throughout the brainstem and any alterations in its functioning leads to decreasing levels of consciousness. The pneumotaxic center, respiratory center, cardiac accelerating and inhibitory centers are also located in this region and any disruptions in their activities are reflected by serious changes in respirations and cardiac rhythm.

Disturbances in hypothalamic functioning also occur in bacterial meningitis. Among other functions, the hypothalamus controls body temperature and regulates body water balance. Fever can be severe in bacterial meningitis. It is partly due to the body's response to inflammatory pyrogens, but it could also be reflective of hypothalamic disruption which could occur secondary to displacement and pressure. The syndrome of inappropriate secretion of ADH has been recognized as a complication of meningitis. The hypothalamus in this case secretes too much ADH which leads to the retention of water and the excretion of sodium.

Seizures frequently accompany meningitis, especially in infants and children. The cause of seizuring varies. It could be due to the toxic effects of the infection, cortical vein thrombosis with venous infarction, empyemas, abscesses, vasculitis, or metabolic problems such as the hyponatremia caused by the syndrome of inappropriate secretion of ADH. Hyperexcited neurons are able to fire at will. Intense local discharges spread and result in a generalized seizure. Fortunately, the seizures resolve as the meningitis clears without leaving residual epilepsy.

Overwhelming bacteremia in association with bacterial meningitis could precipitate septic shock and circulatory collapse. Briefly, in this process, agents released by the bacteria cause hyperpyrexia, peripheral vasodilatation, fluid loss, and a general hypermetabolic state. The vicious cycle of this shock with its continuous demands for oxygen, places excessive demands upon the cardiopulmonary system (see text on Septic Shock). In addition, systemic sepsis may lead to disseminated intravascular coagulopathy.

The necessity for a rapid diagnosis is evident when one considers that untreated bacterial meningitis is 100 percent fatal unless adequate antibiotic therapy is quickly initiated. Examining the cerebrospinal fluid is the only certain way of making a positive identification of the offending organism. An intravenous line must be in place before the lumbar puncture (LP) and a blood glucose must be drawn before the procedure. There is always the possibility that the patient's condition will deteriorate during the LP. If this occurs, intravenous mannitol must be infused over 20 to 30 minutes before the LP needle is withdrawn. All patients must be closely watched after an LP regardless if they deteriorate or not. The blood glucose is compared to the CSF glucose level.

Analysis of the CSF tests can be quite revealing. The opening pressure is usually elevated due to the increased fluid and pressure within the brain. The glucose levels are low secondary to the presence of numerous and possibly various bacteria. The normally clear CSF appears purulent and cloudy due to the elevated number of polymorphonuclear leukocytes within it. A fairly accurate and rapid identification of the offending organism is made on the basis of the Gram stain smear of the fluid. The physician may request additional studies on the CSF to rule out other possible offending organisms. Therapy is begun before the cultures grow out the organism.

In addition to the CSF studies, the physician will want to assess the patient's overall medical status, identify factors that contributed to the patient's development of meningitis, and attempt to find the offending organism in other body fluids. A careful history, physical examination, and other diagnostic tests assist in this differential diagnosis. Baseline laboratory data are a valuable aid in following the patient's response to therapy.

MANAGEMENT

I. Maintain a patent airway and adequate ventilations
   A. Observe and chart respiratory rate, depth and patter q 15 to 30 minutes
   B. Evaluate ability to swallow secretions and integrity of gag reflex
   C. Suction oropharyngeal area prn
   D. Obtain chest x-ray, arterial blood gases, specimens of nose, throat, and sputum for culture and sensitivity testing
   E. Serially assess vital capacity and tidal volume
   F. Assist with passage of a nasogastric tube
   G. Be prepared to insert an oral airway *or* to intubate the patient
   H. Oxygen therapy may be prescribed
II. Maintain adequate circulation to the body's tissues
   A. Record temperature, pulse, respirations, and bp q 15 to 30 minutes

B. Establish an IV line for fluid and drug administration

C. Monitor for signs of septic shock

Early signs: fever and chills, hypotension, warm skin, LOC, tachycardia, leukocytosis, tachypnea

Late signs: hypotension, cool pale extremities, peripheral cyanosis, oliguria, heart failure, respiratory insufficiency, metabolic acidosis

D. Insert an indwelling urinary catheter

E. Record the I & O

III. Identify the offending organism and initiate therapy

A. Assist with the collection of specimens for laboratory analysis

B. Assist with lumbar puncture

1. secure IV line must be in place
2. if done in the presence of a possible mass lesion, a hyperosmolar agent (mannitol) may be administered before or during the tap
3. start high dose steroid therapy
4. be certain that blood glucose is drawn before spinal tap
5. observe patient q 15 minutes posttap for signs of deterioration
6. repeat LP may be performed in 24 to 48 hours after antibiotics are started

IV. Initiate appropriate antibiotic therapy

A. Choice of initial antibiotic depends upon Gram stain, patient's age, predisposing factors, and allergies (to penicillin)

B.

Age	Drug of Choice	Alternative
Infants and children	Ampicillin and chloramphenicol	Chloramphenicol and gentamycin
Adults	Ampicillin *or* penicillin G	Erythromycin and chloramphenicol
Skull fractures or CSF leaks	Ampicillin *or* penicillin G	Erythromycin and chloramphenicol
Immunosuppression or malignancy	Carbenicillin and gentamycin	Erythromycin and gentamycin

C. Antibiotic therapy for known organisms

1. pneumococcus—penicillin G
2. streptococcus, groups A and B—penicillin G
3. streptococcus, group D—penicillin G and gentamycin
4. staphylococcus—oxacillin or methicillin
5. *Listeria monocytogenes*—penicillin G or ampicillin
6. meningococcus—penicillin G
7. *H. influenzae*—ampicillin or chloramphenicol
8. *Pseudomonas aeruginosa*—carbenicillin and gentamycin
9. enteric gram-negative (*E. coli, Proteus, Klebsiella*)—chloramphenicol or ampicillin plus gentamycin

D. Observe for toxicities associated with a high dose of antibiotic therapy

1. observe for hypersensitivity reactions and be prepared to combat ana-

phylactic shock (rash, angineurotic edema, persistent fever, seizures, hypotension).

2. observe for seizures in the patient receiving high dose of penicillin G
3. observe for nephrotoxicity; monitor output, send specimen for repeat urinalysis
4. observe for ototoxicity: headache, nausea, vomiting, vertigo
5. observe for decrease in respirations when aminoglycosides are used; they will cause a neuromuscular blockade
6. observe for monilial overgrowth
7. various antibiotic preparations are sodium or potassium salts—observe for overload of these electrolytes

V. Detect and treat increased intracranial pressure
   A. Observe for signs of impending increase ICP
     1. decreasing LOC; observe for the Cushing reflex (increased bp and bradycardia)
     2. decreasing motor and sensory responses; bilateral Babinski sign, paralysis of upward gaze
     3. decreasing pupillary response, papilledema
     4. if intracranial pressure monitoring device is used, look for characteristic "pressure wave." Intracranial pressure should be kept under 200 mm H_2O

   B. Avoid overhydration by limiting fluid intake
     1. limit fluids to 1200 to 1500 ml/day, IV
     2. avoid hypotonic solutions (e.g., D5W), administer half normal saline solution
     3. subtract amount of dilutant used in antibiotic preparation from 1500 ml
     4. monitor neurologic and vital signs; urinary output, serum osmolarity
     5. elevate head of bed 30 degrees

   C. Reduce cerebral edema
     1. administer steroid preparations
       a. high doses usually initially prescribed; then tapered as infection is brought under control (e.g., stat dose dexamethasone (Decadron) 10 mg IV followed by dexamethasone (Decadron) 4 mg IV q 4 hours. Once infection clears, taper dose to zero over 5 to 10 days.)
       b. observe for the side effects of steroid therapy in 12 to 16 hours
         i. hyperglycemia—monitor blood glucose, urine sugar, and acetone
         ii. hyperacidity—monitor stool guaiacs and gastric upset
         iii. electrolyte imbalances—hypernatremia, hypokalemia, hypocalcemia
         iv. opportunistic infections
     2. administer hyperosmolar agents as prescribed
       a. Mannitol 20 percent solution
         i. 50 g or 1.0 to 1.5 g/kg IV stat may be repeated
         ii. check serum osmolarity after each dose; target level is 300 to 320 mOsm/L

       iii. monitor urinary output, BUN, electrolyte, vital signs

     b. Glycerol 1 to 3 g/kg/day po or instilled in nasogastric tube

       i. 20 percent solution lemon-flavored solution (Osmoglyn) or 50 percent unflavored solution

       ii. dose is divided into 6 doses

       iii. monitor serum osmolarity, urinary output, BUN, electrolytes, vital signs, glucose

   3. hyperventilate patient to produce hypocapnea and metabolic alkalosis which will decrease cerebral blood flow thus reducing intracranial pressure. Maintain P_{CO_2} at 25 torr

   4. consider shunting procedures to correct hydrocephalus (usually deferred until a later date)

VI. Reduce the spread of infectious organisms to others

   A. Carry out respiratory isolation procedure for at least 24 hours with antibiotics

   B. Medical isolation, hand washing and other techniques may be required for longer period in very resistant cases

   C. Treat contacts of patients as described by CDC (include staff, family, friends)

VII. Reduce hyperpyrexia

   A. Place patient in cool environment, limit amount of top linens and clothing

   B. Monitor temperature (rectally)

   C. Administer antipyretic drugs as prescribed

   D. Give tepid sponges as ordered

   E. Be prepared to place patient on hypothermic blanket if temperature rises to 103 °F (40 °C)

   F. Offer oral hygiene frequently to a febrile patient

   G. Increase fluid intake *only* with physician's approval

VIII. Reduce stimuli in patient's environment

   A. Quiet environment and mild analgesic may reduce headache

   B. Darkened, nonstimulatory room reduces photophobia and hypersensitivity

   C. Place patient on complete bed rest; limit visitors

IX. Control seizure activity

   A. Institute seizure precautions

   B. Record all seizuring activity and report; protect patient from injury

   C. Administer anticonvulsant medication as prescribed (e.g., Dilantin)

RATIONALE

In meningitis, as well as in other neurologic conditions, immediate therapeutic measures are initiated to prevent further neurologic damage. Because the brain is unable to store oxygen and because it uses oxygen at a greater rate than other body tissues, it is vulnerable to hypoxia. Deprived of oxygen, glucose, and certain enzymatic substrates, cerebral functioning decreases and catabolic activities ensue with resulting destruction of brain tissue. Disturbances in LOC may be the first direct result of hypoxia and/or decreases in cerebral blood flow. Conversely, respiratory insufficiency and circulatory collapse may be a secondary complication of brain disease. Therefore, rapid correction of hypoxia takes the highest priority in managing this patient. Maintaining an adequate airway and ventilations are prime nursing activities. If systemic shock is present, it should be treated with volume replacement and possibly vasopressors.

Because it is most urgent to begin specific antibiotic therapy in patients with meningitis, all material for bacteriologic examination should be obtained prior to their start. The culture and sensitivity studies of CSF is the only means of making a definitive diagnosis. Cultures of other specimens may fail to identify the offender or report organisms other than those attacking the meninges.

There are certain risks associated with a LP, if intracranial pressure is increased. There are some reports of herniation coincident with or shortly after a LP. This event is probably caused by a continuing leak of CSF through the dural defect and not due to the withdrawal of CSF. Loss of CSF in this manner can disturb intracranial equilibrium leading to herniation through the tentorial notch. Therefore, it is good practice to be alert for this event and prepared to treat it. Before the LP, a secure functioning intravenous line must be in place and a hyperosmolar agent (e.g., mannitol) must be ready for infusion. After all spinal taps, the nurse would closely observe the patient for signs of deterioration (e.g., decreasing LOC, pupillary changes, Babinski, respiratory pattern changes, Cushing reflex).

Once bacteriologic identification of the offending organism is made and the drug sensitivities determined, the precise and appropriate antibiotic(s) can be prescribed. Because of the acuteness of the patient's condition, however, some physicians prefer to begin treatment before the culture results are available. They base their selection of antibiotic(s) on the Gram stain results, age of the patient, predisposing factors, and allergic sensitivities. In the latter case, broad spectrum antibiotics are used.

Adequate treatment of meningitis requires extremely high doses of parenteral antibiotics for 1 to 3 weeks or longer. Only such high doses of the drug(s) cross the meningeal–blood barrier and thus increase the CSF drug levels. However, this places the patient at risk of developing drug toxicities, especially if they have underlying hepatic, renal, or hematologic diseases. The patient must be closely observed for the development of these toxicities.

There have been many attempts to treat meningitis by directly injecting antibiotics into the subarachnoid space (e.g., intralumbar, intracisternal, and intraventricular using an Ommaya reservoir). The rationale for this technique is to expose the offending organism to a higher concentration of antibiotic than can be achieved by intravenous administration. Problems that have arisen using this technique are parasthesias, radiculopathies, myelitis, and arachnoiditis. Additional concerns center around the uneven distribution and diffusion of antibiotics in the CSF following these techniques. Thus, intrathecal administration is reserved for those patients who do not respond to systemic therapy (e.g., gram-negative meningitis, Staphylococcal meningitis, Enterococcal meningitis). This decision need not be made by the emergency department staff and should be deferred to the neurologist who will assume continuing management of this patient once hospitalized.

All efforts are directed at detecting and controlling ICP. Decreasing levels of alertness (LOC) is a very reliable indicator of increasing ICP. It may or may not be accompanied by changes in blood pressure or respiratory pattern. Because papilledema takes up to 24 hours to develop, its absence does not always mean that ICP is normal. Thus, it is not always a reliable sign of acute rises in ICP.

Because the cranial neves originate from the brainstem, any alteration in their afferent or efferent pathways signals changes in ICP. The oculomotor, trochlear, and abducens nerves (III, IV, VI) are most commonly affected by pressure and/or displacement of the brainstem. If uncal herniation is occurring, characteristic changes such as pupillary dilatation and fixation followed by complete ophthalmoplegia is seen. Small reactive pupils with full eye movements on doll's head maneuver is indicated of central herniation. Gaze palsies followed by small reactive pupils and loss of horizontal movements point to cerebellar herniation.

Respiratory functioning is the end product of extensive neuronal integration and is primarily under the control of structures in the brainstem, principally, the pons and the medulla. The inspiratory center and expiratory center in the medulla regulate the contraction of the inspiratory and expiratory muscles. Impulses from the vagus nerve also participate in the reflex regulation of inspiration and expiration (Hering–Breuer reflex). The apneustic and pneumotaxic centers located in the pons enhance the activities of the medulla. The apneustic center when stimulated causes respiration to be deeper and more prolonged. To balance this, the pneumotaxic center when stimulated, accelerates respiratory rate.

The respiratory pattern thus is very helpful in locating a lesion. The nurse should observe the respirations for 1 full minute before identifying the pattern. Some common abnormal patterns are:

1. Cheyne–Stokes: deep and diffuse bilateral hemispheric pathology; basal ganglia and upper brainstem involvement; may be due to metabolic imbalance and not CNS lesion.
2. Central neurogenic: lesion could be between lower midbrain and middle third of the pons; may be seen with midbrain compression or transtentorial herniation but metabolic acidosis and hypoxia must be r/o—poor prognostic sign.
3. Apneustic: lesion probably in the mid or lower pons.
4. Cluster: lesion probably in lower portion of the pons or in the medulla.
5. Ataxic (Biot): lesion probably in the reticular formation of the medulla; event usually precedes respiratory arrest.
6. Depressed: most likely the medulla is depressed—drugs should be ruled out before a lesion is suspected.

Any increase in ICP is reflected in disturbances of the autoregulation of blood volume. As ICP rises and becomes more generalized, systemic blood pressure rises reflexively in an attempt to maintain cerebral perfusion at adequate levels. If the baroreceptor arc is intact, the systemic increase in blood pressure results in a reflex bradycardia. The combination of hypertension and bradycardia is the Cushing reflex and is a sign of critically increased ICP.

Brain swelling and increased CSF pressure are likely to be seen in patients with meningitis. For these reasons it is wise to avoid overhydrating the patient, if hypotension is not a problem. Fluids are restricted and free water avoided to approximately 1200 to 1500 ml/24 hours. Any oral fluid given to the patient or dilutant used to mix the antibiotic must be subtracted from the total prescribed intake.

In the event of rapidly rising ICP, steroid therapy is commonly initiated to reduce the edema. The exact mechanism by which steroids act to reduce cerebral edema awaits elucidation. Some researchers believe that the hormone is capable of stabilizing the endothelial junction of the capillaries and reducing cerebrovascular permeability. Steroids, administered intravenously, act fairly rapidly and positive results are seen in 12 to 16 hours. The nurse must conscientiously observe for the side effects of steroid therapy (e.g., opportunistic infections, carbohydrate intolerance, gastric bleeding, electrolyte imbalances, steroid psychosis).

Hyperosmolar agents are also used to lessen an acute rise in ICP. These drugs rapidly reduce brain water by creating a gradient between the brain and blood plasma. When mannitol is used, a reduction of ICP can be seen in 2 to 4 hours. The nurse must carefully observe for the diuresis that is expected to occur. An indwelling urinary catheter facilitates the measurement of this output. If patients are diabetic, the use of osmotic diuretic agents places them at risk for hyperosmolar hyperglycemic nonketotic coma. Careful observations of serum electrolytes, osmolarity, blood sugar, and blood gases must be done. The goal of using hyperosmolar agents is a serum osmolarity between 300 and 320 mOsm/L. At some point in the repeated use of mannitol, the patient may experience a "rebound" rise in ICP. Concomitant steroid therapy should lessen this effect.

Hyperventilation is another possible approach to decreasing cerebral edema. During this treatment carbon dioxide is blown off from the lungs producing hypocapnea and respiratory alkalosis. The cerebral blood vessels vasoconstrict thus reducing cerebral blood volume. The patient may be hyperventilated until the Pco_2 ranges between 25 and 30 mm Hg. Frequent arterial blood gases are required to monitor this therapy. Suctioning should be limited to 10 to 15 seconds to minimize blood gas alterations.

Additional nursing measures can be taken to reduce ICP. The head of the bed should be elevated 20 to 30 degrees to allow for gravity drainage of the cranium. The head is not hyperextended, flexed, or rotated because these maneuvers might interfere with venous drainage. Efforts are directed toward limiting the Valsalva maneuver (e.g., assist patient to move; direct patient not to strain for anything).

The communicating obstructive hydrocephalus that may complicate meningitis could occur early or late in the course of this illness. It should be suspected when a patient's sensorium fails to clear as the infection lessens. This condition may resolve spontaneously. The decision to lower the pressure in the ventricles by shunting the CSF around the block (ventricle to atrial shunt) may be delayed. However, if the problem is a noncommunicating obstructive hydrocephalus, a medical emergency exists. This problem rapidly leads to brain death unless corrected. In the case of meningitis, constant ventricular drainage might be considered a better option than shunting because the CSF is probably highly infected. The nurse's role is to observe for signs of deterioration and be prepared to assist with this treatment.

Seizuring activity is a frequent occurrence in patients with meningitis. It usually resolves when the meningitis clears and, for the most part, does not indicate a grave prognosis. However, the etiology of the seizuring is quite varied and may indicate a bacterial encephalitis, subdural effusion, occult brain abscess, or metabolic disturbance (e.g., SIADH). If these complications persist, the seizuring requires further evaluation. As a rule, the patient is placed early on anticonvulsant medication. The nurse must observe and carefully chart all seizuring activity and postictal behaviors. She or he must also take measures to protect the patient from injury.

Although the initial fever in the patient with meningitis of a bacterial nature is expected to be high, the temperature should fall as therapy progresses. Continuous high fevers increase the body's metabolic rate and demands for oxygen and in turn produce more heat. When the body temperature reaches 106°F (41°C), the mechanisms to reduce it internally become ineffective and the temperature continues to rise. Control of fever becomes a high priority as well as the search for its cause. Antipyretic drugs are usually prescribed to combat fever. The nurse can use tepid sponges and keep the patient in a cool environment. If these measures are unsuccessful, a hypothermia mattress will be needed. Frequent monitoring of the rectal temperature will detect changes in body temperature. The temperature should not be allowed to exceed 103°F (40°C).

Patients with meningitis of unknown etiology should be placed on respiratory precautions for the first 24 hours of their antibiotic activity or until meningococcal meningitis is ruled out. In addition, medical isolation precautions may be necessary for those cases whose offending organism is resistant to a broad number of drugs, in order to prevent the spread of the infection. Strict hand washing and other protocols established by the hospital or Communicable Disease Center must be adhered to.

If the meningitis is due to meningococcus, contacts of the patient should be treated. One out of every 1000 family members of patients with meningococcus meningitis develop the disease. The number is really quite small because most adults develop their own antibodies to the disease. However, the possibility exists that a family member or close associate of the patient may turn out to be an asymptomatic carrier and in this way, expose other susceptible people to the organism. Close contacts of the patient must be treated as quickly as possible to prevent its spread. Thus, family members, household members, and others in close contact (which includes nurses and doctors) should take sulfadiazine 1.0 g q 12 hours for 2 days. (The doses differ for children and infants.) In some cases, rifampin 600 mg q 12 hours for 4 days is prescribed.

The nurse should offer additional measures that would add to the patient's comfort. A quiet, nonstimulating, darkened room reduces the hyperirritability and photophobia the patient may be experiencing. Visitors should be limited and the patient encouraged to rest. Headache may be relieved with an ice bag or a mild analgesic. The patient must be made to feel free enough to express the fears of the disease and procedures used to detect and/or treat it. Although the stay in the emergency department may be short, hospitalization may be prolonged.

5. Guillain–Barré Syndrome

ASSESSMENT

I. Precipitating and/or contributing factors
  A. History of mild respiratory or GI infection 1 to 3 weeks prior to onset of symptoms
  B. History of preceding viral illness: measles, mumps, rubella, cytomegalovirus, herpes zoster, Epstein–Barr virus, ECHO virus, Coxsackie virus, hepatitis, or immunization of flu vaccine
  C. History of other preceding events or factors include surgery, Hodgkin lymphoma, pregnancy, hyperthyroidism, adrenal insufficiency, and mycoplasma infection
  D. In some patients, no contributing or precipitating factor is found
II. Presenting clinical picture
  A. Neuromuscular system alterations
    1. motor findings
      a. timing: persistent, evolving motor weakness and paresthesias beginning distally in the feet and legs and progressing upward over a period of days
      b. distribution: usually symmetrical losses, feet, legs, arms, trunk, intercostals, neck, and then cranial nerves affected. However, some patients do not follow this pattern
      c. tone and bulk: muscles are hypotonic, eventually becoming flaccid. Patient may present as a flaccid quadriplegic
      d. size: no change in muscle size
      e. reflex status: reduced or diminished deep tendon reflexes are present If later in disease process, patient may be areflexic
    2. sensory findings (minimal)
      a. vibration sense impaired; more so than position or touch
      b. pain experienced by 30 percent of patients. Distal paresthesias common. Some may develop hypesthesia. Muscle tenderness experienced on deep palpation
      c. touch and pressure may be transiently lost
      d. position sense may be transiently lost
    3. cranial nerve findings
      a. facial (VII): facial paralysis, usually bilateral
      b. abducens and oculomotor (VI and III): gaze palsies
      c. hypoglossal (XII): difficulty with tongue movements

   d. trigeminal (V): difficulty in chewing

   e. accessory (IX): difficulty in swallowing

  4. autonomic nervous system findings

   a. fluctuations in bp: hypotension more than hypertension

   b. change in sweating patterns: anhidrosis more than diaphoresis

   c. heart rhythm fluctuations: tachycardia more than bradycardia

   d. skin changes: facial flushing, feelings of warmth

   e. sphincter paralysis: loss of control but could have retention

   f. bronchioles: paralysis of smooth muscles

 B. Respiratory system alterations

  1. may exhibit signs of ventilatory failure

   a. restlessness, anxiety, possibly lethargy, confusion

   b. vital capacity at or below 1000 ml

   c. increased Pco_2 and decreased Po_2 blood gas levels

  2. chest excursions could be shallow. Respiratory rate and pattern is irregular

  3. auscultative findings: perhaps adventitious sounds or rales

 C. Cardiovascular system alteration

  1. ECG changes: transient and sinus tachycardia with flattened T-wave or inverted T-wave in lateral lead

  2. fluctuations occur in bp. Hypotensive episodes are more common than hypertensive episodes

  3. fluctuations in pulse rate

 D. Other findings

  1. vital signs: temperature is usually normal

  2. GI: decreased bowel sounds or paralytic ileus may be found

  3. urinary: possible UTI due to transient retention

III. Alteration in laboratory and other diagnostic studies

 A. Bloods are drawn for RBC, WBC and differential, serum electrolytes, BUN, glucose, muscle enzymes, toxic screen. Moderate leukocytosis is evident. Some patients may have hypokalemia or hyponatremia

 B. Urine studies include routine analysis, porphobilinogen, osmolarity, specific gravity, electrolytes, culture and sensitivity

 C. Sputum and throat cultures are obtained

 D. Pulmonary tests include vital capacity, chest x-ray, and arterial blood gases

 E. Lumbar puncture performed; pressure is normal; cell count is normal; protein may be elevated; culture and sensitivity is negative

 F. Electromyography (EMG) and nerve conduction velocity (NCV) are not usually performed in emergency department but are tested when acute phase of illness is over

PATHOPHYSIOLOGY

Landry–Guillain–Barré–Strohl syndrome may also be called acute idiopathic polyradiculoneuritis, acute inflammatory polyradiculoneuropathy and acute immune-mediated polyneuritis. It is a syndrome characterized by an acute ascending motor paralysis with variable signs of sensory disruption.

The syndrome has been recognized since the mid 1800s but received much attention in 1976, following a sharp rise in the number of cases occurring in people immunized with A/New Jersey, or swine flu, vaccine. Its exact cause continues to remain a mystery. In almost 50 percent of the cases, a mild respiratory or gastrointestinal infection precedes the onset of the symptoms by 1 to 3 weeks. Other reported antecedent and/or predisposing events to the syndrome are surgical procedures, lymphomatous disease (especially Hodgkin lymphoma), hyperthyroidism, adrenal insufficiency, stress, and many other viral illnesses (e.g., measles, mumps, herpes zoster, hepatitis, etc.). It occurs in all seasons and does not appear to be communicable. The illness strikes all age groups, however a rate increase for the older age population is seen. In some studies no sex difference is found whereas in other studies, men appear to be affected more frequently than women. Whites contract the illness more than non-whites.

The pathologic findings are consistent with demyelinated changes in the peripheral nervous system which include the cranial nerves, the spinal nerves, and the autonomic nervous system. The catabolism of axonal myelin sheaths is caused by the perivascular invasion of lymphocytic infiltrates and macrophage which result in the loss of Schwann cells, a widened node of Ranvier (segmental demyelination), and varying degrees of Wallerian degeneration. These infiltrates have been found scattered along the length of the peripheral nerves, the dorsal root ganglia, the ventral and dorsal roots of the cord, and the cranial nerves. At autopsy they can be isolated in the lymph nodes, spleen, heart, and other organs which reflect the widespread involvement of this disease.

Nerve regeneration can occur in Guillain–Barré syndrome. Segmentally demyelinated nerves will recover functioning fairly rapidly. The axon, although denuded, remains intact but transmits impulses much more slowly. The intact Schwann cells, in some manner yet to be elucidated, participate in the remyelinization of the nerve axon. Wallerian degeneration is a classic neurocellular reaction secondary to proximal axonal injury. The myelinated axon undergoes fragmentation and digestion by macrophage. Axonal regeneration in this case is much slower because vigorous axonal proliferation and sprouting must occur which eventually reestablishes continuity with muscle and other structures. Thus, the patient eventually recovers.

Animal and leukocyte studies support the hypothesis of a virus induced cell-mediated autoimmune process aimed at peripheral nerves and/or nerve root ganglia. Two weeks after immunization with peripheral nerve homogenate, animal subjects developed experimental allergic neuritis which is clinically and histologically indistinguishable from Guillain–Barré syndrome. Peripheral blood leukocytes of patients with Guillain–Barré syndrome were shown to be activated on exposure to the P2 protein of peripheral nerves. (This protein of myelin is more specific to peripheral nerves.) The animal studies give support to the probability of a delayed hypersensitivity reaction and the lymphocyte studies suggest that P2 protein is the antigen that lymphocytes have been sensitized to previously. Although attempts to isolate this virus or agent have failed, one must acknowledge that most victims give a history of an antecedent viral infection. Some of these antecedent viruses (e.g., herpes) are capable of establishing latent infections within cells.

The role of humoral antibody formation in the etiology of Guillain–Barré is less clear. There have been reports of positive correlation between circulating immunoblasts and the activity of the disease process. Others have found elevated serum and CSF levels of IgA, IgG, and IgM that return to normal as the patient's condition improves. Still others have found circulating immune complexes. These antibody–antigen complexes could, in some way, alter the brain–nerve barrier thus facilitating antibody or cell-mediated demyelination.

The clinical picture supports an acute evolving process. Muscle weakness develops rapidly and is usually symmetrical beginning with the lower extremities before the upper. The trunk, chest, and neck muscles are next affected and later the cranial nerves. Another consistent finding is diminished deep tendon reflexes progressing to areflexia. This flaccid muscle paralysis has been known to progress so rapidly that death from respiratory failure occurred within a few days. Approximately 50 percent of these patients reach their lowest point of muscle paralysis–weakness in 2 weeks after the onset of the disease. Muscle atrophy is not observed because the progression is so rapid.

Patients may exhibit a variety of other muscular signs. The arms may be less affected and remain stronger than the legs. A facial diplegia occurs in over 50 percent of the patients whereas ocular gaze palsies are found in 10 percent. The cranial nerves most commonly affected are (in sequential order) facial, oculomotor and abducens, hypoglossal, trigeminal, and glossopharyngeal. Cranial nerve dysfunctions lead to difficulty in chewing, swallowing, coughing, and speaking.

Sensory changes are variable. Objective sensory losses are not common and usually restricted to the lower extremities. Pain does occur in over 30 percent of patients. Paresthesias are common. Vibration–sense loss is often greater than position–sense loss or touch–sensory loss. Upon palpating muscles, patients may complain of tenderness. Using skin dermatomes, the nurse can serially assess sensory level responses of the spinal nerves.

In severe cases, autonomic nervous system disruptions occur. Involvement of the sympathetic ganglionic chain or the vagus nerve are responsible for sinus tachycardia (less often bradycardia), facial flushing, hyperpyrexia, hypotensive episodes, anhidrosis more than diaphoresis, sphincter paralysis, and bronchiolar smooth muscle paralysis. Hypertensive episodes probably result from the increased sensitivity of denervated sympathetic receptors to circulating catecholamines.

In some patients extensor Babinski responses and/or papilledema have been reported. These central nervous system signs may occur because of the small amount of P2 protein found in CNS myelin or perhaps because the increased levels of protein in the CSF obstruct the arachnoid villi causing a communicating hydrocephalus. Although headache is rarely seen, a persistent headache should be reported. Nuchal rigidity is rare.

There is no specific diagnostic test for Guillain–Barré syndrome. The usual blood and urine studies are taken as for any acutely ill patient. The body temperature is usually normal unless a coexisting bacterial infection is present. Transient ECG changes in the T-wave are seen. The CSF is usually under normal pressure and is acellular in 90 percent of the cases. However, the CSF protein count is elevated and reaches its peak 4 to 6 weeks after the onset of the symptoms. The EMG and NCV studies are not commonly performed in the emergency department but will show characteristic changes. The pulmonary function studies indicate depressed ventilatory activity if the disease has ascended to the arms and chest muscles.

The physician is further faced with the problem of differentially diagnosing this polyneuropathy from others with similar symptoms. If tests are available they are done to rule out diphtheritic neuropathy, acute intermittent porphyria, botulism, poliomyelitis, heavy metal poisoning, polymyositis, tick bite paralysis, and multiple sclerosis. The mode of evolution, clinical manifestations, and select diagnostic studies help to make the appropriate decision.

In summary, Guillain–Barré syndrome is an acute disease characterized by an ascending flaccid paralysis with weaknesses of the intercostals, muscles of swallowing, and diffuse areflexia. The most important life-threatening complication is respiratory paralysis which may appear in the first 24 hours of onset. Additional complications include gastric dilatation, paralytic ileus, venous thrombosis, pulmonary embolism, and inappropriate secretion of ADH.

MANAGEMENT

I. Maintain and/or support ventilations
    A. Monitor respiratory rate, depth, pattern, and chest excursions q 30 to 60 minutes
    B. Perform spirometric testing at bedside: vital capacity and tidal volumes q 30 to 60 minutes
    C. Assist with drawing bloods for serial blood gas determinations
    D. Assess patient's ability to swallow secretions
    E. Suction oronasal pharynx prn, obtain stat chest x-ray
    F. Report any sudden increase in secretions, difficulty raising secretions, or inability to swallow secretions
    G. Encourage deep breathing and coughing; perform chest physiotherapy
    H. Be prepared to intubate the patient and provide mechanical ventilatory assistance
        1. attach a cuffed endotracheal tube to volume ventilator and oxygen
        2. monitor respiratory rate, airway pressure, position of airway tube, humidifier
        3. set and monitor tidal and minute volume. Minute ventilation equals tidal volume times respiratory rate
        4. offer meticulous care in suctioning and/or tube care
        5. take serial blood gas determinations to evaluate results of therapy
        6. periodically hyperinflate or "sigh" patient
II. Detect and/or treat other pulmonary complications
    A. Atelectasis
        1. keep patient npo if dysphagia or cough reflex is absent

    2. keep secretions moist via humidification

    3. suction frequently; chest physiotherapy; obtain chest x-rays

    4. adequately hydrate patient

  B. Pneumonia

    1. frequently auscultate lung fields; report areas of consolidation

    2. obtain chest x-rays; monitor temperature, pulse, respirations

    3. culture nose and throat and sputum

    4. administer antibiotics as prescribed

  C. Pulmonary emboli

    1. apply antiembolic stockings prophylactically

    2. observe calves for signs of inflammation or tenderness

    3. investigate any complaints of chest pain

    4. obtain chest x-ray and possibly lung scan

    5. be prepared to initiate anticoagulation therapy

III. Maintain adequate circulation to all body tissues

  A. Monitor bp, pulse, LOC q 3 to 6 minutes

  B. Start an IV line to administer fluids and drugs

  C. Obtain a stat ECG and initiate continuous cardiac monitoring. Observe for tachyarrhythmias and T-wave changes

  D. Be prepared to administer vasopressor drugs for hypotension or anticholinergic drugs for bradycardia

  E. Patient may require temporary pacing

  F. Record all I&O and responses to treatment; an indwelling urinary catheter may be needed

IV. Detect changes in the neuromuscular and vasomotor functioning

  A. Evaluate motor functioning q 30 to 60 minutes

    1. peripheral nerves

      a. check ability to extend and flex feet

      b. check ability to bend the knees

      c. check ability to raise and lower the legs, arms, and shoulders

      d. estimate hand grip strength and foot strength

    2. cranial nerves

      a. evaluate facial movements (ability to smile)—facial nerve

      b. test eye movements—oculomotor and abducent nerve

      c. test tongue movements—hypoglossal nerve

      d. estimate chewing capability—trigeminal nerve

      e. evaluate strength of neck and shoulder muscles—accessory nerve

  B. Evaluate sensory functioning q 30 to 60 minutes

    1. using dermatome charts, serially assess responses to touch in

      a. sacral dorsal root segments

      b. lumbar dorsal root segments

      c. thoracic dorsal root segments

      d. cervical dorsal root segments

  C. Observe patient for vasomotor instability

    1. keep accurate record of pulse, noting tachycardia or bradycardia

       2. take bp frequently, noting hypotension or hypertension

       3. note any facial flushing, extreme general warmth, fever

       4. note any diaphoresis or anhidrosis

       5. note excessive bronchial secretions

    D. Observe for signs of central nervous system involvement (rare)

       1. test pupillary responses; report any changes or papilledema

       2. report any complaints of headache

  V. Maintain fluid, electrolyte and nutritional balance

    A. Monitor serum electrolytes, BUN, and glucose serially

       1. report values out of the normal range

       2. on occasion, hypokalemia or hyponatremia has been observed

    B. Assess GI functioning

       1. a nasogastric tube is frequently passed and attached to low suctioning

       2. at a later time, patient may require tube feedings

    C. Plan to adequately hydrate patient

       1. approximately 2500 to 3000 ml/24 hours or more will be required

       2. monitor serum electrolytes; serum osmolarity

       3. observe for signs of fluid overload

    D. Obtain a baseline weight

    E. Observe for the syndrome of inappropriate ADH secretion (rare)

       1. record all urine output accurately; report decreases

       2. monitor serum sodium levels and urine specific gravity

       3. observe closely for pulmonary edema

 VI. Maximize remaining functions and prevent iatrogenic complications

    A. Combat the problems that could arise from immobility

       1. place feet up against a foot board

       2. turn frequently aned massage bony prominences

       3. keep sheets wrinkle free and skin dry

       4. perform passive ROM and stretching

       5. if muscle pain is present, keep bed linens off legs

    B. Meet the hygienic needs of the patient

       1. offer skin care as needed

       2. offer mouth care frequently

       3. protect the eyes from trauma

    C. Provide for emotional support for patient and relatives

       1. explain the importance and reasons for diagnostic tests

       2. interpret the rationale for emergency management activities

       3. allow patient and relatives to ask questions and verbalize their fears

       4. if patient cannot talk, establish some means of communication

       5. provide constant, vigilant attendance

    D. Continue monitoring and consider more definitive therapy

       1. admit patient to intensive care unit for observation and care

       2. refer patient to physician who will assume long-term management

       3. therapies that might be considered are long-term steroids and plasma-pheresis

RATIONALE

Because the etiology of Guillain–Barré syndrome is yet to be elucidated, management strategies in the emergency department focus upon correcting respiratory malfunctioning plus detecting and treating all life-threatening complications. If proper care is offered during this initial phase of the disease, over 95 percent of the patients can be restored to completely normal functioning. The speed of recovery varies but it can occur within a few weeks or months depending upon the extent of nerve damage.

The essence of emergency treatment is the recognition and management of respiratory insufficiency because it is the most life-threatening complication of this syndrome. Up to 24 percent of the patients with Guillain–Barré require artificial ventilatory support. Accurate assessment and management of respiratory depression has reduced the mortality rate of this illness significantly.

Serial spirometric testing is an excellent guide to assess respiratory–pulmonary status. The lungs can normally hold approximately 5 to 6 liters of air depending upon the age, sex, height, and health of the individual. The vital capacity (VC) is the volume of gas that can be expelled from the lungs by forceful effort after a maximal inspiration. The normal VC can be calculated:

Men: VC = 25 ml × height in cm (5′10″ = 70″ = 178 cm × 25 = 4450 ml VC)
Women: VC = 20 ml × height in cm (5′4″ = 64″ − 163 cm × 20 = 3260 ml VC)

The nurse looks for a trend in VC measurements. Frequently when the VC drops to 25 to 30 percent below the normal expected value, intubation or tracheostomy is performed.

The tidal volume (TV) is the volume of gas inspired and expired during a normal respiratory pattern. A general rule for estimating a patient's tidal volume is to multiply the patient's weight by three. Example:

TV = weight × 3 (170 lb × 3 = 510 ml);   average is 500 ml

The dead space must be subtracted from the tidal volume. It is that part of the tidal volume that does not participate in the pulmonary perfusion. It is approximately equal to the weight of the patient in pounds. For example, a 150 lb patient has a 150 ml dead space. Thus, if the average tidal volume is 500 ml, only 350 ml (500 − 150 = 350) reaches the alveolar level. Decreases in tidal volume plus subtraction for dead space indicate hypoventilation which can lead to hypoxia and carbon dioxide retention.

Hemodynamic monitoring of the patient with Guillain–Barré syndrome is another important aspect of emergency care. Dysrhythmias are not infrequent occurrences because of electrolyte, acid–base, or vasomotor abnormalities. Remember that during suctioning, arrhythmias commonly occur. An intravenous line provides an access route for emergency drugs as well as fluids. In the early stages, the patient may exhibit urinary retention, thus an indwelling catheter is inserted. However, some physicians prefer intermittent catheterization to reduce the possibilities of an ascending UTI. Intake and output, weights, and serial blood chemistries help determine responses to therapy and alert the staff to changes.

Frequent monitoring of neuromuscular functioning detects changes in the patient's condition. Very often the paralysis progresses even after admission to the intensive care unit. It usually peaks in 1 to 14 days. Because examiners differ in their interpretations of some of the neurological findings, it is preferred that the same nurse perform these tests to rule out examiner error.

During the patient's time in the emergency department efforts are also directed toward the prevention of complications related to immobility. The nurse guards against foot drop by keeping the feet up against a foot board. Attention is paid to turning, skin massage, clean and wrinkle free bed linens, and so forth to avoid the effects of positional trauma (decubitus ulcer). Passive ROM and gentle stretching keep the joints and muscles mobile. Hygienic needs are offered as the patient's condition warrants with special attention paid to oral and eye care.

This patient must marshall all his or her defense mechanisms to cope with this acute crisis situation. Explanations should be given in language understood by the patient and family. The nurse should be as truthful and supportive as possible and allow the patient to vent anger, resentment, and hostility. The patient may not be able to speak or contact the nurse because of the paralysis. In this situation, the nurse must remain with the patient constantly and establish some means of communication.

The patient will be admitted to the hospital for further study, observation, and care. The average hospital stay is 75 days. It is not common for the emergency department to initiate long-term therapeutic measures (e.g., steroid therapy, plasmapheresis). This is best left to the neurologist who assumes the continuing management of this patient.

6. Myasthenia Gravis

ASSESSMENT

I. Presenting clinical picture
   A. General behavior and mental state
      1. weakened, fatigued individual in respiratory distress
      2. most commonly gives a history of myasthenia gravis
      3. appears tired and somewhat undernourished
      4. may be irritable, restless, anxious
   B. Neuromuscular system alterations
      1. ocular muscles: ptosis of eyelids, impaired rotational eye movements (ocular palsies), diplopia, strabismus
      2. facial and throat muscle weakness
         a. difficulty smiling, "snarled" expression on smiling, possibly expressionless

  b. difficulty chewing or inability to chew

  c. difficulty in swallowing or unable to swallow

  d. choking and/or nasal regurgitation of secretions

  e. swallow and cough reflex absent

  f. jaws that tend to sag; difficulty holding head up

  g. nasal dysarthric speech, dysphonia or aphonia, may only be able to speak in whispered short sentences

 3. respiratory muscle weakness

  a. shallow, depressed respiratory excursions

  b. apparent dyspnea and distress

  c. air passages may be obstructed with secretions

  d. irregularity in respiratory rate, depth, pattern; apneic

 4. other muscle weakness

  a. trunk: may be unable to sit or stand for any length of time

  b. limbs: proximal muscle weakness; may be unable to lift arms or legs; weakness may or may not be symmetrical

  c. abdominal: weak, peristalsis may be decreased

  d. sphincters: loss of tone, relaxed

 5. muscle reflexes: deep tendon reflexes are preserved but fatigue upon repeated tapping

C. Respiratory system alterations (additional findings)

 1. collection of secretions in mouth, oropharynx, and bronchioles

 2. aspiration of secretions due to loss of reflexes

 3. auscultative findings: adventitious sounds, rales, areas of consolidation

 4. decreased vital capacity (below 1000 ml)

 5. inadequate oxygen and carbon dioxide exchange as evidenced by increased P_{CO_2} levels and decreased P_{O_2} levels in blood

 6. may exhibit signs of cyanosis

 7. chest x-ray may reveal atelectasis, pneumonia, thymic enlargement

 8. fluoroscopy may reveal minimal movement of diaphragm

D. Cardiovascular system alteration

 1. bp and pulse may be elevated, if hypoxia severe

 2. cardiac tachyarrhythmias on ECG; possibly anoxic ectopic rhythms; possibly cardiac arrest

E. Gastrointestinal and urinary systems alterations

 1. depressed bowel sounds possible; incontinence of stool

 2. incontinent of urine

F. Other systems alterations

 1. there may be evidence of thyroid hyperfunctioning; the thymus gland may be abnormal

 2. skeletal system may indicate evidence of rheumatoid arthritis

II. Possible precipitating and/or contributing causes

A. Physical stress: overtired, infection (especially pulmonary), trauma, surgery, pregnancy

B. Psychologic stress: wide variety of events

C. Progression and deterioration of disease. History of increasing large doses of medication without improvement in muscle strength. Patient becoming resistant to treatment.

D. Medication problems: underdosage (myasthenic crisis); overdosage (cholinergic crisis)

E. History of beginning steroids, antibiotics, or cardiovascular drugs

F. Coexisting diseases have become active

III. Symptoms suggestive of cholinergic rather than myasthenic crisis

A. In addition to the nicotinic effects on muscle power, these patients exhibit muscarinic symptoms as well

1. eyes: miosis, blurred vision, excessive lacrimation

2. gastrointestinal: nausea, vomiting, abdominal cramps, diarrhea, excessive salivation

3. cardiopulmonary: bradycardia, increased bronchial secretions

4. muscles: fasciculations of eyelids, face, neck, and legs

B. Negative response to Tensilon test

IV. Alterations in laboratory and other diagnostic tests

A. Bloods are drawn for CBC, electrolytes, BUN, glucose, thyroxine levels, and blood gases

B. Sputum, urine, and blood may be sent for culture if fever and/or infection is suspected.

C. Serum may be sent for ACh receptor antibodies (increased) and/or T3 and T4 antibodies, if thyroid problem suspected

D. EMG testing (usually deferred) pathognomic response pattern is one of decremental response to peripheral nerve stimulation followed by a plateau or an increment

E. Endrophonium chloride (Tensilon) test

1. this test is diagnostic for myasthenia in most cases and will differentiate between myasthenic and cholinergic crises

2. this test is not performed on an apneic patient

3. pulse and cardiac monitoring must accompany testing to detect arrhythmias; be prepared for intubation

4. the antidote, atropine 0.4 mg, must be ready to administer if untoward response results

5. placebo testing should also be carried out in the nonacute patient to rule out false positives of a psychogenic origin

6. test procedure: draw up 1 ml (10 mg) of edrophonium in a tuberculin syringe

inject 0.2 ml (2 mg) IV and leave needle in situ

a. observe for a cholinergic reaction: increased muscle weakness; increased salivation, sweating, lacrimation; epigastric distress; perioral, periocular, lingual fasciculations; miosis

b. if above response is seen, the test is discontinued and atropine is administered. The problem is cholinergic crisis

c. if no reaction occurs after 45 seconds, inject the remaining 0.8 ml of

Tensilon. Within 1 to 5 minutes observe for a positive response: marked improvement of striated muscle strength with minimal side effects and the return to pretesting muscle strength in 15 to 20 minutes. A positive response indicates the problem of myasthenia

F. If the Tensilon test is inconclusive, prepare to administer neostigmine (Prostigmine) 0.04 mg/kg body weight (0.5 mg) IM or IV. In 30 minutes, observe for signs of improvement. Atropine, 0.6 mg, usually given simultaneously

PATHOPHYSIOLOGY

The most serious manifestation of myasthenia gravis is severe depression of breathing resulting from progressive paralysis of the diaphragm and intercostal muscles plus airway obstruction due to paralysis of laryngeal and pharyngeal muscles. To understand these events it is necessary to review basic events in neuromuscular transmission.

The anatomy of a neuron-to-muscle synapse is quite remarkable. The peripheral nerve neuron has an inner sheath, neurolemma, and an outer sheath, endoneural sheath. The outer sheath extends beyond the terminal nerve ending and joins with the muscle sheath forming a tentlike structure over this neuromuscular junction.

The terminal cytoplasmic portions of the peripheral neuron axons branch out into many footlike structures called end plates. The end plates invaginate into the folds of the muscle fiber but lie entirely apart from it. The tips of the nerve end plates appear slightly swollen. These structures are called knobs and on close examination, each knob contains many vesicles and mitochondria. The vesicles store acetylcholine (ACh). The membrane around the neuronal knobs is called the presynaptic membrane.

Between the neuronal end plates and the muscle is a space called the synaptic cleft. The synaptic cleft contains gelatinous ground substance through which extracellular fluid diffuses.

The muscle membrane, called the postsynaptic membrane, is structured into many elaborate folds of sarcolemma. This greatly increases the surface area for the action of the excitatory neurotransmitter, ACh. The nicotinic ACh receptors are located on the crests of these folds which lie just beneath the nerve terminals. The receptor substance is a glycoprotein and each receptor molecule appears to have one or more binding sites for ACh. In addition, the enzyme cholinesterase is present along the folds of the muscle sarcolemma in fairly high concentrations.

When a nerve impulse reaches its axon's terminal knob a series of events occur which stimulate muscle contraction. At specialized release sites, the neuronal vesicles release quanta, or packages, of ACh. Some of the ACh crosses the synaptic space and attaches to the receptor molecules. When this connection occurs a transient increase in muscle cell permeability occurs. It appears that ACh opens ionic gates allowing the influx of sodium ions and an efflux of potassium ions. This creates a change in the electrical field of the cell and an action potential, which is called depolarization. The amplitude of the end plate depolarization depends upon the number of ACh molecules that interact with receptor molecules. When sufficient muscle fibers have been stimulated and their threshold reached, the entire muscle contracts. This is called cholinergic transmission. Normally, in a very few millionths of a second, sodium is actively removed from the cell and potassium returned to the cell by the action of the sodium–potassium pump. The cell returns to its normal resting potential or is repolarized.

It has been recognized that certain amounts of ACh are released spontaneously into the synaptic cleft which leads to a local end plate depolarization of small amplitude. This is termed miniature end plate potential (MEPP) and does not result in muscle depolarization. Further research evidence of excess ACh in the synaptic cleft suggests that only a small proportion of the ACh molecules released interact with receptor molecules and that only a small number of receptors are activated at one time. This excess provides us with a "safety margin" of neuromuscular transmission. Any change in this margin, especially a reduction, may result in failure of neuromuscular transmission.

In myasthenia gravis a number of factors operate to produce the clinical picture. There appears to be a reduction in the amplitude of MEPP at the neuromuscular junction which might be due to a decrease in ACh per quantum or a problem with the ACh receptor. It is well documented that many myasthenics have a reduction in the number of their ACh receptors per neuromuscular junction. In the past, it was hypothesized that the number of ACh molecules released was decreased. However, this hypothesis has now been discarded in favor of a receptor site problem(s).

There is much evidence that myasthenic patients have antibodies to their ACh receptors which may block attachment of ACh or in some manner destroy the receptor molecule. These antibodies have been found in close to 90 percent of myasthenics which gives much credence to the humoral immune theory of causality. It must be noted, however, that antibody titers do not always correlate with the clinical picture. There is further evidence that myasthenic immunoglobulins, especially IgG antibody, attaches to the area near the receptor and may be responsible for blocking attachment of ACh or degrading ACh in some manner. The appearance of complement, C-1 and C-3, seems to enhance this effect in myasthenics. The precise basis for the humoral theory is still unknown but it is postulated that a viral invasion of the thymus could injure the ACh nicotinic receptors located in this gland which would induce antibody formation to other ACh receptors. It must be noted, that approximately 75 percent of all myasthenics have thymic abnormalities (e.g., hyperplasia, thymoma).

There is also some evidence that the disease may be a cellular mediated immune process. In animals, peripheral blood lymphocytes increase their cell division in the presence of ACh receptor protein but this is not always evident in humans. Stimulation of lymphocytes in response to a specific antigen dictates that these lymphocytes have previously been sensitized to that antigen. It is known that the percentage of T-lymphocytes is reduced in myasthenics whereas the percentage of B-lymphocytes is increased. Mixed leukocyte cultures in some myasthenics show abnormal leukocyte autoreactivity which further suggests some change in antigenic makeup.

The onset of myasthenia may begin at any age. Peak onset occurs between 20 and 30 years. Women are affected two or three times as often as men, if the disease begins under 40 years of age. In later life, no sex difference is seen. However, the majority of patients who have thymomas are in the older age group and in these cases, more men than women have thymomas.

The course of the illness varies. Rapid spread is not universal. Unexplainable remissions of 1 to 2 months do occur. The danger of death is greatest during the first year after onset and then between the fourth and seventh year of the disease. Myasthenia occurs relatively frequently in patients with other immune disorders (e.g., thyrotoxicosis, rheumatoid arthritis, lupus erythematosus, and polymyositis). Familial occurrence is known but rare. A transitory form of myasthenia has been described in babies born to myasthenic mothers.

Myasthenic patients exhibit fluctuating weakness of certain voluntary muscles. Those innervated by the bulbar nuclei of the brainstem are the most common (e.g., ocular, masticatory, facial, tongue, swallowing). Although 50 percent of the patients initially present with ocular symptoms, very few remain at this stage. A majority display a progression of symptoms over the initial 12 to 18 months of the disease.

The clinical symptoms reflect the muscles affected. Lack of innervation from cranial nerves III, IV, and VI, to the superior levator palpebrae muscles results in ptosis of the eyelids and ocular movement palsies with possible intermittent diplopia and strabismus. The second most common muscle groups that become involved are those muscles innervated by cranial nerves V, VII, IX, X, XI, and XII which affect muscles of the face, chewing, deglutition, and vocalization. The face commonly appears immobile and expressionless or when the patient attempts to smile, a type of nasal snarl results. The patients have fluctuating difficulty in chewing and swallowing their food. Many resort to changes in consistency of foods to sustain nutritional intake. The typical speech is of a high pitched nasal quality which fades with prolonged use almost terminating in a whisper. The flexors and extensors of the neck may be involved resulting in a drooping jaw and inability to hold up the head. Involvement of the shoulder girdle muscles results in fatigue upon combing the hair or performing a facial shave. When the erector spinae muscles of the trunk are involved, the patient has difficulty standing or sitting for any length of time. In advanced cases, all muscles are weakened which would include the diaphragm, abdominals, intercostals, and sphincter muscles to name a few.

Other neurologic functions are usually preserved. Tendon reflexes do not change substantially. Pupillary responses to light and accommodation are normal. In fact, normal pupillary responses found in conjunction with weakness of the extraocular muscles is virtually diagnostic of myasthenia. Sensory losses are minimal. Smooth and cardiac muscle are not generally affected.

The onset of myasthenia may be abrupt or insidious. It has been found that many drugs worsen the disease, unmask an unsuspected case or produce a myasthenic-like syndrome. Cardiovascular drugs (e.g., quinidine, procainamide, propranolol) and quinine, found in tonic water, tend to enhance neuromuscular blockade. Certain antibiotics (e.g., neomycin, kanamycin, cholistin, streptomycin, polymyxin B, and some tetracyclines) impair neurotransmitter release. Tranquilizers and antidepressants (e.g., lithium) and d-penicillamine have also led to muscle weakness. A careful history should detect if the patient has taken any of these medications.

A rapid onset and/or worsening of the condition has been associated with physical and/or psychologic stressors in the patient's life. The symptoms may worsen during pregnancy or the first few weeks postdelivery. The symptoms may appear during recovery from some surgical procedure. Respiratory infections have frequently been a triggering event as have emotional upsets from any number of situations.

Myasthenic crisis is an emergency situation which is usually due to undermedication and/or an abrupt deterioration of the condition. The hallmark is extensive muscle weakness, especially of the respiratory muscles. Respiratory distress is caused by an increase in secretions which pool in the oropharynx, inability to swallow these secretions, aspiration of the secretions because the cough reflex is absent and respiratory muscle weakness which limits lung expansion. All of these problems result in hypoxia which in turn leads to a compensatory tachycardia, increase in blood pressure, extreme restlessness, cyanosis, and possible cardiac arrest. The patient is usually unable to speak. He or she experiences excessive lacrimation and profuse diaphoresis. Incontinence of urine and stool may accompany the crisis. These symptoms may be gradual or abrupt in onset. Atelectasis and pneumonia only compound the insult to the respiratory system.

Respiratory failure could result from an overdose of the medications used to treat myasthenia. Anticholinesterase drugs prolong ACh activity at the neuromuscular junction but can accumulate in the body to the point of serious overdosage because the action of these drugs is indirect and reversible effects are seen with higher doses. This leads to increased muscle weakness and muscle fasciculations from blockage of nicotinic receptors plus prominent muscarinic side effects (e.g., increased salivation and lacrimation, urinary incontinence, diarrhea, bronchial constriction, increased bronchial secretions, nausea, vomiting, diaphoresis, bradycardia, hypotension, miosis, and occasionally unequal pupils).

In summary, the pathophysiologic changes in myasthenia gravis are attributed to a decrease in the number and/or functioning of ACh receptors at the neuromuscular junction. The problem is most likely an immune disorder although precise mechanisms have yet to be determined. Respiratory distress is the most common reason for seeking emergency care. The house staff may or may not elect to distinguish the origin of the crisis (myasthenic or cholinergic) but in either case, respiratory support is a top priority to avoid fatality.

MANAGEMENT

    I. Recognize and manage respiratory failure
       A. Establish a patent airway
          1. position patient on side with head elevated
          2. suction oronasopharynx prn; note increases in secretions
          3. encourage deep breathing and coughing; chart effectiveness

4. perform chest physiotherapy frequently
5. chart the depth, rate, and pattern of respirations q 10 to 15 minutes
6. send sputum specimen to laboratory for culture and sensitivity
   B. Auscultate lungs frequently: report any rales, adventitious sounds, areas of consolidation
   C. Draw serial blood gases and obtain chest x-rays
   Report rising levels of PCO_2 and decreasing levels of PO_2
   D. Assess the vital capacity q 1 to 2 hours; report levels below 1000 ml
   E. Be prepared to insert a cuffed endotracheal tube and to assist ventilations mechanically. Tracheostomy may be deferred until later
   F. Administer oxygen as prescribed. Perform all activities in an aseptic manner to avoid the possibility of iatrogenic infection
II. Detect and correct possible fluid, electrolyte, and acid–base imbalances
   A. Baseline and serial blood specimens are drawn for CBC, BUN, electrolytes, glucose, and blood gases
   B. Monitor temperature, pulse, respirations and bp q 15 to 30 minutes
   C. Obtain a stat ECG and begin cardiac monitoring
   D. Initiate an IV line and administer fluids as prescribed
   E. Keep accurate records of I & O; an indwelling urinary catheter may be required
III. Serially assess the neuromuscular status
   A. Chart neurologic vital signs q 15 to 30 minutes
   B. Monitor muscle strength q 15 to 30 minutes (one or more of these)
      1. score swallowing ability. Patient is asked to identify the type of substance or food thought possible to swallow
         0 = nothing
         1 = saliva
         2 = liquids
         3 = pureed foods
         4 = soft foods
         6 = regular foods
      2. Score the extent of ocular ptosis with patient looking straight ahead
         1 = unable to open eyes, none of iris is visible
         2 = lids open, some of lowermost iris is visible
         3 = lower half of pupil visible
         4 = all of pupil visible, none of uppermost iris visible
         5 = all of pupil visible, some of uppermost iris visible
      3. Eye lid strength: note the length of time patient can maintain an upward gaze before downward drift of eyelids occurs
      4. Lips: note length of time patient can hold a tongue blade between teeth against resistance
      5. Speech: note length of time patient can speak without dysphonia
      6. Legs: note length of time patient can cross and uncross the legs
IV. Maintain nutritional balance
   A. Patients without a swallow or gag reflex are npo

B. A nasogastric tube is frequently passed. This route is used to meet nutritional needs and to give medications

C. Monitor I & O; weight should be recorded

V. Rest the motor end plate from the effects of exogenous drugs

    A. Complete withdrawal of all medications including cholinesterase inhibitors for 24 to 72 hours

    B. Elective intubation or tracheostomy with mechanically assisted ventilations and oxygen for 3 to 10 days

    C. Close monitoring of cardiopulmonary and neurologic status

    D. Offer nutritional support

    E. Protect patient from iatrogenically induced infection

    F. Search for a contributing or precipitating factor(s)

VI. Restore muscle strength (this may be deferred until much later)

    A. Administer cholinesterase inhibitor drugs as prescribed

        1. Neostigmine (Prostigmine) 0.5 to 1.5 mg IM or subcutaneously q 2 to 3 hours along with atropine 0.6 to 0.4 mg

        2. Pyridostigmine (Mestinon) 2 mg IM or IV or 60 mg po q 2 to 3 hours. This drug has a longer duration of action and lower incidence of GI side effects

    B. Note and record muscle strength before, during, and after administration of drug

    C. Assess urinary output

VII. Counteract the effects of excess cholinesterase inhibitors

    A. Withhold all medications. Maintain on artificial ventilatory support

    B. Administer atropine 1.0 mg IV and repeat as prescribed

    C. Closely monitor secretion viscosity; perform chest physiotherapy and auscultate lung fields

VIII. Offer supportive nursing care

    A. Avoid the complications of muscle disuse and weakness

        1. place a sheepskin or air mattress beneath patient

        2. reposition and give skin care to pressure areas q 2 to 3 hours

        3. perform ROM to all joints qid

        4. provide oral and nasal hygiene prn

        5. apply elastic wraps to lower extremities

    B. Establish a means of communication

        1. if strong enough, use paper and pencil or magic slate

        2. if lips can move, try to read them

        3. decide with patient upon a series of signals

        4. remain in constant attendance, especially if there is insufficient strength to use call bell

    C. Decrease fear and apprehension

        1. explain all activities in a calm manner

        2. recognize that although the patient is unable to respond or communicate, he or she can see and hear all that is occurring

        3. provide for constant attendance by nursing staff

RATIONALE

Natural worsening of the disease, changes in response to medication, infection, emotional stress, and/or other coexisting problems could lead to an acute life-threatening situation in the myasthenic patient. Even though many diagnosed individuals carry Prostigmine and use it in the event of respiratory distress, the patient should be under close medical supervision. Likewise, in the undiagnosed patient, the major function of the emergency department is to treat the respiratory insufficiency.

All efforts are directed at recognizing and managing respiratory failure. A functional airway and assisted mechanical ventilatory support are vital to prevent cardiopulmonary collapse and death. The nurse should understand that this patient will not exhibit the classical picture of respiratory distress (e.g., suprasternal retraction, flaring of the nares) because these muscles are also weakened. Important signs of respiratory insufficiency are choking, dysphagia, dysphonia, restlessness, tachycardia, headache, and an increase in blood pressure. Monitoring of the tidal volume, vital capacity, and blood gases are good indices of ventilatory success or failure. If respiratory effort or swallowing ability deteriorate, elective endotracheal intubation is performed before emergency intubation becomes necessary. Assisted mechanical ventilations and oxygen administration will support the patient through this crisis.

Once the airway is secured further diagnostic and monitoring activities are carried out. The history and physical examination are supplemented by laboratory and radiologic investigation in the same manner as is done for any acutely ill patient. Complete blood counts, serum chemistries, blood gases, chest x-ray, ECG, and other tests are all procedures that help to evaluate the total status of this patient.

Whereas it is uncommon for myasthenics to have fluid, electrolyte, and acid–base problems, these could occur because of other existing conditions. Early detection and correction of these problems makes the diagnostic and treatment picture clearer. Proper ventilation and oxygenation corrects the possible respiratory acidosis that the myasthenic may have.

Because infection could trigger a myasthenic crisis, a search is made for the source. Temperature is monitored and specimens of sputum and urine are cultured. An intravenous line is inserted to provide a route for drug and food administration. Accurate intake and output records are required and an indwelling urinary catheter may facilitate output monitoring during the acute stage.

Throughout both the assessment and management phase of this condition, the nurse makes frequent neuromuscular status evaluations. Assessment of swallowing ability is judged subjectively by scoring what the patient believes he or she can swallow. This is probably a safer way to assess swallowing. Because the cough and swallow reflex is weak or missing, offering liquids to this patient might result in aspiration. The degree of eyelid ptosis can also be scored by inspection. Muscle strength is frequently evaluated and can be a fairly accurate indication, if peformed by the same evaluator and not repeated so often that fatigue is reached. Strength of the eyelids, lips, legs, and muscles if the larynx (speech) can be tested as described.

In some emergency departments, the physician will wish to identify the type of crisis the patient is experiencing. Differentiating myasthenic crisis from cholinergic crisis can be done via the Tensilon (endrophonium) test. Intravenous injection of 2 to 5 mg of this drug produces temporary muscle improvement, if the crisis is myasthenic in origin and no improvement, possibly worsening, if cholinergic crisis is the problem. When this test is performed atropine, 1.0 mg, must be ready to be administered in the event that the symptoms worsen. The decision to treat the muscle weakness is a decision that may be deferred until the patient is in an intensive care unit.

It has been well documented that complete withdrawal of all medications for a period of time, as long as the patient is intubated, is quite beneficial. The rationale is to rest the motor end plate from the effects of exogenous drugs. In the past, curare has been used to induce rest, but this is not common today. Some investigators believe that increasing amounts of cholinesterase inhibitors produce ACh resistance or insensitivity and the possibility of a cholinergic hyperpolarization block of the neuromuscular junction. A careful search is made for the possible etiology of this change in response to anticholinergic medication. It has also been reported that some patients treated in this manner, upon recovery have an unexplained remission of the disease.

On the other hand, restoration of muscle strength may be started, if the physician has clearly established that a lack of cholinesterase inhibitor drugs is the basis of the respiratory difficulties. Rapid acting neostigmine may be prescribed. Neostigmine methylsulfate (Prostigmine) intravenously or intramuscularly produces an increase in muscle strength in 15 to 30 minutes reaching its maximum effect in 1 to 2 hours. Because its effects are gone in 3 to 4 hours, the drug may be repeated.

Anticholinesterase drugs are capable of increasing the amount and accumulation of ACh at the neuromuscular synapse because ACh is not immediately hydrolyzed by cholinesterase. Their effect is limited to the cholinergic nerves. However, the receptors for these drugs, as well as ACh, differ. The nicotinic type of receptor, so named because an alkaloid of nicotine mimics the effects of ACh, are found at the skeletal neuromuscular junction and at the synapses of the autonomic ganglia. These receptors are less sensitive to blockade or inhibition by atropine. The muscarinic receptors are found at the synapses of the postganglionic neurons with the effector organ (e.g., sweat glands, lacrimal glands, salivary glands, stomach, intestines, bronchioles). They are called muscarinic because ingestion of a certain mushroom mimics the effects of ACh on these receptors. If these receptors are stimulated, abdominal cramping, excessive salivation and tearing, sweating, diarrhea, and so on occur. These disagreeable muscarinic side effects are controlled by atropine.

Atropine competitively antagonizes ACh at the postsynaptic muscarinic receptor sites. However, it will lead to drying of the oral and bronchial secretions. If these secretions thicken to the point of difficulty in their removal, atelectasis from a mucus plug in the bronchi could result. Vigorous chest physiotherapy, hydration, deep breathing, and coughing are all techniques used to keep the respiratory tract clear.

Throughout the patient's stay in the emergency department supportive nursing care is provided. Progressive weakness and muscle flaccidity severely limit the patient's ability to perform even the slightest task. The nurse takes all measures to avoid the complications of muscle paralysis and bed rest. The nurse must keep in mind that increased anxiety inhibits recovery and thus, institute measures to relieve fear and anxiety.

In most situations, the patient is admitted to hospital once respiratory insufficiency is controlled and a nasogastric tube inserted. A continued search is made for contributing factors by a neurologist. Steroid therapy, plasmapheresis, and thymectomy considerations are best left to the physician who assumes continuing responsibility for this patient.

7. Neurovascular Injuries (Compartmental Syndrome)

ASSESSMENT

I. Presenting clinical picture
   A. Patient with multiple trauma and/or contusions
   B. Fractures of the elbow, wrist, knee, leg, spine
   C. Patients who have lain in one position for a long period of time (e.g., trapped under rubble, overdose victims, ethanol abuser)
   D. Patients who complain of severe pain on passive motion of fingers and toes. Pain appears out of proportion to the injury
   E. Patients who exhibit paresis associated with other injuries and then later signs of puffiness, pallor, and pulselessness of the extremity involved

II. Precipitating and/or contributing causes
   A. Application of excessive traction on a limb
   B. Tight dressings, localized external pressure
   C. Fractures and dislocation
   D. Increased pressure from exercise, bleeding (see Table 5)

III. Alterations in neuromuscular functioning
   A. Depends upon nerves, muscles, and vessels involved (see Table 5)
   B. Assess for neurologic impairment. Motor and/or sensory losses will be found
   C. Common nerves to test (sensation to light touch or two point discrimination is the preferred method)
      1. radial–motor: touch each finger to thumb
         sensory: test web space between thumb and first finger elevation of third finger against resistance with elbow extended causes characteristic point
      2. median–motor: touch fourth finger to thumb
         sensory: test distal surface of index finger
                   pain, tingling, numbness in first three digits suggests carpal tunnel syndrome

3. ulnar–motor: abduction of fingers
        sensory: test distal end of little finger
                     light pressure on cubital tunnel reproduces pain, if nerve trapped near elbow. Burning sensation in fourth and fifth digits, if trapped at the wrist
4. peroneal–motor: dorsiflex ankle and extend toes
         sensory: test web space between first and second toes
                     usually a history of ankle or foot injury
5. tibial–motor: plantar flexion of ankle and flexion of toes
       sensory: medial and lateral surfaces of sole of foot
                     burning pain in toes and foot suggests tarsal tunnel syndrome

IV. Alterations in vasomotor functioning
    A. Depends upon the amount of blood vessel damage and/or compression of structures
    B. Assess for the following being sure to compare limbs
        1. color changes: pink, red, bluish-red, blue, pale
        2. temperature changes; area is cool or hot to touch
        3. pulse changes: charted as normal, diminished or absent—take all pulses in limb affected. Upper limb: axillary, brachial, ulnar and radial. Lower limb: femoral, popliteal, posterior tibialis, dorsal pedis. Portable Doppler flowmeter is helpful in determining pulses
        4. changes in capillary filling: test for blanching of nails, finger pads or toe pads
        5. changes in size: note any swelling, puffiness, edema or, tenseness of compartments

V. Assess for signs of compartmental involvement
    A. Upper extremity compartments
        1. volar compartment—symptoms: weakness of fingers and wrist flexion. Pain on finger and wrist extension. Hypesthesia of volar aspects of fingers. Tenseness of volar forearm fascia. Pulses and capillary filling may be intact
    B. Lower extremity compartments
        1. anterior compartment—symptoms: weakness of toe extension and foot dorsiflexion. Pain on passive toe flexion and plantar flexion of foot. Hypesthesia in dorsal first web space. Tenseness of anterior compartmental fascia. Pulses and capillary filling may be intact
        2. deep posterior compartment—symptoms: weakness of toe flexion and foot inversion. Pain on passive toe extension and foot eversion. Hypesthesia of plantar aspects of foot and toe. Tenseness of deep posterior compartmental fascia (between tibia and Achilles tendon). Pulses and capillary filling may be intact

VI. Detect the extent of the injury and existing of concomitant problems
    A. Collect bloods for: RBC, Hgb, Hct, WBC and differential; electrolytes, glucose, BUN, creatine, creatine phosphokinase
    B. X-ray limb involved; possibly arteriography

TABLE 5. MAJOR PERIPHERAL NERVE ENTRAPMENT SYNDROMES: AN OVERVIEW

Nerve	Motor	Sensory	Causes of Injury	Clinical Manifestations
Radial	Muscle extension of forearm, hand, phalanges, and little finger Abduction of thumb	Sensation to the dorsal aspect of the arm, forearm, and dorsal aspect radial half of hand Isolated area is a small patch of skin between thumb and index finger (thenar space)	Cervical cord injuries Brachial plexus injuries Peripheral branches injured by shoulder dislocations, fractures of humerus, fractures of neck of radius, pressure from crutches, pressure from sleeping for long period of time Violent blows to the area	Motor signs: extensor paralysis of the thumb, proximal phalanges, wrist, and elbow Pronation of hand with wrist and fingers flexed "wrist drop" Adduction of thumb. Unable to grasp an object or adequately make a fist Triceps and radial reflex absent. Sensory: loss is slight; most marked on dorsal radial surface of hand. Pain is rare Vasomotor: findings absent or very slight
Median	Most of the flexor pronator muscles of forearm Most all of the deep and superficial volar muscles Radial flexion of hand. Flexion of middle phalanx of all fingers but thumb Abduction of thumb metacarpal. Opposition of thumb	Supplies skin of palmar aspect of thumb and the lateral two and one half fingers plus distal ends of these fingers	Cervical cord injuries Brachial plexus injuries Lacerations of arm, forearm, wrist, or hand (e.g., auto accident, stab wound, bullet wound, suicide attempt) Prolonged compression (e.g., sleep, anesthesia) Dislocation of ulna Fracture of elbow and lower radius	Motor signs: paralysis of the flexor–pronator and thenar muscles. Patient flexes forearm but holds elbow outward Wrist: weak flexion and abduction Hand: inclined towards ulnar side Thumb: unable to flex or oppose Grip: weak, especially thumb and index finger Sensory: variable loss of sensation. Most constantly seen over distal phalanges of first two fingers. Pain is a common finding Vasomotor: skin of palms frequently dry, cold, discolored, chapped, and keratotic

161

Nerve				
Ulnar	Ulnar flexion of hand. Flexion of terminal phalanx of ring and little finger. Opposition and flexion of little finger	Supplies skin of little finger and medial half of hand and ring finger	Cervical cord lesions. Brachial plexus injuries. Peripheral injuries: fractures and dislocations of the head of the humerus and at the elbow. Direct trauma: lacerating wounds (e.g., stab wounds, auto accidents). Pressure injuries: sleeping for long periods of time	Motor signs: "claw hand" wherein patient is unable to flex proximal or distal phalanges of fourth or fifth digit and first phalanges remains hyperextended. Unable to extend second and distal phalanges. Unable to adduct or abduct fingers or to oppose all fingers to make a cone. Unable to adduct thumb. Wrist flexion is weak. Sensory signs: loss of sensation on ulnar side of hand and especially little finger. Pain is uncommon. Vasomotor signs: skin of little finger is cold, dry, at times discolored. Nail may be deformed
Sciatic	Supplies the hamstring muscles. Flexion of leg. Assists in extension of thigh	Supplies the outer aspect of the leg and foot	Herniation of lumbar disc. Dislocation of hip. Pelvic fractures. Stab or gunshot wounds in the area	Motor signs: hamstring muscle paralysis thus patient is unable to flex leg and there is paralysis of leg and foot muscles. Loss of Achilles and plantar reflexes. Sensory signs: loss of sensation outer side of leg and entire foot excepting instep and internal malleolus. Pain is common. Vasomotor signs: edema of leg and foot is common. Skin is dry, discolored. Plantar hyperkeratosis

(continued)

TABLE 5. (Continued)

Nerve	Motor	Sensory	Causes of Injury	Clinical Manifestations
Peroneal	Dorsiflexion of foot Suppination of foot Extension of toes	Supplies the skin at the upper outer portion of the fibula just below the knee, lateral aspects of the leg and lower front of the leg Branches supply the dorsum of the foot, part of the big toe and ankle. First and second toe web space	Sacral plexus and sciatic nerve lesions Peripheral injuries: direct trauma to area near neck of the fibula Fractures of the leg Compression injuries: (e.g., prolonged kneeling, sitting with crossed knees, compression of legs when in a lying position)	Motor signs: paralysis of extensor–abductor foot muscles. Inability to dorsiflex foot, "foot drop." Inability to abduct or evert foot or to stand on affected heel (steppage gait) Sensory signs: Sensation lost over dorsum of foot and outer side of leg. Pain is rare Vasomotor signs: not marked
Tibial	Plantar flexion of foot Flexion of toes Spreading and closing of toes	Supplies the skin on the dorsolateral portion of the leg and lateral side of the foot Also the plantar surface and ungual phalanges of the toes	Sacral plexus and sciatic nerve lesions Peripheral injuries: in, near or below the popliteal space (e.g., gun shot wounds, stab wounds, auto accidents) Fractures of the leg	Motor signs: unable to plantarflex, adduct, or invert the foot. Unable to flex, abduct (separate) or adduct the toes. Unable to stand on tiptoes. Walking is fatiguing, painful and difficult. The ankle jerk is absent Sensory signs: sensation is lost on the sole of the foot (except inner border), lateral surface of heel, and plantar surface of toes. Plus ungual phalanges. Pain is usually severe and common Vasomotor findings: edema, discoloration, cold are common findings

C. Urine for routine analysis and myoglobin
D. Measure tissue pressure: infusion or Wick techniques (if available)
E. Direct nerve stimulation to test neural functioning

PATHOPHYSIOLOGY

Exterior to the vertebral column, the motor and sensory fibers of a spinal nerve are joined by autonomic fibers. Together these three fibers constitute a peripheral nerve. The distribution of these nerves is characterized by extensive overlapping. As these nerves travel to supply the limbs, they are rearranged into a plexus. The spinal nerve lose their identity once they exit the plexus and emerge as peripheral nerves. The most important peripheral nerves are the median, the radial, the ulnar for the upper limbs, and the sciatic with its peroneal and tibial branches in the lower extremity.

Interruption of a peripheral nerve is followed by motor, sensory, and trophic changes. Motor losses are usually manifested by weakness and/or paralysis. Sensory deficits may be subjective (e.g., pain, numbness), which usually indicates an irritated nerve, or objective, as manifested by anesthesia, upon testing a nerve segment. The trophic changes are related to impaired nutritional and metabolic activities which are partially under neurogenic vasomotor control.

Entrapment neuropathies are most commonly due to mechanical compression of a nerve trunk within a fixed anatomic space. These neuropathies result from acute or chronic trauma. Varying degrees of inflammation, edema, and vasculitis are associated with these injuries which result in ischemia of the nerve and the surrounding tissues. Nerve cells are very susceptible to ischemia and hypoxia. Within 15 to 30 minutes of ischemia, sensory and motor deficits can be detected. Muscle tissue can survive somewhat longer, up to 6 hours, in an hypoxic state, but after this time muscle cells die and acute rhabdomyolysis can occur as well as gangrene.

Compartmental syndrome occurs less frequently than entrapment syndrome but it can result in more serious consequence. Tissues in a compartment (e.g., nerves, blood vessels, muscles) are enveloped by the epimysium, connective tissue which surrounds the muscle, and fascia, the fibrous sheath between muscles. The epimysium and fascia limit the distensibility of the compartment. Compartments are found in the forearm, hands, buttocks, legs, and feet.

The volume in a compartment can rise from a number of sources. A major vessel may be injured resulting in bleeding into the compartment. Exercise, trauma, intraarterial drugs, and burns could cause a postischemic swelling which is the result of increased capillary permeability. Increased capillary pressure and swelling can arise from excessive exercise or venous obstruction. Distraction of bone fragments by traction, snake bites, and infiltrated infusions could also increase compartmental contents and thus increase the pressure within that compartment.

Compartmental syndrome has also occurred when its normal size has been compressed in such a manner that circulation is compromised. Examples leading to this event would be externally applied pressure as occurs in the application of air splints, MAST trousers, compression dressings, arterial tourniquets, casts, and the person who lies on a limb for a prolonged period of time.

Increased compartment pressure leads to a severely decreased capillary perfusion to that compartment, and edema quickly follows. Edema in this limited space increases the pressure further and results in future ischemia of the tissue within the compartment. Progressive muscle and nerve death follows. Persistent hypesthesia, motor weakness, infection, myoglobinuria, contractures, amputation, and possibly death can result from insults to large body compartments.

The physical findings suggest the syndrome, but a high index of suspicion is needed to detect the problem. Time is of the essence if complications are to be avoided. The pain the patient experiences seems out of proportion to the insult. This is significant and should be reported to the physician immediately, especially when analgesia does not control the pain. Whereas there are experimental monitoring devices to measure compartment pressure, the motor and sensory deficits continue to be the best guide to detecting the problem. It must be remembered that the pulse is not always diminished or lost in compartment syndrome because the pressure in the compartment rarely rises high enough to occlude an artery. Thus, peripheral pulses are palpable and capillary filling is present which could give the examiner a false feeling of security.

MANAGEMENT

I. Identify the patients at risk for developing these problems
  A. Patients who have had extremity trauma and complain of pain, and exhibit increasing paresis, puffiness, pallor, and possibly pulselessness of that limb
  B. Patients who have air splints, antishock trousers, vascular clamps, or tourniquets in place on arrival to the emergency room
  C. Patients who have experienced prolonged compression on a limb from lying in one position for a prolonged period of time (e.g., drug overdose victims, inebriated victims)
II. Detect the signs of neuromuscular–vascular compromise
  A. Reevaluate motor, sensory, and vascular status q 30 minutes
  B. Document findings on a flow sheet. Report trends in findings
  C. Perform sensory testing using two-point discrimination and light touch rather than pinprick
  D. Monitor muscle strength and report it using the acceptable grading system:
    Grade 5 (Normal)—Normal power present, muscles can move through full range of motion against full resistance
    Grade 4 (Good)—The muscles can move the joint through a full range of motion against gravity and against some resistance but cannot overcome normal resistance
    Grade 3 (Fair)—The muscle can move the joint through a full range of motion only against gravity
    Grade 2 (Poor)—The muscle can move the joint through a full range of motion only when gravity is eliminated

Grade 1 (Trace)—Contraction of the muscle is felt, but no motion of the joint is produced

Grade 0 (Zero)—Complete paralysis is present with no visible or palpable contractions

E. Palpate compartments for tenderness, tautness, and warmth

F. Assist with measuring compartment pressure, if devices are available

G. If uncertain of pulses, secure a portable Doppler instrument to validate findings

H. Obtain x-rays of involved area

III. Reduce compartmental pressure

A. Remove all external devices causing pressure

B. Elevate extremity above the heart, if syndrome has not begun

C. Keep limb at heart level once syndrome is suspected

D. Obtain a surgical consultation for possible decompression of the compartment. This must be performed within 6 hours of the onset of symptoms to insure positive results

E. Prepare the patient for a fasciotomy

IV. Reduce nerve entrapment

A. Administer diuretics as prescribed to reduce edema

B. Administer steroids as prescribed to reduce the inflammatory response

C. In some situations, area is immobilized. Patient is instructed to avoid traumatizing activities

D. Surgical consultation may be needed to adequately reduce the pressure (e.g., transect offending ligament, transpose the nerve, disengage the nerve from surrounding adhesions or destroy the nerve)

RATIONALE

The ultimate goal of therapy in nerve entrapment and compartmental syndromes is to preserve limb functioning and minimize neurologic deficits thereby preventing unnecessary deformity and possible loss of a limb. Once airway, breathing, and circulation have been established, attention is paid to the limb injury.

Thus, for all patients at risk for developing these compression types of syndromes, nursing vigilance is the key to discovery. Objective measurement of the motor, sensory, and vascular status must be done frequently and documented. Because there is an element of subjectivity in testing, the same nurse should perform the tests and when nurses change, the oncoming nurse must perform the tests with the offgoing nurse to obtain an accurate picture.

The nurse should use two-point discrimination and/or light touch when performing sensory testing. These parameters are better qualifiers and more sensitive than pinprick responses. The specific areas to test depend upon the involved nerve or nerves and their testing is described under the assessment part of this topic. Conscientious documentation is necessary to detect trends in the patient's responses.

The strengths of all potentially involved muscles should be graded and charted. This again gives the reviewer an indication of the trends of deficit in the involved limb. Because passively stretching an ischemic muscle produces pain, this sign must be quickly reported as well as the pain that seems out of proportion to the injury.

The nurse must also palpate the compartment involved because tenseness and tautness are signs of compartmental syndrome. This necessitates that the involved area be free of all encumbrances such as clothing, splints, and dressings. Warm and red skin over the affected compartment suggests an inflammatory process and should be immediately reported.

The vascular assessment of an injured area must be performed systematically to rule out arterial and/or venous insufficiency which compromises circulation and leads to ischemia. Skin color is a rough estimate of circulation and when assessing deeply tanned or dark-skinned patients, color may not accurately reflect the vascular status. Temperature, capillary filling, and pulses of the involved area are more useful parameters. The nurse must remember, however, that the peripheral pulse is frequently normal in the presence of compartmental syndrome.

Whereas entrapped nerves are not life-threatening, they do carry a high morbidity. The patient must be observed for limb complications. In some instances diuretics and steroids might be prescribed to reduce the edema and inflammatory response. Splinting of the limb is used to avoid trauma. If these treatments are unsuccessful, surgery may be indicated at a later date.

Compartmental syndrome is a more devastating problem and permanent injury can occur within 6 hours. Elevation of the affected area is not done if the patient is suspected of having a compartmental syndrome. Keeping the limb at the level of the heart assures that local blood pressure is not compromised by elevation.

There are available experimental devices to measure the pressure within the fascial compartments. The three techniques under study include the infusion technique, the wick technique, and the injection technique. Tissue pressure readings in excess of 40 mm Hg are strongly suggestive of compartmental syndrome. However, these techniques are still experimental and only examiners proficient in their use should employ them. Until precise tools are available to measure tissue pressure, the staff should rely on the history of the injury and the ongoing assessments to establish the proper diagnosis and management plan.

8. Status Epilepticus

ASSESSMENT

I. Presenting clinical picture
   A. Neuromuscular system alteration
      1. body in rigid extension; arms abducted; elbows flexed; hands pronated; legs hyperextended
      2. teeth and jaws may be clenched; frothing, drooling and excessive salivation common and may be blood tinged

3. excessive tonic–clonic movements of all limbs
4. excessive diaphoresis; fever
5. usually unconscious between seizures
6. eyes: pupils usually dilated and nonreactive; conjugate deviation, roving or clonic movements in either direction; papilledema may be observed

B. Respiratory system alteration
1. airway may be obstructed
2. respirations may be labored, slow, apneic periods
3. secretions accumulate in oropharynx
4. pulmonary congestion; hypercarbia; hypoxia; cyanosis

C. Cardiovascular system alteration
1. if seen early, bp will be elevated; if later, bp will be low; hypotensive shock could be present
2. initial tachycardia is followed by bradycardia
3. cardiac arrhythmias common; cardiac arrest a possibility
4. systemic anoxia or hypoxia exists
5. volume depletion could exist

D. Homeostatic system alteration
1. hypovolemia, hyperkalemia, respiratory and metabolic acidosis: could also be hyponatremic, hypocalcemic
2. initial hyperglycemia is followed by hypoglycemia
3. vomiting common; may be incontinent of stool
4. usually incontinent of urine but may be oliguric; myoglobinuria and renal failure a late complication

II. Possible precipitating and/or contributing causes

A. In patients with preexisting epilepsy: discontinuance of their anticonvulsant medications or incorrect dosage to control seizures; alcohol or barbiturate abuse; intercurrent infection; sleep deprivation; stress

B. Acute neurologic insult: infarction, trauma, infection; hypoxia, or cerebral neoplasm (usually frontal lobe)

C. Metabolic factors: fluid, electrolyte, glucose and/or glucose imbalances; liver failure; renal failure; poisonings with heavy metals

D. Drug withdrawal: alcohol, barbiturates, glutethimide, benzodiazapines

III. Alterations in laboratory and other diagnostic tests
The diagnosis usually rests upon the witnessing of frequent generalized tonic–clonic seizures occurring in a patient with a depressed LOC and who does not awaken fully between seizures

A. EEG during a seizure shows generalized spikes. Postictally, it generally is slow and interictally, it may be normal. It may indicate a focal or lateralized abnormality

B. Serum electrolytes may indicate hyperkalemia, hyponatremia, hypocalcemia, azotemia, hyper- or hypoglycemia

C. Blood gases may indicate metabolic and respiratory acidosis

D. CAT scan may indicate hemorrhage, degenerative disease, or major structural abnormality

E. Skull films may indicate fracture
F. Elevations in RBC, Hgb, and Hct may be result of hemoconcentration
G. Toxic screen of blood and urine may indicate heavy metal poisoning, inadequate anticonvulsant levels or high alcohol and/or barbiturate levels
H. WBC and differential and the cultures of blood, urine, and sputum may indicate an infectious process

PATHOPHYSIOLOGY

According to the World Health Organization dictionary, status epilepticus is described as a condition characterized by an epileptic seizure that is sufficiently prolonged or repeated at sufficiently brief intervals so as to produce an unvarying and enduring epiletpic condition. Others describe it as any seizure lasting 30 to 60 minutes or more. Current classifications of status have broadened to include:

1. Convulsive status epilepticus, in which the patient does not recover to a normal alert state between repeated tonic–clonic attacks
2. Nonconvulsive status epilepticus, such as absence status and complex partial status, in which the clinical picture is one of a prolonged "twilight" state
3. Continuous partial seizures (epilepsia partialis continuans) in which consciousness is preserved.

Status epilepticus can occur in any age group and the disease does have a familial nature. In patients with a history of epilepsy, errors in dosage or discontinuance of anticonvulsant medication are the most common cause of status followed by alcohol abuse, intercurrent infection, and other stressful or life-style changes. A febrile state or CNS infection are the most common precipitating events in children. In older children and adults, primary tonic–clonic seizures could be idiopathic or due to metabolic imbalances whereas partial seizures, with or without spread, represent focal brain damage (e.g., hematoma, hemorrhage, infarction, tumor) and carries with it a graver prognosis.

Convulsive status epilepticus is a medical emergency involving a high morbidity and mortality. In prior years, mortality rates of 5 to 50 percent existed. More recent figures indicate a 10 to 12 percent mortality for both children and adults. The patient may succumb to prolonged seizuring activity per se but more often, death is due to the acute precipitating event, cardiac arrest, respiratory failure, or renal failure. The morbidity of prolonged status is manifested in children by mental retardation and in adults by intellectual deterioration, permanent neurologic impairments, cerebral atrophy, and continuing recurrence of seizures.

Status epilepticus is a symptom complex and is not limited to continuous grand mal seizuring. The mechanisms for producing continuous seizures therefore involves differing actions for each type of status and none of these mechanisms is known at the present time. It is recognized that a population of brain cell neurons for some unknown reason continuously fire stimuli which spread synaptically to adjacent neurons, then to the contralateral cerebral cortex, the subcortical nuclei of the brainstem, thalamus, hippocampus, amygdala, and cerebellum. These massive discharges occurring simultaneously in all parts of the motor cortex are responsible for the tonic–clonic movements. The EEG tracing is the only tool to date that can validate the electrophysiologic changes occurring before, during, and after a seizure.

Much research activity is being directed at studying the events that lead to increased excitability of neurons and mechanisms that might cause a loss of normal inhibitory influence. It is possible that there is an increase in the release of excitatory neurotransmitters or a decrease in the amount or release of inhibitory neurotransmitter (e.g., GABA). It could also be possible that postsynaptic receptors are stimulated or enhanced by excitatory neurotransmitters. On the other hand, it could be that postsynaptic receptors are blocked by some substances (e.g., strychnine, bicuculline) or their inhibitory transmitter is blocked. Other researchers are studying mechanisms that directly increase the excitability of the postsynaptic membrane and conversely, mechanisms that block postsynaptic membrane changes initiated by receptor activation.

Experimentally, seizures have been produced by changing cerebral metabolism, modifying neural structures and by altering the internal as well as the external environments of the neuron. Local fluid and electrolyte changes in the milieu of the neurons can trigger a seizure. Imbalances in the inward flow of calcium and sodium into a neuron and the outward flow of potassium have been shown to trigger a seizure. Some neurons are apparently very sensitive to acetylcholine. The muscarinic effect of this neurotransmitter can reduce amounts of both calcium and sodium in the neuronal environment. Thus, any increase in cholinergic activity could result in epileptiform discharges. It seems then, that the seizure threshold of susceptible persons may be lowered by electrolyte changes, water imbalances plus fever, fatigue, stress, and other factors.

The physiopathologic events accompanying status epilepticus result from (1) the massive stimulation of the autonomic nervous system and central nervous system, (2) cumulative hypoxia and anoxia, (3) muscle tissue breakdown, and (4) excessive metabolic activity of vulnerable neurons.

The increased activation of both the sympathetic and parasympathetic branches of the autonomic nervous system have far reaching consequences and explain much of the clinical picture. Massive autonomic discharges result in fever, excessive sweating, increased production of saliva and tracheobronchial secretions, an initial rise in blood pressure and glucose levels, increased cerebral oxygen and glucose consumption, bronchial constriction, and vomiting.

Cardiovascular complications are related to the sympathetic stimulation, hypoxia, and other concomitant metabolic imbalances. Excess epinephrine produces an initial tachycardia and an increase in systemic blood pressure. Cerebrovascular resistance decreases permitting an increase in cerebral blood flow resulting in vasodilatation. In conjunction, cerebrovenous pressure and cerebrospinal fluid pressure rise. However, after 30 minutes of seizuring, arterial blood pressure falls, cerebral blood flow and venous pressure may only be slightly elevated or normal. If cerebrovasodilatation persists in the presence of lower perfusion rates and increases in venous pressure levels, ischemic neurologic damage may result. Prolonged seizuring and sustained hyperkalemia result in irregular cardiac rhythm, cardiac failure, and cardiac arrest. A concomitant lactic acidosis due to hypoxia also adds to cardiac complications.

Respiratory problems during status epilepticus result from a variety of mechanisms. Some researchers believe that neurogenic factors increase pulmonary microvascular pressure, lymphatic flow, and capillary permeability resulting in a transudation of fluid in the pulmonary bed and congestion. The excessive autonomic stimulation results in bronchial constriction and an increase in bronchial secretions. It is also postulated that the brainstem respiratory center is inhibited by the excessive electrical discharges. Regardless of the specific or multiple mechanisms, there are a variety of respiratory patterns exhibited by the patient in status, retention of carbon dioxide, reduced oxygenation of hemoglobin, copious secretions and danger of atelectasis, pneumonia, and respiratory failure.

The cumulative effects of sustained hypoxia have dire metabolic consequences. Deprived of oxygen, the normal oxidative pathway, which produces needed cellular energy in the form of ATP, must switch to the inefficient anaerobic glycolytic pathway. The end result of this short pathway is the combining of pyruvic acid and hydrogen ions to yield lactic acid. The presence of increased quantities of lactic acid under hypoxic conditions shifts the blood pH to below 7.35 resulting in a metabolic acidosis. The lack of the energy of ATP halts the cellular sodium–potassium pump causing sodium to move into the cell and potassium to move out into the extracellular fluid. The lack of sufficient ATP results in decreased cellular chemical activity and eventually, cell death.

The generalized convulsive state with its associated excessive muscular activity could lead to lower nephron nephrosis or acute tubular necrosis. Muscle destruction results in muscle weakness and the release of myoglobin (a conjugated protein similar to hemoglobin), potassium, and other muscle proteins which enter the plasma and are normally excreted in the urine. Myoglobin gives the urine a dark color. In high concentrations, and if the patient is hypovolemic, it could precipitate in the renal tubules leading to obstruction, oliguria, anuria, azotemia, and renal failure.

Experimental studies indicate that permanent neuronal cell damage occurs in the hippocampus, amygdala, cerebellum, thalamus, and cortical layers of the brain after an hour of convulsive seizuring. Cell death of these vulnerable neurons occurs in spite of adequate oxygenation and probably is a reflection of diminished metabolic substrates available to meet the increased demands of these structures and neurons. Regional oxygen insufficiency probably adds an additional insult to neuronal cell damage. The accumulation of toxic amounts of arachidonic acid, arachidonoyl diglycerols, prostaglandins, and leucotrienes in firing neurons leads to cerebral edema and cell death in selected brain regions. Autopsy findings in patients with longstanding epilepsy indicate a neuronal loss, gliosis, and atrophy of such structures as the cerebellum, thalamus, and cerebral cortex.

Clinical and experimental studies to date dictate that convulsive status epilepticus be terminated as rapidly as possible if permanent damage, neurologic sequelae, and secondary metabolic complications are to be avoided.

MANAGEMENT

I. Insure an adequate airway and ventilation
  A. Insert an oral airway; be prepared to intubate patient
  B. Suction oronasal pharynx frequently (during the quiet phase of seizure activity)
  C. Position for maximum oxygenation; administer oxygen
  D. Obtain stat chest x-ray; auscultate lung fields
  E. Obtain blood gas levels and monitor serially
  F. Send sputum specimen for culture and sensitivity
  G. Perform chest percussion to mobilize secretions
II. Support circulation
  A. Record temperature, pulse, respirations and bp q 30 minutes
  B. Obtain stat ECG and prepare for continuous cardiac monitoring
  C. Establish an intravenous line and means for CVP monitoring
  D. Initial IV fluid is usually saline
  E. Administer Thiamine 100 mg IV push or add vitamin B complex to saline solution
  F. Follow above with 50 ml of 50 percent glucose
  G. Insert an indwelling urinary catheter
  H. Chart all I & O and serial CVP measurements
III. Perform a rapid systems survey
  A. Neurologic system
    1. perform a careful neurologic exam ictally and postictally to determine if any focal or lateralizing aspects of the seizure can be found.
    2. note any signs of head trauma or meningeal irritation
    3. keep a record of seizure activity. Note the following: time of onset, duration; appearance of a "cry out"; position of head, trunk, and extremities; sequence of muscle movements; pupillary size and reaction to light; any deviation of eyes or head; skin changes; respiratory rate, rhythm or periods of apnea; frothing and/or drooling about the mouth; LOC; postictal state, if any. (See Appendix B, Seizure Checklist)
  B. Cardiopulmonary systems: performed as airway, breathing, and circulation are being supported. Staff must be prepared for a possible cardiac arrest, defibrillation, or temporary pacing
  C. Gastrointestinal: insert a nasogastric tube to decompress the stomach and attach to low suctioning
IV. Assist with the collection of a history and baseline data
  A. A careful history from relatives, friends to ascertain a past history of seizures, medication regimen, life-style changes, recent injuries or surgery, alcohol and/or barbiturate abuse
  B. Draw blood samples for CBC, serum electrolytes, BUN, glucose, anticonvulsant levels, alcohol levels, toxic screen, liver function, WBC and differential. Blood cultures are taken, if infection is suspected. Blood gases are drawn

C. Send urine samples for routine analysis, culture and sensitivity, toxic screen, myoglobin levels

D. Stat chest x-ray, ECG, skull films, CAT scan, EEG

E. Lumbar puncture is only done when there is strong indication of infection (e.g., bacterial meningitis). It may be deferred until seizures are brought under control

V. Terminate electrical and clinical seizure activity

Selection of initial drugs is dependent upon history and drug protocols.

A. Administer diazepam simultaneously with phenytoin

1. diazepam (Valium) IV is administered at a rate no faster than 2 mg/minute until seizures stop or a total dose of 20 mg is given

   action: sedative–hypnotic drug with brief anticonvulsant action; controls seizures within 5 minutes

   side effects: serious respiratory depression and/or hypotension plus a decrease in LOC

   contraindications: seizures due to head trauma or other neurologic conditions because it makes neurologic evaluation most difficult

   nursing: patient must be monitored for respiratory arrest, hypotension, cardiac arrest

2. phenytoin (Dilantin) IV is administered slowly and simultaneously in another IV line no faster than 50 mg/minute to a total dose of 18 mg/kg of body weight or 1000 mg in 20 minutes

   action: effective anticonvulsant that will not complicate the neurologic picture or affect the EEG

   side effects: hypotension, heart block, respiratory depression

   contraindications: when known heart disease or conduction abnormalities are part of the history but may still be used

   nursing: monitor bp, respiratory rate, and EEG during injection. Drug may be given undiluted in slow IV push because it precipitates out in IV solutions of glucose. If diluted, saline is dilutant of choice. Solution should be placed in a volume control setup and drip rate monitored carefully. Observe patient for bilateral horizontal nystagmus which develops at therapeutic blood levels of 10 to 20 μg/ml

B. After 30 to 40 minutes, if seizures persist, the second line of drugs used are IV phenobarbital *or* diazepam IV drip

1. at this point in management, the patient *must* be intubated

2. phenobarbital is administered no faster than 90 to 120 mg/minute until seizures cease or to a maximum dose of 500 mg in adults

   action: a hypnotic, sedative anticonvulsant which rises seizure threshold and limits seizure spread

   side effects: depresses central nervous system especially respirations

   nursing: closely monitor respiratory rate, depth, and pattern. Be prepared to mechanically assist ventilations. Drug will interfere with accurate neurologic evaluations

3. diazepam drip is prepared by diluting 100 mg of diazepam in 500 ml of

5 percent D/W and administered at 40 ml/hour to ensure blood levels of 0.2 to 0.8 μg/ml

    4. Respiratory rate depth and pattern, bp, ECG, and blood gases must be monitored closely

C. After 50 to 60 minutes, if seizures persist, general anesthesia with halothane and neuromuscular blockade is indicated. If anesthetist is not available, the third line of drugs may be tried. These are paraldehyde *or* lidocaine

    1. paraldehyde: a 4 to 5 percent solution in saline is administered IV at a rate of up to 2.5 ml/kg or 0.5 ml/minute or fast enough to stop seizuring

       action: hypnotic, useful for refractory forms of seizuring

       side effects: respiratory depression

       nursing: drug will dissolve plastic syringes and tubing. Administer in a glass syringe with a metal connector. Patient's blood may turn black on contact with drug. Closely observe for respiratory depression. Have equipment ready to mechanically assist ventilations

    2. lidocaine may be given IV push and if successful, by continuous IV drip by diluting 50 to 100 mg in 250 ml of 5 percent D/W and administering it at a rate of 1 to 2 mg/minute

       action: depresses membrane excitability

       side effects: central nervous system depression and respiratory arrest

       nursing: monitor respirations, bp, ECG, and have emergency drugs and equipment at the bedside

D. After 80 minutes of therapy with first, second, and third line drugs and seizuring still persists, general anesthesia must be given

E. During drug therapy serial EEG monitoring should be performed to assure the cessation of electrical seizure activity which may not be evidenced by clinical manifestations

VI. Correct the secondary metabolic complications of prolonged seizuring

A. Dehydration: administer IV fluids as prescribed. Plan fluids to cover a 12 to 24 hour period. Closely monitor CVP, I&O, and observe for fluid overload

B. Hypoglycemia: administer IV glucose solutions. Monitor serial glucose determinations

C. Electrolyte imbalances: serial electrolytes must be monitored

    Hyperkalemia: insulin and glucose may be prescribed

    Hyponatremia: saline or 3 percent saline may be prescribed

    Hypocalcemia; calcium gluconate may be prescribed

D. Lactic acidosis: bicarbonate or Ringer's lactate solution may be used. Insure adequate oxygenation. Monitor blood gases

E. Respiratory acidosis: adequately ventilate patient. Keep airway clear. Suction frequently. Administer oxygen. Monitor blood gases. Note occurrence of rebound alkalotic state

F. Fever: cooling sponges, few clothes, cool environment. Usually returns to normal once seizuring is stopped. Take rectal temperature every 30 minutes

G. Cerebral edema: mannitol or other hypertonic osmotic diuretic agent may be used. Observe for diuresis following administration. Perform frequent neurologic testing to detect this problem

H. Renal failure: monitor urine output and color. Keep patient adequately hydrated. Report any decrease in output or change in color. Monitor nitrogenous substances in the blood

VII. Protect the patient from injury

A. Place patient in an environment where close observation is possible

B. Thoroughly pad side rails and head of bed

C. Avoid the use of arm or leg restraints as well as constricting clothing

D. Administer basic oral and skin hygiene as needed

VIII. Correct and/or treat the contributing cause

A. Referral to a neurologist for follow-up supervision

B. Referral to a neurosurgeon for possible surgical intervention when seizures do not respond to medical management

C. Admit to intensive care unit for further observation and treatment

---

RATIONALE

The compromised state of the cardiopulmonary system demands immediate priority in managing patients in status epilepticus. An oral airway will facilitate breathing and provide a route for suctioning. A padded tongue blade is of little use and intubation should be considered.

Oxygen is needed to decrease cerebral and systemic hypoxia and to meet increased cerebral neuronal activity requirements. High flow rates can be provided with a bag–valve mask setup. Positioning in the side lying position facilitates drainage of excessive oral secretions and prevents their aspiration. Baseline and serial blood gas determinations detect the severity of the acidosis that is usually present. In addition, they help monitor the patient's responses to therapy.

Pneumonia, atelectasis, and respiratory depression in status epilepticus are due to seizuring and drug therapies. Meticulous lung hygiene and chest percussion keeps secretions mobilized and enhances their removal. The nurse closely monitors the patient's respiratory rate, depth, and effort throughout seizure activity and its treatment. Mechanical ventilatory devices must be within close reach for emergency use.

The cardiovascular system is vulnerable to dysrhythmias, failure, and arrest during status epilepticus. Contributing factors are hyperkalemia, possible hypocalcemia, hypoxia, acidosis, and drugs used to treat the seizures. Continuous cardiac monitoring, serial serum electrolytes and blood gases must be performed to assess the extent of this problem and to initiate timely interventions. Equipment and drugs to perform cardiac resuscitation should be close by.

Fluid imbalances, most commonly a fluid deficit, occur during status epilepticus because of fever, diaphoresis, decreased intake, increased metabolic activity, and vomiting. Fluid imbalances are detected by CVP, blood pressure, clinical, and laboratory assessments. Balance is restored by intravenous administration of fluids because of vomiting and possible intestinal ileus which would prevent the absorption of fluids from the gastrointestinal tract. A nasogastric tube on low suctioning prevents aspiration of vomitus and decompresses the stomach. An indwelling urinary catheter facilitates accurate output. The initial fluid given to patients in status is usually saline.

In the early phase of treatment and before laboratory data is returned, hypoglycemic seizures must be ruled out. The administration of thiamine or vitamin B complex before glucose is necessary to avoid precipitating Wernicke–Korsakoff encephalopathy in the thiamine deficient patient. Glucose requires thiamine for its proper metabolism. A bolus of 25 to 50 ml of 50 percent dextrose would stop the seizures of a hypoglycemic origin.

The diagnosis of status epilepticus is made by clinical observation of seizure activity and history. Frequent and carefully performed neurologic assessments and EEG tracings, if possible, help to classify the type of seizure and guide the physician in planning care. Primary generalized tonic–clonic status responds to first line drugs but tonic–clonic seizures with partial onset generally require multiple drugs. The nurse keeps accurate records of seizure activity and observes the patient for any focal or lateralizing signs. Seizures due to focal brain disease carry a graver prognosis than primary generalized seizures. Skull films and CAT scan are helpful tools that identify focal disease processes.

A careful search is done to identify the precipitating and/or contributing cause(s) of the seizures. Because the patient is usually unconscious, friends and relatives are interviewed to obtain the personal history. Along with the history a physical examination is performed and multiple laboratory tests begun. The data collected should provide the examiner with enough information to establish the type of seizure and the extent of the metabolic consequences of seizuring.

Most patients in status epilepticus are febrile and a possible infectious basis must be ruled out. Blood, sputum, and urine are cultured to detect any offending organism. Lumbar puncture to retrieve cerebrospinal fluid for culture is technically difficult in a seizuring patient and is usually deferred until seizures are controlled unless meningitis is highly suspected.

To rapidly terminate seizuring, potent drugs are administered intravenously to insure effective serum and brain levels of the drug. Diazepam given simultaneously with phenytoin is the first line of pharmaceutic defense, in most cases and at most institutions. However, differing institutions may have differing protocols. Intravenous diazepam stops seizures within 3 minutes in 33 percent of patients and within 5 minutes in 80 percent of patients. Because it is distributed quickly and widely, 10 to 20 minutes after injection, seizures will recur.

To prevent the recurrence of seizures, phenytoin is administered slowly and simultaneously in another intravenous line. Its anticonvulsant action requires 10 to 20 minutes to take effect and is dose related. Approximately 400 mg stops seizures in 30 percent of patients. Most adults require a 1000 mg dose to reach desired blood levels. A good indicator of blood levels of phenytoin is the appearance of bilateral horizontal nystagmus on lateral gaze which should appear when dosage is in the therapeutic range.

The potential hazardous side effects of diazepam on respirations and cardiac activity and phenytoin on blood pressure must be closely monitored. In a controlled environment the dangerous side effects can be dealt with properly and swiftly, if the patient is constantly observed and monitored. Neurologic and metabolic responses to drug therapy is the responsibility of the entire staff.

If seizuring is resistant to the first line of drugs, intravenous phenobarbital or diazepam drip might prove helpful. Administering phenobarbital at this time adds to respiratory depression and interferes with neurologic testing results. A more frequent option is to start an intravenous drip of diazepam and maintain blood levels of this drug. The patient must be intubated, if this approach is decided upon because of the high probability of respiratory depression.

Seizuring persisting over 60 minutes carries a grave prognosis. Anesthesia with neuromuscular blockade or lidocaine or paraldehyde might be considered. It is unfortunate that at the present time there is no one drug that stops seizuring, remains in the brain long enough to prevent recurrence and is free from undesirable effects.

While controlling seizures, efforts are directed at correcting secondary metabolic consequences of prolonged seizure activity. Because even minor imbalances in fluid, electrolyte, and glucose make seizure control difficult, special efforts are directed at correcting imbalances. Fluid replacement is restored with saline or free water depending upon the neurologic findings, laboratory data, and output.

Intravenous glucose is required to combat the hypoglycemia which occurs 30 minutes after prolonged seizuring. Hypoglycemia results from increased metabolic activity during seizuring.

Insulin plus glucose drives potassium back into the cells and thus reduces the hyperkalemia. However, once seizures are reduced potassium levels should return to normal providing renal functioning is adequate.

It must be kept in mind that seizures could result from hyponatremia or hypocalcemia. A serum sodium of below 120 mEq/L and a history of compulsive water drinking or head trauma should raise suspicion of hyponatremia. Before laboratory results are at hand a prolonged QT interval on the ECG is suggestive of hypocalcemia. The patient should be given 1 to 2 ampules of calcium gluconate. Serial electrolyte determinations help guide the physician in determining the patient's needs.

The respiratory and metabolic acidosis is combatted with oxygenation, assisted ventilations, and by possibly administering intravenous alkalinizing solutions (e.g., bicarbonate, Ringer's). Serial blood gases are necessary to monitor responses to this therapy.

Papilledema and other pupillary changes are usually indicative of increasing intracranial pressure. Appropriate therapy in this instance is the administration of intravenous osmotic diuretics (e.g., mannitol, dextran). Extremely careful delivery of these drugs plus accurate renal output monitoring must be performed when these drugs are prescribed.

The patient must be constantly observed for signs of impending renal failure, such as oliguria, increasing BUN, rising serum potassium, and myoglobinuria. If these signs are detected early, appropriate actions can be taken. Adequate hydration should avoid renal failure associated with precipitation of myoglobin in the renal tubules.

Throughout the patient's stay in the emergency department all efforts are directed toward the patient's safety and avoidance of injury. Side rails and head board must be thoroughly padded. In some instances, a helmet is provided to avoid head trauma. No attempt should be made to restrain the patient because a seizuring patient can be severely injured and/or physically exhausted from struggling against the restraints. Frequent change of position, skin care, and oral hygiene can be provided during the "quiet phase" of seizure activity.

Referral to a neurologist for follow-up supervision is needed once the patient stops seizuring. The patient should be admitted to hospital for further study, observation, and treatment. A neurosurgeon may need to be consulted, if seizuring has a focal basis which is amenable to surgical intervention.

Neuromuscular Emergencies References

CEREBROVASCULAR ACCIDENT

Ball, P. Preventing stroke through non-invasive carotid artery assessment. *Journal of Neurosurgical Nursing*, 1982, **14**, 182.

Davis, J., & Mason, C. *Neurologic critical care.* New York: Van Nostrand Reinhold, 1979, pp. 229–234.

Dembo, M. Arteriovenous malformation of the brain: A review of the literature since 1960. *Archives of Physical Medicine and Rehabilitation*, 1982, **63** (11), 565.

Doolittle, N. Arteriovenous malformations: The physiology, symptomotology, and nursing care. *Journal of Neurosurgical Nursing*, 1979, **11**, 175.

Gary, R. Cerebral vasospasm: Process, trends and interventions. *Journal of Neurosurgical Nursing*, 1981, **13**, 256.

Greenfield, N. Subclavian steal: A review. *Heart and Lung*, 1982, **11** (4), 327.

Greer, M. Current concepts in managing TIA's and stroke. *Geriatrics*, 1979, **34** (4), 53.

Heros, R. Cerebellar hemorrhage and infarction. *Stroke*, 1982, **13** (1), 106.

Hickey, J. *Quick reference to neurological nursing.* Philadelphia: J. B. Lippincott, 1984, chap. 24, pp. 409–424.

Hinton, R. C. Treatment of cerebral ischemia. *Comprehensive Therapy*, 1981, **7**, 24.

Jones, G. Glasgow coma scale. *American Journal of Nursing*, 1979, **79**, 1551.

Maida, M. J. Regional cerebral blood flow: Patient correlations. *Journal of Neurosurgical Nursing*, 1982, **14** (6), 309.

Miller, M. Emergency management of the unconscious patient. *Nursing Clinics of North America*, 1981, **12**, 145.

Miller, V. T. Lacunar stroke: A reassessment. *Archives of Neurology*, 1983, **40** (3), 129.

Raichle, M. E. The pathophysiology of brain ischemia. *Annals of Neurology*, 1983, **13** (1), 2.

Sherman, D. G., & Easton, J. D. Cerebral edema in stroke. *Postgraduate Medicine*, 1980, **68** (1), 107.

Stroke by strangulation. *Emergency Medicine*, 1981, **13**, 126.

Stroke from a sharp twist. *Emergency Medicine*, 1981, **13**, 101.

Tilton, C., & Maloof, M. Diagnosing the problems in stroke. *American Journal of Nursing*, 1982, **82**, 596.

Walleck, C. Neurological assessment for nurses—A part of the nursing process. *Journal of Neurosurgical Nursing*, 1978, **10** (1), 13.

CRANIOCEREBRAL TRAUMA

Adelstein, W. Chronic subdurals. *Journal of Neurosurgical Nursing*, 1980, **12** (1), 36.

Blacker, H. M. Head injury: Move quickly to avert permanent brain damage. *Consultant*, 1982, **22**, 163.

Connolly, R., & Zewe, G. Update: Head injuries. *Journal of Neurosurgical Nursing*, 1981, **13** (4), 195.

Dagrosa, T. Brainstem damage associated with cerebral injury. *Journal of Emergency Nursing*, 1976, **2**, 9.

Fuller, E. Coma: Evaluating depth of consciousness. *Patient Care*, 1981, **15**, 127.

Gennis, P. Coma. *Topics in Emergency Medicine*, 1982, **4**, 47.

Hanlon, K. Description and uses of intracranial pressure monitoring. *Heart and Lung*, 1976, **5**, 277.

Head trauma. *Emergency Medicine*, 1980, **12**, 103.

Jones, C. Outcomes following closed head injuries. *Journal of Neurosurgical Nursing*, 1981, **13** (4), 178.

Marshall, L. F. Mannitol dose requirements in brain injured patients. *Journal of Neurosurgery*, 1978, **48**, 169.

Ricci, M. M. Intracranial hypertension: Barbiturate therapy and the role of the nurse. *Journal of Neurosurgical Nursing*, 1979, **11**, 247.

Rimel, R. W. Emergency management of the patient with central nervous system trauma. *Journal of Neurosurgical Nursing*, 1978, **10**, 185.

Rimel, R., Jane, J., Edlich, R. Care of CNS trauma at the site. *Critical Care Quarterly*, 1979, **2** (1), 1.

Roberts, J. Pathophysiology, diagnosis and treatment of head trauma. *Topics in Emergency Medicine*, 1979, **1** (1), 41.

Spector, R. H. Ocular clues to neurologic disease. *Emergency Medicine*, 1981, **13**, 66.

Ward, J. D. Central nervous system trauma. *Topics in Emergency Medicine*, 1982, **4** (3), 11.

Zeegeer, L. J. Nursing care of the patient with brain edema. *Journal of Neurosurgical Nursing*, 1982, **14** (5), 268.

CERVICAL CORD INJURY

Albin, M. S. Resuscitation of the spinal cord. *Critical Care Medicine*, 1978, **6**, 270.

Almond, B. Management of cervical and thoracic spinal cord injured patients. *Journal of Neurosurgical Nursing*, 1981, **13** (2), 97.

Cloward, R. Acute cervical spine injuries. *Clinical Symposia*, 1980, **32** (1), 2.

Diving injuries . . . splint 'em where they float. *Emergency Medicine*, 1982, **14**, 140.

Donovan, W., & Bedbrook, G. Comprehensive management of spinal cord injury. *Clinical Symposia*, 1982, **34** (2), 2.

Fedlum, P. Tethered cord syndrome. *Journal of Neurosurgical Nursing*, 1982, **14** (3), 144.

Ginnity, S. Assessment of cervical cord trauma by the nurse practitioner. *Journal of Neurosurgical Nursing*, 1978, **10** (4), 193.

Giubilato, R. Acute care of the high-level quadriplegic. *Journal of Neurosurgical Nursing*, 1982, **14** (3), 128.

Hummelgard, A., & Martin, E. Management of the patient in a halo brace. *Journal of Neurosurgical Nursing*, 1982, **14** (3), 113.

Pfaudler, M. Care of the patients with severe cord injuries. *Current Practices in Critical Care*, 1979, **1**, 216.

Roberts J. Trauma of the cervical spine. *Topics in Emergency Medicine*, 1979, **1** (1), 63.

Stauffer, E. S., & Kelly E. G. Fracture dislocations of the cervical spine. *Journal of Bone and Joint Surgery*, 1977, **59-A**, 45.

Thompson, R. A., & Green, J. R. *Critical care of neurologic and neurosurgical emergencies.* New York: Raven Press, 1980.

Young, J. S. Spinal cord injury: Associated general trauma and medical complications. *Advances in Neurology*, 1979, **22**, 255.

MENINGITIS

Bell, W. E. Treatment of fungal infection of the central nervous system. *Annals of Neurology*, 1981, **9**, 471.

Belshe, R. Commonly misdiagnosed viral infections. *Hospital Medicine*, 1980, **16**, 29.

Cefotaxime sodium (Claforan). *Medical Letter on Drugs and Therapeutics*, 1981, **23**, 61.

Feigin, R. D., & Dodge, P. R. Bacterial meningitis: Newer concepts of pathophysiology and neurologic sequelae. *Pediatric Clinics of North America*, 1976, **23**, 541.

Gaddy, D. S. Meningitis in the pediatric population. *Nursing Clinics of North America*, 1980, **15**, 83.

Goodstein, R. S. The pathogenesis of gram-negative bacillary meningitis: Review of the literature. *Journal of the American Osteopathic Association*, 1982, **38** (12), 749.

Heerema, M. Diagnosis: Meningitis. *Hospital Medicine*, 1982, **18**, 13.

Moxalactam disodium (Moxam). *Medical Letter on Drugs and Therapeutics*, 1982, **24**, 13.

Newer drugs for enteric gram-negative bacillary meningitis in adults. *Medical Letter on Drugs and Therapeutics*, 1981, **23**, 73.

Sibbald, W. Bacteremia and endotoxemia: A discussion of their roles in the pathophysiology of gram-negative sepsis. *Heart & Lung*, 1976, **5** (5), 765.

Smith, D. H. The challenge of bacterial meningitis. *Hospital Practice*, 1976, **12**, 71.

Swartz, M. N. Intraventricular use of aminoglycosides in the treatment of gram-negative bacillary meningitis: Conflicting views. *Journal of Infectious Diseases*, 1975, **131**, 543.

The choice of antimicrobial drugs. *Medical Letter on Drugs and Therapeutics*, 1982, **24**, 21.

GUILLAIN–BARRÉ SYNDROME

Cooksley, P. Guillain–Barré syndrome: Fading away. *Nursing Mirror*, 1981, **152**, 38.

Giesser, B. Landry–Guillain–Barré syndrome. *Medical Times*, 1983, **3** (7), 87.

Kealy, S. Respiratory care in Guillain–Barré syndrome. *American Journal of Nursing*, 1977, **77** (1), 58.

Kim, S. Segmental demyelinating disease: Guillain–Barré syndrome. *Archives of Physical Medicine and Rehabilitation*, 1980, **61**, 210.

Mills, N., & Plasterer, H. Guillain–Barré syndrome: A framework for nursing care. *Nursing Clinics of North America*, 1980, **15** (2), 257.

Samonds, R. J. Guillain–Barré syndrome: The acute stage. *Critical Care Update*, 1981, **8**, 38.

Samonds, R. J. Guillain–Barré syndrome: Helping the patient in the acute stage. *Nursing '80*, 1980, **10** (8), 35.

Swash, M. Clinical aspects of Guillain–Barré syndrome: A review. *Journal of the Royal Society of Medicine*, 1979, **72** (9), 670.

Tikkanen, P. L. Landry–Guillain–Barré–Strohl syndrome. *Journal of Neurosurgical Nursing*, 1982, **14** (20) 74.

MYASTHENIA GRAVIS

Anchie, T. Plasmapheresis as a treatment of myasthenia gravis. *Journal of Neurosurgical Nursing*, 1981, **13**, 23.

Barry, L. The patient with myasthenia gravis really needs you. *Nursing '82*, 1982, **12**, 50.

Blount, M., Kinney, A. B., Stone, M. Plasma exchange in the management of myasthenia gravis. *Nursing Clinics of North America*, 1979, **14**, 173.

Drachman, D. B. Myasthenia gravis: Part I. *New England Journal of Medicine*, 1978, **298** (3), 136.

Drachman, D. B. Myasthenia gravis: Part II. *New England Journal of Medicine*, 1978, **298** (4), 186.

Gooder, E. Myasthenia gravis: Life transforming treatments. *Nursing Mirror*, 1981, **153**, 40.

Hrovath, M. Myasthenia gravis: A nursing approach. *Journal of Neurosurgical Nursing*, 1982, **14**, 7.

Lisak, R. Myasthenia gravis: Mechanisms and management. *Hospital Practice*, 1983, **19** (3), 101.

Sorriano, V. Myasthenia gravis. *International Journal of Neurology*, 1980, **14** (1), 6.

The alliance against myasthenia gravis. *Emergency Medicine*, 1982, **14**, 26.

Zenk, K. E. Drugs used for neurological disorders. *Critical Care Update*, 1979, **6**, 19.

NEUROVASCULAR INJURIES

Bicknell, J. N. Nerve compression syndrome: Every active person is at risk. *Consultant*, 1980, **22**, 279.

Crossland, S., & Deyerle, W. M. Compartmental syndrome. *Nursing '80*, 1980, **10** (11), 51.

Extremity trauma. *Emergency Medicine*, 1980, **12**, 127.

Hackett, C. Limbering up your neurovascular techniques. *Nursing '83*, 1983, **13** (3), 40.

Lupien, A. E. Head off compartment syndrome before it's too late. *RN*, 1980, **43** (12), 38.

Matsen, F. A. III. Compartmental syndrome. *Clinical Orthopedics*, 1976, **113**, 8.

Matsen, F. III, Winquist, R., Krugmire, R. Diagnosis and management of compartmental syndrome. *The Journal of Bone and Joint Surgery*, 1980, **62-A** (2), 286.

Mubarak, S., Owen, C., Hargens, A., et al. Acute compartment syndromes: Diagnosis and treatment with the aid of the Wick catheter. *The Journal of Bone and Joint Surgery*, 1978, **60-A** (8), 109.

Stein, J., & Warfield, C. Two entrapment neuropathies. *Hospital Practice*, 1983, **19** (1), 100a.

STATUS EPILEPTICUS

A single drug approach to seizures. *Emergency Medicine*, 1982, **14**, 218.

Aminoff, M. J., & Simon, R. P. Status epilepticus: Causes, clinical features and consequences in 98 patients. *American Journal of Medicine*, 1980, **69**, 657.

Browne, T. R. Therapy of status epilepticus. *Comprehensive Therapy*, 1982, **8** (5), 28.

Curry, H. B. Fits and faints: Causes and cures. *Emergency Medicine*, 1982, **14**, 70.

Delgado-Escueta, A. V., & Westerlain, C. G. Current concepts in neurology: Management of status epilepticus. *New England Journal of Medicine*, 1982, **306** (22), 1337.

Hauser, W. A. Status epilepticus: Frequency, etiology and neurological sequelae. In A. V. Delgado-Escueta, C. G. Wasterlain, D. M. Treiman, & R. J. Porter (Eds). *Advances in neurology. Vol. 34 Status epilepticus*. New York: Raven Press, 1983, pp. 3–14.

Hurken, M. Seizures: Etiology, classification, intervention. *Journal of Neurosurgical Nursing*, 1979, **11**, 166.

Husk, G. T. Seizures. *Topics in Emergency Medicine*, 1982, **4**, 59.

Lovely, M. P. Identification and treatment of status epilepticus. *Journal of Neurosurgical Nursing*, 1980, **12** (2), 93.

Norman, S., & Browne, T. Seizure disorders. *American Journal of Nursing*, 1981, **81**, 984.

Penry, J. K., & Newmark, M. E. The use of antiepileptic drugs. *Annals of Internal Medicine*, 1979, **90**, 207.

Waddell, G. Status epilepticus: Nursing management. In A.V. Delgado-Escueta, C. G. Wasterlain, D. M. Treiman, & R. J. Porter (Eds.). *Advances in neurology. Vol. 34. Status epilepticus.* New York: Raven Press, 1983, p. 405.

Woodward, E. The total patient: Implications for nursing care of the epileptic. *Journal of Neurosurgical Nursing*, 1982, **14** (4), 166.

B. RESPIRATORY EMERGENCIES

1. Acute Upper Airway Obstruction: Food and Foreign Objects

ASSESSMENT

I. Initial assessment data
  A. Identify events prior to onset of symptoms
  B. Rule out history of previous conditions
    1. heart disease
    2. asthma
    3. laryngeal carcinoma
    4. epiglottitis
    5. thoracic aneurysm
    6. congestive obstructive pulmonary disease
II. Alterations in respiratory function (laryngeal foreign bodies)
  A. partial obstruction
    1. hoarseness
    2. stridor
    3. use of accessory muscles of respiration
    4. coughing
    5. gagging
  B. Complete obstruction
    1. severe dyspnea (air hunger)
    2. stridor
    3. arterial hypoxia
    4. cyanosis
    5. severe anxiety
    6. loss of consciousness
    7. asphyxia

    C. Inflammatory symptoms
       1. pain
       2. tenderness
       3. swelling
       4. fever
III. Alteration in respiratory function (bronchial foreign object)
    A. Initial coughing episode
    B. Silent or asymptomatic period (varying from hours to months or years depending on whether object is organic or nonorganic)
    C. Obstructive symptoms
       1. cough
       2. wheezing
       3. atelectasis
       4. hypoxia
       5. cyanosis
    D. Inflammatory symptoms
       1. pain in affected area
       2. fever
       3. infection
       4. possibly obstructive emphysema
    E. Radiographic findings
       1. posteroanterior and lateral x-rays of neck and chest
          a. reveal nature of object ⎫
                                  ⎬ if opaque material
          b. reveal location of object ⎭
       2. fluoroscopy
          a. reveal diminished diaphragmatic movement ⎫
          b. mediastinal shift ⎬ all might suggest a foreign object
          c. focal emphysema ⎪
          d. atelectasis ⎭
          e. rule out
             i. pneumonia
             ii. lung abscess
             iii. bronchiectasis
             iv. tuberculosis

PATHOPHYSIOLOGY

A variety of foreign objects including boluses of food may obstruct the airway and lodge in the hypopharynx, larynx, trachea, or bronchi, however, most lodge in either the larynx or the bronchi. A variety of instances may predispose to this situation such as rapid eating, carelessness while holding something in the mouth, sudden inspiration triggered by surprise, impairment of normal mouth sensations by full dentures, and states of unconsciousness.

Foreign objects lodged between the larynx and the carina may precipitate a life-threatening condition, and if complete obstruction of the air passages is present, asphyxia and death are imminent. If the airway obstruction is below the carina, only one lung or a portion thereof is affected; the condition, although serious, is not as life-threatening, and the presenting symptoms are not as dramatic. The severity of the clinical signs and symptoms depends on the size of the foreign object, its relation to the obstructed lumen, the location of the obstruction, the shape of the object, which often determines whether the obstruction is partial or total, and the amount of edema or inflammatory swelling.

Other conditions arising from the walls of the airway (laryngeal carcinoma, epiglottitis, laryngeal edema, peritonsillar abscesses), from collapse of the airway walls (aneurysm in thoracic area, retrosternal goiter, mediastinal lymph node enlargement), and thickened secretions may lead to acute airway obstruction. An initial history may be helpful in identifying or ruling out these conditions as major upper airway obstructors.

It is critical that the upper airway pathway remain patent at all times, and that the swallowing and cough reflex, as well as the muscle tone of the pharynx and larynx, remain intact to insure this patency. Any disruption in the upper air passage causes impairment of gas exchange and increases the work of breathing. If uninterrupted, these changes result in compromised respiratory efficiency and development of hypoxemia. Delayed emergency management allows the problem to progress. Alveolar ventilation is inadequate to cope with carbon dioxide production; hypercapnea will develop in conjunction with hypoxemia; and death may ensue. Rapid assessment and management is vital for the survival of the patient.

MANAGEMENT

I. Initial management measures
  A. Open mouth and examine for visible obstruction
  B. Position patient
    1. tilt head backward and push mandible forward
    2. place in Trendelenberg position
    3. clear secretions and particulate matter from mouth and pharynx
    4. suction secretions, if necessary
  C. Remove visible object by hand or with forceps, if available
  D. For nonvisible objects
    1. give four quick back blows
      a. deliver with heel of rescuer's hand
      b. deliver between the shoulder blades
    2. Heimlich maneuver (abdominal thrust)
    3. chest thrust (for obese or pregnant women)
      a. heel of rescuer's hand over lower mediastinum
      b. four rapid thrusts administered
II. Promote measures to reestablish airway (In those individuals for whom the above maneuvers have proven inadequate.)

    A. Evaluate ventilatory status

        1. check air flow at mouth and nose

            a. listen for air

            b. feel for air with dorsum of hand in close proximity to nose and mouth

        2. observe for absence of chest wall movement with each ventilation

        3. observe for absence of abdominal wall movement with each ventilation

        4. auscultate chest to identify focal area of wheezing or other abnormality

    B. ventilatory apparatus

        1. resuscitator bag and mask (use prior to intubation and mechanical ventilation)

        2. oral airway (use in conscious patients when head positioning is not adequate to clear airway)

        3. nasopharyngeal tube (use in semiconscious patients and those with clenched jaws)

        4. endotracheal tube (method of choice for emergency care)

            a. for those nonresponsive to above methods

            b. for comatose patients unable to maintain own respirations

        5. surgical approaches to ventilation

            a. cricothyrotomy

                i. when upper airway continues to be obstructed

                ii. when endotracheal tube cannot be passed

            b. tracheostomy

                i. when passing of endotracheal tube is not possible or feasible

                ii. in the presence of facial trauma or laryngeal edema

                iii. when access to airway is needed on a long-term basis

        6. mechanical ventilators

III. Institute measures to extract foreign bodies not amenable to initial management maneuvers

    A. Laryngoscopy ⎤ with use of specialized forceps. Performed under general an-

    B. Bronchoscopy ⎦ esthesia

    C. Thoracotomy—to remove foreign objects in periphery of lung (e.g., straight pin). Performed under general anesthesia

IV. Institute any of the following measures to support management modalities if necessary

    A. Intravenous line

    B. Arterial line

    C. Indwelling urethral catheter, if indicated

    D. Electrocardiographic monitoring

    E. Endotracheal suctioning

    F. Blood gases and blood pH

    G. Electrolytes as indicated

    H. Additional x-rays, fluoroscopy as needed

V. Monitor continuously for trends and responses to management modalities especially in those with continual air flow obstruction

    A. Vital signs

    B. Skin quality and appearance

    C. Blood gases and blood pH
    D. Respiratory status
    E. Cardiac status
    F. Development of hypoxemia
        1. anxiety, restlessness, confusion
        2. tachycardia
        3. dysrhythmias
        4. insomnia or altered mentation
        5. diaphoresis
        6. central cyanosis
        7. cardiac and renal failure
        8. coma
VI. Establish measures to promote physical and emotional well-being
    A. Instruct and discuss all aspects of care with conscious patient
    B. Frequent positioning to prevent pneumonia
    C. Coughing and deep breathing exercises as often as possible
    D. Maintain adequate fluid intake
    E. Aseptic technique
        1. at all infusion sites
        2. during suctioning
        3. with tracheostomy care
        4. with indwelling urethral catheter care
    F. Techniques to provide emotional support
    G. Techniques to allay anxiety of family members or significant others

RATIONALE

Acute airway obstruction of any degree requires immediate attention and management. The major concern is to reestablish the airway either by removing or bypassing the obstruction. The first step undertaken by the rescuer at the scene or at an emergency station is to examine the posterior mouth for any visible object causing the obstruction. If found, the patient should be placed on his or her side and the mouth wiped out with a piece of material. If the individual continues to choke or if the object is not visible, any of the identified maneuvers, or a combination thereof may be used. If pregnant women or obese individuals, the chest thrust is the technique of choice.

    In those patients for whom these maneuvers have proven inadequate, immediate emergency management is necessary and vital. Arterial hypoxemia rapidly ensues in the acutely obstructed person, followed by loss of consciousness, asphyxia, and death.

    Once in the emergency room, ventilatory status is evaluated and appropriate ventilatory support is begun in order to reestablish an airway. Techniques to remove foreign bodies are instituted. Laryngeal foreign bodies are generally removed with a grasping forceps through a direct laryngoscope while the patient is positioned in a Trendelenberg position and under local or general anesthesia. Bronchial foreign objects are removed through a bronchoscope and under general anesthesia. In some instances, when the object lies in the lung periphery, a thoracotomy may be necessary to retrieve it. It is necessary that bronchial foreign bodies be identified and that exhaustive measures be instituted to make that identification. Unrecognized foreign bodies in the bronchi may lead to severe and progressive pulmonary infections (e.g., abscesses, empyema, pneumonia).

In the event that an endotracheal tube cannot be passed for the reasons identified, surgical approaches in the form of cricothyrotomy or tracheostomy may be performed. The lumen of the cricothyrotomy catheter can be used not only for ventilatory support, but also for suctioning. If an artificial airway is needed for longer than 48 hours, and an endotracheal tube still cannot be passed, a tracheostomy must be performed. If at all feasible, it is a good tactic to insert an endotracheal tube prior to performing a tracheostomy for the following reasons: to control ventilation during the procedure and to prevent aspiration during the procedure. The presence of inadequate respiratory effort despite the open airway may necessitate the intervention of mechanical ventilation, especially in the face of nonspontaneous breathing. Ventilatory support is guided through such parameters as the need for assist or controlled ventilation, blood gas determinations, tidal volumes, percentage of oxygen needed, maximum pressure, sigh frequency, sigh volume, and required dead space. Blood gases and blood pH determinations must be assessed frequently to address the adequacy of this ventilatory intervention.

Appropriate measures must be instituted to support the emergency modalities. Baseline data related to vital signs, physical changes in appearance, system checks, and signs and symptoms of developing hypoxemia must be initially gathered so that continual monitoring throughout the emergency period will indicate trends and responses of the patient to the prescribed management.

Physical and emotional well-being are important to the care of all individuals, however, the sense of impending death from possible asphyxia and the anxiety it produces weighs heavily on the individual with acute upper airway obstruction. Every possible effort and technique must be made to promote physical and emotional support, and to allay anxiety. Those identified measures are only some of the ways of achieving such ends; and it is hoped that all members of the professional emergency team will consider the emotional component of management as well as the physical component.

2. Croup

ASSESSMENT

I. Initial asessment data
  A. Age of child
  B. Recency of upper respiratory infection
  C. Time of onset

      D. Frequency and length of spasm
      E. Presenting conditions
         1. temperature
         2. status of hydration
         3. unable to lie down
         4. frightened appearance
         5. struggling for breath

II. Alterations in respiratory status
      A. Utilization of accessory muscles of respiration
         1. flaring of nostrils
         2. suprasternal retractions
         3. subcostal and/or intercostal retractions
      B. Mouth breathing
      C. Harsh inspiratory stridor
      D. Hoarse or barking-like cough
      E. Possible cyanotic changes (first noted in lips and nails)
      F. Symptoms of hypoxia
         1. anxiety, restlessness, confusion
         2. tachycardia
         3. dysrhythmias
         4. insomnia and/or altered mentation
         5. diaphoresis
         6. central cyanosis
         7. cardiac and/or renal failure
         8. coma
      G. Viscous mucus

III. Alterations in central nervous system
      A. Obtunded ⎫ CNS failure
      B. Hypotonic ⎭

IV. Assess laboratory and other diagnostic parameters
      A. Electrolytes
      B. Blood gases and pH
      C. Blood culture
      D. Sputum culture
      E. Chest film

V. Assess croup severity via croup score (e.g., Downes Croup Score). (See Fig. 3.)

PATHOPHYSIOLOGY

The term croup is a generalized term for inflammation of the larynx. It is quite common in children with a susceptible or small airway and those that suffer from a cold or upper respiratory infection. The clinical picture of this inflammatory manifestation is spasm of the laryngeal muscles, partial respiratory obstruction, and the classic respiratory signs and symptoms listed.

    Croup is specific to very young children, usually between the ages of two and

	0	1	2
Inspiratory breath sounds	Normal	Harsh with rhonchi	Delayed
Stridor	None	Inspiratory	Inspiratory and expiratory
Cough	None	Hoarse cry	Bark
Retractions and flaring	None	Flaring and supersternal retractions	As under 1, plus subcostal and intercostal retractions
Cyanosis	None	In air	In 40 percent oxygen

Figure 3. Clinical croup score. (*After J. J. Downes. Emergency Medicine, Jan. 15, 1982, p. 141.*)

five, and there may be an individual or familial predisposition to this syndrome. Croup attacks are acute, dramatic, usually appear at night, and may occur more than once during the same night. In the presence of upper respiratory infection, changes of temperature from one room to another may precipitate a spasm. These spasms cause difficult inspiration with concomitant inspiratory stridor, use of accessory muscles of respiration, the sudden sitting up position, and in severe spasm, the appearance of impending asphyxia. Except for complications, croup is rarely fatal. It is important once the child is seen in the emergency room to assess the severity of croup as objectively as possible. The Downes Croup Score is a convenient and objective measure which allows the physician or nurse to assess each of the five categories included on the score chart according to an assigned numerical value (see Fig. 3). A score of five or more points is generally a cause for concern. This assessment should be done several times during the observation period, and especially following initial therapy to determine the status of the child's response.

If the child is to be hospitalized because of progressive symptomatology, e.g., continued cyanosis, increase in the Downes Croup Score, nonresponsiveness to initial therapy, he or she must be carefully monitored for impending hypoxemia, respiratory, and central nervous system failure, so that more aggressive management may be instituted.

MANAGEMENT

I. Institute measures to reduce bronchial spasm and viscous mucus
   A. High mist therapy
   B. Oxygen via mist mask
   C. Croupette
   D. Intravenous fluids
   E. Antispasmodic drugs (e.g., syrup of Ipecac, especially in infants, ½ tsp q 15 minutes until 3 doses ingested)
   F. Racemic epinephrine (via inhalation), 0.5 ml of a 25 percent solution in 25 ml normal saline q 1 hour, prn
   G. Steroids (if artificial airway indicated)
II. Institute measures to support management modalities by establishing
   A. Intravenous line
   B. Arterial line, if needed

   C. Intravenous fluids
   D. Laboratory tests
      1. serum electrolytes
      2. blood gases and pH, as indicated
      3. blood and sputum cultures
   E. ECG monitoring
   F. Chest films
III. Monitor continuously for trends and responses to management modalities
   A. Temperature, pulse, respirations, and bp
   B. Level of consciousness
   C. Skin quality and appearance
   D. Electrolytes and gases, specifically P_{CO_2}
   E. Hydration status
   F. ECG for dysrhythmias when sympathomimetic therapy utilized
   G. Croup score chart
IV. Promote and institute measures to prevent respiratory and central nervous system failure
   A. Nasotracheal intubation
   B. Tracheostomy
   C. Indicators for artificial airway
      1. rising croup score
      2. rising P_{CO_2}
      3. persistent cyanosis
      4. use of racemic epinephrine more frequently than indicated
 V. Promote measures to combat infection
   A. Chemotherapy for severe infections
   B. Aseptic technique for intubation or tracheostomy care
VI. Initiate measures to promote comfort
   A. Encourage frequent parent visits
   B. Attendance by nurse other than at treatment time
   C. Emotional support to parents and child
   D. Small doses of phenobarbital for extreme anxiety in children

---

RATIONALE

Initial management is directed toward relieving the laryngeal spasm, and liquefying and eliminating the viscous mucus. The child is started on high mist therapy. Various means may be employed to administer the moist air such as a croupette, mist under compressed air, or with a high mist oxygen mask. In addition, intravenous fluids may be administered to maintain optimal hydration and to compensate for lack of oral fluids taken because of difficult swallowing.

   To achieve vasoconstrictive effects on the swollen laryngeal tissues, racemic epinephrine may be introduced via inhalation in the dose recommended. Caution must be exercised when using this drug because of the possibility of rebound vasoconstriction 2 to 3 hours after administration. Sympathomimetic drugs carry with them myocardiotoxicity. If the child is hypoxic, the use of racemic epinephrine may trigger dysrhythmias, therefore the child must be placed on a cardiac monitor.

A variety of antispasmodic drugs are available for preventing or relieving the laryngeal spasms. Among them is syrup of Ipecac. When given in recommended doses, especially in infants, it will promote emesis, and at the same time expulsion of the mucus.

The use of steroids is still controversial in the treatment of croup, but may be indicated for those children who have not responded to initial therapy and in whom there is continual laryngeal swelling. Steroids are employed usually when artificial airway is anticipated.

Baseline data must be gathered regarding electrolyte imbalances, acid–base disturbances, hydration status, vital signs, skin color and quality, radiologic films of the chest, and blood and sputum samples for culture and sensitivity, so that additional management modalities may be instituted if indicated.

Despite a variety of intervention modalities, there are those children who have progressive respiratory failure and if obtunded or hypotonic, experience central nervous system effects. Rising croup score, elevated P_{CO_2}, persistent cyanosis, frequent use of sympathomimetic drugs, coupled with the central nervous system effects are imminent danger signs, and an indicator for securing an artificial airway. Whether the child is intubated with a nasotracheal tube or a tracheostomy is performed, it is critical that it be performed by a specialist with ENT or anesthesia experience. Frequent blood gas studies are necessary to identify and treat any hypoxemia that may be present. Once an airway is established, constant care and observation of the airway is of fundamental importance to identify changes in respiratory status, child's reaction to treatment, bleeding, or signs of infection. In addition to scrupulous aseptic technique in caring for artificial airways, antibiotics may or may not be indicated depending on the results of blood and sputum cultures, presence of otitis media, or infiltrates identified on x-rays.

All possible measures must be used to allay the anxiety of, to promote the comfort of, and to provide emotional support for both child and parents.

3. Acute Epiglottitis

ASSESSMENT

I. Initial assessment data
   A. Age of onset (3 to 7 years of age; may be seen in adults)
   B. Abrupt onset
   C. Elevated temperature
   D. Drooling, precipitated by difficult swallowing
   E. Severe sore throat

    F. assumes classical positioning
      1. sits upright
      2. jaw thrust forward
      3. arms back
    G. Anxious in appearance
    H. Dysphonic
    I. Fiery red and swollen epiglottis
      1. identified in child by depression of tongue while in upright position
      2. identified by direct or indirect laryngoscopy in adults
II. Alterations in respiratory status
    A. Rapid and progressive airway obstruction
    B. Dyspnea
    C. Distress on inspiration
    D. Minimal or no difficulty on expiration
III. Alterations in acid–base imbalances
    A. Hypoxic state
      1. anxiety, restlessness, confusion
      2. tachycardia
      3. dysrhythmias
      4. insomnia and/or altered mentation
      5. diaphoresis
      6. central cyanosis
      7. cardiac and/or renal failure
      8. coma
    B. Hypercapneic state
      1. headache
      2. papilledema and/or miosis
      3. confusion; changes in mentation
      4. diaphoresis
      5. hypertension progressing to hypotension
      6. somnolence
      7. muscle twitching
      8. asterixis
      9. coma
      10. cardiac failure and renal failure
IV. Laboratory diagnostic studies
    A. Blood culture
    B. Cultures from epiglottal surface
    C. Examination for ampicillin and chloramphenicol sensitivity
    D. CBC and differential
V. X-ray diagnostic studies
    A. Lateral, anterior, and posterior neck
      1. swollen aryepiglottis folds
      2. swollen epiglottis
    B. Chest film for infiltrates (pneumonia)

PATHOPHYSIOLOGY

Epiglottitis is an inflammatory process involving the epiglottis, the aryepiglottic folds, and the ventricular folds. It is characterized by cellulitis and gross edema of these structures due to a bacterial infection usually *Hemophilus influenzae*, type B. The majority of cases of epiglottitis occurs in children 3 to 7 years of age, although there appears to be a rise in the incidence of this condition in adults. The exact mechanism by which the organism infects the epiglottis is not known, but it is suspected that the infection follows direct invasion by *H. influenzae.*

Presenting symptomatology is directly related to progressive obstruction of the airway when all the tissues in and around the epiglottis begin to swell. With progressive edema and infection, the epiglottis begins to curl posteriorly and inferiorly. The process of inspiration continually aggravates this situation by pulling the edematous epiglottis down into the laryngeal inlet, thus producing the signs and symptoms of inspiratory distress.

High fever, inspiratory difficulties, drooling, dysphagia, severe sore throat, and the classic positioning identified are the clues to the diagnosis of acute epiglottitis. Inadequate air flow caused by the progressively obstructed airway results in inadequate oxygenation as well as increased carbon dioxide concentration in the arterial blood which leads to hypoxic and hypercapneic states.

Direct examination, which identifies a fiery red and swollen epiglottis, should never be attempted unless an airway team is standing by to provide an artificial airway in case of cardiorespiratory arrest. Controversy exists as to whether or not to instrument a child even with a tongue blade unless an airway team is present, and the child is placed under anesthesia. In older children and adults, it may be necessary to use either direct or indirect laryngoscopy to confirm the diagnosis.

Laboratory studies to confirm the diagnosis should include a white blood cell count and differential, blood, and epiglottal mucus cultures to identify the *H. influenzae* type B organism, as well as sensitivity studies to determine if β-lactamase is present. β-lactamase indicates that the identified organism is ampicillin-resistant.

Radiologic studies of the neck may be indicated when examination of the epiglottis has not been conclusive. The use of this medium may, however, delay definitive emergency management and possibly heighten the risk of respiratory embarrassment. Despite the possible initial delay in management, x-rays of the neck involving anterior, posterior, and lateral views taken during inspiration are considered a reliable alternative to examining the edematous epiglottis and the aryepiglottic folds.

MANAGEMENT

I. Establish measures to insure adequate oxygenation and patency of airway
   A. Oxygen therapy
   B. Endotracheal intubation
   C. Tracheostomy

II. Institute measures to maintain airway humidity and to liquefy secretions
   A. Periodic suctioning of tracheal secretions
   B. Frequent positioning changes
   C. Postural drainage
   D. Cold water nebulization
III. Establish measures to support management modalities
   A. Intravenous line
   B. Arterial line (if necessary)
   C. Laboratory data
      1. serum electrolytes
      2. blood gases and blood pH, as indicated
      3. blood and epiglottal mucus cultures
      4. sensitivity studies for β-lactamase production (ampicillin-resistant *H. influenzae* type B)
   D. ECG monitoring, if necessary
IV. Promote measures to insure hydration and prevent acidosis
   A. IV fluids (120 to 140 ml/100 cal)
   B. Maintenance sodium (3 mEq/100 cal) in children
   C. Potassium (3 mEq/100 cal)
V. Promote measures to combat infection
   A. ampicillin (200 to 400 mg/kg daily q 4 hour intervals, IV)
   B. chloramphenicol (50 to 100 mg/kg daily q 6 hour intervals, IV for a maximum of 4 g daily)
   C. Sterile tracheal care
VI. Monitor continuously for trends and responses to management modalities
   A. Temperature, pulse, respirations, bp
   B. Mentation; anxiety level
   C. Skin quality and appearance
   D. Blood pH, electrolytes and gases, especially P_{CO_2}
   E. Hydration status
VII. Initiate measures to promote comfort
   A. Emotional support
   B. Attendance by nurse other than at treatment time

RATIONALE

The success of all management modalities in the treatment of epiglottitis is based on securing an airway and in administering antibiotics. Once an airway is established, humidified oxygen is given to maintain airway humidity as well as to liquefy secretions. The periodic suctioning, frequent positioning changes, and the possible use of postural drainage all assist in maintaining airway patency.

Intravenous fluids are necessary to maintain adequate hydration. If abnormal laboratory values so indicate, electrolytes and other chemical elements may be given in the intravenous fluids; these, in association with oxygen therapy, are used to alleviate a developing acidotic state.

Measures to combat infection are of paramount importance and should be initiated immediately. Ampicillin and chloramphenicol is the combination drug therapy of choice against the *H. influenzae* type B organism. Even though some strains of *H. influenzae* type B are resistant to ampicillin, the literature does not at this time record any strains recovered from those ill with the disease that are resistant to both of these drugs. Careful and meticulous aseptic technique in suctioning and in handling tracheal secretions will be a deterrent to furthering the infection.

Continuous monitoring of vital signs, mentation, skin quality and color, blood gases, pH, electrolytes, status of hydration, and other assessment parameters is necessary to identify trends and responses to the emergency management modalities.

Acute epiglottitis is a frightening disease. The rapid progression of the airway obstruction gives rise to the presenting signs and symptoms. These signs and symptoms can be exacerbated by the child's or adult's anxiety; therefore, measures to promote comfort and allay anxiety will prove most beneficial.

4. Status Asthmaticus

ASSESSMENT

I. Initial assessment data
  A. Possible precipitating episodes
    1. recent history of asthmatic over- or undermedication
    2. presence of upper respiratory infection
    3. progression of respiratory symptoms prior to admission
    4. psychologic crisis or emotional stress prior to attack
    5. history of present medications
  B. General appearance and demeanor
    1. anxious and apprehensive
    2. unable to assume recumbent position
    3. flushing or perspiration of face and upper torso
    4. monosyllabic speech
II. Alterations in respiratory status
  A. Shortness of breath
  B. Wheezing
  C. Tightness in chest and dyspnea
  D. Difficult inspiration
  E. Coughing with inability to raise sputum
  F. Tenacious sputum
  G. Use of accessory muscles of respiration
  H. Tachypnea
  I. Auscultative findings
    1. hyperresonance
    2. low-lying diaphragm

    3. hyperinflation

    4. distant, loud, and coarse breath sounds

    5. prolonged respiration

    6. coarse, musical rhonchi

    7. focal rales ⎫

    8. areas of consolidation ⎬ ? atelectesis or pneumonia

    9. paradoxically silent chest (ominous sign)

III. Alterations in cardiovascular status

    A. Hypertension ⎫ reflect increased catecholamine output

    B. Tachycardia ⎭

    C. Rapid pulse (greater than 130/minute indicative of hypoxia)

    D. Pulsus paradoxus (pulmonary hyperinflation)

IV. Alterations in acid–base and fluid imbalances

    A. Respiratory alkalosis

        1. tachypnea

        2. headache

        3. vertigo

        4. syncope

        5. paresthesias of hands and face

        6. tetany

        7. carpopedal spasms

        8. altered sensorium

    B. Hypoxemia

        1. anxiety, restlessness, confusion

        2. tachycardia

        3. dysrhythmias

        4. insomnia and/or altered mentation

        5. diaphoresis

        6. central cyanosis

        7. cardiac and renal failure

        8. coma

    C. Respiratory acidosis

        1. headache

        2. papilledema and/or miosis

        3. confusion; changes in mentation

        4. diaphoresis

        5. hypertension progressing to hypotension

        6. somnolence

        7. muscle twitching

        8. asterixis

        9. coma

      10. cardiac failure and renal failure

    D. Dehydration

        1. thirst (in mentally alert patient)

        2. poor skin turgor (especially over forehead and upper chest)

3. dryness of skin and mucous membranes
4. dry and furrowed tongue
5. soft and sunken eyeballs
6. weight loss
7. increased temperature
8. apprehensive and restless
9. oliguria progressing to anuria
10. coma (severe dehydration)
11. renal shutdown (severe dehydration)
12. concentrated urine with elevated specific gravity above 1.030
13. urine sodium less than 10 mEq/L
14. elevated hematocrit
15. serum sodium above 150 mEq/L

V. Alterations in laboratory and other diagnostic studies
  A. Sputum (gross and microscopic exam)
    1. pathology
    2. Curschmann spirals (indicative of asthma)
    3. tenacious, white, mucoid sputum (indicative of allergic insults)
    4. purulent sputum (indicative of infection)
    5. high eosinophil count
  B. Blood tests
    1. WBC and differential
    2. blood chemistries
    3. immunoglobulin concentration
    4. blood gases and pH
      a. respiratory acidosis
        i. pH below 7.35
        ii. P_{CO_2} below 40 mm Hg
        iii. P_{O_2} normal (90 to 100) or decreased (90 to 60 mm Hg)
        iv. HCO_3 above 21 to 28 mEq/L (partial or complete compensation) HCO_3 normal (21 to 28 mEq/L) if compensated
      b. respiratory alkalosis
        i. pH above 7.45
        ii. P_{CO_2} below 40 mm Hg
        iii. P_{O_2} generally normal (90 to 100 mm Hg)
        iv. HCO_3 normal (21 to 28 mEq/L) uncompensated HCO_3 below 21 mEq/L if compensated
  C. Urine analysis
  D. X-ray
    1. hyperlucency of lung tissue
    2. widening of costal interspaces
    3. depressed diaphragm
    4. increased air retrosternally
  E. Electrocardiogram
    1. sinus tachycardia (severe hypoxemia)

    2. right bundle branch block $\Big\}$ severe asthmatic attack
       prominent right atrial P waves

    3. myocardial ischemia $\Big]$ asthmatic episodic distress in elderly and with car-
       other dysrhythmias diac stimulating drugs

VI. Assess for and rule out other biophysiologic disruptions
    A. Pleurisy
    B. Atelectesis
    C. Heart failure
    D. Pneumonitis
    E. Pulmonary emboli
    F. Pneumothorax

PATHOPHYSIOLOGY

Asthma, a clinical term of long standing, is an aggregate of concurrent symptoms arising from a wide spectrum of etiologic factors. It is characterized by an augmented response of the trachea and bronchi to a variety of stimuli, demonstrated by a narrowing of the airways. A number of theories have been generated concerning the causation of the airway obstruction and the presenting clinical picture. These theories consider the hyperactive airway response to be a result of one of three reasons: (1) exaggeration of the normal defenses within the respiratory tract, (2) abnormal tissue reactions in the bronchioles, which may have been induced immunologically, or (3) as an imbalance of the normally balanced responses.

Two basic pathophysiologic pathways are offered in the literature for this reactive response. One involves a reflex action in which the autonomic nerves are triggered by irritants, and, as a result, stimulate a hypersecretion of mucus and capillary dilation. In this situation, it is believed that the individual has a deficit in the sympathetic nerves that innervate the bronchi. These β-adrenergic end plates fail to produce both smooth muscle relaxation and a decrease in mucous secretion in the presence of bronchial hypersensitivity as a response to stimulants. The second pathway is concerned with antigen–antibody reaction. In this instance, the bronchial hypersensitivity is generated by the exceptional ability of susceptible individuals to form abnormally large amounts of IgE when they are first exposed to specific allergens. The immunoglobulin IgE attaches itself to the bronchial mast cells, and upon a further encounter with the same allergen, causes the mast cells to degranulate and release a number of chemical mediators, specifically histamine and the slow-reacting substance of anaphylaxis (SRS-A). Both of these chemical mediators produce bronchospasm.

Factors other than immunologic reactions may precipitate an asthmatic attack. Such factors may include severe emotional states, psychologic crises, respiratory infections, exercise, exposure to cold air, as well as adverse reactions or intolerance to certain medications.

Despite the specific mechanisms that may produce the asthmatic episode, the effects of airway obstruction on respiratory function and on blood gases and blood pH are similar, giving rise to the symptoms of respiratory distress and the concomitant respiratory acidosis and hypoxemia. Impaired air flow causes impaired ventilation. In addition, bronchospasms, hypersecretion of mucus, edema, and inflammatory response all contribute to the narrowing and obstruction of the bronchi and bronchiolar structures. The obstruction not only impairs the distribution of gases to alveoli and ventilation, but also causes the muscles of respiration to produce greater chest expansion to increase the inspiratory driving force. The muscles of respiration are also called upon to play a greater role in the process of expiration because of the lungs' decreased recoil capacity.

In the early stages of a severe attack when hypocapnia and hypoxemia are first noted, respiratory alkalosis is evident by blood gas determinations (Pa_{O_2} between 55 to 70 mm Hg; Sa_{O_2} between 85 to 90 percent; Pa_{CO_2} less than 30 mm Hg; and blood pH > 7.50). As the obstruction progresses and the expiration is increasingly prolonged, air becomes trapped. The trapped air increases the residual volume and causes the individual, as a compensatory response, to breathe at higher lung volumes thus producing hyperinflation. The work of breathing is increased as respiration effectiveness is decreased, and dyspnea, tachypnea, and cyanosis become markedly pronounced.

As a result of alveolar hypoventilation and the pronounced ventilatory–perfusion disturbances, hypoxemia becomes a primary gas exchange defect in asthma. In addition, the increased work of breathing increases the oxygen needs, increases carbon dioxide production and rentention, and is directly responsible for the development of respiratory acidosis. The presence of hypoxemia and respiratory acidosis causes a reactive pulmonary hypertension. Further failure in ventilation, in combination with the pulmonary hypertension, are responsible for the development of cardiac arrhythmias and respiratory failure.

Status asthmaticus is said to exist when conventional therapy is noneffective for an acute asthmatic attack. It is an extreme emergency situation and hospitalization is critical because of the intense medical and nursing care required for management and monitoring.

MANAGEMENT

    I. Establish measures to insure adequate oxygenation and airway humidity
       A. Nasal cannula with humidified oxygen
       B. Venturi mask with humidified oxygen
       C. Oxygen at 4 L/minute and adjust to Pa_{O_2} results
    II. Institute measures to mobilize secretions, clear airway, and promote hydration
       A. Remove secretions
          1. coughing
          2. frequent position changes
          3. pulmonary toilet
          4. suctioning (especially when obtunded or with endotracheal tube)

     5. bronchoscopy and lavage (when suctioning is unsuccessful)

B. Fluids

    1. oral, if possible

    2. intravenous

       a. D5W in quarter

          percent normal saline } maintain urine output at 50 ml/hour

       b. 3 to 4 L/24 hour

C. Pharmacologic agents

    1. expectorants

       a. potassium iodide solution, po

       b. ammonium chloride solution, po

       c. glyceryl guaiacolate, po

    2. mucolytics

       a. *N*-acetylcysteine (Mucomyst, Respaire)

         i. via nebulization or endotracheal instillation

        ii. 3 to 5 ml of 5 to 10 percent *N*-acetylcysteine mixed with 0.5 ml of 1:200 isoproterenol

        iii. monitor for possible increased bronchospasm

       b. desoxyribonuclease (Dormavoc)—50,000 to 100,000 units tid, via aerosol for 2 to 6 days

III. Promote measures to relieve bronchial spasms

A. Catecholamines

    1. aqueous epinephrine 1:1000

       a. children: 0.01 ml/kg, sc, repeated at 30 to 60 minute intervals times 2 doses

       b. adults: 0.2 to 0.3 ml, sc repeated at 30 to 60 minute intervals times 2 doses

    2. isoproterenol

       a. nebulizer: 0.25 to 0.5 ml of 1:200 solution with 2 ml saline, q 6 hours

       b. intravenously: 1 to 4 mg/minute continuous drip

       c. not recommended for children

       d. assess for dysrhythmias

B. Xanthines

    1. aminophylline

       a. initial dose: 6 mg/kg IV in 100 ml D5W over 20 minutes

       b. reduce or eliminate initial dose for those taking aminophylline previously

       c. use ideal weight for dose calculation in overweight patients

       d. FDA recommended schedule for continuous intravenous infusion

         i. children and young adult smokers: 1 mg/kg/hour for 12 hours, then reduce to 0.8 mg/kg/hour

        ii. healthy nonsmoking adults: 0.7 mg/kg/hour for 12 hours, then reduce to 0.5 mg/kg/hour

        iii. older patients and those with cor pulmonale: 0.6 mg/kg/hour for 12 hours, then reduce to 0.3 mg/kg/hour

   iv. CHF and liver failure: 0.5 mg/kg/hour for 12 hours, then reduce to 0.1 to 0.2 mg/kg/hour

   v. subsequent doses determined by serum concentration (10 to 20 μg/ml recognized therapeutic range)

   vi. not to exceed 2 g daily

   vii. assess for theophylline side effects

    (a) abdominal pain

    (b) seizures

    (c) nausea, vomiting, diarrhea

    (d) coma

    (e) death

  2. choline theophylline (Choledyl)

  3. theophylline (Aqualin, Elixophyllin)

 C. Corticosteroids

  1. prednisone: 40 to 80 mg IV (initial dose)

   a. adult: 300 to 400 mg daily

   b. child: 2 mg/kg/24 hours

  2. methylprednisolone sodium succinate

   a. adult: 250 mg IV as loading dose

   b. reevaluate q 6 hours for succeeding doses

  3. corticosteroid monitoring

   a. hypokalemia

   b. hypoglycemia

   c. suprarenal suppression

   d. aggravation of diabetes mellitus

   e. hypertension

IV. Institute measures to prevent or treat acid–base imbalances

 A. Respiratory alkalosis

  1. use of rebreathing mask

  2. encourage breathing techniques

  3. if hyperventilating because of vigorous mechanical ventilation, reduce output of ventilator to appropriate minute volume

 B. Respiratory acidosis

  1. suction as necessary

  2. chest physiotherapy

  3. be alert to increase pulse rate or respiratory distress

  4. maintain O_2 flow as per order

  5. if on ventilator, reduce output to appropriate minute volume

  6. sodium bicarbonate administration

   a. 45 to 90 mEq/L, IV over 5 minutes, followed by repeated arterial gases

   b. repeat q 30 minutes until acidemia corrected (pH between 7.35 and 7.40)

 C. Metabolic acidosis (especially in infants and children)

  1. maintain I&O for planning fluid replacement

       2. sodium bicarbonate

       3. evaluate for signs of cardiovascular collapse

       4. evaluate for progressive hypoxemia

       5. observe for diarrheal episodes

       6. observe for signs and symptoms of dehydration

       7. administer pharmacologic agents based on biochemical assessments and clinical events

    D. Metabolic alkalosis

       1. maintain I&O to determine chloride and potassium ion depletion (vomiting, diuretics, nasogastric suctioning, diarrhea, or chronic corticosteroid therapy)

       2. appropriate electrolyte replacement

       3. evaluate clinical changes indicative of metabolic alkalosis

       4. seizure precautions for possible convulsions or tetany

V. Establish measures to support management modalities

    A. Intravenous line

    B. Arterial line

    C. Laboratory data

       1. serum electrolytes

       2. blood gases and blood pH

       3. glucose levels

    D. Electrocardiographic monitoring

    E. Indwelling urethral catheter

VI. Monitor continuously for trends and responses to management modalities

    A. Temperature, pulse, respirations, bp

    B. Mentation; anxiety level

    C. Skin quality and appearance

    D. Blood gases and pH

    E. Electrolytes

    F. Glucose level (especially if on corticosteroid therapy)

    G. Hydration status

    H. Patency of airway

    I. Cardiac status

    J. Renal status

VII. Institute mechanical modalities for support of respiratory system

    A. Indications for mechanical intervention

       1. rising CO_2 tension and other biochemical observations

       2. apnea

       3. coma

    B. Modalities

       1. endotracheal intubation

       2. mechanical ventilator

    C. Specific parameters for monitoring ventilator effectiveness

       1. arterial blood gases and pH

       2. vital signs

3. ECG, chest films
4. sputum (volume, characteristics, and culture results)
5. lung compliance
6. body weight
7. I&O
8. CVP, if indicated
VIII. Promote measures to combat infection
    A. Aseptic technique when suctioning
    B. Antibiotics as indicated by culture results
  IX. Initiate measures to promote emotional well-being
    A. Develop rapport and open communication with patient
    B. Adequate instruction and information on patient's condition
    C. Physical and emotional comfort

RATIONALE

Oxygen administration is a basic and immediate intervention for the patient in status asthmaticus. If the arterial oxygen tension is allowed to fall below 20 to 25 mm Hg for more than a few minutes, it may lead to irreversible damage to the brain, heart, kidneys, or possible death. In less severe oxygen tension ranges, the degree of hypoxia may result in a variety of biophysiologic and metabolic disruptions, including cardiac failure, pulmonary hypertension, hepatic injury, encephalopathy, or increased airway resistance. Humidification is necessary to reduce the drying of mucosal secretions and the resultant bronchial irritation.

A variety of measures have been identified to assist in the mobilization of secretions and in clearing the airway. The rationale for such is to facilitate the raising of secretions and to ultimately help in diminishing or terminating the asthmatic attack. One major modality that assists in this process is the insurance of adequate hydration. It has been found that many patients in status asthmaticus are in a dehydrated state because of a variety of factors (e.g., reduced fluid intake, diaphoresis, vomiting) and, as a result, the secretions become thick and tenacious. Hydration assists in thinning out the mucus and renders it easier to mobilize for coughing and suctioning. In addition, adequate hydration prevents the development of hypovolemia, which has been reported as a cause of death in status asthmaticus. Expectorant and mucolytic drugs may be used concurrently with humidification and hydration for the loosening and possibly breaking down of mucus, especially when purulent secretions are present.

Relief of bronchospasms is paramount in the emergency management of status asthmaticus. Three categories of pharmacologic agents may be employed to relieve and reverse this problem. Initial therapy begins with the use of catecholamines, namely, epinephrine and isoproterenol, which act by stimulating the β-adrenergic receptors. Harmful adverse responses may be noted, however, such as refractoriness to management, decrease in arterial oxygen tension, and progressive airway obstruction. The patient must be continuously monitored for these responses. At times, the nonresponse to epinephrine therapy is related to the presence of respiratory acidosis, which can be corrected by administration of sodium bicarbonate and other intervention modalities which reduce the arterial carbon dioxide level. Isoproterenol may occasionally cause severe bronchospasm. This bronchospasm may be a result of a formation of a metabolite with a β-blocking action. Both drugs may have to be discontinued if the patient's condition worsens.

A second group of drugs, the xanthines, have been found more beneficial in the treatment of status asthmaticus. Of this group, aminophylline appears to be the most potent and most effective. Aminophylline acts specifically by inhibiting phosphodiesterase, which results in higher cellular concentrations of cyclic adenosine monophosphate (AMP). This higher concentration of cyclic AMP prevents bronchocontractions, and ultimately, relaxation of the bronchiolar musculature.

A third group of drugs, the corticosteroids, have been shown to play a lifesaving role in the patient with status asthmaticus. The pharmacologic effects of the corticosteroids includes the enhancement of the catecholamine effect on β-adrenergic receptors in the bronchioles and on the inhibition of the enzyme phosphodiesterase—an enzyme that interferes with the diffusion of cyclic AMP into the cell where it activates the mechanism that prevents contraction of the bronchiolar musculature. Corticosteroid therapy must be maintained until clinical improvement is noted. Doses must be tapered gradually to prevent suprarenal suppression, especially when used in children. Prolonged therapy with corticosteroids can lead to serious multisystem effects.

The progression of airway obstruction and the refractoriness to conventional therapy leads to serious ventilation–perfusion disturbances. The impaired gas exchange in combination with electrolyte imbalances or depletions, cardiovascular collapse, hypovolemia resulting from dehydration, and other biophysical and metabolic disruptions may cause serious acid–base imbalances. Constant monitoring for these disturbances is vital so that measures, such as those mentioned, may be employed to prevent or treat these serious and often life-threatening sequelae to status asthmaticus.

In the face of ventilatory failure, it is necessary to institute mechanical modalities for support of the respiratory system. This consists of endotracheal intubation and the use of a mechanical ventilator. Indications for such interventions are made on the basis of progressive clinical deterioration and on blood gas and blood pH determinations. Specific assessment parameters have been identified to evaluate the effectiveness of mechanical ventilation on improving the patient's clinical status.

Antibiotics are not administered as a routine protocol in status asthmaticus. Appropriate antibiotic therapy is begun when specific infecting organisms are isolated from sputum and/or blood cultures. In the event of infection, every measure should be taken to reduce the potential of that infection, which includes the use of aseptic technique when suctioning, especially in endotracheal suctioning.

The psychologic and emotional impact of status asthmatics on the patient is overwhelming. Both physician and nurse must develop a rapport and open communication with the patient from the onset of admission and adequately instruct and inform the individual regarding the intervention strategies and expected outcome. Physical and emotional comforting helps alleviate this major stress.

5. Near Drowning

ASSESSMENT

I. Alterations in respiratory status
  A. Hypoxia
  B. Acidosis
  C. Aspirated contaminants
  D. Pulmonary insufficiency
  E. Pulmonary edema
  F. Rales, rhonchi
  G. Cyanosis
II. Alterations in consciousness
  A. Alert and wakeful
  B. Drowsy
  C. Stupor
  D. Coma
III. Alterations in fluid, electrolyte, and acid–base status
  A. Hypertonic (saltwater) aspirations
    1. hypernatremia
    2. hyperkalemia
    3. hyperchloremia   } uncommon and depends on amount aspirated
    4. hypercalcemia
    5. hypermagnesemia
  B. Hypotonic (freshwater) aspirations
    1. hyponatremia
    2. hyperkalemia
    3. hypochloremia   } uncommon and depends on amount aspirated
    4. hypocalcemia
    5. hypomagnesemia
  C. Metabolic (lactic) acidosis
IV. Alterations in cardiovascular status
  A. Dysrhythmias
  B. Possible falsely elevated central venous pressure
  C. Low cardiac output
V. Alterations in central nervous system status
  A. Psychomotor retardation
  B. Cervical injury
  C. Intracranial injury
  D. Increased intracranial pressure

      E. Nonpurposeful or random muscle activity
  VI. Alterations in hemopoietic system status
      A. Hemolysis
      B. Coagulation disorders
        1. abnormal prothrombin
        2. abnormal partial prothrombin
        3. abnormal platelet count
      C. Disseminated intravascular coagulopathy (possible)
 VII. Alterations in renal status
      A. Oliguria
      B. Hemoglobinuria
      C. Renal failure
VIII. Assess laboratory and other diagnostic parameters
      A. CBC
      B. Electrolytes including magnesium
      C. BUN
      D. Urine analysis
      E. Serum and urine hemoglobin (freshwater)
      F. Blood gases and pH
      G. PT, PTT and platelets
      H. Thrombin time, fibrinogen level, fibrin degradation products, and euglobulin lysis if PT, PTT, and platelet count deranged
      I. Gram stain of blood, urine, and tracheal secretions
      J. EEG
      K. ECG
      L. True temperature, via rectal probe (if hypothermia suspected)
      M. Radiologic studies of chest, skull, and cervical spine

PATHOPHYSIOLOGY

Drowning is suffocation or asphyxiation caused by immersion in a liquid. Near drowning implies that a state of survival has occurred following the initial immersion. Drowning and near drowning can be further delineated as "wet" when aspiration of liquid has occurred or "dry," postulated to be a result of asphyxia brought on by laryngospasm.

    The extent of injury or trauma depends on a variety of factors which include the tonicity of the liquid aspirated, the temperature of the liquid, duration of submersion, the nature and amount of contaminants or foreign material, and the duration of hypoxia. Animal studies have demonstrated significant physiologic differences, e.g., electrolyte abnormalities, hemoglobinuria, and blood volume changes between hypotonic and hypertonic liquid aspirations (Figs. 4 and 5). Studies of near drowning in humans demonstrate that despite the tonicity of aspirated fluid, the clinical picture is quite similar.

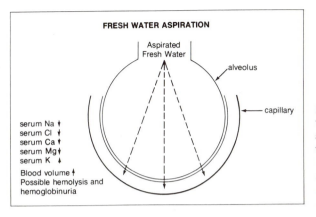

Figure 4. Fluid passes through the alveolus to the vascular space (freshwater is hypotonic to plasma). (*From Knopp, R. Near drowning. Journal of the American College of Emergency Physicians, 1978, 7 (6), 250.*)

Injury to the respiratory system is the major problem in near drowning and it is multifaceted. Immediately following the injury is the development of respiratory acidosis, metabolic lactic acidosis, and hypoxemia. Frequently, by the time the individual reaches an emergency service, the respiratory acidosis may have reversed either by artificial respiration administered at the scene and/or by spontaneous hyperventilation. Pulmonary edema may ensue as a result of hypertonic aspiration which pull fluids out of the circulation into the lung, decreased surfactant secondary to hypotonic fluid aspiration, contaminants that irritate the alveoli resulting in deposits of proteinaceous fluid into the alveoli, and from direct injury to the lungs or small vessels. The resultant pulmonary insufficiency precipitates hypoxia, cyanosis, rales, and rhonchi (Fig. 6).

Altered states of consciousness are directly related to cerebral anoxia. The longer the individual is immersed, the greater the chances are for the development

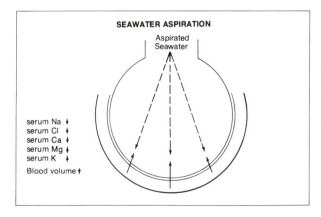

Figure 5. Fluid passes to the alveolus and, because it is three and one-half to four times more concentrated then plasma, draws protein-rich fluid from the vascular space to the alveolus. (*From Knopp, R. Near drowning. Journal of the American College of Emergency Physicians, 1978, 7 (6), 250.*)

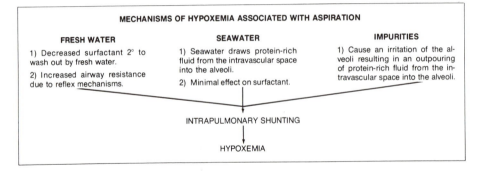

Figure 6. Proposed causes of hypoxemia associated with freshwater seawater, and impurities. (*From Knopp, R. Near drowning. Journal of the American College of Emergency Physicians, 1978, 7(6), 250.*)

of cerebral edema and anoxic encephalopathy. Water temperature also affects the conscious state. Immersion in cold fluid stimulates hyperventilation which in turn results in hypocapnea, altered mentation, and coma.

As previously mentioned, major electrolyte disturbances are not common in humans mainly because of the minimal amount of aspirate that enters the system. However, theoretical changes are possible with increased amounts of hypertonic or hypotonic aspiration (Figs. 4 and 5). Compensatory anaerobic metabolism develops because of increased oxygen demands, decreased oxygen transport, and decreased cardiac output. This lactic acidotic state may be intensified by cold water immersion which causes various vascular beds to cool at different rates thus decreasing the amount of circulating blood through the coronary and other vessels.

Alterations in cardiac status, namely, ventricular dysrhythmias and/or cardiac arrest are attributed to lactic acidosis, hypoxia, and hypothermia caused by cold water immersion, and possibly to electrolyte disturbances. Central venous pressure readings may be falsely elevated or unreliable in individuals demonstrating increased pulmonary–vascular resistance from the hypoxic–acidotic state, in individuals with right-sided heart failure, and in those with cardiovascular or pulmonary instability.

All near drowning victims must be carefully assessed for central nervous system damage because most of these individuals have some neurologic dysfunction. Neurologic pathology begins at the onset of hypoxia. Ischemic brain tissue rapidly becomes acidotic and is accompanied by cerebral edema, which, in turn, compromises cerebral perfusion and intensifies the possibility of cellular damage. Increased intracranial pressure results from cerebral edema and is probably responsible, in conjunction with increased oxygen consumption, for the nonpurposeful and/or random muscle activity observed. Additional neurologic assessment and observation must be made to identify cervical spinal injury or intracranial injuries which may be ameliorated by surgical intervention.

Hemopoietic disorders in the form of coagulation problems and hemolysis may be associated with both hypotonic and hypertonic near drowning immersions. These disorders may be initiated by a variety of factors including hypoperfusion, sepsis, hypoxia, or acidosis.

Renal failure is not a common finding in near drowning although oliguria is usually present during the first hours of admission. If renal failure is to occur it usually will not be noted for a few days. The pathology of renal insufficiency and renal failure is usually caused by acute tubular necrosis resulting from the hypoxemia. On occasion the failure may be due to large amounts of aspirated hypotonic fluid causing hemolysis and hemoglobin deposits in the renal tubules with a resultant hemoglobinuria.

MANAGEMENT

 I. Provide on-the-scene measures to support follow-up emergency management (Figs. 7 and 8)
    A. Monitor ABCs (airway, breathing, circulation, and vital signs)
    B. CPR (if indicated)
    C. Position to drain water from lungs
    D. IV line
    E. Oxygen (100 percent)
    F. Nonrebreathing mask for spontaneous respirations
    G. Intubation (if apneic)
    H. Sodium bicarbonate, 1 mEq/kg (if comatose or in severe respiratory distress)
    I. Cervical collar and spine board for transportation

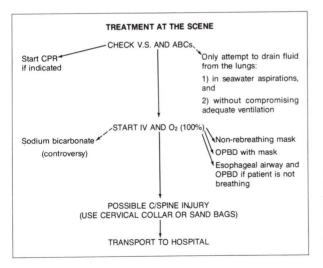

Figure 7. Protocol for treatment of submersion victim at the scene. (*From Knopp, R. Near drowning. Journal of the American College of Emergency Physicians, 1978, 7 (6), 252.*)

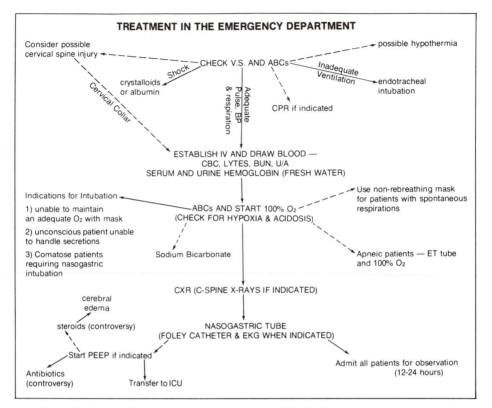

Figure 8. Protocol for treatment of submersion victim in the emergency department. (*From Knopp, R. Near drowning. Journal of the American College of Emergency Physicians, 1978,* **7** *(6), 253.*)

II. Institute measures to provide optimal pulmonary function and relieve hypoxia
   A. Oxygen via standard mask for responsive hypoxia
   B. CPAP via mask (continuous positive airway pressure)
      1. indicated for those patients not able to maintain PaO_2 greater than 50 torr via standard mask
      2. contraindicated for obtunded patients
      3. contraindicated for unconscious patients
      4. contraindicated for those with CO_2 retention
   C. Tracheal intubation with mechanical ventilator
      1. indicated for those with increased $PaCO_2$ above 50 torr despite adequate arterial oxygenation
      2. indicated for those unable to tolerate mask
      3. indicated in those when PaO_2 is not attained by other measures
      4. indicated for those with altered states of consciousness
      5. indicated for those who require CPR

    D. Fiberoptic bronchoscopy to remove minute material from bronchi

    E. Sodium bicarbonate to maintain pH above 7.25

    F. IV infusion of albumin (controversial)

    G. Diuretics

III. Institute measures to provide baseline data to support management modalities

    A. Intravenous lines

      1. peripheral

      2. central

    B. Foley catheter

    C. X-rays (chest, skull, and cervical spine)

    D. Nasogastric tube (if necessary)

    E. Laboratory tests

      1. CBC

      2. BUN

      3. urine analysis

      4. serum and urine hemoglobin (freshwater)

      5. electrolytes including magnesium

      6. blood gases and pH

      7. prothrombin time, partial prothrombin time, and platelet count

      8. thrombin time, fibrinogen level, fibrin degradation products, euglobulin lysis (if indicated)

    F. Rectal probe (if hypothermia suspected and for true temperature)

    G. ECG

    H. EEG

    I. Nasogastric intubation, if indicated

    J. Cultures of blood, urine, and tracheal secretions

IV. Monitor continuously for trends and responses to management modalities

    A. Temperature, pulse, respirations, and bp

    B. Central venous pressure

    C. Level of consciousness

    D. Skin quality and appearance

    E. Signs of shock

    F. Arterial pH and arterial gases

    G. Bicarbonate levels

    H. Kidney function (hourly output, character, quality and specific gravity)

    I. Cardiac function (Swan–Ganz determinations)

    J. Laboratory tests indicated

    K. Subjective responses

V. Promote and institute measures aimed at restoring fluid balance

    A. Normal saline

    B. Ringer's lactate

    C. Albumin (controversial)

    D. Blood, if indicated

  VI. Restore, maintain, and support cardiac function
     A. Swan–Ganz catheterization
     B. Inotropic support
       1. dopamine (3 to 10 μg/kg/minute)
       2. dobutamine (2.5 to 10 μg/kg/minute)
       3. isoproterenol (0.015 to 0.04 μg/kg/minute)
 VII. Restore, maintain, and support renal function
     A. Mannitol   (0.2 g/kg over 3 to 5 minutes; test dose)
                         (50 to 200 g in 24 hours)
     B. Dialysis (peritoneal)
VIII. Restore, maintain, and support central nervous system
     A. CAT scan
     B. Cerebral angiography
     C. Treat cerebral edema
       1. monitor increased intracranial pressure
       2. urea and/or mannitol, IV
       3. hyperventilation to reduce Pa_{CO_2} (range 25 to 30 torr)
       4. barbiturate, IV and guided by
         a. bp
         b. cardiac output
         c. intracranial pressure
       5. dopamine, IV   ⎫
       6. isoproterenol, IV ⎬ to support cardiovascular system against negative
       7. calcium, IV   ⎭ effects of barbiturates
     D. Control hyperpyrexia
       1. surface cooling
       2. antipyretics
     E. Neuromuscular blockers for random muscle activity
       1. valium
       2. barbiturates
       3. phenothiazine
  IX. Restore, maintain, and support hemopoietic system
     A. Fresh frozen plasma
     B. Platelets
   X. Institute measures for rewarming
     A. Surface rewarming
     B. Peritoneal dialysis with warmed solutions
     C. Rewarming guided by stringent monitoring of
       1. cardiac status (development of dysrhythmias)
       2. acid–base variables (development of lactic acidosis)
       3. electrolyte variables (development of hyperkalemia)
       4. hemodynamic variables (development of coagulation problems)
  XI. Promote measures designed to combat infection
     A. Antibiotics, if indicated
     B. Meticulous aseptic technique

RATIONALE

Management of near drowning victims must begin at the scene, and with the availability of telecommunications and emergency technicians, initial support management can be supervised from an emergency department. Those measures listed are the first lines of intervention modalities that effect follow-up emergency care.

Optimal pulmonary function and relief of hypoxia are priority objectives. Administration of oxygen via mask or by intubation is necessary to relieve the pulmonary inefficiency. Continuous positive airway pressure by mask and tracheal intubation with mechanical ventilator may be instituted and tailored to individual needs depending on arterial blood gas values, level of consciousness, responsiveness, and on other physiologic variables. Fiberoptic bronchoscopy may be indicated to remove aspirated minute particles that may be helping to compromise pulmonary efficiency. It must be noted that when CPAP or mechanical ventilation are used continuously cardiac output may be impeded or reduced. A controversial modality, namely the infusion of albumin, is being used for the purpose of slowing down the transudation of fluid into the lungs. The albumin, in effect, raises the plasma oncotic pressure and thereby maintains the fluid within the vascular spaces. Diuretics may or may not be used concomitantly with albumin to assist with the removal of fluids from the body. Sodium bicarbonate, guided by arterial blood gases and arterial pH levels, is used in those individuals in extreme respiratory distress, and who are exhibiting signs and symptoms of respiratory acidosis and metabolic lactic acidosis.

Numerous measures are necessarily instituted to support the management of near drowning victims. The measures indicated provide baseline data. Central and peripheral lines are established for fluid and drug administration, access to the general circulation, and in the case of the central line, venous pressure readings. A Foley catheter with urimeter allows for the continuous monitoring of urine with respect to character, output, specific gravity, and is a fairly reliable measure for adequacy of hydration, and, indirectly of vital organ perfusion. Radiologic studies of the chest, skull, and cervical spine are performed to rule out other specific injuries or trauma. The laboratory tests suggested are drawn several times during the first 24 hours, for example, to estimate kidney function, coagulation derangements, electrolyte imbalances, or acid–base imbalances. Cultures of blood, urine, and tracheal secretions are performed to identify infectious organisms. In those individuals who have suffered prolonged hypothermia or in those in whom hypothermia has been induced to promote central nervous system stabilization, the hypothermia suppresses the immune system and masks the signs and symptoms of infection. These results along with other identified parameters must be monitored continuously in terms of trends and responses to management modalities and corrective measures employed.

Shock and hypovolemia may be present in near drowning, especially in hypotonic immersion (freshwater). If present, normal saline, Ringer's lactate, albumin, or blood may be infused depending on the specific requirements of the individual.

Individuals with multisystem trauma, such as in near drowning, require astute and frequent observations of cardiac status. Central venous pressure readings may not be a stable indicator of cardiac stability. For this reason Swan–Ganz catheterization has become a major tool in the management of individuals with severe cardiorespiratory problems and provides more exacting measures of cardiac output, oxygen transport, and other hemodynamic parameters. Inotropic support may be necessary in treating a depressed myocardium in the presence of acidosis and hypoxia. Dopamine, dobutamine, and isoproterenol are effective inotropes that increase contractility of the myocardium, increase cardiac output, and increase renal blood flow without significant increases in peripheral resistance. Of these three drugs, isoproterenol may increase myocardial oxygen consumption to the greatest degree. Diuretics may be employed to lower hydrostatic pressure and ultimately decrease the crossing of fluid into the lung tissue.

The maintenance or restoration of renal perfusion and circulating volume is critical, and the administration of mannitol promotes adequate volumes of urine and prevents the renal tubules from being plugged with free hemoglobin. In cases of renal failure, peritoneal dialysis may be instituted, especially in the presence of acidotic and shock states when cardiac output is already compromised.

Because some form of central nervous system injury is present in most near drowning victims, radiologic studies must be performed as quickly as possible so that if surgical intervention is indicated, it may be carried out without delay. Increased intracranial pressure monitoring must be maintained in all patients with central nervous system dysfunction. The use of mannitol or urea can minimize the evolving cerebral edema. Hyperventilation, a technique that lowers the $Paco_2$ can be used along with the osmotic diuretics to assist in reducing the cerebral edema.

Intravenous barbiturate administration is an experimental modality instituted when osmotic diuretics have not been effective in reducing the elevated intracranial pressure. It is recommended that intravenous barbiturates only be administered when the patient is intubated and on mechanical ventilation. If cardiac output falls because of the negative inotropic effect of the barbiturates, inotropic agents must be used.

Extremely elevated body temperatures, a common accompaniment of near drowning, cause increased cerebral oxygen consumption. Antipyretics and surface cooling are indicated in the early management, especially in those with central nervous system trauma. Nonpurposeful or random muscle activity is often associated with cerebral edema and increased intracranial pressure. Neuromuscular blocking agents may be used to alleviate these symptoms, but it must be remembered that these agents may mask ongoing neurologic assessment.

Hemopoietic derangements in the form of coagulation disorders may develop as a result of acidosis, hypoxemia, hemolysis, and a variety of other factors related to the clotting mechanism. Fresh frozen plasma, platelets, and in some instances, whole blood are recommended to treat and prevent bleeding.

Following stabilization of cardiovascular and central nervous systems it may be necessary to consider rewarming the patient. Such a decision necessitates scrupulous observation in terms of the development of cardiac dysrhythmias, lactic acidosis, coagulation problems, and electrolyte imbalances, particularly hyperkalemia.

Appropriate antibiotics are indicated when cultures taken identify specific pathogenic organisms. Special attention must be paid to asepsis, especially when invasive techniques are performed, to combat and prevent infection or sepsis.

6. Adult Respiratory Distress Syndrome

ASSESSMENT

I. Initial assessment data
  A. Recent history of possible precipitating events
    1. trauma
      a. contusion of lung
      b. fat embolism
    2. intrinsic or extrinsic pathologic events
      a. shock states
      b. infections (bacterial, viral, fungal, mycoplasmal, parasitic)
      c. toxins (inhaled, ingested, injected)
      d. CNS disorders or insults (especially with increased intracranial pressure)
      e. allergic reactions (anaphylaxis)
      f. blood problems (DIC, multiple transfusions)
      g. aspiration complications (water or acid, e.g., gastric secretions)
      h. multiple metabolic disorders (pancreatitis, hepatitis, acute renal failure with uremia)
  B. Appearance and symptomatology
    1. anxious and apprehensive
    2. complaints of
      a. difficulty in breathing
      b. tightness in chest
      c. respiratory effort increased over hours or days
      d. general aches and pains
      e. low grade fever
II. Alterations in respiratory status
  A. Physical findings
    1. tachypnea
    2. dyspnea
    3. cyanosis (if severely hypoxic)
  B. Chest auscultation
    1. possibly normal chest sounds initially
    2. basilar fine rales and/or rhonchi possibly
III. Alterations in cardiovascular status
  A. Tachycardia
  B. Rapid pulse
  C. Elevated bp

IV. Alterations in laboratory and other diagnostic studies
  A. X-ray findings
    1. interstitial infiltrates (patchy)
    2. alveolar infiltrates (patchy)
    3. possible areas of consolidation
  B. Routine blood chemistries and hematology
    1. initially nondiagnostic
    2. necessary to provide baseline profile
    3. necessary to rule out deviations from normal
  C. Blood gases and pH
    1. pH above 7.45
    2. $PaCO_2$ below 40 mm Hg
    3. HCO_3 normal, 21 to 28 mEq/L, if uncompensated; below 21 mEq/L, if compensated
    4. CO_2 content 23 to 25 mEq/L
    5. PaO_2 room air 60 mm Hg
      PaO_2 on 100 percent $O_2 \times 10$ minutes (250 mm Hg)
    6. Base excess +1
V. Alterations in acid–base balance
  A. Hypoxemia (initially moderate, progressing rapidly to severe)
    1. anxiety, restlessness, confusion
    2. tachycardia
    3. dysrhythmias
    4. insomnia and/or altered mentation
    5. diaphoresis
    6. central cyanosis (as hypoxemia progresses to severe state)
    7. cardiac and renal failure
    8. coma and death
  B. Respiratory alkalosis (mild to moderate)
    1. tachycardia
    2. headache
    3. vertigo
    4. syncope
    5. paresthesia of hands and feet
    6. tetany
    7. carpopedal spasms
    8. altered sensorium

PATHOPHYSIOLOGY

Adult respiratory distress syndrome (ARDS) is a pathologic process that collectively characterizes a group of signs and symptoms representing a number of conditions or biologic insults that present with a similar clinical picture. It is a commonly seen entity with a high mortality rate that not only occurs in patients in medical or surgical intensive care units, but can be frequently seen in previously healthy adults without lung problems. Although multiple etiologic events are associated with the development of ARDS, it is obvious that lung injury or insult is either delivered to the lungs via the circulation or through the airways. (See Table 6 and Fig. 9.) The common denominator, despite the inciting event, is damage to the alveolar–capillary membrane. As a result, the permeability of this membrane is increased allowing water, protein, and other solutes to pass through, accumulate in the interstitial space, and eventually pass into the alveolar spaces producing pulmonary edema and hypoxemia. Additionally, the continual flux of these substances into the interstitial and alveolar spaces disrupts the function of surfactant, a phospholipid substance present in the lungs that assists in controlling the surface tension of air–liquid emulsion and in lowering surface tension. Disruption of the surfactant function is correlated with the development of atelectasis. These major physiologic changes lead to the physical and clinical findings in ARDS: decreased compliance, progressive hypoxemia, dyspnea, tachypnea, cyanosis, tachycardia, rales, rhonchi, blood gas changes, and other related signs and symptoms.

Several theories or mechanisms have been proposed as to causations of alveolar–capillary membrane damage. The first mechanism is related to direct lung injury by such agents as oxygen. In the case of very high oxygen concentrations, every organ in the body has a chance of being damaged. The lung, however, will be damaged in oxygen concentrations of less than one atmosphere of pressure, and the injury in this case is due to superoxide radicals (negatively charged, short-lived oxygen radicals that increase in number as oxygen tension increases), hydroxyl groups, and hydrogen peroxide. Normally these superoxide radicals are metabolized by a protective catalytic enzyme in the lung, however, with very high oxygen concentrations, these radicals accumulate faster than they can be metabolized, resulting in toxicity and diffuse alveolar damage.

A second mechanism is related to decreased perfusion to lung tissue which is

TABLE 6.   PARTIAL LIST OF CONDITIONS ASSOCIATED WITH ARDS

Shock	**Aspiration of gastric contents**
Septicemia	**Drug overdose**
Trauma	Heroin
Fat emboli	Methadone
Lung contusion	Barbiturates
Nonthoracic trauma (especially head	Ethchlorvynol
trauma)	**Disseminated intravascular coagulation**
Infection	**Near-drowning**
Viral pneumonia	Fresh or salt water
Bacterial pneumonia	**Miscellaneous**
Fungal pneumonia	Pancreatitis
Tuberculosis	Uremia
Inhalation of toxic gases	Postcardiopulmonary bypass
Oxygen (FIO$_2$ > 0.5)	Postcardioversion
Smoke	Multiple transfusions
Nitrous oxide	

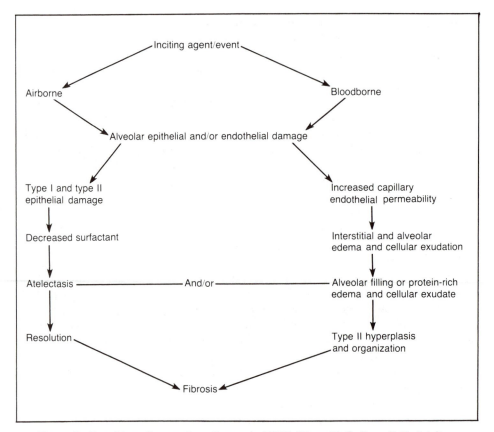

Figure 9. Possible pathogenetic pathways in ARDS. (*From McCaffree, D. R. Adult respiratory distress syndrome: Pathogenesis and pharmacologic management. Hospital Formulary, 1982, **17**(2) 1584.*)

evidenced by shock, a frequently seen event in the development of ARDS. It has been demonstrated in the literature that hypoxia in and of itself does not impair alveolar–capillary function, but its presence may initiate other physiologic or compensatory events that directly interrupt the integrity of the alveolar–capillary membrane.

A third hypothesis is that of alveolar–capillary damage through injury by humoral agents. Evidence is mounting to implicate the complement system in lung injury. If the entire complement system through C8 and C9 is activated, especially when it occurs on a cell surface, it radically alters the function of the cell membrane. In sepsis, for example, another precursor of ARDS, endotoxins activate complement. With the activation of C5, there is attraction of leukocytes which eventually results in pulmonary leukostasis. Superoxide radicals and lysosomal enzymes are produced as end products of leukocyte metabolism and these agents damage the endothelium and alter alveolar–capillary permeability.

A fourth theory implicates cellular components of blood and abnormal coagulation problems as a cause of alveolar–capillary injury.

The fifth and final mechanism suggests that increased intracranial pressure can, in many cases, be associated with the rapid development of pulmonary edema related to marked elevation of the pulmonary arteriole pressure. With the reduction of the increased intracranial pressure, pulmonary edema may exist for some time, and as a result, possibly alter the alveolar–capillary membrane.

Whether one or a combination of mechanisms is operating, significant pathologic processes are involved. Lung compliance diminishes; hyaline membranes line damaged alveoli and alveolar ducts; functional residual capacity is reduced because of increased recoil of the lung; venous blood shunted through nonventilated areas of the lung produces an extremely widened differential between oxygen tension in alveolar gas and arterial blood; and profound hypoxemia worsens with rapid deterioration and death unless the condition is diagnosed and appropriate intervention instituted.

The clinical course of this syndrome develops very rapidly and has been characterized by four rather distinct phases. The first phase follows the initial lung insult and is represented by subtle clinical signs with x-ray findings relatively normal. Phase two (latent phase) demonstrates some abnormal physical and x-ray findings such as hyperventilation, tachypnea, fine crackling lung sounds, and beginning of reticular patterning on chest film although the individual appears "stable." Phase three, an explosive phase in terms of clinical findings, is characterized by pulmonary edema and severely reduced arterial oxygen tension. The final phase, known as the terminal phase, reveals itself in terms of persistent and refractory hypoxemia, and carbon dioxide retention. Rapid deterioration and death may ensue. Despite aggressive therapy, the mortality rate is at least 50 percent.

MANAGEMENT

  I. Establish measures to insure respiratory support
     A. Continuous positive airway pressure (CPAP)
        1. nonventilator technique
        2. provides increased inspired oxygen concentrations at a constant positive pressure
        3. range of pressure up to about 10 cm H_2O
     B. Positive end expiratory pressure (PEEP)
        1. if Pao_2 of 60 mm Hg cannot be maintained with inhaled oxygen concentration less than 50 percent
        2. begin at 4 to 5 cm H_2O, not to exceed 20 cm H_2O
        3. increase incrementally according to blood gas determinations until adequate Pao_2 is achieved
     C. Packed red blood cells to maintain hemoglobin at a minimum of 10 g
 II. Institute measures to maintain fluid balance
     A. Restrict fluids to 15 to 25 ml/kg daily body weight
     B. Fluids to maintain pulmonary capillary wedge pressure (PCWP) between 5 and 10 mm Hg
     C. Diuretics (e.g., furosemide, IV, if necessary)

III. Institute pharmacologic measures to diminish lung damage
   A. Corticosteroids (especially during early stages)
     1. A-methaPred
     2. Solu-Medrol
   B. Anticoagulants
     1. Lipo-Hepin
     2. Liquaemin sodium
     3. Panheparin
   C. Vasodilators (e.g., nitroprusside)
   D. Diuretics (e.g., furosemide, ethacrynic acid)
   E. Experimental pharmacologic agents
     1. prostaglandin synthesis inhibitors
       a. ibuprofen (Motrin, Rufin) ⎫
       b. indomethacin (Indocin) ⎬ cyclooxygenase inhibitors
       c. meclofenamate (Meclomen) ⎭
     2. artificial surfactant or surfactant stimulators
IV. Establish measures to support management modalities
   A. Peripheral intravenous line
   B. Arterial line
   C. Swan–Ganz catheter into pulmonary artery
   D. Laboratory data
     1. routine blood chemistries and hematology
     2. arterial and venous blood gas determinations and pH
     3. base excess or deficit
     4. lactate levels
   E. Endotracheal intubation
   F. Ventilatory support (CPAP, PEEP) (See Tables 7 and 8)
   G. ECG monitoring
   H. Indwelling urethral catheter
   I. Nasogastric tube
   J. Blood, sputum, and ventilator cultures
V. Monitor continuously for significant clinical changes, trends, and response to management modalities
   A. Vital signs including bp
   B. Skin quality and appearance
   C. Swan–Ganz readings
   D. Level of consciousness
   E. Arterial and venous blood gases and pH
   F. Bicarbonate levels
   G. Hemoglobin levels
   H. Serum electrolytes
   I. Hydration status
   J. Deterioration of physiologic state
     1. decreasing respiratory efficiency and lung compliance
     2. increase in amount and tenaciousness of pulmonary secretions

TABLE 7. MANAGING THE PATIENT ON A VENTILATOR

Type of ventilator	1. Volume-controlled ventilator (MAI; Ohio 560, Emerson). Will deliver set tidal volume with varying pressures 2. Pressure-controlled ventilator. Preset pressure is achieved at varying tidal volumes
Fraction of inspired oxygen (F_1O_2)	Interpretation of PO_2 will depend upon the concentration of inspired O_2. Normal values: 1. F_1O_2—room air 21 percent O_2 PO_2—100 mm Hg or 105 minus half of patient's age 2. $F_1O_2 = 100$ percent $PO_2 = 500$ mm Hg
Tidal volume (V_T)	10–15 ml/kg body weight
Respiratory rate	10–12/minute
Sensitivity setting	1. Increased sensitivity indicates that very low negative pressure is required to trigger machine 2. Do not allow patient to generate more than −2 cm H_2O to trigger the ventilator
Type of ventilation	1. Controlled. The machine ventilates the patient according to set tidal volumes and respiratory rate. These patients usually require medication with morphine, curare, or pancuronium 2. Assist control. The patient triggers the machine
Inspiration to exhalation ratio	1. Should be 1:3, 1:2 or 1:1 (1 second of inspiration to 3 seconds of exhalation, etc.) 2. Inspiration should never be longer than exhalation, because venous return to the right side of the heart occurs on exhalation. Prolonged inspiration prevents venous return and may cause hypotension 3. Patients with obstructive lung disease need longer exhalation time to keep the bronchi open and allow exit of more air
Minute volume (V_E)	Tidal volume × respiratory rate/minute Normal = 6–8 L/minute
Airway pressure	Normal = 15–20 cm/H_2O Low airway pressure is seen with air leak High airway pressure is seen in: 1. Increased secretions 2. Airway obstruction 3. Bronchospasms 4. Pulmonary edema 5. Pneumothorax 6. Flail chest 7. Patient out of phase with respirator
Sigh	1. The lungs are hyperinflated periodically to open collapsed alveoli 2. The sigh is given by machine or manual hand-bag ventilation 3. Sigh volume is 3 times tidal volume every 5–10 minutes
Mechanical dead space	Refers to the volume of tubing from endotracheal or tracheostomy tube connector to the Y piece *Purpose:* 1. To rebreathe exhaled CO_2 2. Serves as a pliable connector from tracheostomy tube to Y piece; thus prevents discomfort when patient moves

(continued)

TABLE 7. (Continued)

	Caution: The volume of mechanical dead space should not be larger than one third of the set tidal volume, especially at 21 percent of F_1O_2, because hypoxic oxygen concentrations may result due to exhaled CO_2 dilution. Should not be used to correct metabolic alkalosis
Flow rate	*Slow* 1. Opens up more alveoli because of a more even air flow distribution within the respiratory tract 2. If flow rate is too slow it will prolong inspiration and may hinder venous return *High* 1. Shortens inspiratory time 2. Preferential flow of gases to alveoli with least resistance and may not open atelectatic alveoli at all
Expiratory retard	1. Used only when prescribed by physician 2. Keeps the terminal bronchioles patent, preventing early closure on exhalation; thus, more air can be exhaled
Humidity and temperature	1. Heated humidity is provided for all intubated and tracheotomized patients to avoid thick and viscid secretions 2. Daily clinical evaluation of the viscosity of the patient's secretions provides a guideline for the effectiveness of humidification and nebulization
Positive end expiratory pressure	1. A positive pressure of 5, 10, or 15 cm H_2O is maintained at the end of exhalation instead of a normal 0 cm H_2O pressure 2. Increases functional residual capacity
Synchronization of patient with ventilator	1. Inspiratory and expiratory time of the patient and respirator should be synchronized 2. Asynchrony (out of phase) with ventilator will result in altered cardiopulmonary hemodynamics and cause arrhythmias, hypotension, and increased airway pressure

(From Brunner, L.S., & Suddarth, D. S. Textbook of Medical–Surgical Nursing. Philadelphia: J. B. Lippincott, 1980, p. 457.)

       3. diffuse rhonchi

       4. rust-colored sputum

       5. falling Pao_2 despite increased percentage of oxygen

       6. rising $Paco_2$

       7. demonstrable base deficit

       8. decreasing cardiac output, bp, pulse

       9. pulmonary edema

     10. diffuse consolidation or white out on chest films

   K. Pharmacologic intervention side effects

      1. diuretics

         a. monitor for hypokalemia

         b. monitor for hyperkalemia (if diuretic potassium sparer)

         c. monitor for hypochloremia

TABLE 8. FACTORS THAT MAKE THE PATIENT FIGHT THE VENTILATOR

Problem	Nursing Action
1. Increased secretions Volume ventilator—airway pressure is increased but tidal volume is maintained Pressure ventilator—secretions will make the patient cough or generate increased intrapulmonary pressure, which will oppose the preset pressure on the ventilator; thus the inspiratory volume is reduced. The reduced tidal volume will promote progressive atelectasis and shunting	1. Suction as often as necessary 2. Hourly, hand ventilate with self-inflating bag for 5–10 minutes 3. Chest physical therapy 4. Frequent change of position 5. Adequate humidification and nebulization 6. For pressure ventilator—adjust flow rate and preset pressure to maintain an adequate chest expansion and satisfactory air entry heard on auscultation 7. If suctioning of trachea does not improve phasing with ventilator call the physician
2. Low F_1O_2—may manifest initially with tachycardia, hyperventilation, or arrhythmias	1. Measure inspired oxygen concentration and arterial blood gases 2. Call respiratory therapist to check accuracy of delivered F_1O_2 3. Call physician for differential diagnosis and management
3. Hypercarbia—may be manifested initially by hyperventilation, tachycardia, arrhythmias, increased blood pressure, and increasing drowsiness	1. Measure arterial blood gases 2. Call respiratory therapist to check mechanical dead space, accuracy of valves and ventilator performance 3. Call physician for differential diagnosis and management
4. Inadequate minute volume $V_E = V_T \times RR$	1. Measure exhaled tidal volume and respiratory rate if minute volume is lower than 6 L/minute. Increase delivered tidal volumes to 10–15 ml/kg at a rate of 10–12/minute 2. Call respiratory therapist for accuracy of ventilator performance 3. Call physician for differential diagnosis and management
5. Pulmonary edema—may be manifested as follows: High airway pressure Poor compliance Tracheal secretion foamy or pink frothy secretions abundant watery, and bright red fluid Engorged neck veins Dusky, cyanotic color Chest, full of wet rales Tachycardia, hypotension Marked restlessness	1. 100 percent F_1O_2 2. Hand ventilate with self-inflating bag. Use volume controlled respirator and PEEP (positive and expiratory pressure) 3. Suction trachea 4. Elevate head of bed (sitting up position) 5. Call physician. Give specific drug therapy as directed

(From Brunner, L. S. & Suddarth, D. S. Textbook of Medical–Surgical Nursing. Philadelphia: J. B. Lippincott, 1980, p. 458.)

      d. monitor for ototoxicity with ethacrynic acid use and in the presence of decreased renal function

  2. corticosteroids

    a. monitor for development of peptic ulcer and bleeding

    b. monitor for development of thrombosis and embolic formation

    c. monitor for development of infectious processes

  3. anticoagulants

    a. observe for

      i. petechiae

      ii. purpura

      iii. nose bleeds

      iv. bleeding from gums

      v. blood in stool or urine

  4. vasodilators (e.g., nitroprusside and other antihypertensive drugs acting on vascular smooth muscle to cause dilation)

    a. epigastric distress

    b. bradycardia

    c. hypotension

    d. respiratory depression

    e. vascular collapse

L. Mechanical ventilator complications

  1. abdominal distention

  2. alterations in tidal volume and minute ventilation

  3. tension pneumothorax

  4. oxygen toxicity when concentrations of O_2 is 50 percent or more

  5. decreased cardiac output

  6. pneumomediastinum

  7. systemic hypotension

  8. subcutaneous emphysema

  9. ventilator pneumonia

  10. fluid retention due to IADH syndrome

M. Electrolyte imbalances resulting from nasogastric suctioning

VI. Promote measures to combat infection or treat underlying conditions

A. Infection

  1. specific antibiotic therapy for identified organism(s)

  2. aseptic technique at all catheter sites

  3. aseptic technique with suctioning endotracheal tube

  4. frequent culturing of sputa (especially while on ventilator)

  5. attention to antisepsis in machine circuits

  6. change ventilator and humidifier every 24 hours

  7. bronchoscopy with peripheral brushings, especially in the immunocompromised patients, to identify fungal infections

B. Bleeding from stress or steroid therapy

  1. prophylaxis for stress ulcer and/or corticosteroid use

    a. antacids q 1 to 2 hours (to keep gastric pH > 5)

    b. cimetidine (Tagamet), IV (to prevent gastrointestinal hemorrhage)

    c. test for occult bleeding
      i. guaiac stools and emesis
      ii. monitor hematocrit values
  C. Disseminated intravascular coagulation (DIC)
    1. monitor frequently
      a. platelet counts
      b. fibrinogen level
      c. partial prothrombin and prothrombin times
    2. observe and assess
      a. bleeding from intravenous sites
      b. bleeding from mucous membranes
      c. bleeding during endotracheal suctioning
      d. skin for petechiae and bruises
  D. Other underlying conditions
    1. observe, assess, and identify other presenting pathologic or disease processes
    2. select management modalities appropriate to treatment
VII. Institute measures to promote physical and emotional well-being
  A. Keep patient, family, or significant other apprised of what is being done in terms of management modalities and why
  B. Identify specific source of anxiety within the patient and attempt to dispel it
  C. Enlist patient's cooperation and participation in care
  D. Attend to small details and demonstrate skill and confidence in carrying out care
  E. Frequent positional changes contribute to physical comfort and relieve muscular tension accompanying anxiety
  F. Continual emotional support to family or significant other

RATIONALE

The emergency management of ARDS must be directed toward maintaining arterial oxygenation and ventilation, and in treating underlying causes or conditions precipitating this syndrome. Correction of the hypoxemic state is of high priority. Introduction of high concentrations of oxygen via face mask may be used initially; however, if the intrapulmonary shunt fraction is greater than 25 to 30 percent or if a PaO_2 of 55 mm Hg cannot be achieved, additional ventilatory support is indicated, and continuous positive airway pressure (CPAP) can be instituted. This technique prescribes the patient to breathe an increased inspired oxygen concentration at a constant fixed positive pressure in the range of 10 cm H_2O, and as a result, produces a high end expiratory pressure. If poor or inadequate oxygenation is still a presenting problem, the individual must be intubated and mechanical ventilation with positive end expiratory pressure (PEEP) instituted. The use of PEEP is intended to increase the functional residual capacity of the lungs, improve gas exchange and ventilation, reduce the degree of right-to-left shunting of blood flow (mixed venous blood shunted to left atrium despite nonventilated zones of lung injury), and improve tissue oxygenation. Careful and continual patient assessment must be observed when mechanical ventilation is used. Blood gases should be determined at regular intervals so that modalities may be altered accordingly. With the additional use of PEEP, frequent monitoring of systems is necessary to identify associated complications. These include tension pneumothorax (may develop as a result of small pleural tears that are not able to seal against the continuous positive pressure), decreased cardiac output (pulmonary arterial pressure causes an increase in mean thoracic pressure resulting in reduced cardiac output by decreasing venous return to the chest), oxygen toxicity (from high oxygen concentrations), and the syndrome of inappropriate antidiuretic hormone (atrial receptors sensitive to decreased venous return to the chest stimulate secretion of antidiuretic hormone, and thus, retention of water).

The introduction of the Swan–Ganz catheter into the pulmonary artery provides accurate information related to cardiac output and arterial oxygen content. From this data, oxygen delivery can be calculated and altered according to findings. In addition, with use of the Swan–Ganz catheter, fluid assessment and fluid administration can be determined, and pulmonary capillary wedge pressure can be maintained at optimal pressures. To maintain optimal pressure, the patient is usually kept "dry" but not dehydrated, and fluid administration should not exceed 25 ml/kg of body weight per day. Diuretics may be used to achieve optimum pulmonary capillary wedge pressure if pulmonary edema or fluid retention is present. If fluid is necessary to maintain cardiac output, crystalline solutions are generally used rather than colloids because colloids are thought to leak into the pulmonary interstitium thereby initiating an osmotic stimulus for increasing pulmonary edema. To maintain adequate hemoglobin levels to support adequate tissue oxygenation, packed red blood cells may be administered as a possible method of volume replacement.

Pharmacologic interventions in combination with ventilatory support modalities are being used in ARDS to interrupt the pathogenetic mechanisms in the early emergency management. The use of corticosteroids is intended to stabilize lysosomes, and, thus prevent membrane deterioration. Because of the adverse effects and complications of prolonged corticosteroid therapy, careful monitoring of those parameters identified is of great importance. Anticoagulant therapy may be instituted as an intervention strategy if evidence of abnormal clotting and fibrinolytic activity is developing. Awareness of and assessment for bleeding manifestations is a vital part of this management. Administration of diuretics as a modality in maintaining optimal pulmonary capillary wedge pressure and in treatment of pulmonary edema may be indicated, and assessment for signs and symptoms of electrolyte imbalances must be ongoing so that appropriate interventions may be instituted to ameliorate these conditions. Antihypertensive drugs such as nitroprusside sodium, a potent direct acting vasodilator, must be used cautiously, and effort must be made to identify its many side effects throughout its administration.

Combatting infection must be instituted early in the course of emergency management. This is especially true in the immunocompromised individual. Specific measures identified must become an integral part of emergency care and an aggressive approach to identifying and treating infections is fully warranted.

In the immediate period following diagnosis, measures to support management modalities and laboratory and x-ray information to serve as baseline data must be established. Monitoring parameters, as identified, must be assessed on a continual basis in order to evaluate significant clinical changes and for trends and responses to emergency intervention strategies. It must be remembered that throughout the care of this seriously ill individual, every possible effort must be expended to promote physical and emotional comfort. Treatment of this respiratory distress syndrome is supportive as opposed to curative. Those surviving this illness can expect to return to a relatively normal state within a year following the onset and diagnosis.

7. Pulmonary Embolism

ASSESSMENT

  I. Alterations in general appearance
    A. Apprehensiveness
    B. Pallor or cyanotic
    C. Sweating (moderate to severe)
 II. Alterations in respiratory/pulmonary status
    A. Changes in respiratory rates
    B. Chest pain (pleuritic or constant)
    C. Use of accessory muscles of respiration
    D. Tachypnea
    E. Dyspnea
    F. Retractions (intercostal, suprasternal, supraventricular)
    G. Splints
    H. Decreased vocal fremitus
    I. Reduced or abnormal breath sounds (involved side)
    J. Friction rub
    K. Hiccoughs
    L. Hemoptysis (possible)
    M. Small tidal volume
    N. Rales
    O. Hypoxia
III. Alterations in cardiovascular status
    A. Cardiac output reduction
      1. decreasing bp
      2. tachycardia
      3. vertigo
      4. changes in mentation (confusion)
      5. angina
    B. Symptoms of right-sided heart failure
      1. atrial dysrhythmias
      2. distended neck veins

3. engorgement of liver
4. elevated CVP readings
5. peripheral edema
6. accented pulmonary sounds (P2)
7. tachycardia
8. gallop rhythm
9. pulmonic murmurs
C. Air embolism
   1. sudden and severe dyspnea
   2. signs and symptoms of shock
   3. cyanosis
   4. churning sound in right ventricle
D. Fat embolism
   1. petechiae (axillary folds, anterior neck, anterior chest)
   2. signs and symptoms of cor pulmonale
   3. decreasing cardiac output
IV. Alterations in laboratory and other diagnostics
   A. Blood gases and pH
      1. pH < 7.35
      2. P_{CO_2} > 40 mm Hg
      3. P_{O_2} normal or decreased (between 90 and 60 mm Hg)
      4. HCO_3 > 21 to 28 mEq/L (partial or complete compensation); normal (if uncompensated)
   B. Other blood studies
      1. serum LDH, normal or elevated
      2. serum bilirubin, normal or elevated
      3. fibrin degradation products, normal or elevated
      4. leukocyte count, normal or elevated
   C. Possible ECG findings
      1. deep S wave in lead I
      2. prominent Q wave in lead III
      3. inverted T wave in lead III
      4. tall P waves in lead II
      5. right axis deviation
      6. inverted T wave in V_{1-4}
      7. transient incomplete right bundle branch block
      8. displacement of transitional zone to the left
   D. Possible x-ray, lung scan, and pulmonary angiography findings
      1. decreased pulmonary vascularity
      2. enlargement of main pulmonary artery
      3. elevation of a hemidiaphragm
      4. pleural effusion
      5. pulmonary densities
      6. filling defect (pulmonary angiography)
      7. lobar or multiple segmental defects (perfusion lung scan)

PATHOPHYSIOLOGY

Pulmonary embolism is a life-threatening emergency condition that not only may complicate the course of acutely ill hospitalized patients, but may also affect healthy ambulant individuals. The clinical picture presented by the patient is primarily a result of pulmonary artery occlusion and spasm, reduction in cardiac output, and a diminishing in the filling of the coronary artery. It is thought that most pulmonary emboli arise from intravascular clots in the peripheral veins (veins of the lower extremities and pelvic veins) or from the chamber of the right side of the heart. The exact reasons why these clots dislodge is not certain, but conditions that cause blood stasis (e.g., immobilization, CHF, obesity), conditions that arise from abnormalities of the venous wall (e.g., trauma, atherosclerosis, IV punctures), and conditions initiating hypercoaguability (e.g., dehydration) increase one's risk of developing a pulmonary embolism. Additional risks of thrombus formation are increased during pregnancy, with use of oral contraceptives, with cardiovascular conditions, peritonitis, sickle cell anemia, cancer, and with any prolonged period of inactivity. The signs and symptoms that are manifested are dependent on the impact of the embolism on the circulatory system in terms of its size and location. Not all patients exhibit all signs and the emergency team should not wait for positive clinical proof of pulmonary embolism, but should proceed with management on suggestive evidence. It is possible for some individuals not to exhibit any symptom and suffer immediate death from a massive pulmonary embolism which probably originated in the femoral or iliac trunk and occluded the pulmonary artery.

Oxygen deprivation is probably responsible for many of the altered clinical states and the resultant cerebral ischemia produces symptoms of restlessness, vertigo, syncope, or convulsions. Ventricular hypertension, which decreases the gradient of blood flowing in the right coronary artery, initiates the anginal-type chest pain. Patients may exhibit gastrointestinal symptoms which arise as a reflex stimulated by chest pain and apprehensiveness. Decreased coronary artery perfusion causes possible ischemia to myocardial tissue and the precipitation of diminished cardiac output and other cardiac alterations. If an embolus has occluded either the left or right branch of the pulmonary artery, severe cardiopulmonary symptomatology develops. The effect is that of right-sided heart failure (cor pulmonale). Concomitant with this failure is a precipitous drop in cardiac output and arterial pressure which results in hypoxemia and shock. On cardiopulmonary examination there might be an audible pleural friction rub. It is thought that the rub arises from a very dilated pulmonary artery which subsequently rubs against the pericardium. The patient may also exhibit a systolic murmur caused by a partially stenosed pulmonary artery. A diastolic murmur, if present, may exist because of a thrombus extending from the right ventricle through the pulmonary valve. If an embolus has occluded either the left or right branch of the pulmonary artery, reduced breath sounds are elicited on the involved side.

Large pulmonary emboli usually present with sudden onset of dyspnea and anxiety, with or without substernal pain. Signs of acute right heart failure and circulatory collapse may shortly follow. In the case of pulmonary infarction, there is sudden dyspnea, pleuritic pain, cough, hemoptysis, and x-ray density on the lung. Gradual development of unexplained dyspnea, with or without x-ray densities, may indicate repeated minor embolization to the lungs.

The clinical and laboratory manifestations often depend on the level at which the obstruction occurs. The findings may be minimal or absent if the embolism is in a terminal artery, and will not be evident until repeated embolization has occurred. In a medium-sized artery, pulmonary signs and symptoms and x-ray densities predominate. In a large artery, signs of acute right heart failure progress to shock, syncope, cyanosis, and sudden death. Hemoptysis, pleuritic pain, and infiltrates on x-ray are a result of lung infarction which appears approximately 12 to 36 hours postembolism.

Chest x-ray is most often negative; however, following large emboli, an area of decreased pulmonary vascularity may be apparent, and may demonstrate enlargement of a main pulmonary artery, elevation of a hemidiaphragm, and plueral effusion. Pulmonary densities, when they do occur, are generally of various configuration, and are usually adjacent to a pleural surface. These densities are due to infarction and appear 2 to 3 days following the embolism. A more definitive procedure for confirming the diagnosis of pulmonary embolism and estimating the extent of involvement of pulmonary vasculature is pulmonary angiography. This is, however, a very drastic procedure and should only be considered when major embolism is suggested, and x-ray and scanning procedures are not diagnostic.

Electrocardiographic findings are often transient and when they do occur, they usually evolve rapidly. Significant findings appear in approximately 10 to 20 percent of the cases.

In addition to emboli arising from the vascular bed, different types of emboli, such as air, fat, and pieces of polyurethane tips from long line intravenous catheters, may predispose to this acute emergency condition. Specific signs and symptoms related to these forms of emboli are included so that emergency care providers are aware of these clinical findings if they should appear during assessment and monitoring.

MANAGEMENT

    I. Employ measures to insure adequate oxygenation and airway humidity
       A. Humidified oxygen via face mask or nasal cannula
       B. Oxygen in sufficient concentrations to achieve or maintain Pa_{O_2} between 60 to 70 mm Hg
   II. Institute measures to support management modalities
       A. Intravenous line
       B. Central venous pressure line
       C. Electrocardiographic monitoring
       D. Oxygen therapy
       E. Chest films; lung scan; pulmonary angiography, as indicated
       F. Serum electrolytes

G. Serum LDH

H. Serum bilirubin

 I. Fibrin degradation products

 J. Leukocyte count

K. Blood gases; blood pH; and bicarbonate levels

L. Partial thromboplastin time; thrombin time; Lee and White clotting time; whole blood euglobulin levels; lysis time

III. Institute measures to inhibit blood coagulation and prevent recurrences

A. Heparin administration

    1. initial priming dose: 5000 to 10,000 U, IV bolus

    2. maintenance dose: 1000 U/hour/24 hours via continuous infusion

B. Monitoring parameters for desired effect

    1. partial thromboplastin time: maintain at 1.5 to 2 times baseline control level

    2. Lee and White clotting time: maintain at 2 to 3 times baseline control level

C. Assess for side effects

    1. bleeding

    2. thrombocytopenia

D. Anticoagulant antagonists

    1. protamine for heparin overdose

    2. vitamin K for warfarin overdose

VI. Employ thrombolytic agents to enzymatically remove the obstruction

A. Streptokinase

    1. priming dose: 250,000 U, IV over 30 minutes
maintenance dose: 100,000 U/hour for 24 to 72 hours via continuous infusion

    2. monitoring parameters for desired effects

        a. whole blood euglobulin

        b. lysis time

        c. thrombin time

        d. partial thromboplastin time

        } performed prior to therapy and q 3 to 4 hours after initiation of therapy

B. Urokinase

    1. priming dose: 4400 U/kg, IV over 10-minute period
maintenance dose: 4400 U/kg/hour times 12 to 24 hours via continuous infusion

    2. monitoring parameters for desired effects

        a. whole blood euglobulin

        b. lysis time

        c. thrombin time

        d. partial thromboplastin

        } performed prior to therapy and q 3 to 4 hours after initiation of therapy

C. Monitor for the following complications and side effects of thrombolytic therapy

    1. hemorrhage

    2. fever

      3. allergic reactions (rarely with urokinase; in approximately 10 percent of those using streptokinase)
         a. pruritis
         b. urticaria
         c. anaphylactic reactions (in 2 percent of patients treated)
   D. Pharmacologic interventions to reverse allergic reactions
      1. epinephrine (first line drug in anaphylaxis)
      2. parenteral corticosteroids
      3. antihistamines
   E. Modalities to reverse coagulation abnormalities from thrombolytic therapy
      1. fresh whole blood
      2. packed red blood cells with either of the following
         a. fresh frozen plasma
         b. cryoprecipitate

 V. Institute measures to relieve hypotension and increased pulmonary vascular resistance
   A. Hypotension
      1. dopamine: 200 mg in 500 ml of normal saline initially titrated at a rate of 2.5 μg/kg/minute } titrated at a rate to maintain a systolic pressure of 90 mm Hg
      2. isoproterenol: 4 mg/L
   B. Pulmonary vascular resistance
      1. correction of hypoxemic state
      2. isoproterenol, IV

 VI. Employ measures to sustain and support vital functions
   A. Cardiovascular drug management, if indicated
      1. to treat dysrhythmias
      2. to treat cardiac failure
      3. to treat circulatory collapse
   B. Fluid replacement or restoration, if indicated
      1. to maintain fluid balance
      2. to treat shock
   C. Medications to relieve pain and reduce anxiety
      1. morphine: 1 mg at a time up to 5 to 10 mg, subcutaneously or IV q 3 to 4 hours
      2. meperidine (Demerol): 50 to 100 mg, subcutaneously or IV q 3 to 4 hours
      3. codeine for mild to moderate pain
      4. monitor the following as complications of narcotic therapy
         a. hypotensive effects
         b. depressive effects on CNS and respiratory system

 VII. Monitor continuously for trends and responses to management modalities
   A. Temperature, pulse, respirations, and bp

   B. Skin quality and appearance
   C. Blood gases, blood pH, and bicarbonate levels
   D. Serum electrolytes
   E. Tests for blood clotting determinations
   F. Hydration status
   G. Metabolic status
   H. Cardiac status
   I. Renal status
   J. Respiratory status
   K. Hematologic states in relation to bleeding or coagulation
   L. Central venous pressure readings
   M. Signs of further embolization or pulmonary infarction
VIII. Institute measures to prevent further embolization
   A. Bed rest
   B. Elastic stockings or leg wraps (toe to groin)
   C. Instruct patient not to cross legs
   D. Elevate legs 10 to 15 degrees
   E. Bed activities
      1. active leg exercises (flexion and extension)
      2. frequent positioning and turning
   F. Stool softeners
   G. Breathing exercises
   H. Routine and frequent inspection of lower extremities (especially calf and popliteal areas) for
      1. tenderness
      2. pain
      3. redness
      4. swelling
   I. Doppler test (ultrasound technique) to identify deep vein thrombosis in iliofemoral and popliteal veins
 IX. Institute surgical intervention modalities to remove the embolus or prevent further embolization
   A. Indications for pulmonary embolectomy
      1. refractory clinical state to heparin and thrombolytic therapy
      2. when anticoagulant therapy absolutely contraindicated
   B. Indications for vena caval interruption
      1. when anticoagulant therapy contraindicated
      2. recurrent embolization during anticoagulant therapy

RATIONALE

The management of pulmonary embolism is supportive because there is no cure for an embolism once it has occurred. Therapeutic management modalities are directed toward three approaches (1) surgically or enzymatically removing the obstruction, (2) inhibiting blood coagulation to prevent recurrences, or (3) surgically interrupting the inferior vena cava.

Oxygen is administered in fairly high concentrations by mask or nasal cannula to overcome any existing hypoxia or hypoxemia, to help prevent cardiorespiratory failure, and to promote oxygenation of the tissues. In the immediate period following diagnosis, measures to support management modalities must be instituted, and information from laboratory, x-ray, and other diagnostics must be obtained to establish a physiologic data base profile. Monitoring parameters, as identified, must be assessed on a continual basis for the purpose of evaluating significant clinical changes and for trends and responses to emergency intervention strategies.

Heparin is administered in large doses to inhibit blood coagulation and prevent recurrences. The priming dose is given as an intravenous bolus and the maintenance therapy is aimed at administering 24,000 units in a 24-hour period by continuous infusion. Laboratory tests for monitoring clotting activity should be performed approximately 6 hours after the priming dose, and once or twice more within the first 24 hours. These test results are to be compared to the blood samples obtained prior to instituting management so that appropriate dosing of heparin and optimal effects can be achieved. Check the patient at frequent intervals for bleeding, and if excessive, heparin antagonists are to be administered.

Thrombolytic agents, in the form of exogenous plasminogen activators, may be introduced into management to improve right heart and pulmonary circulation hemodynamics, lyse clots, and to improve pulmonary microvasculature circulation by breaking down and absorbing microemboli within this microstructure. The use of thrombolytic agents is absolutely contraindicated when there is active internal bleeding, a history of cerebrovascular or coagulation disorders, or a recent history of trauma, fractures, or surgical procedures within the past 2 months. Both streptokinase and urokinase are administered in terms of priming doses and continuous maintenance infusion. Coagulation tests, established as part of baseline data, are to be monitored every 2 to 4 hours during infusion to insure the objective of therapy, namely, prolongation of coagulation time to more than twice baseline data results. Hemorrhage, fever, and allergic reactions are the possible complications and side effects of thrombolytic therapy. Although hemorrhage and fever are the complications shared by both streptokinase and urokinase, allergic reactions from urokinase are rare. Throughout this therapy, careful monitoring is in order so that if any of these side effects or complications appear, appropriate pharmacologic interventions can be instituted.

If hypotension develops, pressor amines are used to relieve this situation rather than administering large amounts of fluid. Aggressive fluid therapy would only further compromise an already existing state of failure. Arterial vasodilators such as isoproterenol and modalities to correct hypoxia are usually sufficient to relieve increased pulmonary vascular resistance.

The nurse and physician must be alert in identifying parameters indicative of shock or alterations in cardiovascular status. Immediate intervention with use of pharmacologic agents, fluids, or blood are usually in order. In using fluids or blood in shock management, quantities should be limited because patients suffering from pulmonary embolism already have increased congestion in the peripheral venous system and too much fluid may cause circulatory overload. If narcotic therapy is used to relieve pain and to reduce anxiety and apprehension, careful monitoring is necessary to identify the major complications of this therapy, namely, central nervous system and respiratory center depression. It must be noted that narcotic therapy is to be avoided in the presence of shock and that all intramuscular injections must be avoided in heparinized individuals.

Measures to prevent further embolization and reduce circulatory demands are instituted at the beginning of emergency management. Bed rest is indicated to prevent further embolism, to reduce demands on the heart and circulatory system, and to conserve oxygen. The use of elastic wraps from foot to groin may help prevent thrombus formation in the deep veins of the lower extremities by giving added support to the veins and facilitate venous return from the legs. Elevation of the legs and active flexion and extension leg exercises also helps to promote venous return. Stool softeners are administered to prevent the patient from straining during bowel evacuation which may stimulate the Valsalva effect, and in turn, be a cause in thrombus dislodgement. Breathing exercises in combination with frequent positioning and turning assist in reducing pulmonary complications. Routine and frequent inspection of lower extremities for the cardinal signs of inflammation, and use of the Doppler test for deep vein tenderness, are ideal ways of detecting the development of thrombosis.

In massive embolism, or in individuals in whom heparin or thrombolytic therapy is either refractory or contraindicated, surgical intervention is necessary to remove the embolus or to prevent further embolization. If this is considered, preoperative preparations are made rapidly, and the patient is transferred to surgery.

8. Facial Trauma

ASSESSMENT

I. Physical examination
   A. Determine adequacy of airway
   B. Examine oral airway for obstruction
     1. blood
     2. mandibular fragments
     3. broken dentures
     4. teeth
     5. other foreign bodies
   C. Control bleeding (site, amount, type)
   D. Check for occlusion/malocclusion of teeth

   E. Evaluate for integrity of cranial nerves III to VII
   F. Examine ear for presence of blood behind tympanic membrane
   G. Examine for Battle sign (basilar skull fracture; lacerations of ear canal)
   H. Look for central nervous system drainage via nasal passage
   I. Examine for limitation of jaw motion (trismus)
   J. Determine visual acuity
   K. Other observations
      1. dyspnea
      2. crepitus
      3. palpate facial bones for
         a. tenderness
         b. nonalignment
      4. anesthesia (chin and lower lip area)
      5. diplopia (may be masked by edema)
      6. pain (type, location, duration)
   L. Associated injury assessment regarding
      1. altered ventilatory capacity
         a. pneumothorax
         b. hemothorax
         c. fractured ribs
      2. shock (excessive blood loss)
      3. cardiovascular injury
      4. altered mental state
         a. craniocerebral injury
         b. metabolic disorders
II. Laboratory studies
   A. Hematocrit
   B. Hemoglobin
   C. Prothrombin and partial prothrombin time
   D. Type and crossmatch
III. Radiographic studies
   A. Stereoscopic posterior/anterior ⎱
   B. Stereoscopic lateral
   C. Stereoscopic basal
   D. Mandibular views   ⎰ depending on area of injury
   E. Temporomandibular joints
   F. Maxillary laminographs

PATHOPHYSIOLOGY

Facial bone fractures can be classified according to the type and location of the fracture (Fig. 10):

1. Fractures of upper third of face—including frontal bone, frontal sinuses, and supraorbital ridge

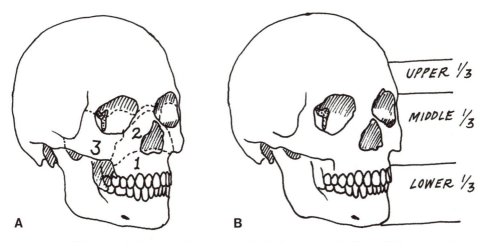

Figure 10. **A.** Facial bone fractures according to type: Le Fort I, II, and III fractures of the middle third of the face. **B.** Facial bone fractures according to location.

2. Fractures of the middle third of face—nasal bones, zygoma, zygomatic arch, or bital bones and maxillary fractures (Le Fort I, II, III)
3. Lower third of the face—mandibular fractures

FRACTURES OF THE UPPER THIRD OF THE FACE

These are most often seen as the result of automobile and motorcycle accidents. Periorbital ecchymosis is the most common finding. Diplopia is evident because of edema and hematoma within the orbit or because of injury to the superior oblique or superior rectus muscles. Anesthesia over the distribution of the supraorbital nerve may be noted. Palpation may elicit tenderness, crepitation, and depression over the frontal area or notching of the supraorbital ridge.

FRACTURES OF THE MIDDLE THIRD OF THE FACE

There are three mechanisms of injury that lead to nasal fractures: blunt blow to one side of the nose, heavier blow that breaks both nasal bones, and a greater force which results in comminuted fracture. Trauma to the nose without epistaxis is a fairly good indicator that there is no fracture. Epistaxis is a likely result from concomitant septal fractures and mucosal laceration. The nose may or may not be deformed. Fractures of the zygoma or zygomatic arch are usually caused by trauma to the lateral side of the face and upper cheek. This particular fracture can be identified when trismus occurs on opening or closing the jaw. The zygomatic arch forms a weak protective shield for the temporomandibular joint and the impaction on the arch fragment causes trismus. Traumatic force to the eyeball increases the intraocular pressure suddenly and drastically. As the pressure is propelled in all directions, the orbital floor which is the weakest part of the orbit, gives way and fractures downward into the maxillary sinus. There is a resultant subconjunctival hemorrhage, periorbital edema, and hematoma. These symptoms occur due to the rapid increase of intraocular pressure. Diplopia occurs because of the inferior displacement of the ocular globe and occasionally because the fracture fragments trap the eye's herniated inferior rectus muscle. Enophthalmos is a common presenting symptom and occurs due to a loss of infraorbital fat or dislocation of the fracture floor. It takes a great disruptive force to fracture the maxilla and usually stems from automobile accidents or massive beating.

Classifications (According to Le Fort, a French Anatomist)

- Type   I—Transverse alveolar fracture
- Type   II—Fracture line is higher and the result is a pyramidal fragment that includes the central part of the maxilla on both sides and extends to the nasal area so that the nose moves with the distal arch when the fragment is shifted
- Type III—Includes a tripod fracture

A tripod fracture is caused by a blunt trauma that fractures the zygomatic arch, infraorbital rim, and frontozygomatic suture.

Maxillary fractures frequently result from a direct anteroposterior blow to the middle third of the face, depending upon the magnitude, direction, and site of the blow. The upper dentition, the maxillary sinus, the orbital floor, and the maxillary division of the fifth cranial nerve are important anatomic structures to be considered. A displaced maxillary fracture is characteristically manifested by gross malocclusion. Anesthesia over the cheek and upper lip, which are areas innervated by infraorbital nerve, may be demonstrable. Enophthalmos with depression of the globe is an important diagnostic finding. Subcutaneous emphysema with palpable crepitus over the cheek suggests communication between the antrum and subcutaneous space through the fracture site. False motion may be demonstrated by palpatation or grasping of the upper teeth and noting movements separate from the cranium.

FRACTURES OF THE LOWER THIRD OF THE FACE

The mandible is the most fequently fractured bone within the facial complex. About 60 percent of mandibular fractures are bilateral. The powerful muscles of mastication inserting on the mandible may account for continuing displacement of the fractures unless fixation is achieved by treatment. The complex temporomandibular joint, lower teeth, and mandibular division of the fifth cranial nerve are important anatomic structures related to fractures of the mandible. Examination may reveal deformity or malocclusion, with crepitation and swelling as characteristic signs. Anesthesia over the chin and lower lip suggest injury to the inferior alveolar nerve.

MANAGEMENT

  I. Establish measures to maintain adequate airway
    A. Extend head, pull mandible forward
    B. Place patient on either side to facilitate adequate gravitational drainage
    C. Oral airway or endotracheal intubation
 II. Institute measures to control bleeding and hemorrhage
    A. Direct pressure on bleeding site
    B. Foley catheter with 30 cc bag seated in naso-pharynx
    C. Anterior and posterior nasal packing with nonadherent gauze.
    D. Electrocoagulation (bleeding points in septum or turbinates).
    E. Ice packs to minimize bleeding and edema
    F. External carotid artery ligation
    G. Anterior ethmoid artery ligation (medial wall of orbit) in extreme cases
III. Initiate measures to control shock and provide volume replacement
    A. Establish intravenous line (possibly central venous)
    B. Ringer's lactate
    C. Whole blood or packed cells if required
IV. Initiate specific management modalities for fractures of the upper third of the face
    A. Fractures of the upper third of the face usually require open reduction. Exploration is often necessary to adequately evaluate the extent of the injury as well as to reduce the fragments. An overlying laceration can often provide access for exploration and reduction of these fractures. The combined abilities of both the neurosurgeon and the plastic surgeon are sometimes needed when an upper facial fracture extends into the cranial vault resulting in hematoma, dural tear, or cerebral injury. Fractures without overlying lacerations can be approached through normal forehead skin lines or an eyebrow incision to minimize scarring. When reducing these fractures unstable fragments may require interosseous fixation with small gauge stainless steel wire
 V. Initiate specific management modalities for fractures of the middle third of the face
    A. Nasal fractures
      1. Closed reduction with intranasal manipulation as soon as possible before swelling
      2. In case of swelling, wait several days for swelling to subside
      3. Comminuted fractures require open reduction and direct wiring of fracture fragments
      4. Pack nose without manipulation to control bleeding
      5. External molded plaster of paris splint is applied with strip of adhesive and left in place 14 days
    B. Fracture of zygomatic arch
      1. Unless edema has set in, closed reduction after evaluation of fragments is done

          Type   I—Intermaxillary fixation alone using the dental occlusion

          Type   II—Requires a more extensive reduction

          Type III—Full craniofacial detachment calls for open reduction and may require external stabilization

    2. Avoid nasal packing, if possible

    3. Prophylactic antibiotic, if indicated

    4. Surgical intervention

    5. Minimal blow out fractures may require no surgery. If the patient has no diplopia, they can be followed on an out-patient basis. Displacement fractures require open reduction

VI. Fractures of the lower third of the face

    A. Mandibular fractures require open or closed reduction. It will depend on the location and angle of the fracture

---

RATIONALE

Primary efforts should be directed toward initial life support (airway, bleeding, circulation.) Hemorrhage can usually be controlled through direct, local pressure. Blood may be aspirated and because blood is an irritant, pneumonitis may develop which can be controlled with prophylactic antibiotics. Evidence of shock warrants a complete systems assessment as bleeding from facial trauma is occasionally a cause of a shock state. Because facial injuries often present with massive bleeding and edema, facial bone fractures may sometimes be overlooked. It is important to obtain appropriate radiologic studies which will help to avoid missing less obvious facial fractures. An IV line with Ringer's lactate assists in monitoring fluid replacement and provides a line for medication administration. Management modalities are implemented relative to the mechanism of injury and disruption or displacement of facial bones, with or without nerve involvement. Once the integrity of bones, muscles, and nerves are ensured, efforts should be directed toward any cosmetic, reconstructive surgery which may be indicated. Patients with closed reductions should be carefully monitored to insure adequate nutritional intake, and protein and vitamin supplements should be administered throughout the course of therapy.

Respiratory Emergencies References

ACUTE UPPER AIRWAY OBSTRUCTION

Burrell, R. O. & Burrell, Z. L. Critical care. St. Louis: C. V. Mosby, 1982, pp. 185–200.

First aid for foreign body obstruction of the airway. Washington, D.C.: The American National Red Cross, 1976.

Gann, D. S. Emergency management of the obstructed airway. Journal of the American Medical Association, 1980, 243, 1141.

Hoffman, J. R. Treatment of foreign body obstructions of the upper airway, *Western Journal of Medicine*, 1982, **136**, 11.

Krupp, M. A., & Chatton, M. J. (Eds.). Foreign bodies in the air and food passages. *Current medical diagnosis and treatment—1983*, Los Altos, Calif.: Lange Medical, 1983, pp. 109–110.

Linscott, M. S., & Horton, W. C. Management of upper airway obstruction. *Otolaryngological Clinics of North America*, 1979, **12**, 351.

Redding, J. S. The choking controversy: Critique of evidence on the Heimlich maneuver. *Critical Care Medicine*, 1979, **7**, 475.

Webb, W. R. Airway obstruction. In H. F. Conn, et al. (Eds.), *Current therapy.* Philadelphia: W.B. Saunders, 1983, p. 86.

CROUP

Giammona, S. T. Croup syndrome. In S. S. Gellis, & B. M. Kagan (Eds.), *Current pediatric therapy.* Philadelphia: W. B. Saunders, 1978, pp. 112–114.

Voyles, J. B. Pulmonary problems in infants and children. *American Journal of Nursing,* 1981, **81**, 509–32.

Whaley, L., & Wong, D. L. *Nursing of infants and children.* St. Louis: C. V. Mosby, 1979, pp. 1250–1251.

ACUTE EPIGLOTTITIS

Bass, J. W., Steele, R. W., & Wiebe, R. A. Acute epiglottitis: A surgical emergency. *Journal of the American Medical Association*, 1974, **229**, 671.

Cantrell, R. W., Bell, R. A., & Marioka, W. T. Acute epiglottitis: Intubation vs. tracheostomy. *Laryngoscope*, 1978, **88**(6).

Faden, H. S. Treatment of hemophilus influenzae type B: The etiologic agent in epiglottitis. *Pediatrics*, 1979, **64**, 402.

Hawkins, D. B., Miller, A. H., & Sachs, G. B. Acute epiglottitis in adults. *Laryngoscope*, 1973, **53**, 1211.

Hirschmann, J. V., & Everett, E. D. Hemophilus influenzae infections in adults: Report of nine cases and a review of the literature. *Medicine*, 1979, **58**, 80.

Lewis, J. K., Galvis, A. G., & Michaels, R. H. A protocol for management of acute epiglottitis: Successful experience with 27 consecutive instances treated by nasotracheal intubation. *Clinical Pediatrics*, 1978, **117**, 494.

Pilrog, J. E. Acute supraepiglottitis (epiglottitis in children). *Topics in Emergency Medicine*, 1981, **3**, 53–56.

Rapkin, R. H. The diagnosis of epiglottitis: Simplicity and reliability of radiographs of the neck in the differential diagnosis of the croup syndrome. *Journal of Pediatrics*, 1972, **80**, 96.

Voyles, J. B. Pulmonary problems in infants and children. *American Journal of Nursing,* 1981, **81**, 509–32.

Weber, M. L., Desjardins, R., Perreault G., et al. Acute epiglottitis in children—Treatment with nasotracheal intubation: Report of 14 consecutive cases. *Pediatrics*, 1976, **57**, 152.

STATUS ASTHMATICUS

Brenner, B. E., et al. Acute asthma: Management and therapy. *Topics in Emergency Medicine*, 1980, **2**, 1–11.

Fireman, P. Status asthmaticus in children. In E. Middleston, C.E. Reed, & E.F. Ellis (Eds.), *Allergy: Principles and practice*. St. Louis: C. V. Mosby, 1978, chap. 42.

Hudgel, D. W., & Madsen, L. A. Acute and chronic asthma—A guide to intervention. *American Journal of Nursing*, 1980, **80**, 1791–95.

Paige, P. Treatment of the asthmatic child. *Respiratory Therapy*, 1979, **9**, 57–60.

Petty, T. L. Ventilatory care of status asthmaticus. In E.B. Weiss, & M.S. Segal (Eds.), *Bronchial asthma: Mechanics and therapeutics*. Boston: Little, Brown, 1976, chap. 61.

Petty, T. L. Status asthmaticus in adults. In E. Middleton, C.E. Reed, & E. F. Ellis (Eds.), *Allergy: Principles and practice*. St. Louis: C. V. Mosby, 1978, chap. 41.

Rushing, J. L. Respiratory tract and mediastinum. In M. A. Krupp, & M. J. Chatton (Eds.), *Current medical diagnosis and treatment*, 1982, chap. 6, pp. 111–114.

Weiss, E. B. Status asthmaticus. In E.B. Weiss, & M.S. Segal (Eds.), *Bronchial asthma: Mechanisms and therapeutics*. Boston: Little, Brown, 1976, chap. 60.

Wray, B. B. Management of acute asthma and status asthmaticus. *Respiratory Therapy*, 1980, **10**, 57–59.

NEAR DROWNING

Conn, A. W., Edmonds, J. F., & Barker, G. A. Near drowning in cold fresh water: Current treatment regime. *Journal of the Canadian Anesthesia Society*, 1978, **25**, 259.

Fandel, I., & Bancalari, E. Near drowning in children. *Pediatrics*, 1976, **58**, 573–579.

Hoff, B. H. Multisystem failure: A review with special reference to drowning. *Critical Care Medicine*, 1979, **7**(7).

Hunt, P. K. Never say drowned. *Emergency Medicine*, 1975, 136–137.

Modell, J. H., & David, J. H. Electrolyte changes in human drowning victims. *Anesthesiology*, 1969, **30**, 414–420.

Modell, J. H., Graves. S. A., & Ketover, A. A clinical course of 91 consecutive near drowning victims. *Chest*, 1976, **70**, 127.

Modell, J. H., Giammona, S. T., & Davis, J. H. Blood gas and electrolyte changes in human near drowning victims. *Journal of the American Medical Association*, 1968, **203**, 99–105.

Pace, N. L. Positive end-expiratory pressure (PEEP) in treating salt water near drowning. *Western Journal of Medicine*, 1975, 122, 167.

Rivers, J. F., Orr, G., & Lee, H. H. Drowning: Its clinical sequelae and management. *British Medical Journal*, 1970, **2**, 157–161.

Knopp, R. Near drowning. *Journal of the American College of Emergency Physicians*, 1978, **7**, 249–254.

Weaver, D. W., et al. Pulmonary effects of albumin resuscitation for severe hypovolemic shock. *Archives of Surgery*, 1978, **113**, 387.

ADULT RESPIRATORY DISTRESS SYNDROME

Cooper, J. D., McDonald, J. W. D., Ali, M., et al. Prostaglandin production associated with the pulmonary vascular response to complement activation. *Surgery*, 1980, **88**, 215–21.

Gracey, D. R. Adult respiratory distress syndrome. *Heart and Lung*, 1975, **4**, 280–3.

Hammerschmidt, D. R., Weaver, L. J., Hudson, L. D., et al. Association of complement activation and elevated plasma C5$_a$ with adult respiratory distress syndrome. *Lancet*, 1980, **1**, 947–9.

Hammerschmidt, D. E., White, J. G. Craddock, P. R., Jacob, H. S. Corticosteroids inhibit complement-induced granulocyte aggregation: A possible mechanism for their efficacy in shock states. *Journal of Clinical Investigation*, 1979, **63**, 798–803

Hopwell, P. C. Adult respiratory distress syndrome. *Basics of Respiratory Distress*, 1979, **7**, 1.

Keren, A., Klein, J., & Stern, S. Adult respiratory distress syndrome in the course of myocardial infarction. *Chest*, 1980, **77**, 161.

McCaffree, D. R. Adult respiratory distress syndrome: Pathogenesis and pharmacologic management. *Hospital Formulary*, 1982, **17**, 1582–8.

Murray, J. F. Mechanisms of acute respiratory failure. *American Review of Respiratory Diseases*, 1977, **115**, 1071.

Petty, T. L., & Ashbaugh, D. C. The adult respiratory distress syndrome: Clinical features, factors influencing prognosis and principles of management. *Chest*, 1971, **60**, 233–9.

Rinaldo, J. E., et al. Adult respiratory distress syndrome: Changing concepts of lung injury and repair. *New England Journal of Medicine*, 1982, **306**, 900.

Sibbald, W. J., Anderson, R. R., Reid, B., et al. Alveolo-capillary permeability in human septic ARDS. *Chest*, 1981, **71**, 133–42.

Spragg, R. C. Adult respiratory distress syndrome. *Hospital Medicine*, 1979, **15**(3), 31–42.

Vaage, J. Intravascular platelet aggregation and acute respiratory failure. *Circulatory Shock*, 1977, **4**, 279–90.

PULMONARY EMBOLISM

Bernstein, E. F. The role of operative inferior vena cava interruption in the management of venous thrombosis. *World Journal of Surgery*, 1978 **2**, 61

Cudkowicz, L., & Sherry, S. Current status of thrombolytic therapy. *Heart Lung*, 1978, **1**, 97.

Dexter, L. Pulmonary embolism and acute cor pulmonale. In J. W. Hurst, & R. B. Logue (Eds.), *The heart* (4th ed.). New York: McGraw-Hill, 1978, pp. 1472–1481.

Griner, P. F., et al. Application of principles of test selection and interpretation. *Annals of Internal Medicine*, 1981, **94**, 571.

Groër, M. E., & Shekleton, M. E. *Basic pathophysiology: A conceptual approach.* St. Louis: C. V. Mosby, 1979.

Holloway, N. M. *Nursing the critically ill adult.* Menlo Park: Addison-Wesley, 1979.

Hirsh, J. Pulmonary embolism. In H. F. Conn (Ed.), *Current therapy: Latest approved methods of treatment for the practicing physician.* Philadelphia: W. B. Saunders, 1983, pp. 120–25.

Marder, V. J. The use of thrombolytic agents: Choice of patient, drug administration, laboratory monitoring. *Annals of Internal Medicine*, 1979, **90**, 802.

Moser, K. M., et al. Deep venous thrombosis and pulmonary embolism: Frequency in a respiratory intensive care unit. *Journal of the American Medical Association*, 1981, **246**, 1422.

Robin, E. D. Overdiagnosis and overtreatment of pulmonary embolism: The emperor may have no clothes. *Annals of Internal Medicine*, 1977, **87**, 775.

Rushing, J. L. Pulmonary embolism. In M. A. Krupp, & M. J. Chatton (Eds.), *Current medical diagnosis and treatment.* Los Altos, Calif.: Lange Medical, 1983, pp. 142–46.

Sharma, G. V. R. K., et al. Pulmonary embolism: The great imitator. *Disease A Month*, 1976.

Sharma, G. V. R. K., et al. Thrombolytic therapy. *New England Journal of Medicine*, 1982, **306**, 1268.

FACIAL TRAUMA

Baker, S. P., & Schultz, R. C. Recurrent problems in emergency room management of maxillofacial injuries. *Clinics in Plastic Surgery*, 1975, **2**, 65–71.

Braintigan, C. O., & Grow, J. B., Sr. Cricothyroidotomy: Elective use in respiratory problems requiring tracheotomy. *Thoracic and Cardiovascular Surgeon*, 1976, **71**, 72.

Schultz, R. C. *Facial injuries*. Chicago, Ill.: Year Book Medical, 1970.

Schultz, R. C. One thousand consecutive cases of major facial injury. *Review of Surgery*, 1970, **27**, 394–410.

Schultz, R. C. Supraorbital and glabellar fractures. *Plastic and Reconstructive Surgery*, 1970, **45**, 227–233.

Schultz, R. C. The changing character and management of soft tissue windshield injuries. *Journal of Trauma*, 1972, **12**, 1.

Schultz, R. C. The nature of facial injury emergencies. *Surgical Clinics of North America*, 1972, **52**, 99.

Schultz, R. C. The management of common fractures. *Surgical Clinics of North America*, 1973, **53**, 3–32.

Schultz, R. C. Frontal sinus and supraorbital fractures from vehicle accidents. *Clinics in Plastic Surgery*, 1975, **2**, 93–106.

Schultz, R. C. *The management of fractures of the upper third of the face and their subsequent reconstruction with alloplastic material.* Paris: Proceedings of the 6th International Confederation of Plastic Surgery, 1975.

Schultz, R. C. *Facial injuries* (2nd ed.). Chicago, Ill.: Year Book Medical, 1977.

Schultz, R. C., & Carbonell, A. T. Midfacial fractures from vehicle accidents. *Clinics in Plastic Surgery*, 1975, **2**, 173–189.

Schultz, R. C., & DeVillers, Y. T. Nasal fractures. *Journal of Trauma*, 1975, **15**, 319–327.

Schultz, R. C., & Oldham, R. J. An overview of facial injuries. *Surgical Clinics of North America*, 1977, **57**, 987.

Schultz, R. C., & Wood, J. R. Facial fractures. *Primary Care*, 1976, **3**(4), 47–68.

Zook, E. G., et al. *The primary care of facial injuries.* Littlejohn, Mass.: PSG Publishing, 1980.

C. CARDIOVASCULAR EMERGENCIES

1. Angina

A. Oppressive substernal chest pain, radiating to neck, jaws, or down left arm
B. Pain lasting from 30 seconds to 10 minutes
C. Precipitating factors—stress, heat, cold, or exercise
D. Diaphoresis
E. Tachycardia
F. Pallor
G. Laboratory values—mostly inconclusive
   1. ECG may show signs of ST elevation or depression
   2. no enzyme changes
H. Future diagnostic tests
   1. stress ECG
   2. stress thallium-201 scanning
   3. echocardiography
   4. cardiac catherization

PATHOPHYSIOLOGY

Myocardial ischemia can be defined as a myocardial oxygen deficit resulting from reduced coronary perfusion. This deficit occurs when myocardial oxygen demands exceed the capacity of the coronary artery supply. The ischemic process may be transient and produce signs and symptoms that are reversible. Angina pectoris is an example of reversible myocardial ischemia. Severe or prolonged ischemia may result in necrosis and myocardial dysfunction. Acute myocardial infarction is an example of irreversible myocardial ischemia.

Clinical manifestations of myocardial ischemia include electrical instability, hemodynamic compromise, and extension of the infarcted area. Electrical instability often appears as ventricular fibrillation, a common cause of sudden cardiac death. Hemodynamic compromise often manifests itself as pulmonary edema or cardiogenic shock. Since early assessment and intervention may salvage myocardium destined for infarction, it is important to assess myocardial infarction in the emergency department. In order to make the diagnosis, a combination of physical examination and history, electrocardiogram, chest x-ray, and cardiac enzyme determinations must be used.

Angina pectoris results from an imbalance between myocardial oxygen demand and supply. Activities that produce angina produce hemodynamic changes such as an increase in heart rate, blood pressure, and, perhaps an increase in left ventricular filling pressure.

The location of ischemic pain or discomfort is classically in the anterior chest with radiation to the shoulders and arms. Pain may also radiate to the neck and/or jaw. Duration of pain is an important assessment tool. Though no exact guidelines are available, anginal attacks rarely last longer that 15 minutes. Circumstances surrounding the onset, worsening, and remission of symptoms are also important. Emotional stress, physical exertion, eating a large meal and/or going out into the heat or cold may precipitate anginal attacks.

Laboratory values are usually inconclusive in establishing the diagnosis of angina. There are usually no cardiac enzyme changes associated with angina. The electrocardiogram may show ST deviations; a depression of ST segments occur in about two thirds of patients, and an elevation is seen in the remaining one third.

To make the diagnosis of ischemic coronary artery disease, stress electrocardiogram, stress thallium-201 scanning, echocardiography, and cardiac catherization need to be performed.

MANAGEMENT

  I. Monitor assessment parameters noting any trends or changes
    A. Pulse rate
    B. Bp
    C. Respiratory rate
    D. Continued cardiac monitoring
 II. Determine appropriate pharmacologic regimen
    A. Nitrates
      1. short-acting
      2. moderate
      3. long-acting
    B. Beta-blockers
    C. Calcium antagonists

RATIONALE

Patients should be observed and monitored in the emergency department for a period of time prior to disposition. Trends in their parameters, pulse rate, blood pressure, respiratory rate, and cardiac monitoring for arrhythmias and ST deviations should be noted. The decision to admit patients with anginal symptoms is based on history, and physical and laboratory findings.

Patients may be placed on a variety of medications. A brief explanation of each group of medications follows. Specific dosages and types vary greatly, and the reader is referred to a pharmacology text for further information.

NITRATES

I. Mechanism of action—vasodilation of vascular smooth muscle
   A. Decreases venous tone, reducing the return of blood to the heart (preload) and ventricular dimensions, which in turn reduces wall tension and afterload
   B. Reduces the heart's mechanical activity, volume, and oxygen consumption, which leads to increased exercise capacity
   C. Increases blood flow to the myocardium in areas perfused by stenotic coronary arteries (especially subendocardial arteries)
   D. Allows for increased heart rate before angina occurs
   E. Improves ventricular wall motion
   F. Reduces left ventricular end-diastolic pressure, which can decrease the resistance to coronary blood flow

II. Types of preparations

Fast-Acting	Transdermal	Long-Acting
Nitroglycerin	Transderm	Cartadid
Nitrobid	Nitrodisc	Isordil
Nitroglyn	Nitrol ointment	Sorbitrate
Nitrospan		Peritrate
Nitro-SA		Cardilate
Nitrong		

III. Most common side effects
   A. Headache
   B. Flushing
   C. Tachycardia
   D. Dizzyness
   E. Postural hypotension

BETA-BLOCKERS

I. Mechanism of action
  A. Block β-adrenergic receptor sites as a result of specific competition with β-adrenergic receptor stimulating agents, thus blocking sympathetic nervous system stimulation
  B. Decrease cardiac index, stroke index, heart rate, bp, and tension time index
  C. Reduce myocardial oxygen consumption per minute per beat in the setting of increased concentration of circulating catecholamines
  D. Are indicated for patients in a hyperdynamic state: sinus tachycardia, hypertension, and no evidence of heart failure
  E. Are indicated for patients with a supraventricular tachyarrhythmia, especially those related to excessive sympathetic stimulation
  F. Are indicated for arrhythmia
    1. recent onset of atrial fibrillation
    2. digitalis-induced arrhythmias
    3. reciprocating tachycardias in Wolff-Parkinson-White syndrome
II. Types of preparations—propranolol, most common
III. Most common side effects
  A. Hypotension
  B. Tachycardia
  C. Congestive heart failure

CALCIUM ANTAGONISTS

I. Mechanism of action
  A. Ischemia-related
    1. dilate coronary arteries and arterioles, increase coronary artery blood flow
    2. inhibit coronary artery constriction and platelet aggregation
    3. reduce myocardial oxygen demand by systemic arteriolar dilatation (reduces afterload)
Calcium channel blockers work to decrease coronary artery spasm, inappropriate coronary arteriolar constriction, and platelet aggregation, and to increase oxygen supply delivery.
  B. Antiarrhythmic
    1. slow conduction and prolong refractoriness of the A-V node. Are useful in the termination of A-V nodal reentrant tachyarrhythmia and in slowing ventricular responses in atrial flutter and fibrillation
II. Types of preparations—verapamil, nifedipine, diltiazem
III. Most common side effects
  A. Hypotension
  B. Headache
  C. Dizziness
  D. Flushing

E. Nausea

F. Leg edema

2. Myocardial Infarction

ASSESSMENT

I. History and physical findings
  A. Oppressive midsubsternal chest pain lasting longer than 30 minutes, radiation to arms, neck, jaw
  B. Accompanying nausea, vomiting and diaphoresis, dyspnea, syncope
  C. Auscultation of an S4 gallop
II. Laboratory studies
  A. Enzymes

	SGOT	LDH	CPK (MB)
elevates	8–12 hr	24–48 hr	6–8 hr
peaks	18–36 hr	3–6 days	24 hr
falls to normal	3–4 days	8–14 days	3–4 days

  B. ECG changes
    1. **Area of Infarct ----------→ ECG Changes**

Anterior	ST ↑, Q waves	Leads I, AVL, V2–V6
Anteroseptal	ST ↑, Q waves	Leads V2–V6
Anterolateral	ST ↑, Q waves	Leads I, AVL, V5–V6
Inferior	ST ↑, Q waves	Leads II, III, AVF
Inferolateral	ST ↑, diminished R waves	Leads V5–V6
Posterior	Tall R waves	Leads V1–V2
Subendocardial	ST ↑, loss of R waves, T wave inversion	

    2. Dysrhythmias and/or conduction disturbances
III. Changes in hemodynamic status
  A. Pulmonary edema/cardiogenic shock
    1. hypotension
    2. dyspnea and rales
    3. cold clammy skin
    4. oliguria
    5. elevated pulmonary capillary wedge pressure
    6. decreased cardiac output

PATHOPHYSIOLOGY

Myocardial infarction occurs as a result of coronary artery disease. It may be due to severe atherosclerosis, acute thrombosis, and/or spasm of one of the main coronary arteries. Necrosis of some degree of heart muscle is involved due to inadequate blood supply. Alterations in left ventricular function invariably accompany an acute infarct. The degee of power failure is proportional to the amount of infarcted tissue. Evidence of left ventricular pump failure develops when about 25 percent of the myocardium is infarcted, severe pump failure or cardiogenic shock when about 40 percent is infarcted.

Acute myocardial infarction is suggested by oppressive midsubsternal chest pain that usually lasts longer than 30 minutes and is not relieved by nitroglycerin. Pain may radiate down both arms or to the jaw and neck. It is usually accompanied by nausea, vomiting, diaphoresis, dyspnea and/or syncope. Silent myocardial infarctions may occur especially in diabetics and hypertensives. History is very important in making a diagnosis. Physical examination may be normal except for the presence of an S4 gallop. An S4 gallop is usually associated with high ventricular filling pressures.

Myocardial cells that are irreversibly injured release enzymes. Lactic dehydrogenase (LDH), serum glutamate oxaloacetate transaminase (SGOT), and creatine phosphokinase (CPK-MB) levels are drawn each day. Time of elevation, peak time and when enzyme levels fall back to normal can be found in the preceding assessment section.

The characteristic electrocardiogram signs of myocardial injury are ST elevation, Q waves, reciprocal ST depression, and inversion of the T wave. Myocardial infarction can be pinpointed by where the changes occur. Localization of the infarct is clinically important because the incidence and significance of complications can vary with the site of infarction. (See electrocardiogram changes in the preceding assessment section.)

The most frequent complications of a myocardial infarction are rhythm and conduction disturbances, left ventricular failure, and cardiogenic shock. The most common rhythm disturbances are premature ventricular contractions, which occur in nearly 90 percent of all patients and may lead to the development of ventricular fibrillation. Premature atrial contractions are reported in 15 to 50 percent of patients and usually precede the development of atrial fibrillation. Assessment of arrhythmias depends mainly on detection.

Conduction disturbances include first degree heart block, which occurs in about 10 percent of patients; Wenckebach (Mobitz I), which occurs in about 6 percent; and Mobitz II, which occurs in 0.6 percent of patients and is usually associated with anterior wall infarction. Complete heart block develops in about 5 to 8 percent of patients. Pacemaker insertion is usually necessary for both Mobitz II and complete heart block.

Left ventricular failure and cardiogenic shock in myocardial infarction result in increased pulmonary capillary pressure and diminished cardiac output. Assessment parameters include a pulmonary capillary wedge pressure about 18 to 20 mm Hg, cardiac output less than 2.24 minute/meter^2, hypotension, fatigue, obtundation, tachycardia, oliguria, and cold clammy skin.

MANAGEMENT

    I. Establish intravenous lines; peripheral and central D5W to keep vein open
   II. Monitor cardiac activity
      A. Continuous monitoring
      B. Serial ECGs
  III. Administer oxygen
      A. 40 percent FIO_2
      B. Blood gas determinations
  IV. Correct acid–base disorder
   V. Treat dysrhythmias (Table 9)
  VI. Relieve pain
      A. Nitrates
      B. Morphine, 2 to 5 mg intravenously
 VII. Monitor and treat hemodynamic complications
      A. Pulmonary edema/cardiogenic shock
         1. provide ventilation and oxygenation
         2. correct acid–base
         3. reduce circulatory demands
            a. diuretics
            b. vasodilators
         4. inotropic agents
            a. dopamine
         5. intra-aortic counterpulsation

RATIONALE

Patients suspected of having a myocardial infarction should be placed in a controlled atmosphere as soon as possible. Continuous cardiac monitoring for potential arrhythmias and/or conduction disturbances is the most important management modality. Insertion of a large-bore peripheral catheter, central venous catheter, and, if necessary, Swan-Ganz catheter should be completed as quickly and with as little induced patient anxiety as possible. A solution of 5 percent dextrose in water is generally begun to keep the lines patent. Oxygen should be administered by mask, concentration about 40 percent depending on blood gas values. It has been shown that the administration of oxygen reduces the degree of ST segment elevation and the size of the infarct. If hypoxia occurs, endotracheal intubation may be necessary. Hypoxia has been shown to be a significant factor in the development of cardiac arrhythmias. Arrhythmias should be treated with appropriate pharmacologic agents (see Table 9). Underlying acid–base or electrolyte abnormalities must be corrected since they may contribute to the development of rhythm disturbances.

    Relief of pain is an important management modality. Severe pain may indicate

TABLE 9. ARRHYTHMIAS AND DRUG MODALITIES

Drug	Mechanism of Action	Dosage and Administration
Quinidine Atrial and ventricular arrhythmias, atrial fibrillation	Acts at the cell membrane to block the fluxs of sodium and potassium, decreasing conduction velocity, increasing automaticity. In addition quinidine also paradoxically has an atropine-like effect increasing A-V conduction	Maximal effects 1–3 hours Duration of action 6–8 hours Dose: usual 200–300 mg q 6 hours PO: maximum 1.6 gm/day
Procainamide Atrial and ventricular arrhythmias	Same as quinidine	PO: 250 mg q 4–6 hours, maximum Maximum effects PO: 1 hour Duration of action: 3–6 hours IV: 100 mg q 5 minutes slowly to 1 gm then continuously infused at a rate of 2–3 gm/day (2–4 mg/minute)
Disopyramide Atrial and ventricular tachyarrhythmias	Same as quinidine	PO: 100–200 mg q 6 hours Onset of action: within 2 hours Duration of action: 4–8 hours (with normal renal function)
Propranolol Atrial and ventricular tachyarrhythmias, supraventricular tachycardia with high bp	β-Adrenergic blockade results in decreased conduction velocity, increased refractory period, and decreased automaticity	PO: 20–30 mg q 6 hours IV: 1 mg q 10 minutes up to 1 g for supraventricular tachycardia

Drug	Indications	Action	Dosage
Lindocaine	Ventricular arrhythmias only, prophylaxis in myocardial infarctions	Poorly understood, but probably acts to stabilize membranes in the Purkinje fibers. This causes increased conduction velocity, decreased refractory period and decreased automaticity	Load: 50–100 mg IV push (1 mg/kg) Maintenance: 2–4 mg/minute continuous IV infusion Because of a decrease in blood levels 20–30 minutes after infusion is started, it may be necessary to give bolus dose
Phenytoin	Atrial and ventricular arrhythmias	Phenytoin appears to act on the cell membrane enhancing the entrance of sodium during depolarization, and potassium during repolarization	IV: 100 mg q 5 minutes to a PO: 1 g during first day, then 300 mg/day
Bretylium	Life-threatening ventricular arryhthmias that have not responded to lidocaine or phenytoin	Post ganglionic sympathetic blocking agent. Initially causes a release of stored catecholamines then blocks further release of β-adrenergic amines producing a sympathectomy-like state. Causes decreased conduction velocity, increased refractory period, and decreased automaticity	IV: 5–10 mg/kg rapidly, may repeat q 15–30 minutes to a maximum 30 mg/day, then 1–2 mg/minute continuous infusion

an extending infarct and may in itself aggravate an infarction due to the increase in release of catecholamines during periods of increased anxiety and pain.

The management of left ventricular failure and cardiogenic shock is complex. The ultimate goal is to improve coronary perfusion and cardiac output by reducing circulatory demands. Preload (ventricular end-diastolic volume) can be reduced by the use of diuretics, rotating tourniquets, morphine, and nitrates. Afterload (the resistance against which the heart must pump) can be reduced by the use of vasodilators (e.g., sodium nitroprusside), and the use of intra-aortic counterpulsation techniques.

3. Hypertensive Emergencies

ASSESSMENT

    I. Hypertensive encephalopathy
      A. Diastolic bp greater than 140 mm Hg
      B. Retinopathy and papilledema
      C. Change in mental status
      D. Generalized headache
      E. Vomiting
      F. Drowsiness, confusion
      G. Focal neurological deficits
      H. Coma and death
   II. Malignant hypertension
      A. Diastolic bp greater than 140 mm Hg
      B. Severe headache
      C. Blurred vision
      D. Retinal changes with papilledema
      E. End organ damage
         Cardiac—left ventricular hypertrophy, cardiomegaly
         Renal—hematuria, proteinuria
         Hematologic—microangiopathic hemolytic anemia
  III. Aortic dissection
      A. Diastolic bp greater than 130 mm Hg
      B. Chest pain that radiates to the back
      C. Strong upper extremity pulse and bp
      D. Weak lower extremity pulse and bp
      E. Depending on vessels involved
         1. cerebral ischemia
         2. aortic insufficiency
         3. paraplegia and anesthesia below the level of cord ischemia
         4. renal ischemia
      F. Aortography

IV. Hypertension with congestive heart failure
    A. Diastolic bp greater than 130 mm Hg
    B. Dyspnea
    C. Rales
    D. Elevated central venous pressure
    E. Peripheral edema
    F. Angina
 V. Toxemia of pregnancy
    A. Elevation of prepregnant bp
       Systolic greater than 20 mm Hg
       Diastolic greater than 10 mm Hg
    B. Visual disturbances, headaches
    C. Edema of face and hands
    D. Proteinuria
    E. Seizures
VI. Catecholamine excess due to pheochromocytoma, monoamine oxidase inhibitors, discontinuation of clonidine (Catapres)
    A. Diastolic bp greater than 130 mm Hg
    B. Tachycardia
    C. Tremulousness
    D. Diaphoresis
VII. Other laboratory parameters
    A. Blood urea nitrogen
    B. Creatinine
    C. Urinalysis—for additional protein and blood
    D. Electrocardiogram—hypertensive changes
    E. Chest x-ray
    F. CSF

PATHOPHYSIOLOGY

Hypertension is not a disease in itself but an end result of multiple disease processes. The most common type is essential hypertension; specific cause unknown, though factors such as heredity, age, race, obesity, and sodium ingestion contribute to the development of hypertension. Two theories are offered as to why physiologic changes occur; the first states that hypertension occurs secondary to alterations of the contractile properties of smooth muscle in the arterial walls. The second theory states that failure of the normal autoregulatory mechanisms occurs resulting in low plasma renin levels and ineffective autonomic blockade which leads to a secondary alteration of arterial smooth muscle.

    Other causes beside essential hypertension include primary renal disease, unilateral renal artery stenosis, coarctation of the aorta, atherosclerosis, excessive glucocorticoids, pheochromocytomas, and excessive catecholamine release.

    Specific pathophysiology involved is discussed for the following etiologies. Hypertensive encephalopathy occurs when there is an abrupt, sustained rise in blood pressure which exceeds the limits of cerebral autoregulation. Above a mean arterial pressure of 150 to 200 mm Hg, autoregulation is unable to control cerebral blood flow which leads to vasospasm, ischemia, increased vascular permeability, and brain edema. Assessment parameters include headaches, vomiting, confusion, and change in mental status. Papilledema and retinopathy is also present. Focal neurologic deficits occur. Seizures may develop and the patient may lapse into a coma. There may be elevated levels of blood urea nitrogen, creatinine and hematuria may be noted. The cerebral spinal fluid is clear, increased pressure and protein is noted. Hypertensive encephalopathy is acute in onset and reversible.

Malignant hypertension is either found in a patient with persistent blood pressure elevation or as an initial presentation of a hypertensive patient. The importance of the malignant phase of hypertension is that rapid, progressive, and serious damage is being done to the various organ systems of the body especially the renal, cardiac, and cerebral systems. Physical findings include headache, blurred vision, dyspnea, rales at the lung bases, enlarged left ventricle, chest pain, retinal changes, uremia with elevated levels of blood urea nitrogen and creatinine, hematuria, and proteinuria.

Aortic dissection usually begins with a tear in the aortic intima with blood dissecting within the aorta through the media. Approximately 50 percent of dissections begin in the ascending aorta, 30 percent in the arch, and 20 percent in the descending aorta. Specific symptoms depend on the major vessels involved. Severe cerebral ischemia is usually found with involvement of the carotid arteries. If the coronary arteries are involved myocardial infarction may occur. If spinal arteries are involved subsequent paraplegia and parasthesia may result and if the renal arteries are affected renal ischemia may occur.

Aortography is required to confirm the diagnosis; ECG and chest X-ray may be helpful.

Most patients with congestive heart failure have a certain degree of increased peripheral vascular resistance and resultant hypertension. As a response to the hypertension, myocardial hypertrophy occurs. In the face of severe hypertension, myocardial hypertrophy is insufficient, the left ventricle begins to fail and dilate. Ventricular dilatation can lead to both pulmonary edema and aortic insufficiency. Angina type pain occurs along with rales, dyspnea, and elevation of central venous pressure.

Toxemia of pregnancy is defined as the onset of hypertension, edema and proteinuria during the late stages of pregnancy. Seizures (eclampsia) may be present or absent (preeclampsia). The cause of hypertension in the pregnant woman is questionable but it appears to be due to a combination of vasoconstriction and volume expansion. One does not wait for a diastolic of greater than 130 mm Hg. Treatment begins if there is an elevation of 20 mm Hg systolic and/or 10 mm Hg diastolic from the prepregnant level. Symptoms include proteinuria, edema, headache, visual disturbances, and convulsions.

In pheochromocytomas, the tumor produces catecholamines. Those patients who are on drugs that inhibit monoamine oxidase find that in the presence of tyramine (found in cheeses, wines, coffee, and chocolate) excess amounts of norepineph-rine are released. Lastly, abrupt discontinuation of clonidine allows unopposed α-receptors to circulate catecholamines with resultant vasoconstriction and hyperten-sion.

In all of the above, catecholamine excess usually produces symptoms of palpi-tations, tachycardia, malaise, apprehension, and sweating.

MANAGEMENT

I. Rapid reduction of bp with pharmaceutical agents (Table 10)
  A. Insertion of lifelines
    1. peripheral intravenous
    2. central venous catheter
    3. arterial catheter, monitoring
    4. Foley catheter
  B. Monitor trends and responses
    1. bp
    2. pulse
    3. respirations
    4. temperature
    5. central venous pressure
    6. arterial pressure
    7. urine output
    8. blood urea nitrogen
    9. creatinine
    10. proteinuria
    11. peripheral edema
    12. level of consciousness
  C. Specific therapies
    1. hypertensive encephalopathy
      a. nitroprusside therapy
      b. diazoxide and furosemide therapy
    2. malignant hypertension
      a. nitroprusside therapy
    3. aortic dissection
      a. trimethaphan or nitroprusside with propranolol
      b. surgical management
    4. hypertension with congestive heart failure
      a. nitroprusside
      b. morphine, oxygen, furosemide
    5. toxemia of pregnancy
      a. hydralazine, 10 to 25 mg in 500 ml D5W
      b. magnesium sulfate, 4 to 6 g in a 10 percent solution over 20 minutes
      c. darkened room

    d. sedation

    e. restricted salt diet to 500 to 1000 mg/day

  6. catecholamine excess due to pheochromocytoma, monoamine oxidase inhibitors, discontinuation of clonidine (Catapres)

    a. phentolamine, 5 mg IV repeat in 5 to 6 hours

RATIONALE

The hypertensive crisis is a life-threatening condition that requires immediate intervention and prompt reduction of blood pressure. Any of the above mentioned conditions may be associated with this crisis, the major problem is the elevation of blood pressure not the etiologic basis for the hypertension.

All patients must be monitored closely; arterial monitoring should be established prior to using any of the fast-acting antihypertensives. Monitoring of other parameters, i.e., cardiac monitoring, respirations, temperature, urine output, central venous pressure, should be done accurately every half hour. Determining any change in the patient's level of consciousness, focal neurologic signs including pupillary response and movement of extremities should also be done initially every half hour. Laboratory values of special interest are blood urea nitrogen, creatinine, hematuria, and proteinuria. Renal function must be maintained.

The major management thrust in a patient in hypertensive crisis is to immediately decrease the blood pressure. A variety of pharmaceutical agents may be used (see Table 10).

Specific modalities are as follows for hypertensive encephalopathy:

- Nitroprusside (Nipride) is a direct vasodilator, with an extremely rapid rate of onset, duration of action very short, 100 percent effective in lowering blood pressure, and must be given as a continuous intravenous infusion. The usual adult dose is 0.5 to 10 mg/kg/minute.
- Diazoxide (Hyperstat) decreases peripheral resistance and increases cardiac output. The usual adult dose is 300 mg intravenously given as a bolus, onset of action is extremely rapid, and the duration of action can last from 3 to 12 hours. Diazoxide should be used cautiously in patients with congestive heart failure because the drug causes a marked sodium and water retention. Because of this effect, 20 to 40 mg of Furosemide should be given intravenously. Rapid lowering of the blood pressure with either of two mentioned therapies should result in reversal of most of the symptoms within minutes.

The treatment of malignant hypertension consists of the judicious lowering of the blood pressure by 30 to 40 percent. The agent used depends on the clinical condition. If a rapid result is necessary nitroprusside or diazoxide can be used. Patients with a less severe clinical picture can have their blood pressure lowered over a 24- to 48-hour period (see Table 10).

For a patient with an aortic dissection, it is necessary to diminish the force of ventricle systole as well as to keep the blood pressure at the lowest level while providing adequate organ perfusion. Therefore, drugs of choice should decrease myo-

TABLE 10. DRUGS USED IN THE TREATMENT OF HYPERTENSIVE EMERGENCIES

Drug	Indications	Contraindications	Mechanism	Dose/Route	Onset	Comment
Nitroprusside (Nipride)	Hypertensive encephalopathy, malignant high bp, high bp with ASHD, aortic dissection (after giving propranolol)		Arterial and venous dilatation	0.5–8.0 μg/minute IV by I-Med	1–2 minutes	Wrap in tinfoil. Always use I-Med, never gravity drip. Requires constant bp monitoring
Diazoxide	Hypertensive encephalopathy, malignant high bp	Aortic dissection, high bp with ASHD	Arterial dilatation	150–300 mg rapid IV push, may be repeated in 15 minutes if needed. May be given with Lasix 40 mg IV	1–10 minutes	Have Levophed or Aramine drip ready
Trimethaphan (Arfonad)	Aortic dissection		Ganglionic blockade	0.25 mg/minute IV drip	5–10 minutes	Tilt head of bed up
Hydralazine	Toxemia of pregnancy, asymptomatic high bp without ASHD	Aortic dissection, acute or chronic ASHD	Arterial dilatation	5–10 mg IM q 1–2 hours	10–20 minutes	In toxemia, use after MgSO$_4$
Methyldopa (Aldomet)	Chronic asymptomatic high bp	Encephalopathy, acute CVA with altered mental status	False CNS neurotransmitter	250–500 mg po or IV (slowly)	2–3 hours	Watch for lethargy, postural bp changes
Phentolamine (Regitine)	Pheochromocytoma		β-adrenergic blockade	2.5–5.0 mg IV q 5 minutes		
Clonidine (Catapres)	Clonidine withdrawal, asymptomatic severe high bp		Central β-adrenergic blockade	0.2 mg po, then 0.1 mg q 1 hour (average total dose. 0.5 mg)	30–60 minutes	Do not use if patient unreliable

cardial contractility as well as peripheral vascular resistance. The drug of choice is trimethaphan (Arfonad) given intravenously at 1 to 10 mg/minute. Propranolol is used in conjunction with trimethaphan to reduce cardiac rate and to lower systolic ejection. The dose is usually 1 to 3 mg intramuscularly.

For the hypertensive patient with accompanying conjestive heart failure, the objective is to lower the blood pressure in hope of preventing a myocardial infarction by decreasing cardiac work and oxygen consumption. The drug of choice is sodium nitroprusside. Diazoxide is contraindicated because of its side effect of retaining salt and water. Other therapeutic modalities can be used including morphine, nitrates, oxygen, and furosemide.

The treatment of toxemia is aimed at its prevention and early detection by proper prenatal care. Management modalities should include bedrest in a darkened room, salt restriction to 500 to 1000 mg daily and sedation with phenobarbital. If seizures occur or blood pressure is greater than 140/90 mm Hg, magnesium sulfate should be given. Dosage is initially 4 to 6 g in a 10 percent solution over 20 minutes with continued infusion at a rate of 1 g/hour with constant monitoring. If the blood pressure is greater than 120 mm Hg diastolic, an intravenous drip consisting of 10 to 25 mg hydralazine in 500 ml of D5W should be started. Nitroprusside should be avoided because of its potential side effects on the fetus. As soon as the patient's condition has stabilized, the delivery of the fetus is indicated.

Phentolamine is the α-receptor blocking agent used to treat patients who are hypertensive due to catecholamine excess. The dosage is 5 mg intravenously which may be repeated in 4 to 6 hours.

4. Noncardiovascular Trauma

PNEUMOTHORAX

ASSESSMENT

A. Chest pain referred to the shoulder or arm on the involved side
B. Dyspnea
C. Hyperresonance
D. Decreased chest wall movement
E. Decreased breath sounds
F. Chest x-ray findings: retraction of lung from the parietal pleura, mediastinal shift away from the involved side

PATHOPHYSIOLOGY

The intrapleural pressure is slightly below atmospheric pressure, and the presence of this partial vacuum between the parietal and visceral pleural surfaces is responsible for normal respiratory function. As the diaphragmatic, intercostal, and other

muscles of inspiration contract to enlarge the thoracic cage, the lungs passively follow the diaphragm and the chest wall because of the increased negative pressure
thus produced. Conversely, when the respiratory reflexes halt the inspiratory effort,
the diaphragm and chest wall return passively to the resting condition of expiration.
When there is loss of this *negative pressure*, either due to a blunt or a penetrating
injury which allows air to accumulate in the pleural space, the lung contracts.
Pneumothorax can be caused by penetration of the chest wall, laceration of the
lung, perforation of the bronchus or trachea, and rupture of the alveoli secondary to
blunt trauma.

MANAGEMENT

   I. Maintain adequate airway
     A. O$_2$ mask
     B. Endotracheal intubation, if necessary
  II. Establish the following lifelines
     A. Peripheral intravenous line
     B. Central intravenous line
 III. Monitor continuously for trends and response
     A. Chest wall movement
     B. Percussion of chest sounds bilaterally
     C. Auscultation of breath sounds bilaterally
     D. Bp
     E. Pulse
     F. Respiratory role
     G. Arterial blood gases
     H. Central venous pressure
     I. Routine blood work
     J. Serial chest x-rays
     K. ECG
 IV. Maintain fluid balance
     A. Crystalloid solution (lactated Ringer's, normal saline) depending on moni-
       toring parameters
  V. Reestablish negative pressure within the pleural space
     A. Insertion of argyle chest catheter connected to underwater seal drainage
       and suction
 VI. Prophylactic tetanus and antibiotic immunization

RATIONALE

The first priority must always be the patient's airway. An adequate airway must be
identified or established and oxygen initiated. A 40 percent high-humidity mask is
usually placed on the patient until arterial blood gas results are obtained. With a
simple mask, oxygen is usually sufficient. If endotracheal intubation is necessary, al-

ways remember that neck injuries may be present, therefore avoid unnecessary movement of the head and neck. A patient in stress has oxygen requirements one to two times normal. Try to keep the patient's arterial oxygen tension between 80 and 100 mm Hg.

A large bore peripheral venous catheter should be established immediately. A second one, to monitor central venous pressure, should be inserted to assess the ability of the right heart to accept a fluid load. Ringer's lactate is the initial fluid replacement choice. It is the safest physiologic solution available for infusion in large volumes. One half of the lactate is metabolized in the liver and changed to bicarbonate, the other half is excreted by the kidneys unchanged. Second choice for fluids would be normal saline, though it is usually adequate for fluid replacement, one runs the risk of placing the patient in an hyperchloremic acidosis. The amount of fluid given to a patient is determined by constant monitoring of the patient's vital signs, assessment of the patient's respiratory status, and blood test results. Assessment parameters should include blood pressure, pulse, respiratory rate, chest wall movement, bilateral percussion, and auscultation of chest sounds. Routine blood work should include complete blood count, serum electrolytes, type and crossmatch, and arterial blood gases. In addition, all chest trauma patients should have a CPK isoenzyme drawn. Positive results of the latter would indicate the presence of a myocardial contusion. Patients should be monitored and reassessed initially every 10 minutes until stable.

To reestablish negative pressure within the pleural space, a thoracostomy tube is inserted and connected to an underwater seal drainage suction system. An argyle chest catheter (32 to 36 French) is inserted in the fourth or fifth intercostal space at the midaxillary line on the affected side. Small anterior chest tubes are usually not as effective and are generally not used in trauma patients. For a patient with a spontaneous pneumothorax, one may use an anterior chest tube placed in the second intercostal space.

Prophylactic broad spectrum antibiotics are generally used for all trauma patients. They should be given as soon as possible after the injury to obtain adequate blood levels prior to surgery. Antibiotics are usually given for 48 hours posttrauma or surgery.

Tetanus prophylaxis should not be forgotten. Tetanus immunization is as follows:

- No history obtainable: 0.5 ml absorbed toxoid IM
                             0.250 units tetanus immune globulin IM
- Last immunization greater than 10 years: 0.5 ml absorbed toxoid IM
- Last immunization less than 5 years: no immunization necessary

HEMOTHORAX

ASSESSMENT

A. Pleuritic chest pain
B. Dyspnea

C. Dullness on percussion

D. Decreased breath sounds

E. Chest x-ray findings: opacification of the involved hemithorax, air–fluid levels if patient is in an erect position

F. Circulatory insufficiency—hypotension, tachycardia, decreased tissue perfusion, decreased urine output

PATHOPHYSIOLOGY

Accumulation of blood within the pleural space may be due to blunt or penetrating injuries of the lung, chest wall vessels, intercostal vessels, and/or heart. Accumulation of blood within the pleural space results in collapse of the ipsilateral lung and depending upon the extent of the bleeding, respiratory and circulatory insufficiency may occur. Hemothorax is classified according to the amount of blood, minimal 350 ml, moderate 350 to 1500 ml, or massive 1500 ml or more. With a moderate or massive hemothorax circulatory changes result from a loss of systemic volume, decrease in blood pressure, increase in pulse rate, decrease in urine output, decrease in central venous pressure, and other signs of decreased organ and tissue perfusion.

MANAGEMENT

I. Maintain adequate airway
   A. O₂ mask
   B. Endotracheal tube intubation, if necessary
II. Establish the following lifelines
   A. Large bore peripheral line
   B. Central venous line
   C. Foley catheter
III. Monitor continuously for trends and responses
   A. Chest wall movement
   B. Percussion of chest sounds bilaterally
   C. Auscultation of breath sounds bilaterally
   D. Bp
   E. Pulse
   F. Respiratory rate
   G. Urine output
   H. Arterial blood gases
   I. Serial chest x-ray
   J. Routine blood values
   K. Chest tube output
   L. ECG
IV. Maintain fluid balance
   A. Crystalloid solution—lactated Ringer's
   B. Replace blood volume lost

   V. Reestablish negative pressure within the pleural space
      A. Insertion of argyle chest catheter—underwater seal drainage
      B. Surgical intervention, if necessary
  VI. Prophylactic antibiotics and tetanus immunization

RATIONALE

The first priority must always be the establishment or identification of an adequate airway. Once accomplished, nasal prong or face mask oxygen is usually adequate. The goal is to maintain arterial oxygen tension between 80 and 100 mm Hg.

Establishment of effective large bore peripheral catheter line and central line must be done immediately. Depending on the type of hemothorax, the patient may have lost in blood volume from 350 ml in a minimal hemothorax to greater than 1500 ml in a massive hemothorax. Initial fluid resuscitation is done with lactated Ringer's or normal saline. Crystalloid fluid replacement is accomplished by assuming that two thirds of all fluid given will be lost into the interstitial spaces and only one third will remain in the plasma. As soon as possible blood replacement should begin. In life-threatening situations, type-specific blood can be given without proper crossmatch. If type-specific blood is not available then type O blood may be used. All blood should be given through a macropore filter to decrease platelet and fibrin aggregate accumulation.

Continuous monitoring of the patient's vital signs, urine output, and chest tube drainage are excellent indicators of the amount of fluid replacement needed. A urine output of at least 50 ml per hour in an adult patient should be maintained.

Drainage of the hemothorax is done by the insertion of a 36 French argyle catheter into the fourth or fifth intercostal space midaxillary line. This chest catheter is attached to an underwater seal and suction. If there is a great deal of bleeding, an additional chest tube is placed posterior to the first catheter to prevent a loculation of the hemothorax. Blood in the pleural space remains liquid for an extended period of time due to the movement of the heart and lungs. This produces defibrination, which when coupled with fibrinolytic substances secreted from the pleural mediastinum, inhibits clotting. If a hemothorax is not treated adequately, the blood ultimately clots, resulting in the formation of loculated hemothorax which can only be removed surgically.

Chest tube drainage must be monitored hourly. When the rate of bleeding is greater than 100 ml per hour surgical exploration of the chest to ligate the edges of a lacerated lung or a bleeding chest wall vessel, or to remove a large intrathoracic clot, is indicated.

Patients are started on prophylactic broad spectrum antibiotics immediately upon arrival to the emergency department. Antibiotics are usually continued for 48 hours postinjury.

Tetanus prophylaxis should be given as follows:

• No history obtainable. Never immunized: 0.5 ml absorbed toxoid IM
                                           250 units tetanus immune globulin IM

- Last immunization greater than 10 years: 0.5 ml absorbed toxoid IM
- Last immunization less than 5 years: no immunization necessary

TENSION PNEUMOTHORAX

ASSESSMENT

A. Decreased chest wall movement on affected side
B. Hyperresonance by percussion on affected side
C. Decreased breath sounds on affected side
D. Marked dyspnea
E. Trachea deviated to the opposite side
F. Distended neck veins
G. Displacement of cardiac impulse away from injured side
H. Chest x-ray findings—pneumothorax with displacement of mediastinal structures

PATHOPHYSIOLOGY

Accumulation of air in the pleural space with no release of pressure results in an ipsilateral collapse of the affected lung with an additional displacement of the mediastinal structures toward the unaffected side. This occurs when there is no free communication in the pleural space during inspiration, but due to the type of injury air is inhibited in its return to the lung during expiration. The resulting respiratory and circulatory embarrassment makes a tension pneumothorax, one of the most life-threatening chest injuries. The picture includes a totally collapsed lung, displacement of mediastinal structures and heart to the contralateral side, and total venous return impaired by the increased pressure and distortion of the vena cava.

MANAGEMENT

I. Maintain adequate airway
   A. O$_2$ mask
   B. Endotracheal intubation, if necessary
II. Immediate release of pressure within the pleural space
   A. Needle 15 or 16 gauge to aspirate the air
III. Establish the following lifelines
   A. Peripheral venous line
   B. Central venous line
   C. Foley catheter
IV. Monitor continuously for trends and responses
   A. Chest wall movement

B. Percussion of chest sounds bilaterally
C. Auscultation of breath sounds bilaterally
D. Auscultation of heart sounds
E. Bp
F. Pulse
G. Respiratory rate
H. Central venous pressure
I. Arterial blood gases
J. Routine blood tests
K. Serial chest x-rays
L. Neck vein distention
M. Tracheal deviation
N. ECG
V. Maintain fluid balance
 A. Crystalloid solution (lactated Ringer's, normal saline) depending on monitoring parameters
VI. Reestablish negative pressure within the pleural space
 A. Insertion of argyle chest catheter connected to underwater seal drainage
VII. Prophylactic tetanus and antibiotic immunization

RATIONALE

Tension pneumothorax is a life-threatening emergency that demands immediate decompression of the hemothorax. This should be done as soon as the patient's airway is established. Oxygen should be delivered at 12 liters per mask or under positive pressure with a bag–valve mask device.

A needle thoracentesis should be performed by inserting a needle (3 to 6 cm in length) into the second intercostal space, midclavicular line on the affected side. Needle should be attached to a 50 ml syringe and air should be aspired until the patient's acute symptoms are alleviated. As soon as possible an argyle chest tube or mushroom catheter should be placed in the same anterior second intercostal space at the midclavicular line. The chest tube should be attached to an underwater suction to reestablish negative pressure within the pleural space.

A large bore peripheral venous catheter should be established immediately. A second central venous catheter should also be inserted. Central venous pressure monitoring is a valuable tool in assessing venous return. A rising CVP may indicate a deterioration of the tension pneumothorax. Ringer's lactate is the initial choice for fluid replacement. It is the most nearly physiologic solution available for infusion in large volumes. The second choice for fluid replacement is normal saline. Although it is usually adequate, one runs the risk of placing the patient in a hyperchloremic acidosis.

Monitoring of the patient's vital signs, central venous pressure, and urine output are all good parameters in determining the amount of fluid needed. Additionally, the patient must be constantly assessed for any change in respiratory pattern, neck vein distention, tracheal deviation and breath sound auscultation, and percussion.

Routine blood work should be drawn, and serial x-rays and arterial blood gases taken. Baseline determination should be documented and any alteration should be noted and acted on.

Prophylactic broad spectrum antibiotics are generally given to all trauma patients immediately upon arrival to the emergency department. In this way adequate blood levels can be reached prior to surgery. Antibiotics are usually given for the first 48 hours.

Tetanus prophylaxis should not be forgotten.

- If no history is obtainable and/or patient has never been immunized, 0.5 ml absorbed toxoid IM and 250 units tetanus immune globulin IM
- Last immunization more than 10 years prior: 0.5 ml absorbed toxoid IM
- Last immunization less than 5 years prior: no tetanus immunization necessary

FLAIL CHEST

ASSESSMENT

A. Paradoxical chest wall movements during respirations
B. Pleuritic chest pain
C. Crepitus
D. Pain and splinting of affected side
E. Hypoxia
F. Hypercapnea
G. Chest x-ray findings—may show fractured ribs, pneumothorax or hemothorax, pulmonary contusions

PATHOPHYSIOLOGY

Fracture of two or more adjacent ribs anteriorally or laterally, segmental fracture and/or bilateral rib fractures, result in a "flail chest." Effective ventilation depends upon the presence of a stable wall in order for air to move in and out of the lungs as the result of diaphragmatic descent and elastic recoil of the lungs. When the chest wall is damaged, ventilatory effectiveness is impaired. The damaged portion of the chest wall responds paradoxically; during inspiration, when the rest of the thorax is expanding the portion that is flail sinks in, and on expiration, when the rest of the thorax is contracting, the flail portion moves outward. These paradoxical movements result in a decreased total volume. Other physiologic effects are probably due to the underlying pulmonary contusion, atelectasis, hypercapnia, and hypoxia, which increase the alveolar–arterial gradient and decrease the oxygen carrying capacity of the blood volume.

MANAGEMENT

I. Maintain adequate airway
   A. O_2 mask
   B. Intubate and ventilate
      1. Pao_2 less than 60 mm Hg
      2. $Paco_2$ greater than 45 mm Hg
II. Establish the following lifelines
   A. Peripheral venous line
   B. Central venous line
   C. Swan–Ganz catheter
   D. Foley catheter
III. Monitor continuously for trends and responses
   A. Chest wall movement
   B. Arterial blood gases
   C. Bp
   D. Pulse rate
   E. Respiratory rate
   F. Temperature
   G. Urine output
   H. Level of consciousness
   I. Pulmonary artery and capillary wedge pressures
   J. Routine blood work including MB–CPK isoenzyme to rule out myocardial contusion
   K. Serial chest x-rays
   L. ECG and cardiac monitoring
IV. Provide for adequate fluid resuscitation
   A. Replace blood loss
   B. Fluid restriction to 50 ml/hour
   C. Colloids for serum albumin less than 3
   D. Diuretic therapy—Lasix 40 mg IV
V. Decrease alveolar–arterial O_2 difference
   A. Volume ventilator with PEEP
   B. Intensive pulmonary toilet—suctioning, cupping, posturing, humidification
VI. Stabilize chest wall
   A. External stabilization—splinting, intercostal nerve block, and analgesics
   B. Internal stabilization—endotracheal intubation and mechanical stabilization
VII. Promote methods to stabilize alveolar insult and injury
   A. Broad spectrum antibiotics
   B. Steroids
VIII. Alleviate and control pain
   A. Morphine sulfate IV in small doses

RATIONALE

Immediate treatment of a flail chest is necessary to decrease the morbidity and mortality of this injury. The patient should be admitted to an intensive care area as soon as possible. A baseline set of x-rays, blood laboratory work, including complete blood count (CBC), blood urea nitrogen (BUN) and electrolytes, type and cross-match, arterial blood gases, and liver enzyme (especially MB–CPK) should be drawn. An adequate airway must be established. Initially, patients will usually do well with a high-humidity mask, but as the muscles tire and the overall fatigue experienced by a patient who is working hard to maintain adequate ventilation increases, more aggressive methods may be needed. If the PaO_2 falls below 60 mm Hg on room air or if the PaO_2 rises above 45 mm Hg, endotracheal intubation and mechanical ventilation should be done.

A peripheral venous catheter should be placed immediately. A central venous catheter should be inserted to assist in monitoring the patient's ability to accept a fluid load. In addition, as soon as possible a Swan–Ganz catheter, for measurement of pulmonary artery and capillary wedge pressures, should be inserted. A Foley catheter should be in place to help monitor urine output, an excellent indicator of adequate organ perfusion.

It is very difficult to fluid resuscitate these patients without causing overhydration. Initial blood loss must be replaced. Afterward, crystalline fluid is usually restricted to approximately 50 ml/hour. Patients are usually started on colloid therapy to increase serum oncotic pressure and thereby decrease the incidence of fluid sequestration in the interstitial tissues (alveoli). Administration of a diuretic to also decrease interstitial edema is often advocated. Lasix (furosemide) 40 mg intravenously is usually given especially if the patient shows evidence of fluid overload, i.e., elevated pulmonary artery wedge pressure.

To decrease alveoli–arterial oxygen difference patients are usually placed on volume ventilator with PEEP (positive end expiratory pressure). The use of PEEP enables one to use lower F_IO_2, improve ventilation of nonventilated alveoli, and prevent further alveoli filling or collapse. These measures should work to decrease alveoli–arterial oxygen difference.

A flail chest victim with adequate arterial blood gases can usually be managed with external stabilization, analgesia, good pulmonary toilet, and careful fluid resuscitation. A severe flail chest victim must be internally stabilized. This is accomplished by endotracheal intubation and volume ventilation. The lungs act as a splint and stabilizes the rib fractures in an "out" position.

Other therapeutic modalities used in treating a patient with a flail chest include the use of prophylactic antibiotics, steroids, and analgesics. Pain can be controlled with small doses of intravenous morphine or with intercostal nerve blocks. Broad spectrum antibiotics are started immediately and continued for a minimum of 5 days. Appropriate blood cultures are taken and patients are started on specific antibacterial agents as needed. Methyl prednisolone is given immediately and every 6 hours for 2 or 3 days. Steroids are given in the hope of mitigating cellular injury.

Patients should be watched closely for at least 2 to 3 days because underlying pulmonary contusions may not become clinically evident. Other complications one should be aware of are myocardial contusions, hemothorax and pneumothorax, and/or bronchial or tracheal tears.

5. Cardiovascular Trauma

MYOCARDIAL CONTUSIONS

ASSESSMENT

   I. Associated injuries
     A. One to three rib fractures
     B. Sternal fracture
  II. Retrosternal chest pain
     A. Usually delayed 24 hours to 3 days
 III. Abnormalities in the ECG
     A. Persistent tachycardia
     B. ST elevations, T wave inversions
     C. Right bundle branch block
     D. Atrial flutter, fibrillation
     E. Premature ventricular contractions
 IV. Development of a new cardiac murmur
  V. Pericardial friction rub (late)
 VI. Diagnostic tests
     A. CPK–MB isoenzyme levels
     B. Radionuclide scanning
     C. Coronary artery catherizations

PATHOPHYSIOLOGY

Blunt cardiac trauma is an often missed clinical entity. In this age of high speed automobiles, any patient involved in a motor vehicle accident should be observed for blunt injury to the chest. A myocardial contusion produces cellular injury but not death. On autopsy, tissue of a contused heart shows a well demarcated area of hemorrhage. Hemorrhage may be confined to the myocardium or may lacerate areas of the epicardium or endocardium, resulting in hemopericardium. Microscopic examination reveals a varying degree of muscle damage and additional vascular damage to the capillaries. Small pericardial effusions occur within 2 weeks in about 50 percent of patients. A fibrinous reaction at the contusion site may occur and lead to a delayed rupture of the myocardium and/or ventricular aneurysm.

The clinical picture of a myocardial contusion is often vague and nonspecific. Associated injuries to the bony structure of the chest, first to third rib fractures, and sternal fractures should lead to a high index of suspicion. Chest pain is usually delayed up to 24 hours; it is retrosternal in location and original in character. The most common sign is persistent tachycardia despite successful resuscitation of hypovolemia and hypoxemia. Tachycardia is probably due to the reduced cardiac output (myocardial injury) and a normal blood pressure.

The electrocardiogram obtained after injury is usually nonspecific; the most common arrhythmias are premature ventricular contractions, atrial flutter, and fibrillation. The site of the chest injury may determine the type of cardiac arrhythmia seen. Blunt injury to the right side of the chest effects the right atrium and conduction system and leads to atrial arrhythmias, sinoatrial block, and a high degree of atrioventricular block. An injury to the left side results in primarily ventricle rhythm disturbances, premature ventricular contractions, and right bundle branch block.

Isoenzyme levels of CPK–MB become elevated when myocardial tissue is damaged. Serial enzymes show a peak level in 12 hours and return to normal within 72 hours.

An aid to establish a diagnosis may be the use of radionucleotide imaging with Tc–Sn polyphosphate. The reliability of these tests is still being studied.

MANAGEMENT

I. Maintain adequate airway
  A. Face mask O_2
II. Establish the following lifelines
  A. Peripheral intravenous
  B. Central venous line
III. Cardiac monitoring
IV. Decrease workload of the heart
  A. Bedrest
  B. Analgesics
V. Administer appropriate antiarrhythmic drugs

RATIONALE

The patient with a myocardial contusion should be treated in a similar fashion to the patient with a myocardial infarction. The main management objectives are reduction of oxygen demands of the heart, and early detection and treatment of life-threatening arrhythmias.

At rest, the myocardium normally extracts nearly all available oxygen from arterial blood. The main determinant of oxygen demand is the metabolic requirement of the heart. Measures should be taken to decrease the metabolic need of the heart and to increase oxygen available for consumption. Oxygen by face mask, 4 to 6 liters/minute, may provide some relief of chest pain and may increase tissue oxygenation in marginally ischemic areas of the myocardium.

A patent peripheral line should be available for at least 24 to 48 hours. The amount of fluid given should not be limited until normal vascular volume has been replaced. A good indicator for volume status remains the central venous catheter.

The patient should be attached to continuous cardiac monitoring in order to recognize and be able to treat cardiac dysrhythmias.

In order to prevent enlargement of the ischemic area, myocardial oxygen demands should be reduced. A patient with a myocardial contusion should be placed on bed rest for at least 2 days. Analgesics should be given; morphine sulfate in small intravenous doses is usually effective in reducing pain. Pain causes an increase in oxygen consumption and levels of circulating catecholamines which may also decrease oxygen availability to the myocardium by constriction of the coronary arteries.

Arrhythmias should be treated with appropriate antiarrhythmic drugs. Prior to instituting drug therapy, hypovolemia and hypoxemia should be corrected. Specific dosage of antiarrhythmic agents should be determined by patient's clinical response.

The prognosis of a patient with myocardial contusion depends on the extent of the initial trauma, size and location of the contusion, any involvement of the coronary arterial system, and any other system trauma. The majority of patients with a myocardial contusion do extremely well. The difficulty lies in misdiagnosing these patients and allowing them to go home untreated. Complications of myocardial contusion include life-threatening arrhythmias, ruptured ventricle, and cardiac tamponade.

CARDIAC TAMPONADE

ASSESSMENT

A. Hypotension
B. Neck vein distention—Beck triad
C. Muffled heart sounds
D. Tachycardia
E. Respiratory distress
F. Pulsus paradoxus (inspiratory fall in bp 10 mm Hg)
G. Elevated central venous pressure 15 cm H_2O

PATHOPHYSIOLOGY

Cardiac tamponade most commonly results from a penetrating injury, either a small caliber bullet or a thin "ice pick" knife. Blunt injury rarely causes a tamponade. The diagnosis should be suspected in any patient with wounds near or over the precordium or epigastric. Because one is never sure of the trajectory of a bullet or thrust of a knife wound, a high index of suspicion is needed to prevent marked deterioration.

As fluid accumulates inside the pericardial sac, intrapericardial pressure and volume increases. As the volume of pericardial fluid increases, the atria and ventricles are unable to fill adequately. Ventricular filling is reduced causing a decrease in stroke volume. This results in a decreased cardiac output which leads to a decrease in arterial blood pressure. Concomitantly, on the right side, there is a mechanical back up of blood which causes an increase in central venous pressure and distended neck veins. Muffled or absent heart sounds are caused by a decrease in blood traveling through the heart valves.

The most reliable sign of a cardiac tamponade is an elevated central venous pressure because it is concomitant with hypotension and tachycardia. Beck triad—hypotension, neck vein distention, and muffled heart sounds—becomes evident only in an advanced stage of cardiac tamponade.

Pulsus paradoxus is defined as a drop in systolic blood pressure of greater than 10 mm Hg during normal inspiratory effort. It is usually more pronounced after volume replacement as is the central venous pressure.

Electrocardiographic changes are varied; electromechanical dissociation, sinus tachycardia, and ventricular irritabilities are not diagnostic of a cardiac tamponade.

Radiographic studies usually do not show an enlargement of the cardiac silhouette.

MANAGEMENT

   I. Maintain an adequate airway
      A. Nasotracheal intubation
      B. Orotracheal intubation
  II. Replacement of blood volume
      A. Lactated Ringer's
      B. Whole blood and packed cells
      C. MAST trousers
 III. Establish the following lifelines
      A. Peripheral intravenous catheter
      B. Central venous catheter
      C. Foley catheter
  IV. Monitor trends and responses
      A. Bp
      B. Pulse rate
      C. Respiratory rate
      D. Central venous pressure
      E. Urine output
      F. Heart sounds

V. Prophylactic antibiotics and tetanus immunization
VI. Definitive therapy
    A. Pericardiocentesis
    B. Thoracotomy

RATIONALE

Establishing and maintaining an adequate airway remains the first priority, with control of hemorrhage second. Endotracheal intubation remains the definitive form of airway management. If there is any evidence of a cervical spine injury, nasotracheal intubation should be attempted. Nasotracheal intubation maintains cervical spine immobilization and is usually tolerated better by those patients who are conscious. Once intubated, the patient should be given oxygen as either supportive therapy or ventilation therapy to keep arterial oxygen tension between 80 and 90 mm Hg and arterial oxygen hemoglobin saturation at 95 percent.

Replace lost blood volume immediately. By increasing venous pressure, one may temporarily sustain ventricular filling. Ringer's lactate, 1 to 2 liters, should be given over 15 to 30 minutes. A transfusion of O-negative blood can be given to those patients in hemorrhagic shock. Type specific blood may be used while waiting for a complete crossmatch. Type specific blood offers the advantage of rapid availability and a low incidence of transfusion reactions. Whole blood is preferable to packed cells because it provides more volume in addition to the red blood cell mass. MAST trousers may be helpful in facilitating resuscitation, especially in those patients in whom it is difficult to start peripheral lines.

Patients should be carefully monitored throughout for blood pressure, pulse rate, respiratory rate, and urine output, and these should be taken and checked every 10 to 15 minutes. Changes in central venous pressure, neck vein distention, and heart sounds may be an indication of a worsening tamponade. Any pneumothorax or hemothorax must be assessed and treated during resuscitation of a cardiac trauma victim.

A pericardiocentesis should be done for both diagnostic and therapeutic reasons. A subxiphoid approach is used, aiming toward the right shoulder with a 16 or 17 gauge pericardiocentesis needle at a 30 to 45 degree angle. The pericardiocentesis needle should be connected to a metal three-way stopcock, one end attached to the syringe and one end to an alligator clamp leading to the V-lead on the electrocardiogram. As the needle is inserted, the ECG is able to pick-up any precipitation of arrhythmia, i.e., enter the ventricular sac, the needle should then be withdrawn. Aspiration of 10 to 20 ml of blood may be enough to dramatically show a clinical improvement. The procedure should be repeated until the clinical picture becomes stabilized. Normally, pericardial blood will not clot, unlike intracardiac blood which should clot.

If pericardiocentesis is unsuccessful, the clinical status deteriorates (blood pressure and CVP fail precipitously), bradycardia with electromechanical dissociation occurs, and an immediate open thoracotomy in the emergency department should be performed.

Any patient with a penetrating injury should receive tetanus immunization; if never immunized 0.5 ml of tetanus toxoid plus 250 units of human tetanus immune globulin should be given. If they have been immunized 5 years prior, 0.5 ml of tetanus toxoid should be given.

Antibiotics should be started preoperatively. Septic complications are common after penetrating injuries and may increase the patient's chance of developing post-traumatic complications including local infection and pulmonary insufficiency. Broad spectrum antibiotics should be used until blood cultures are available.

Prognosis of patients with cardiac tamponade depends on their clinical status on arrival. Patients with a blood pressure greater than 50, who have been aggressively treated, have a 95 percent survival rate. The survival rate decreases markedly for patients with an exsanguinating hemorrhage, no palpable blood pressure, and no evidence of tamponade. Cardiac rupture usually develops after massive blunt trauma and explains why cardiac tamponade is rarely seen in these cases.

TRAUMATIC AORTIC RUPTURE

ASSESSMENT

A. Retrosternal or interscapular pain
B. Dyspnea
C. Dysphagia
D. Ischemic pain of the extremities
E. Upper extremity hypertension along with absent or diminished femoral pulses
F. Harsh systolic murmur over the precordium or interscapular region
G. Radiographic findings
    1. blurring or obliteration of the aortic knob
    2. widened mediastinum
    3. deviation of trachea to the right
    4. presence of a pleural cap
    5. depression of left main stem bronchus
    6. obliteration of space between the pulmonary artery and the aorta
    7. deviation of the esophagus to the left
H. Positive aortography

PATHOPHYSIOLOGY

Rupture of the thoracic aorta is usually caused by blunt trauma either as a result of a motor vehicle accident or from a high fall. Of the 15 percent of cases sustaining these accidents, 85 to 90 percent die instantaneously. The remaining 10 to 15 percent survive at least temporarily because the aortic blood is tamponaded by surrounding mediastinal soft tissue. About 50 percent of these survivors usually die within 24 hours of reaching the hospital.

Aortic dissection is caused by separation of the aortic intima and media by the progressive force of blood entering the media through a small intimal tear. This tear may be due to the effect of high speed deceleration on different portions of the aorta, especially at points of fixation and the increased intraluminal pressure that results from the impact. If this thinned outer layer ruptures, it may lead to acute tamponade or exsanguination.

The most common site of rupture is the descending aorta at the isthmus just distal to the left subclavian artery. Ruptures of the ascending aorta are much less common, although they carry an even higher mortality. The ascending aorta usually ruptures into the pericardium causing a tamponade.

A high index of suspicion is necessary in diagnosing an aortic injury. Approximately one third to one half of reported cases in the literature have had no external evidence of thoracic injury. Concomitantly, these patients usually have other extensive system injuries that mask the signs and symptoms of an aortic injury.

The patient usually complains of retrosternal or interscapular pain. Other symptoms include dyspnea (due to tracheal compression and deviation) and dysphagia (as a result of compression of the esophagus). Parasthesia of the extremities resulting from an impairment of the arterial supply to the cord, may also be evident.

An important clinical sign is the acute onset of upper extremity hypertension along with absent or diminished femoral pulses. This symptom is caused by a hematoma that compresses the aortic lumen.

A harsh systolic murmur may be heard over the precardium or posterior interscapular area and is probably due to the turbulent flow across the dissection.

Radiographic findings are invaluable in assessing an aortic rupture. Findings include a blurring or obliteration of the aortic knob, widened mediastinum, deviation of the trachea to the right, deviation of the esophagus to the left, presence of a pleural cap, depression of the left main stem bronchus, and obliteration of space between the pulmonary artery and the aorta.

Aortography is the only definitive technique for establishing the diagnosis of acute disruption and dissection.

MANAGEMENT

I. Maintain an adequate airway
   A. Nasotracheal intubation
   B. Orotracheal intubation
II. Establish the following lifelines
   A. Large bore peripheral catheter
   B. Central venous catheter
   C. Foley catheter
   D. Nasogastric tube

III. Replacement of blood volume
    A. Lactated Ringer's
    B. Whole blood and packed cells
IV. Monitor trends and responses
    A. Bp in upper and lower extremities
    B. Pulse rate
    C. Central venous pressure
    D. Urine output
    E. Respiratory rate
  V. Antihypertensive medications
 VI. Prophylactic antibiotic therapy and tetanus immunization
VII. Definitive therapy
    A. Surgery—repair of the aorta or resection of the injured area and grafting

RATIONALE

Maintenance of an adequate airway remains the first priority. The goal is to keep the arterial oxygen tension at 80 mm Hg or better, resulting in an arterial oxygen hemoglobin saturation of about 95 percent. In most patients this can be accomplished by administering oxygen via nasal prongs or face mask. However, if significant arterial desaturation occurs (Pao_2 less than 60), tracheal intubation is necessary. Nasotracheal intubation should be attempted first, to prevent any cervical spine injuries.

Volume replacement should be given dependent on assessment parameters. A patient who presents in hemorrhagic shock should have two peripheral and one central line inserted. Lactated Ringer's should be started, 1 to 2 liters of fluid within 15 to 30 minutes. If needed, a transfusion of O-negative blood followed by type specific may be given until a complete crossmatch is available. In case of an abdominal aortic dissection, MAST trousers may be very helpful in containing the hemorrhage.

Patients should be monitored continuously for any change in blood pressure (upper and lower extremities), pulse rate and strength, central venous pressure, respiratory rate, and urine output. Any deviation from baseline values should be assessed and appropriate intervention should be instituted to prevent deterioration of the patient.

In some cases, patients present in hypertensive crisis due to thoracic aortic dissection. In these patients it is important to maintain blood pressure below 120 mm Hg systolic. The objective in lowering the blood pressure is to decrease the shearing effect of the pulse and thus to decrease the possibility of continued adventitial dissection. This can be accomplished with a variety of agents: nitroprusside, trimethaphan, hydralazine, and guanethidine, to name a few (see Table 10). The drug should rapidly lower the blood pressure, and the patient should be monitored at all times with an intraarterial pressure monitor. Nitroprusside is often used because of its short half-life, 3 to 5 seconds; if hypotension occurs the medication can be quickly discontinued.

Prophylactic antibiotic therapy should be started preoperatively. Broad spectrum antibiotics should be given until specific blood culture results are available. In the multiply-injured patient, tetanus immunization should be instituted. For a patient never immunized, 0.5 ml of tetanus toxoid plus 250 units of human tetanus immune globulin (hypertet) should be given. If immunization has occurred more than 5 years before, 0.5 ml of tetanus toxoid should be administered.

The repair of the lesion should be performed as soon as the diagnosis has been made, to prevent the sudden lethal rupture. An end-to-end anastamosis may be done, however, most probably a synthetic graft will be used because of the extensive damage done to the ends of the vessel. The mortality rate of those who survive long enough to get to the operating room varies from 20 to 35 percent. The high mortality may be due to excessive bleeding during surgery and/or organ damage sustained during periods of tissue anoxia preoperatively.

Cardiovascular Emergencies References

Atcheson, S., & Fred, H. L. Complications of cardiac resuscitation. *Journal of the American Heart Association*, 1975, **89**, 263.

Becker, C. E., & Benowitz, N. L. Hypertensive emergencies. *Medical Clinics of North America*, 1979, **60**, 127.

Brunner, H. R., & Gavras, H. *Clinical hypertension and hypotension*. New York: Marcel Dekker, 1982.

Byron, F. B. *The hypertensive vascular crisis*. New York: Grune & Stratton, 1969.

Cohen, A. S. *Medical emergencies: Diagnostic and management procedures from the Boston City Hospital* (2nd Ed.), Boston: Little, Brown, 1983.

Curtis, P. Family practice grand rounds. Spontaneous pneumothorax: A dilemma of management. *Journal of Family Practice*, 1978, **6**, 367.

Doty, D. B. Cardiac trauma: Clinical and experimental correlations of NYO cardial contusion. *Annals of Surgery*, 1974, **180**, 452.

Gifford, R. W., Jr. Hypertensive crises. In G. R. Schwartz, et al. (Eds.), *Principles and practices of emergency medicine* (Vol. 2). Philadelphia: W. B. Saunders, 1978.

Kaplan, N. H. Hypertensive crises. In: *Clinical hypertension* (2nd Ed.). Baltimore: Williams & Wilkins, 1976.

Kirsh, M. M., & Shoan H. *Blunt chest trauma: General principles of management*. Boston: Little, Brown, 1977.

McIntyre, K. M., & Parken, M. R. Standards and guidelines for cardiopulmonary resuscitation and emergency cardiac care. *Journal of the American Medical Association*, 1980, **244**, 453.

Mills, J. *Current emergency diagnosis and treatment*. Los Altos, Calif.: Lange Medical, 1983.

Oren, A., Bar-shom, B., & Stern, S. Acute coronary occlusion following blunt injury to the chest in absence of coronary arteriosclerosis. *Journal of the American Heart Association*, 1976, **92**, 501.

Rosen, P. *Emergency medicine concepts and clinical practice* (Vols. I & II). St. Louis: C. V. Mosby, 1983.

Schwartz, G. R. *Principles and practices of emergency medicine* (Vols. I & II). Philadelphia: W.B. Saunders, 1978.

Wackers, F. J. Coronary artery diseases in patients dying from cardiogenic shock or congestive heart failure in the setting of acute myocardial infarction. *British Heart Journal*, 1976, **38,** 906.

D. GASTROINTESTINAL EMERGENCIES

1. Gastrointestinal Hemorrhage

ASSESSMENT

  I. Assess the amount of blood loss
    A. Decreased bp, postural hypotension
    B. Tachycardia
    C. Decreased urine output
    D. Skin changes
    E. Change in level of consciousness
    F. Decreased central venous pressure
    G. Volume of hematemesis
    H. Volume of melena
 II. Obtain an accurate history
    A. Ulcer disease
    B. Liver disease
III. Abdominal and rectal examination
    A. Palpation
    B. Percussion
    C. Auscultation
 IV. Diagnostic procedures to determine site of bleeding
    A. Nasogastric insertion
    B. Esophagogastroduodenoscopy
    C. Arteriography
    D. Barium radiography
  V. Laboratory studies
    A. Decreased hemoglobin and hematocrit
    B. Abnormal coagulation studies
    C. Liver function tests

PATHOPHYSIOLOGY

Assessing the severity of the hemorrhage should be done as soon as the patient enters the emergency department. The clinical effects of the bleed depend on the amount of blood lost and the rapidity of the bleeding. Signs or symptoms of hemorrhagic shock include a drop in blood pressure, widening of pulse pressure, tachycardia, pale and sweating skin, decreased urine output, and restlessness. Postural hypotension represents a postural (supine to upright) drop in systolic blood pressure by greater than 10 mm Hg with an accompanying increase in pulse rate greater than 20 per minute. These changes may indicate a 20 to 25 percent decrease in circulating blood volume. An estimate in continuing blood loss can be judged by the volume of hematemesis and bloody bowel movements. The gastrointestinal tract reacts with irritability to the presence of blood and the patient vomits until the stomach has been emptied. This hematemesis should be measured as accurately as possible. The absence of bright red blood does not rule out active upper gastrointestinal bleeding because bright red blood may turn in the stomach (presence of hydrochloric acid) very quickly. In 25 percent of the cases of a duodenal bleed, nasogastric aspirate is negative. The effects of blood on the stool again depends on the rapidity and amount of the bleed. Melena is defined as liquid, tarry, foul smelling black stools. Melena is usually due to bleeding from a source in the upper gastrointestinal tract and indicates that at least 500 ml of blood has been lost in the last 24 hours. Grossly bloody stools may be seen in upper gastrointestinal bleeding if the blood loss is quick and massive and the transit time is rapid. A fall in the hematocrit or hemoglobin is the least sensitive indicator of acute blood loss due to the fact that hemodilution is only one third complete in 2 hours and one half complete in 8 hours. It would take about 12 to 18 hours to get an accurate reading.

A history of peptic ulcer, ingestion of antacids, and pain suggesting a duodenal ulcer may suggest ulcer disease. A history of alcoholism with accompanying symptoms of hepatic disease, jaundice, hepatosplenomegaly, spider angiomas, ascites may indicate esophageal varices. A history of ingestion of aspirin and nonsteriod inflammatory agents may indicate gastritis. Lastly, a history of recent vigorous emesis may suggest a Mallory–Weiss tear.

Abdominal examination may provide some clues as to the source of bleeding. Inspect the abdomen for surgical scars to indicate any previous intervention. Palpate the abdomen for any masses, hepatosplenomegaly and ascites. Pain and tenderness are common findings in gastritis and ulcer disease but rare in patients with varices. Auscultation of the abdomen may provide an indication of bleeding. Severe upper gastrointestinal bleeding usually leads to hyperactive bowel sounds due to the strong laxative effect of blood.

Diagnostic procedures to determine the site of bleeding should be started as soon as the patient's cardiovascular status is stabilized. Esophagogastroduodenoscopy has become the primary method of identifying the site of upper gastrointestinal hemorrhage. In order to improve visualization the procedure should be performed when the lavage returns shift from red to pink. Diagnostic accuracy falls between 85 and 95 percent with a low morbidity.

Arteriography may be successful in locating the site of bleeding, especially when the stomach cannot be adequately cleared for visualization. The procedure has an additional advantage of being diagnostic and therapeutic because once a lesion is identified control of upper and lower gastrointestinal bleeding may be achieved by selective arterial infusion of vasopressin.

Barium studies are not useful in diagnosing the actively bleeding patient. Barium adheres to the mucosa and prevents further diagnostic testing, i.e., endoscopy or angiography. Its usefulness lies in providing helpful information for the nonbleeding patient in stable condition.

Laboratory studies may offer additional clues to the site and amount of upper gastrointestinal bleeding. Bloods should immediately be drawn for hematocrit and hemoglobin, type, and crossmatch. Liver function tests, bilirubin, SGOT, SGPT, alkaline phosphatase and serum protein electrophoresis should be drawn and may help diagnose liver disease and varices as a source of bleeding. Coagulation studies, bleeding time, prothrombin, partial thromboplastin time, and platelet count should be drawn. In addition, arterial blood gases should be serially obtained.

MANAGEMENT

I. Maintain adequate blood volume
   A. Lactated Ringer's
   B. Whole blood and packed cells
II. Establish the following lifelines
   A. Large bore peripheral lines
   B. Central venous catheter
   C. Foley catheter
   D. Nasogastric tube
   E. Oxygen catheter
III. Monitor continuously for trends and responses
   A. Abdominal bleeding
   B. Melena
   C. Hemoglobin, hematocrit
   D. Bp
   E. Pulse rate
   F. Urine output
   G. Respiratory rate
   H. Central venous pressure
IV. Management of specific etiologies of gastrointestinal bleeding
V. Peptic ulcer disease
   A. Ice saline nasogastric lavage
   B. Intraarterial vasopressin—0.1 to 0.4 U/minute
   C. Cimetidine—300 mg q 6 hours

    D. Antacids—Maalox alternate with Mylanta 30 ml/hour

    E. Surgery

VI. Esophageal varices

    A. Balloon tamponade

    B. Intravenous vassopressin—0.1 to 0.4 U/minute

    C. Vitamin K—5 to 10 mg IM

    D. Injection sclerotherapy

    E. Shunt therapy

RATIONALE

Restoration of blood volume is the main objective in managing the patient with upper gastrointestinal hemorrhage. Ringer's lactate is the initial fluid replacement of choice. It is the most nearly physiologic solution; it gives the emergency personnel time to get the patient typed and crossmatched and decreases blood viscosity thereby improving resuscitation at the microcirculatory level. Two liters of fluid are given within 20 to 30 minutes. Physiologic parameters are monitored: blood pressure, pulse pressure, pulse rate, respiratory rate, central venous pressure, and urine output. Replacement with blood products should begin as soon as possible. In life-threatening situations, type O blood may be given, followed by crossmatched blood when available. Each unit of whole blood should raise the hematocrit 3 to 4 percent.

    The necessary lifelines are a large bore peripheral intravenous, a central venous catheter, a Foley catheter, a nasogastric tube, and an oxygen catheter.

    Oxygen should be administered to keep the patient's arterial oxygen tension between 80 and 100 mm Hg.

    The amount of hematemesis and melena should be monitored along with any color changes which may indicate fresh bleeding.

    Specific management modalities for peptic ulcer disease and esophageal varices follow initial modalities and are the same regardless of the etiology of the upper gastrointestinal bleed.

    Peptic ulcer disease is responsible for almost half of all episodes of upper gastrointestinal bleeding. About 95 percent of all duodenal ulcers occur in the duodenal bulb or cap; gastric ulcers are usually found within 6 cm of the pylorus. Signs and symptoms include epigastric distress, nocturnal pain, sudden and massive bleeding with accompanying shock. Restoration of blood volume was discussed previously in this chapter and will not be rediscussed. Specific management modalities for hemorrhage from peptic ulcer disease are enumerated and discussed. First, a large bore tube (at least 1 cm in diameter) is passed into the stomach. Gentle lavage with iced saline is done until clear. The therapeutic value of iced saline has not been proven but it is thought to cause a local vasoconstriction and thereby decreased bleeding. Cimetidine is usually started though it does not directly decrease bleeding. Cimetidine inhibits gastric acid secretion stimulated by food, gastrin, histamine, and caffeine. The dosage is usually 300 mg given intravenously every 6 hours. Along with cimetidine, when acute bleeding ceases, antacids should be begun. Hourly antacids, magnesium hydroxide–aluminum hydroxide mixtures (Maalox, Mylanta) 30 ml/hour dosage should be effective in neutralizing acidic stomach secretions.

Selective arterial infusion of vasopressin has not been shown to be effective but may be tried in patients who are considered a high surgical risk. The dosage is 0.1 to 0.4 units of vasopressin per minute.

If the patient continues to bleed or rebleed, surgery is necessary (stabilization usually occurs within 72 hours). Patients should be operated on if there is exsanguinating hemorrhage, bleeding that requires more than 5 units of blood with accompanying circulatory compromise, and rebleeding during the same hospitalization.

Esophageal varices carries with it a mortality rate of 50 percent. Variceal hemorrhage does not occur unless there is significant portal hypertension. Portal hypertension in this case is due primarily to cirrhosis. In cirrhosis, collaterals develop to increase blood flow between the portal and systemic venous systems. The most common area for bleeding varices is at the gastroesophageal junction, probably due to a combination of increased venous pressure and the exaggerated pressure gradients located in that region. Signs and symptoms include massive gastrointestinal hemorrhage, cirrhosis, hepatomegaly, jaundice, vascular spiders, splenomegaly, ascites, and a history of a recent alcoholic binge. Laboratory values include an elevated bilirubin, serum albumin below 3 g/dl, abnormal prothrombin time and partial thromboplastin time, and anemia.

Although blood volume is being restored, other management modalities should be instituted. Initially, the stomach should be irrigated through a large bore nasogastric tube with iced saline. The nasogastric tube is replaced by the Minnesota tube. This tube has a gastric and an esophageal balloon plus four lumens, two to fill the balloons, the third permits aspiration of gastric contents, and the fourth aspirates fluid above the esophageal balloon. The tube is passed into the stomach; the gastric balloon is inflated with air (450 to 500 ml) and attached to traction to provide a snug fit between the balloon and the gastroesophageal junction. If bleeding continues, the esophageal balloon should be distended using manometer control, 45 to 50 mm Hg. Complications include aspiration, asphyxiation, esophageal ruptures, and atelectasis.

Continuous peripheral intravenous infusion of low dose vasopressin should be started immediately. Vasopressin lowers mesenteric blood flow by constricting mesenteric arterioles. Vasopressin is given intravenously at 0.4 to 0.6 U/minute for 12 hours and halved for the next 12 hours. The cardiovascular complications of vasopressin therapy should be monitored. These include a decrease in cardiac output and a decrease in coronary blood flow. Vitamin K can be given especially to patients with an elevated prothrombin time. Other therapies should include measures to treat or prevent encephalopathy.

Injection of the varices with a sclerosing agent can be performed through an esophagoscope. A sclerosant (sodium morrhuate, ethanolamine oleate) is injected into each varix. A dose of 3 to 4 ml is used for each varix. Local compression of the

TABLE 11. TYPES OF SHUNTS AVAILABLE

Portasystemic shunts	Selective shunts
End-to-side	Distal splenorenal
Side-to-side	Left gastric venacaval
Side-to-side portacaval	
Mesocaval	
Central splenorenal	
Denosplenic	

submucosa and inflammation causes the varix to thrombose. This procedure is repeated biweekly until all remaining varices are injected. About 80 percent of acute bleeding episodes can be stopped. Overall mortality rate has not been improved. Complications of this procedure include esophageal perforation, stricture, ulceration, and the formation of gastric varices.

Medical management is successful in controlling bleeding in 50 to 80 percent of all cases. The surgical measures for the acutely bleeding patient include emergency portal caval shunts and, if time allows, side-to-side and selective shunts (splenorenal) (Table 11). The portal caval shunt is effective in stopping variceal bleeding in about 95 percent of the cases. Some of the other shunts do not totally disconnect the liver from the portal system therefore patients experience less encephalopathy.

2. Inflammations

PERITONITIS

ASSESSMENT

   I. Systemic responses
      A. Hypotension
      B. Fever
      C. Malaise
      D. Nausea and vomiting
  II. Abdominal signs
      A. Pain and tenderness
      B. Muscle rigidity
      C. Paralytic ileus
      D. Absence of liver dullness
III. Laboratory values
      A. Leukocytosis
      B. Metabolic acidosis
      C. Respiratory alkalosis

IV. Positive abdominal paracentesis
    A. WBC count 300/WBC/mm
    B. Elevation of polymorphonuclear cells
    C. Elevated protein concentration
V. X-ray findings
    A. Gas and fluid collection in large and small bowel

PATHOPHYSIOLOGY

Peritonitis is the most serious complication of a wide variety of acute abdominal disorders. Peritonitis may be caused by perforation or necrosis of the gastrointestinal tract. Another form of peritonitis, chemical peritonitis, is caused by acute pancreatitis, introduction of bile, gastrointestinal fluid, and blood. Bacterial peritonitis can be due to decompensated cirrhosis, trauma, intraabdominal infection, mesenteric vascular insufficiency, neoplasms, and postoperative sites. Common organisms found are *Escherichia coli, Bacteriodes fragilis,* anaerobic streptococci, *Streptococcus pneumonia, Staphylococcus aureus,* and *Neisseria gonorrhoeae.*

Depending on the extent of the disease process, systemic responses vary. The massive loss of fluid into the peritoneum, as a result of peritoneal irritation, leads to varying degrees of hypovolemic shock. A drop in blood pressure, increase in pulse and respiratory rate, decrease in central venous pressure, and urine output are usually seen in patients with peritonitis. Pyrexia is usually found due to leukocyte production of endogenous pyrogens which circulate to the thermoregulatory center.

Nausea and vomiting are usually present with any type of peritoneal irritation, though not dominant without an area of obstruction.

The most obvious signs of peritonitis are found during the abdominal examination. Abdominal rigidity is usually found only in cases of peritonitis; the rectus abdominis muscle remains rigid throughout the respiratory cycle. Abdominal tenderness may be localized initially in early peritonitis and may give a clue as to the involved area but becomes diffuse as the inflammation spreads.

If there has been a perforation of a hollow viscus with air under the diaphragm, there may be diminished or absent liver dullness.

Within the first hour of injury, patients will develop a paralytic ileus. Again, total absence of audible peristalsis is usually seen only in cases of diffuse peritonitis.

Leukocytosis is usually seen as a systemic response to bacterial infection. Metabolic acidosis develops because of poor perfusion at the cellular level. Respiratory demands are usually increased because of fever, pain, and elevation of the diaphragm, which reduces ventilatory capacity and respiratory exchange.

An abdominal paracentesis usually shows an increase in the white blood cell count, an elevation of polymorphonuclear cells, and an elevated protein concentration. Microscopic examination of the fluid may reveal the causative organism; fluid should be cultured in both aerobic and anaerobic media.

Flat and upright films of the abdomen usually show distention of both large and small bowels. The presence of free air under the diaphragm is indicative of a perforated viscus, i.e., perforated gastric or duodenal ulcer; free air under both diaphragms indicates colonic perforation. A thickened appearance to the loops of the bowel may indicate the presence of fluids. The swallowing of barium should be avoided; the use of angiograms, ultrasound, and CAT scan are safer and provide more valuable information.

MANAGEMENT

    I. Correction of hypoxia
   II. Replacement and maintenance of adequate blood volume
      A. Blood products
      B. Crystalloids
      C. Colloids
      D. Vasoactive agents
  III. Determination of laboratory values
      A. CBC
      B. Electrolytes and BUN
      C. Arterial blood gases
  IV. Decreased effects of the paralytic ileus
      A. Bed rest
      B. Nasogastric suctioning
      C. npo
   V. Antibiotic therapy
      A. Initially broad spectrum
      B. Specific antibiotic therapy after results of cultures
  VI. Relief of pain
      A. Morphine sulfate 2 to 4 mg IV
 VII. Surgical intervention
VIII. Prevention of further complications
      A. Abscess formation
      B. Adhesions

RATIONALE

The maintenance of adequate ventilation and circulatory function should be the first concern in treating the patient with peritonitis.

Respiratory demands are usually increased as previously mentioned and patients should be provided with supplemental oxygen. A patient in shock has an increased oxygen requirement of one and a half to two times normal. Supplemental oxygen by face mask, intubation, volume ventilation should be given in order to maintain arterial oxygen at 90 to 100 mm Hg.

Access to the vascular system must be promptly maintained. A large bore peripheral line plus a central venous line should be inserted. If possible, a Swan–Ganz catheter should be inserted to provide a better index of left ventricular function. A Foley catheter to monitor urine output should be in place. Initial fluid therapy is Ringer's lactate, anywhere from 500 to 2000 ml depending on central venous pressure and wedge pressure readings.

Crystalloids do not sustain plasma volume, as a result of fluid loss into the interstitial spaces, and the use of colloids will probably be necessary. Fresh-frozen plasma, albumin 5 percent in saline, and 25 percent albumin can be given, especially to those patients who are third-spacing and/or whose albumin level is less than 3 g/dl. Electrolytes should be replaced depending on laboratory findings.

Vasoactive drugs should be avoided until restoration of blood volume, correction of hypoxia and fluid, and electrolyte disturbances are completed. Dopamine hydrochloride 400 to 800 μg/ml can be given. It stimulates the dopaminergic receptors to increase the renal blood flow and urinary output. Second, the β-adrenergic cardiac receptors are stimulated which increase the cardiac output.

Nasogastric suctioning should be started to prevent gastrointestinal distention as soon as the patient enters the emergency department. If a paralytic ileus persists, the stomach can be more adequately decompressed with a Miller Abbott tube. Abdominal distention leads to marked respiratory compromise. Other maneuvers to decrease distention include keeping the patient on bed rest and NPO.

Broad spectrum antibiotics should be given until cultures are available and specific antibiotics can be chosen. A combination of clindamycin and chloramphenicol and gentamicin should be given. Doses are as follows:

- Gentamicin, 5 mg/kg/day IV
- Chloramphenicol, 3 mg/day IV
- Clindamycin, 1.8 g/day IM

Narcotics should be given intravenously to relieve pain. Small doses of morphine do not mask symptoms and insure comfort.

Operative procedures to close perforations, removal of gangrenous bowel or inflamed appendix, and draining of abscesses should be done as promptly as possible. If the cause of peritonitis can be corrected, the accompanying infection, ileus, and metabolic disruptions will be corrected.

Principal late complication is intraperitoneal abscess formation. Abscesses usually occur in the subdiaphragmatic, subhepatic, and pelvic areas. Adhesions are another complication that can lead to internal obstruction. If fever, leukocytosis, toxemia, or ileus fails to respond to general measures, an abscess should be suspected. Surgical drainage is usually necessary.

PANCREATITIS

ASSESSMENT

A. Agonizing midepigastric pain—pain is centered close to the umbilicus, may radiate to the back

B. Vomiting may be persistent, does not relieve abdominal pain
C. Abdominal rigidity
D. Loss of bowel sounds
E. X-ray—dilated small bowel adjacent to the pancreas (sentinel loop)
F. Fever 102°F
G. Involvement of lung bases—Po_2, Pco_2
H. Laboratory values
    1. serum amylase
    2. serum lipase
    3. urine amylase
    4. hyperglycemia
    5. calcium
    6. magnesium
    7. glucagon level
    8. SGOT
    9. SGPT
    10. WBC 15,000 cu/mm
I. Evidence of jaundice, 25 percent of all patients

PATHOPHYSIOLOGY

There are two main types of pancreatitis. In interstitial pancreatitis, which is usually short lived, the patient complains of abdominal pain, and an elevated serum amylase level which rapidly falls to normal within 24 to 48 hours. In hemorrhagic pancreatitis, the second type, you have entire portions of the pancreas becoming hemorrhagic and necrotic, the course of the disease is usually complicated with a high mortality.

In both cases, patients complain of acute epigastric pain unrelieved by vomiting. Pain is usually caused by an irritation of the sphincter of Oddi, spasm, and increased biliary duct pressure and drainage of the panceatic enzymes down the abdominal gutter which produces local fat necrosis.

All of the above leads to abdominal rigidity, loss of bowel sounds, and tenderness. On x-ray, distended loop of small bowel adjacent to the pancreas (sentinel loop) is found.

Jaundice may appear in 25 percent of all acute pancreatitics due to a functional obstruction of the common duct because of edema at the head of the pancreas.

In severe hemorrhagic pancreatitis, assessment parameters would include those of shock and respiratory failure. Spillage of pancreatic enzymes into the peritoneal cavity produce a "burn" with concomitant loss of fluid and electrolytes.

Respiratory failure with accompanying dyspnea, cyanosis, and hypoxemia is probably due to an increased lecithinase release with resultant impaired pulmonary surfactant activity.

Increased amylase levels are a good diagnostic signal of acute pancreatitis. The height of serum amylase levels bears no relation to the severity of the disease. Lower levels of serum amylase may represent a partially fibrotic pancreas. Levels usually rise significantly within the first few hours and return to normal within 1 to 2 days.

Urinary amylase levels remain increased for at least a week because of the increase renal clearance of amylase during pancreatitis, therefore the serum levels do not remain high for very long but the amount in the urine remains elevated.

Hyperglycemia occurs in about 20 percent of all patients and is probably due to an excess of glucagon rather than a lack of glucose.

The level of calcium in the serum usually falls due to the sequestration of calcium by fat necrosis in the peritoneum. It may be associated with hypomagnesia.

A rise in the SGOT and SGPT is probably due to external compression of the common bile duct as it passes through the edemation head of the pancreas.

MANAGEMENT

   I. Reduction of pancreatic stimulation
      A. Removal of hydrochloric acid
          Nasogastric tube to intermittent suction
      B. H_2 blocker—Cimetidine
  II. Relief of pain
      A. Demerol, 50 to 100 mg q 4 to 6 hours
 III. Replacement of fluid and electrolytes
      A. Third—spacing
      B. Lactated Ringer's 200 ml/hour
      C. Albumin infusions—serum albumin is less than 3 g/dl
      D. Ca gluconate 1 g daily, Ca 9.0 mg/dl
      E. $MgSO_4$
  IV. Glucose and insulin infusion
   V. Prophylactic antibiotics
      A. If indicated for febrile patients; broad spectrum, i.e., ampicillin 1 g q 6 hours gentamicin 1.7 mg/kg/q 8 hours
  VI. Prevent further complications
      A. Pancreatic abscess
      B. Pseudocyst

RATIONALE

The mortality rate of acute pancreatitis depends on the severity of the pathologic process, 5 to 10 percent in interstitial pancreatitis and up to 50 to 80 percent in hemorrhagic or necrotic pancreatitis. Aggressive therapy is essential to decrease morbidity and mortality.

Whatever the cause of pancreatitis, obstruction of the pancreatic ducts is certainly present, therefore treatment is primarily directed at reducing pancreatic secretion. Hydrochloric acid and food are two such stimulants. Patients are placed on continuous nasogastric suctioning, nothing by mouth and on bed rest.

Demerol, 50 to 100 mg, is given intramuscularly to control pain. Morphine is contraindicated because it usually causes spasms in the sphincter of Oddi.

In conjunction with the above, maintenance of an adequate circulating volume is essential. Initially, lactated Ringer's should be given at a rate of 200 ml/hour. The pancreatic enzymes, which spill into the peritoneal cavity, produce a "burn" with a concomitant fluid and electrolyte loss. It may be necessary to give colloids in addition to crystalloids to decrease the amount of fluid being lost into the peritoneal cavity due to "third-spacing." Colloids increase the oncotic pressure inside the vascular system, decreasing the loss of fluid into the interstitial spaces.

Calcium gluconate, 10 ml of a 10 percent solution, should be given. The amount is determined by the patient's clinical response and the serum calcium level.

Other medications include H_2 blockers (i.e., Cimetidine), which also help to decrease gastric acid secretions. Antibiotics are ordinarily not required for a patient with acute pancreatitis unless there is damage to the bowel wall or direct drainage of the peritoneal cavity. Broad spectrum antibiotics should be given to any patient who remains febrile. Blood, urine, and sputum should be cultured.

A combination of insulin and glucose is sometimes beneficial to patients. It is theorized that a lipase present in fat cells activated in acute pancreatitis leads to fat necrosis and this same enzyme is inhibited by glucose and insulin.

Most patients should respond to the aforementioned therapeutic maneuvers. About 10 percent of patients may develop complications, i.e., abscesses or pseudocyst abscesses occur as collections within the pancreas and pseudocysts as collections outside the pancreas. Surgery and immediate drainage of the abscess is necessary, although unless the patient is symptomatic, most pseudocysts resolve on their own with continued medical treatment.

HEPATITIS

ASSESSMENT

I. Systemic reactions
  A. General malaise
  B. Myalgia
  C. Arthralgia and occasionally arthritis
  D. Upper respiratory symptoms
  E. Severe anorexia
  F. Nausea and vomiting
  G. Fever 39.5°C (103.1°F)
  H. Distaste for smoking
II. Hepatic
  A. Abdominal pain—right upper quadrant
  B. Clinical jaundice
  C. Hepatomegaly

      D. Liver tenderness

      E. Splenomegaly

III. Laboratory findings

      A. SGOT

      B. SGPT

      C. WBC—normal or decreased

      D. Proteinuria

      E. Bilirubinuria

      F. Serum bilirubin

PATHOPHYSIOLOGY

Hepatitis A is a viral infection, usually transmitted by the fecal–oral route, though occasionally by contaminated needles. Incubation period is 2 to 6 weeks and blood and stools are infectious throughout the incubation period and until peak transaminase levels are achieved.

Hepatitis B is a viral infection, transmitted by inoculation of infected blood or blood products. Hepatitis B antigen can also be spread by oral or sexual and fecal contact. Incubation period is 6 weeks to 6 months.

There is also evidence of the existence of a non-A and non-B hepatitis. Occurrence of these infections usually follows a blood transfusion. The same population is usually effected as in hepatitis B, primarily drug addicts and homosexuals.

In most patients with acute viral hepatitis, the onset of jaundice is preceded by nonspecific systemic reactions and gastrointestinal symptoms. The patient complains of general malaise, anorexia, fatigue, myalgia, and arthralgia. He or she develops an aversion to cigarettes. Gastrointestinal symptoms may include nausea, vomiting, diarrhea, epigastric discomfort, and right upper quadrant pain.

Prior to the development of jaundice, the patient's urine darkens and the stool lightens. Once jaundice appears, the gastrointestinal symptoms begin to abate. Jaundice lasts from 6 to 8 weeks. Liver enlargement and tenderness begin to decrease in 1 to 2 weeks after the onset of jaundice.

After the jaundice subsides, it takes anywhere from 2 to 6 weeks for the patient to stop feeling fatigued. Complete recovery is expected within 3 to 4 months.

Mild leukopenia is occasionally seen during the initial phase. Liver enzymes both the serum glutamic-oxaloacetic transaminase (SGOT) and the serum glutamic-pyruvic transaminase (SGPT) elevate 7 to 14 days prior to jaundice. These enzymes reflect hepatic cell necrosis and altered cell permeability with enzyme leakage into the blood. SGPT values are usually higher than SGOT. Serum bilirubin in clinically jaundiced patients is usually 3 mg/100 ml or greater. Urine urobilinogen may increase during the preicteric phase and then declines with the appearance of alcoholic stools. The prothrombin time may be increased during the period of jaundice.

The metabolic functions of the liver are too numerous to present. These include carbohydrate, fat, and protein metabolism. The liver is also involved in formation of bile, storage of vitamins, coagulation process, storage of iron, and removal or excretion of drugs, hormones, and other substances.

MANAGEMENT

  I. Prevention of further infection
     A. Hand washing techniques
     B. Stool precautions
     C. Disposal of needles, blood products
 II. Decrease workload of the liver
     A. Bed rest
     B. Avoid hepatotoxic agents
     C. Avoid alcohol
     D. Diet
III. Prophylaxis
     A. Gamma globulin, 0.2 ml/kg
     B. Hepatitis B immune globulin, 0.6 ml/kg
     C. Repeat in 1 month
     D. Hepatitis B vaccine
 IV. Prevention of further complications
     A. Fulminant hepatic failure
     B. Chronic hepatitis
     C. Hepatic encephalopathy

RATIONALE

Preventing the spread of hepatitis should be one of the major management modalities. Type A hepatitis is usually spread by the fecal–oral route. Good hand washing techniques and isolation of stools should be done during the first 2 to 3 weeks of clinical illness.

To prevent the spread of hepatitis B, good hand washing techniques, gloves worn when handling body fluids, and disposable needles and syringes should be used. All bloods sent on this patient should be properly labeled.

For non-A, non-B hepatitis isolation measures similar to hepatitis B should be employed.

The general treatment of a hepatitis patient is the same regardless of type. Measures should be taken to enable the liver to regenerate. No specific diet has been proven to be more effective though patients usually tolerate a high calorie, balanced diet. If anorexia is severe, the patient may require intravenous feeding. Ambulation should be related to how easily the patient fatigues. Any medications, which have hepatic toxicity, should be avoided, i.e., alcohol, until liver chemistries have a chance to return to normal.

Prophylaxis against hepatitis depends on the type. For hepatitis A, immune globulin administered before exposure and during early incubation is effective in 90 percent of the exposed patients.

In hepatitis B, hepatitis B-immune globulin (HBIG), should be given to individuals who have been in direct contact via mucous membrane inoculation, following a needle stick or oral ingestion of blood from a patient with a positive diagnosis of hepatitis B.

For non-A, non-B type hepatitis immune globulin is recommended, though effectiveness is questionable.

Vaccination with Heptavox B should be given to medical and laboratory personnel, hemodialysis patients, male homosexuals, neonates of infected mothers, and spouses of chronic hepatitis B carriers. Dosage of the vaccine is three 20 μg doses, the first two spaced 1 month apart and the third at 6 months.

Less than 1 percent of patients with viral hepatitis progress within 4 weeks to fulminant hepatic failure. Assessment parameters include increasing jaundice, shrinkage of the liver, clotting abnormalities, and hepatitic encephalopathy. Once coma ensues, mortality is 80 to 90 percent. Treatment is supportive; high protein and carbohydrate diets, salt restriction and multivitamins. Patients are placed on bed rest. Fresh-frozen plasma is given for clotting abnormalities; medications that are toxic to the liver are withheld. Other measures have been tried though effectiveness has been questionable. These include exchange transfusions, plasmaphoresis, saline washout, charcoal hemoperfusion, and extracorporeal pig liver perfusion.

Chronic hepatitis is defined as hepatitis which lasts for at least 6 months. It can develop from hepatitis A, B, and non-B viruses. A liver biopsy must be done prior to therapy. The therapy for chronic hepatitis is similar to that mentioned above with the addition of corticosteroid therapy. Prednisone is usually started at 60 mg/day and tapered to a dose of 20 mg/day until remission is obtained.

Hepatic encephalopathy represents a state of altered cerebral metabolism produced by the accumulation of various metabolic products from protein breakdown. Normally these products are cleared by the liver, i.e., ammonia which is normally converted to urea by the liver. Therapy is mainly directed at reducing nitrogenous substrates in the gastrointestinal tract. Modalities include removal of any blood in the gastrointestinal tract, dietary protein reduced to zero, removal of fecal material from the colon, and administration of lactulose (60 to 160 g/day) and neomycin (1 to 2 mg in 100 to 200 ml of isotonic saline enema).

3. Abdominal Trauma

ASSESSMENT

   I. Inspection of abdomen
     A. Penetrating injuries

    B. Contusions

    C. Ecchymotic discoloration of the flanks (Grey–Turner sign)

  II. Percussion of abdomen

    A. Loss of liver dullness (bowel perforation)

    B. Loss of gastric tympany (splenic injury)

    C. Flank dullness (retroperitoneal hematoma)

  III. Palpation of abdomen

    A. Muscular guarding

    B. Rebound tenderness

  IV. Ausculation of abdomen

    A. Peristaltic sounds in the chest

    B. Absent or decreased bowel sounds

  V. Pain

    A. Referred pain to shoulder (Kehrer sign)

    B. Testicular pain (retroperitoneal injury)

  VI. Radiographic studies

    A. Upright and supine

    B. Ingestion of water soluble radiopaque medium

    C. IVP

    D. Angiography

    E. CAT scan

  VII. Paracentesis and peritoneal lavage

    A. Gross blood

    B. Blood aspirate

    C. 100,000 RBC/cc mm

    D. 500 WBC/cc mm

    E. Elevated amylase

    F. Bile

    G. Bacteria

    H. Fecal material

  VIII. Blood chemistries

    A. Not usually helpful for initial evaluation of abdominal injuries

PATHOPHYSIOLOGY

Abdominal trauma is found in 1 percent of all trauma related admissions. Mortality rate is about 5 percent in penetrating abdominal trauma and around 10 to 30 percent in blunt abdominal injury. Signs and symptoms found in a patient with an abdominal injury are a result of blood loss, contusion, or laceration of a solid or hollow organ. Examples of solid organs are spleen, liver, kidney, and pancreas; hollow organs are stomach, small and large intestines, and bladder.

In the emergency department time should not be spent trying to decide which organ is injured. A high index of suspicion and willingness to act quickly and decisively will decrease morbidity and mortality.

There are two basic types of injury; penetrating and blunt. Penetrating injury usually results in hemorrhage from the penetration of a major vessel, liver, spleen, or perforation of the segment of the bowel. In blunt injury damage is done by either compression of the abdominal contents against the vertebral column, by direct transfer of energy to an organ, or by rapid deceleration with resultant tearing of structures. As in penetrating trauma, the onset of symptoms may be rapid because of hemorrhage or insidious due to peritonitis.

The abdomen should be inspected for signs of penetrating injuries, contusions, and ecchymotic areas. The anterior and posterior walls of the abdomen, flanks, and lower chest should be inspected.

The abdomen should be percussed for any changes. Loss of liver dullness may indicate a bowel perforation due to leakage of air. Splenic injury results in a loss of gastric tympany due to the accumulation of blood. Evidence of dullness noticed in the flank region could indicate a retroperitoneal hematoma.

Auscultation of the entire abdomen should be carefully completed. Absence or diminished bowel sounds are usually due to either blood, bacteria, or chemical irritants invading the peritoneal cavity and causing an ileus.

Palpation of the abdomen is done to ascertain any muscular guarding or rebound tenderness. Muscular guarding is defined as spasm of the body wall musculature in an effort to prevent deep palpation. Inflammation or injury to the abdominal wall produces muscular guarding as found in peritonitis. Deep abdominal injury can be palpated after the abdominal wall is relaxed.

Rebound tenderness is felt with evidence of intraabdominal inflammation. Damage of the abdominal viscera is often found in blunt trauma and is often missed.

The abdomen may be divided in three parts for palpation. The intrathoracic abdomen is the portion protected by the bony thorax. This area contains the spleen, liver, stomach, and diaphragm. Fractures of the lower ribs can produce a laceration of the liver on the right and/or spleen on the left.

The true abdomen consists of the small and large intestines and bladder. Abdominal findings, muscular guarding and rebound tenderness in conjunction with positive abdominal x-rays and peritoneal lavage, can lead to an early diagnosis. Bladder injury is usually suspected when hematuria is noted on catherization. Any evidence of blood around the urinary meatus should delay catherization until urethra integrity is confirmed by intravenous pyelogram (IVP).

Rectal and vaginal examination should not be forgotten. Palpating the prostate for evidence of sogginess may indicate a retroperitoneal hematoma. Vaginal and rectal tenderness may indicate peritonitis.

The last part can be called the retroperitoneal abdomen and is the most difficult to assess. Palpation for tenderness and rebound tenderness leads to negative results especially during early examination. A high index of suspicion is essential to avoid increased morbidity and mortality.

Radiographic studies are a useful adjunct to the diagnosis of abdominal trauma. All patients should initially have an upright and supine film. Any bony fractures should be investigated from underlying visceral injury. An elevated diaphragm on the right may be the liver protruding into the chest or may indicate a ruptured lobe of the liver.

Air from a ruptured stomach, duodenum, or colon can usually be found free in the peritoneal cavity or limited to the lesser sac with perforation of the stomach or stripping the area behind the duodenum.

The spleen, liver, or kidneys may be enlarged indicating a hematoma or hemorrhage. Loss of the psoas shadows indicates a retroperitoneal bleed.

Any displacement of neighboring viscera and/or accumulation of fluid between the gas shadows of the bowel loops may indicate solid viscera rupture.

Other diagnostic procedures should be done depending on patient's specific signs and symptoms. IVP should be performed for any evidence of gross or microscopic hematuria. Angiography of the celiac, superior and inferior mesenteric arteries may be done to indicate individual organ injury including visceral bleeding, hematomas, and arteriovenous shunting.

The CAT scan can be useful to detect injuries to the liver, spleen, pancreas, and kidneys. It should only be done on hemodynamically stable patients and on those patients where abdominal findings are equivocal.

Peritoneal lavage is another tool for assessing abdominal trauma. An abdominal tap should be done on all patients with suspected blunt abdominal traumas. Patients who have an altered level of consciousness, spinal cord injuries, are intoxicated, have a head injury with questionable abdominal trauma, and those patients with equivocal findings are all good candidates for a peritoneal lavage.

Positive findings include grossly bloody aspirate, bloody lavage fluid, greater than 100,000 red blood cells per cubic millimeter, greater than 500 white blood cells per cubic millimeter, an elevated amylase and presence of bile, bacteria, or fecal material.

Negative peritoneal lavage results do not rule out retroperitoneal injuries to the pancreas, duodenum, and genitourinary tract.

MANAGEMENT

    I. Maintain adequate blood volume
       A. Lactated Ringer's
       B. Whole blood and packed cells
       C. MAST trousers
   II. Establish the following lifelines
       A. Large bore peripheral lines
       B. Central venous catheter
       C. Foley catheter
       D. Nasogastric tube
       E. Oxygen catheter
  III. Monitor continuously for trends and responses
       A. Abdominal signs—rigidity, rebound tenderness
       B. Hemoglobin, hematocrit
       C. WBC
       D. Urine output
       E. Central venous pressure

      F. Serial x-rays

      G. Bp

      H. Respiratory rate

      I. Pulse rate

      J. Temperature

IV. Sterile dressings for any penetrating injury

V. Antibiotic therapy

      A. Clindamycin, 60 mg/kg/day IV, 3 to 4 divided doses, and

      B. Tobramycin, 5 mg/kg/day IV, 3 divided doses, or

      C. Gentamicin, 5 mg/kg/day IV, 3 divided doses

VI. Tetanus immunization

      A. Prior immunization—0.5 ml absorbed toxoid

      B. No past immunization—0.5 ml absorbed toxoid, 250 units of tetanus immune globulin

VII. Management of specific abdominal injuries

      A. Penetrating injuries

          1. peritoneal lavage

          2. "mini-lap"

          3. contrast media into wound site

      B. Blunt injuries

          1. peritoneal lavage

          2. radiographic studies

              a. water-soluble radiopaque swallow

              b. intravenous pyelogram

              c. arteriogram

              d. upright and supine films

          3. serial blood chemistries

              a. BUN, electrolytes, CBC, liver enzymes, amylase

RATIONALE

As mentioned earlier a patient with abdominal trauma either experiences signs and symptoms of hemorrhagic shock and/or peritonitis. In either case, restoration of blood volume is the main objective. Ringer's lactate is the initial fluid replacement of choice. It is the most nearly physiologic solution, there are no known allergic responses, and it gives emergency personnel time to get the patient typed and crossmatched. Two liters of fluid are given while the physiologic parameters are monitored, blood pressure, pulse rate, respiratory rate, central venous pressure, and urine output. Replacement of blood should be started as quickly as possible. In lifethreatening situations, type O blood may be given until crossmatched blood becomes available. In managing hypotension in patients with abdominal trauma the MAST (military antishock) trousers are a very important adjunct to therapy. MAST trousers work by increasing the peripheral resistance of the vascular bed, by diminishing the size of those vessels under inflation, and by increasing the patient's preload. In abdominal trauma, MAST trousers are especially effective in tamponading intraabdominal bleeding, i.e., retroperitoneal hematoma and traumatic abdominal aneurysm.

Patients should be monitored continuously and watched for changes in vital signs, abdominal pain and rigidity, and results of x-ray studies. Any evidence of fever, tachycardia, diffuse abdominal pain and tenderness and an ileus would suggest peritonitis.

Most patients with penetrating abdominal injury are explored. If the injury is due to a gunshot wound and the bullet enters the peritoneal cavity, surgery is indicated. It is extremely difficult to determine the trajectory angle or the amount of dissipated kinetic energy of a bullet, therefore gunshot wounds should be operated on. Penetrating injuries caused by arrows or knives cause injury by local tissue disruption in the track of the weapon and therefore one can better predict the extent of internal injuries. If penetrating injury is not obvious on inspection (an ice pick implanted in the abdomen), other management modalities can be instituted prior to any decision to operate. Peritoneal lavage can be performed. Local exploration of wound ("mini-lap") to determine if the wound has penetrated the peritoneum. Adjunctive tests, radiopaque studies, CAT scans, arteriography can be performed to determine if surgery is necessary. Liver, stomach, and small and large intestines are the most common organs injured in penetrating trauma.

Patients with blunt injury to the abdomen are often difficult to diagnose because of the insidious clinical manifestations that occur. One should look for signs and symptoms of hemorrhagic shock, peritonitis, and any associated injuries (i.e., rib fractures, pelvic fractures). An accurate history is often helpful in making the diagnosis. Careful examination of the abdomen, including inspection, palpation, percussion, and auscultation, should be performed at regular intervals. Adjunct diagnostic tests include peritoneal lavage, radiographic studies, CAT scans, and intravenous pylogram.

A rectal and vaginal exam should not be forgotten. Serial blood chemistries including BUN, electrolytes, liver enzymes, and complete blood count should be drawn at regular intervals. Laparotomy should be perfomed if any of the test results are abnormal, if there is unexplained persistent abdominal pain, and hypotension. The most commonly injured organs in blunt trauma are spleen, pancreas, and duodenum.

Prior to any operative intervention, tetanus and antibiotic prophylaxis should be started as stated in the management modalities. Antibiotics given should be active against both aerobic and anaerobic bacteria.

Gastrointestinal Emergencies References

1. Avery Jones, F. Hematemesis and melena: With special reference to causation and to the factors influencing the mortality from bleeding pectic ulcers. *Gastroenterology*, 1956, **30**, 166.

2. Bishop, R. P. The diagnosis of pancreatic disease. *Gastroenterology,* 1968, **49,** 112.

3. Bloomer, J. R. & Waldmann,T. A. Relationship of serum alpha fetoprotein to the severity and duration of illness in patients with viral hepatitis. *Gastroenterology,* 1975, **68,** 342–50.

4. Cohen, A. S., et al. *Medical emergencies: Diagnostic and management procedures from the Boston City Hospital* (2nd ed.). Boston: Little, Brown, 1983.

5. Galambos, J. T. Alcoholic hepatitis. In F. Schaffner, S. Shenlock, C. M. Leevy (Eds.), *The liver and its diseases.* New York: Intercontinental Medical, 1974.

6. Hornyak, S. W., & Shaftan, G. W. Value of inconclusive lavage in abdominal trauma management. *Journal of Trauma,* 1979, **19,** 329.

7. Levitt, M. D., Rapoport, M., & Cooperbank, S. R. The renal clearance of amylase in renal insufficiency, acute pancreatitis and macroamylasemia. *Annals of Internal Medicine,* 1969, **71,** 919.

8. Mason, J. H. The expectant management of abdominal stab wounds. *Journal of Trauma,* 1964, **4,** 210.

9. Moore, E. E. Mandatory laboratory for gunshot wounds penetrating the abdomen. *Journal of Surgery,* 1980, **140,** 847.

10. Olsen, W., & Hilbarth, D. Abdominal paracentesis or peritoneal lavage in blunt abdominal trauma. *Journal of Trauma,* 1971, **11,** 824.

11. Ranson, J. H. C. Acute pancreatitis. *Current Problems in Surgery,* 1979, **16,** 1.

12. Rosen, P. E. *Emergency medicine concepts and clinical practice* (Vols. I & II), St. Louis: C. V. Mosby, 1983.

13. Salzman, E. W., & Bartlett, M. K. Pancreatic duct exploration in selected cases of acute pancreatitis. *Annals of Surgery,* 1963, **158,** 859–863.

14. Thomson, H. Abdominal wall tenderness. *Lancet,* 1977, **2,** 1053.

15. Warren, W. D., Zeppa, R., & Fomon, J. J. Selected transplenic decompression of gastroesophageal varices by distal splenorenal shunt. *Annals of Surgery,* 1967, **166,** 437.

16. Yajko, R. D., Norton, L. W., & Eiseman, B. Current management of upper gastrointestinal bleeding. *Annals of Surgery,* 1975, **181,** 471.

E. GENITOURINARY EMERGENCIES

1. Acute Renal Failure

ASSESSMENT

   I. Initial assessment data
     A. Rule out urinary tract obstruction
       1. recent history of decreased urinary output
       2. presence of distended bladder
       3. physical and sonography findings
         a. residual urine
         b. urinary calculi
         c. tumors
         d. papillary necrosis with obstructed ureters
         e. renal size
         f. presence of hydronephrosis
     B. Rule out prerenal azotemia
       1. recent history of
         a. hypotension
         b. shock
         c. extracellular volume depletion as in
           i. burns
           ii. hemorrhage
           iii. severe vomiting and/or diarrhea
       2. laboratory findings
         a. urine osmolality >500 mOsm/kg H_2O
         b. BUN: creatinine concentrations >10:1
         c. urine sodium concentration <20 mEq/L
         d. fractional excretion of filtered sodium <1
       3. identify other precipitating factors

   a. dehydrated states
      i. pre- and postsurgery
      ii. diagnostic studies requiring dehydration
   b. transfusion reaction
   c. progressive infections or septic condition
   d. patients with indwelling catheters
   4. general appearance and demeanor
      a. appears critically ill
      b. lethargic
      c. nausea, vomiting, diarrhea
      d. skin and mucous membranes, dry
      e. odor of urine on breath
II. Alterations in urinary function and laboratory data
   A. Urinary output 400 ml/day
   B. Specific gravity (1.010)
   C. Rise in serum concentration of the following
      1. urea
      2. creatinine
      3. uric acid
      4. organic acids
      5. potassium
      6. magnesium
   D. Urinalysis
      1. urine Na concentration >60 mEq/L
      2. urine osmolality ratio <1.2
      3. urine urea to plasma urea ratio of 3 or less
      4. urine creatinine to plasma creatinine ratio of 10 or less
      5. presence of Bence Jones protein ⎫ possible parenchymal failure
      6. RBC and Hgb casts   ⎭
      7. WBC casts
III. Alterations in electrolyte and acid–base status
   A. Hyperkalemia
      1. electrocardiographic changes
         a. tented T waves
         b. elevated T waves
         c. widened QRS complex
         d. prolonged QT interval
         e. flattening to absent P waves
         f. ST segment depression
      2. physical findings
         a. weakness
         b. possible flaccid paralysis
         c. twitching
         d. hyperreflexia progressing to possible paresthesias or paralysis

   e. bradycardia progressing rapidly to cardiac arrest

   f. oliguria

 B. Hypermagnesemia

  1. reduced nerve and muscle activity

  2. impaired respirations due to reduced nerve and muscle activity

  3. lethargy and/or coma

  4. cardiac arrest

 C. Hyponatremia

  1. weakness

  2. restlessness

  3. delirium

  4. hyperpnea

  5. oliguria

  6. elevated temperature

  7. flushed skin

  8. abdominal cramps

  9. convulsions

  10. vasomotor collapse

   a. hypotension

   b. rapid, thready pulse

   c. cold, clammy skin

   d. cyanosis

  Hypernatremia

  1. pitting edema

  2. increased blood pressure

  3. dyspnea

  4. dry, sticky mucous membrane

  5. flushed skin

  6. intense thirst

  7. oliguria

 D. Metabolic acidosis

  1. headache

  2. drowsiness

  3. nausea, vomiting, diarrhea

  4. coma

  5. twitching

  6. convulsions

  7. hyperpnea (Kussmaul respirations)

 E. Hypoxemia

  1. anxiety, restlessness, confusion

  2. tachycardia

  3. dysrhythmias

  4. insomnia or altered mentation

  5. diaphoresis

  6. central cyanosis

  7. cardiac and renal failure

  8. coma

IV. Alterations in cardiovascular status

 A. Increased cardiac output

 B. Hypertension

 C. Pulmonary edema

 D. Dysrhythmias

 E. Left ventricular failure

V. Alterations in integumentary status
   A. Ecchymosis
   B. Pruritis
   C. Pigmentation
   D. Terry's nails (possible)
   E. Uremic frost
VI. Alterations in gastrointestinal status
   A. Stomatitis
   B. Anorexia
   C. Nausea, vomiting
   D. Abdominal pain
   E. Duodenal ulcer
   F. Bleeding
VII. Alterations in hematologic status
   A. Hemolysis
   B. Anemia
   C. Bleeding defect
VIII. Alterations in neurologic (central nervous and peripheral) status
   A. Headache
   B. Muscle twitching
   C. Convulsions
   D. Coma
   E. Uremic manifestations
      1. fatigue
      2. loss of appetite
      3. apathy and/or mental dullness
      4. elevated bp
      5. itching, pruritus
      6. restlessness
      7. asterixis
      8. continued decrease in urinary output
      9. seizures
      10. decreased vibratory sense
      11. loss of deep tendon reflexes (ankles more than knees)

PATHOPHYSIOLOGY

Acute renal failure (ARF) is a clinical syndrome characterized by a sudden decrease in glomerular and tubular function. Associated with this condition are multiple biochemical changes as well as acute uremia. Acute renal failure is usually associated with urine volumes of less than 400 ml/day, and is related to the consequences of reduction in glomerular rate such as increases in blood urea nitrogen and serum creatinine. Various etiologic factors may precipitate acute renal failure, but, in general, the most common causes are related to nephrotoxic agents or prolonged renal ischemia.

Acute renal failure is often identified according to prerenal, renal, and post-renal causes. Prerenal etiology includes those factors causing a reduction in blood flow to the kidneys, or in which the renal function is disrupted by overt systemic change(s). In this prerenal state, urine sodium levels are markedly decreased. Renal (intrarenal) causes are those factors primarily related to pathophysiologic processes occurring within the kidney structures. In this situation, damaged tubules are unable to concentrate urine or excrete nitrogenous waste produced by protein metabolism. Postrenal causes are primarily a result of obstruction or disruption of the urinary tract.

Multiple theories have been postulated to explain the pathophysiology of acute renal failure once the causative factor has been identifed. These include:

- *Back Leak Theory.* The interruption in the integrity of tubular epithelium allows glomerular filtrate to leak into intestitial tissue where it is reabsorbed by renal capillaries.
- *Tubular Obstruction Theory.* This theory is usually applicable to acute renal failure as seen in those individuals who have suffered crushing injuries which would allow the release of large amounts of myoglobin. As a result of the traumatic edema, the accumulation of myoglobin and hemoglobin breakdown end products and other intraluminal debris, causes renal tubular obstruction to occur.
- *Vascular Theory.* The systemic or nephrotoxic causes may either vasoconstrict the afferent arteriole or vasodilate the efferent arteriole, which, in any case, would precipitate poor renal perfusion. Included as well in this theory is the consideration that any factor decreasing glomerular membrane permeability adversely affects renal perfusion.
- *Cell Swelling Theory.* This theory assumes that any ischemic event, which would reduce the quantity of metabolic energy necessary to actively transport and pump sodium out of the cell, would cause an elevation in cellular osmolarity. Rising osmolarity triggers an osmotic movement of water into the cell causing the cell to swell. This swelling reduces renal blood flow, and thus promotes the persistence of ischemia and poor renal perfusion.
- *Renin–Angiotensin Theory.* Renal tubular dysfunction brought on by either toxic or ischemic injuries causes sodium ion concentration within the intraluminal areas of the renal structures. This sodium ion concentration, sensed at the macula densa, triggers the stimulation and release of renin which in turn activates the renin–angiotensin system. As a result, renin and angiotensin II constrict the afferent arteriole, thus leading to poor renal perfusion.

This discussion is limited to those changes found in acute tubular necrosis, the most common cause of acute renal failure. Despite the multiple causes (Table 12), the effects on the patient and the emergency management are applicable to all types of acute renal failure. The clinical course of acute renal failure is usually divided into three stages: oliguric stage, diuretic stage, and recovery stage. The focus is on the oliguric phase. As soon as acute renal failure is considered, diagnostic measures and urologic consultation must be obtained and instituted immediately with the goal of excluding treatable causes of oliguria such as prerenal obstruction and prerenal azotemia.

TABLE 12. CAUSES OF ACUTE TUBULAR NECROSIS

Drug Related	Illness or Systemic Injury Related
Antimicrobials	Crushing injuries
Sulfonamides	Major operative procedures
Gentamicin	Severe blood loss
Kanamycin	Severe hypertension
Streptomycin	Rhabdomyolysis (from any cause)
Amphotericin	Myoglobinuria (from any cause)
Bacitracin	Heat stroke
Colistin	Heroin overdose
Neomycin	Severe febrile illnesses
Vancomycin	Gram-negative sepsis
Cephaloridine	Gram-positive sepsis
Polymixin	Lactic acidosis
Organic iodonated x-ray contrast media	Major extracellular fluid volume losses
Methoxyflurane (anesthetic)	Burns
Nephrotoxic agents	Complicated pregnancies
organic solvents	Incompatible blood transfusions
carbon tetrachloride	Intravascular hemolysis
tetrachloroethylene	
ethylene	
diethylene glycol	
inorganic mercurials and other heavy metals	
bismuth	
uranium	
lead	
organic mercurials (rare)	
methylalcohol	
salicylates	
paraldehyde	

(Adapted from Beeson, P. B., & McDermott, W. Textbook of Medicine. Philadelphia: W. B. Saunders, 1975, pp. 1107–1114.)

Acute renal failure can be considered a multisystem problem because almost every part of the body is affected when renal regulatory mechanisms are altered. Laboratory studies of blood and urine give valuable information in establishing the differential diagnosis of acute renal failure. In addition, thorough assessment serves as the foundation for planning and implementing therapeutic management modalities to relieve the effects of acute renal failure, and, hopefully, to prevent its complications.

Any individual with acute renal failure has a decreased ability to excrete potassium. The end products of protein catabolism, possible blood in the gastrointestinal tract, food intake, blood transfusion, intravenous infusions, drug constituents, e.g., potassium, penicillin, and the results of extracellular shifts in response to metabolic acidosis, are all responsible for a hyperkalemic state. Magnesium, a predominantly intracellular ion, and essential in many enzymatic systems, is also retained as kidney function decreases.

The disruption of water, electrolytes, and acid–base balance as a result of the kidney's inability to concentrate urine leads to severe extracellular volume deficits, via sweating, vomiting, fever, and diarrhea, and ultimately the development of hypernatremia. Therefore careful and continual assessment of electrocardiographic readings and serum electrolyte determinations are of utmost importance. As renal function further deteriorates, the kidneys become unable to excrete hydrogen ions. As a result, the decreased elimination of acids in the urine, the rising levels of ketones produced by the body's mobilization of fat to combat catabolism, the depletion of the bicarbonate ion, the decreased reabsorption of bicarbonate by the kidney, and the failing ability of the kidneys to acidify phosphate salts, produces a metabolic acidotic state.

Although fluid and electrolyte changes are of grave importance, nitrogenous wastes including urea, creatinine, and uric acid are retained. As the plasma levels of these substances rise, significant changes occur in oxygenation, metabolism, and the immune response which renders the individual subject to infections, altered perceptions, and other central and peripheral nervous system signs and symptoms.

Extracellular fluid volume excesses during the oliguric phase can lead to circulatory overload. As renal failure progresses, the kidney is no longer able to produce erythropoietin, and as a result, anemia develops. Anemia, in concert with the hypervolemic state, increased cardiac output and increases blood pressure, which in turn causes the development of pulmonary edema and left ventricular failure. Other major cardiovascular findings are primarily related to potassium and calcium imbalances. Bleeding disorders, when apparent, are usually related to a drop in platelets; and any anemia that may be present will be aggravated by blood loss from gastrointestinal hemorrhage, a very real threat because up to one third of all uremic patients develop duodenal ulcers, all of which are capable of bleeding from any site along the gastrointestinal tract. Additional causes of bleeding might be folate deficiency, iron deficiency, and hypersplenism.

With proper understanding of the pathophysiology of acute renal failure and the immediate identification of appropriate assessment parameters, emergency management modalities may be initiated quickly in the hope of reversing the renal failure.

MANAGEMENT

    I. Establish measures to support modalities
      A. Intravenous line
      B. Arterial line
      C. Indwelling catheter
      D. ECG monitoring
      E. Oxygen therapy, if indicated
      F. Nasogastric suctioning, if indicated
      G. X-rays of chest and abdomen
      H. Laboratory data baselines
         1. serum electrolytes including magnesium and phosphates
         2. blood gases and pH
         3. BUN

    4. glucose
    5. creatinine concentration
    6. uric acid and urea levels
    7. CBC and differential
    8. urinalysis for
       a. sodium concentration
       b. urine osmolality
       c. urea level
       d. creatinine level
       e. RBC, WBC, Hgb, and casts
       f. specific gravity

II. Monitor continuously for trends and responses to management modalities
  A. Temperature, pulse, respirations, and bp
  B. Skin quality and appearance
  C. Blood gases and pH
  D. Serum electrolytes and other determinants, as indicated
  E. Hydration status
  F. Metabolic status
  G. Respiratory status
  H. Cardiac status
  I. Renal status
  J. Daily weight changes
  K. CVP measurements

III. Institute measures to treat or prevent electrolyte, acid–base, and fluid imbalances
  A. Hyperkalemia
    1. 10 ml of 10 percent calcium gluconate solution for potassium >6.5 mEq/L and major electrocardiographic abnormalities (absent P waves, wide QRS complexes, or ventricular dysrhythmias)
    2. potassium level >6.5 mEq/L without ECG abnormalities
       a. 100 ml of 50 percent glucose with or without 25 units of regular insulin
       b. alternatively
          i. 2 ampules (44 mEq/ampule) sodium bicarbonate, IV, or
          ii. 1000 ml isotonic sodium bicarbonate, IV
    3. potassium level between 5.5 and 6.5 mEq/L
       a. sodium polystyrene sulfonate resin (Kayexalate)
       b. sorbitol
          i. orally
             15–20 g resin
             20 ml of 70 percent sorbitol } 3 to 4 times/day
          ii. retention enema
             50 g resin
             50 ml of 70 percent sorbitol } administered, retained for 30 to 45
             100 ml tap water } minutes, and expelled

    4. peritoneal dialysis
      a. indications for
         i. refractory hyperkalemia
        ii. refractory acidosis
       iii. ECG changes not responsive to conservative therapy
      b. solutions utilized
         i. 2000 ml 1.5 percent glucose solution (warmed)
        ii. 4.25 percent glucose solution, if necessary to enhance osmosis
       iii. potassium and other electrolyte replacements as indicated by serum determinations
      c. monitor for the following complications
         i. hypoventilation
        ii. atelectasis
       iii. pneumonia
       iv. hyperglycemia ⎫
        v. hypernatremia ⎬ especially if obtunded
       vi. disequilibrium syndrome
          nausea and vomiting
          cramps
          headache
          irritability
          muscle twitching
          convulsions
      d. measures to prevent possible complications
         i. assess for symptoms of overload
        ii. assess for symptoms of dehydration
       iii. precise dialysis recordings
       iv. elevate head of bed to minimize pressure on diaphragm
        v. frequent ECG and nervous system assessment
       vi. coughing, deep breathing, and frequent position changes

B. Hypermagnesemia
   1. calcium salts, parenterally
   2. dialysis

C. Hyponatremia and hypernatremia
   1. extracellular fluid excess (excess sodium in presence of increased sodium and water)
      a. administer diuretics
      b. restrict sodium and fluid intake
   2. extracellular fluid deficit
      a. isotonic saline solution, IV ⎫
      b. hypertonic saline solution, IV ⎬ depending on severity of deficit
   3. intracellular fluid deficit
      a. water replacement, po
      b. 5 percent dextrose in distilled water, IV
   4. intracellular fluid excess
      a. fluid intake restricted

TABLE 13. GENERAL PRINCIPLES OF DIALYSIS MANAGEMENT IN ACUTE RENAL FAILURE

A. With frequent dialysis (peritoneal or hemodialysis)
   1. moderate salt restriction
   2. moderate water restriction
   3. moderate protein restriction (40 to 60 g/day)
B. With infrequent dialysis
   1. extremely careful regulation of sodium, water, and potassium to minimize volumetric and chemical abnormalities of body fluid
   2. fluid restriction to effect ½ lb of body weight per day
   3. approximately 400 to 500 ml of water allowed per day in addition to the amounts lost via urine and the gastrointestinal tract
   4. if able to tolerate food by mouth, a 2000-calorie diet that is protein and potassium free, and essentially sodium free (some physicians favor the inclusion of 20 g of protein a day which contains the minimal daily requirements of essential amino acids)
   5. parenteral alimentation (if necessary)
      a. dextrose—100 g/day with vitamins (IV)
      b. fat emulsions to fulfill calorie requirements (IV)
      c. if glucose is utilized, it must be hyperosmotic (because of fluid restriction requirement) (IV)

(Adapted from Beeson, P. B., & McDermott, W. Textbook of Medicine. Philadelphia: W. B. Saunders, 1975, pp. 1107–1114.)

    D. Metabolic acidosis
        1. measures to reduce protein catabolism
            a. protein restriction
            b. utilization of carbohydrates
        2. supportive oxygen therapy
        3. sodium bicarbonate, IV
        4. dialysis (Table 13)
    E. Fluid balance restoration
        1. assess for fluid overload or dehydration
        2. replacement based on
            a. daily weight loss (0.5 to 1.0 kg/day)
            b. urinary and extrarenal losses
                i. urinary output per 24 hours
                ii. 600 to 800 ml insensible loss per 24 hours
IV. Institute measures to combat additional complications of ARF
    A. Hypoxemia, dyspnea and volume overload
        1. oxygen via nasal cannula at 4 to 5 L/minute
        2. clonidine 0.1 mg po q 2 to 4 hours
            or — for hypertension
            sodium nitroprusside, IV drip — Maintain blood pressure no lower than 150/100 mm Hg
            (50 mg in 500 ml 5 percent D/W at a rate of 0.5 to 8.0 μg/kg/minute)
        3. packed red blood cells for Hct <30 percent (especially in elderly)
        4. fluid restrictions

    5. phlebotomy of 500 ml if pulmonary edema attributable to over administration of parenteral fluids and Hct >35 percent

    6. digoxin 0.25 mg q 6 hours to total of 1 mg with continued maintenance dose for CHF associated with primary cardiac disease

    7. dialysis for uremic problems and fluid overload

      a. hemodialysis with ultrafiltration

      b. peritoneal dialysis with hyperosmolar dialysate

  B. Gastrointestinal bleeding

    1. management directed toward

      a. cause

      b. amount, rate, and location

    2. gastric lavage

    3. volume replacement

    4. vigorous dialysis

    5. emergency surgery

  C. Anemia

    1. maintenance of nutrition

    2. packed red blood cells

  D. Neurologic symptoms usually rapidly controlled via dialysis

V. Promote measures to maintain appropriate nutrition

  A. High caloric, low protein diet

    1. protein of high biologic value

    2. protein to contain essential amino acids (20 g of essential amino acids needed daily for tissue maintenance)

  B. Possible sodium or potassium restrictions

  C. Avoid magnesium-containing antacids

  D. Aluminum hydroxide gel (Amphogel) 30 ml with meals

  E. Frequent oral hygiene

  F. Give reasons to patient for special diet

  G. Plan diet around patient's food preferences, if possible

  H. Hyperalimentation if unable to tolerate po intake

    1. assess for nonketotic, hyperosmolar, hyperglycemic coma

    2. assess for secondary hyperchloremic acidosis

  I. Tube feedings

VI. Promote measures to combat infection

  A. Monitor carefully for infectious processes

  B. Design nursing care to prevent infection in high-risk areas

    1. respiratory tract

    2. mouth

    3. wounds

  C. Aseptic technique

    1. at all infusion sites

    2. with each peritoneal dialysis infusion

    3. with indwelling catheter care

VII. Institute measures to promote emotional well being

A. instruct and discuss all aspects of care with patient
B. encourage patient to verbalize questions, anxieties, and fears
C. involve family members and significant others in patient care
D. administer physical and emotional comfort

RATIONALE

The kidney has an outstanding ability to recover after injury or insult; therefore, the primary goal of management of acute renal failure is to establish as soon as possible a normal homeostatic environment which will allow repair of kidney tissue and restoration of renal function. In the early minutes following diagnosis, measures to support management modalities and laboratory data to serve as baseline data must be established. Monitoring parameters, as identified, must be assessed on a continual basis to evaluate the patient's clinical status in terms of trends and responses to treatment.

Concentrated effort is made to treat or prevent electrolyte, acid–base, and fluid imbalances. Hyperkalemia is probably considered the most dangerous imbalance because no elevated serum potassium is safe in the patient with acute renal failure. A variety of measures may be utilized depending on the severity and refractoriness of the hyperkalemic state. Calcium gluconate, when administered, opposes the action of potassium on myocardial tissue, but because of its transitory effect, it is essential to initiate other modalities to control hyperkalemia. The intravenous infusion of 100 ml of 50 percent glucose with or without 25 units of regular insulin, or 1000 ml of isotonic bicarbonate solution lowers potassium levels by causing the intracellular movement of potassium. This treatment modality is not without complications. The use of bicarbonate solution expands extracellular fluid volume possibly inducing cardiac failure. If glucose is infused, especially if insulin is used, reactive hypoglycemia may develop within approximately 3 hours after administration. Cation exchange resins may be administered orally or rectally to facilitate the excretion of potassium. Sorbitol is given along with the resin to increase the rate of passage of resin through the gastrointestinal tract, to prevent impaction, and to eliminate the sodium released by the exchange resins. Because of this last fact, assessment for sodium overload must be vigilant during the cation exchange treatment.

Refractory hyperkalemia with electrocardiographic changes that do not respond to the identified therapies is an indication for immediate dialysis. Peritoneal dialysis can be rapidly instituted, especially in an emergency setting. The objective of dialysis is to establish a negative balance, and in so doing, the patient loses fluids in addition to the toxic nitrogenous waste products that have accumulated in the blood. Dialysate solutions must be warmed to body temperature to increase urea clearance and to cause the least amount of discomfort to the patient.

Throughout the dialysis process, additional electrolyte, acid–base, and fluid imbalances, as well as other complications may occur, and must be observed for on a regular basis. Respiratory complications such as hypoventilation, pneumonia, and atelectasis can be prevented by elevating the head of the bed, thus minimizing pressure on the diaphragm and allowing for lung expansion. Instituting coughing and deep breathing exercises allows for a greater gas exchange. The neurologic signs and symptoms occurring during dialysis, known as disequilibrium syndrome, are attributed to rapid dialysis. Small doses of sedatives and reduction of flow rate usually corrects this situation.

Magnesium excesses depress the central nervous system, diminish muscle cell irritability by blocking acetylcholine at the myoneural junction, decreases blood pressure by its direct vasodilating effect, and increases conduction time through its cardiac inhibitory effect. Hypermagnesemia is treated with parenteral doses of calcium salts, which are magnesium antagonists, or via dialysis.

Because variations in sodium concentrations reflect a change in either intracellular or extracellular fluid concentration, treatment is geared toward altering these two variables as indicated within the management modalities for hyponatremia and hypernatremia. Careful attention must be paid to various points in the emergency management of this condition when sodium excesses or deficits may be most prominent. In the initial stages of acute renal failure, hyponatremia may cause fatigue and possibly seizures. Infusion of hypertonic saline may be administered to correct this imbalance. In the obtunded patient receiving hypotonic fluids, hypernatremia may develop, and should be assessed for periodically. Rapid loss of body fluids during dialysis causes fluid volume deficits, and signs and symptoms of hypernatremia can occur.

Metabolic acidosis accompanies the oliguric phase of acute renal failure because the kidney cannot eliminate a sufficient amount of hydrogen ions produced by the metabolic process. This is reflected by a drop in CO_2 combining power and in blood pH. Appropriate measures such as protein restriction, utilization of carbohydrate, supportive oxygen therapy, sodium bicarbonate, and dialysis may be used to correct this acid–base disturbance.

Fluid balance is also disrupted in acute renal failure, and every effort must be made through as many assessment parameters as possible (e.g., daily weight loss, accurate intake and output, changes in vital signs, skin turgor, mucous membranes, and central venous pressure readings) to detect and correct this imbalance. Fluid replacement should approximate the 24-hour urinary output plus the 600 to 800 ml of insensible fluid loss over the same time period. Peritoneal dialysis can increase the fluid imbalance problem, and patients should be observed for the occurrence of fluid overload or dehydration. In addition, laboratory determinations for blood glucose levels must be ongoing because hyperglycemia can occur from the glucose in the dialysate.

The major cardiovascular symptoms or complications are generally related to extracellular volume excess and electrolyte disturbances. It is not usual for a previously normal heart to develop failure; however, it may develop along with hypertension and pulmonary edema from circulatory overload and from the increased cardiac demands brought on by the anemia. Suggested therapeutic modalities such as those identified may be instituted to combat these complications.

Gastrointestinal bleeding usually results from the stress ulcers that occur as a complication of acute renal failure, and from the increased gastric acid secretion produced by the parathyroid hormone excess that is usually noted in uremia. Gastric lavage, volume replacement, vigorous dialysis, or emergency surgery may be needed.

Management of anemia is directed toward restoration of folate and iron levels, maintenance of nutrition, and possibly tranfusion of packed red blood cells. Present research is looking at supplying histidine as an intact essential amino acid, because, during uremia, some unknown alteration prevents histidine formation. Histidine deficits increase the severity of the anemia.

Appropriate nutrition for the patient with acute renal failure is a diet high in carbohydrates and low in protein. Carbohydrates reverse the process of gluconeogenesis, and the intake of high biologic protein containing the essential amino acids is necessary to reduce nitrogenous waste products. Food preferences should be taken into consideration whenever possible, as a means of encouraging adequate intake. Limitations of foods containing sodium or potassium may be indicated. Because of the frequency of stomatitis in acute renal failure, scrupulous mouth care is needed several times a day, and especially before and after meals. Magnesium-containing antacids as well as citrus juices are to be avoided to prevent hypermagnesemia and hyperkalemia. In those individuals unable to tolerate oral feedings, or whose oral intake is not sufficient to meet nutritional requirements, tube feedings or hyperalimentation may be necessary. Two major problems may arise in the individual who is receiving hyperalimentation. Nonketotic, hyperosmolar, and hyperglycemic coma may result from an intolerance to the high carbohydrate content of the feeding. Secondary hyperchloremic acidosis may develop as a result of an excess of chloride ions being ingested or retained. With the excess of chloride ions, bicarbonate ions are released in the kidney tubule, and this lowers the base bicarbonate circulating in the extracellular fluid.

Nursing care measures must be designed to combat or prevent infection in individuals with acute renal failure, because infection is the most frequent cause of death in these individuals, and to promote physical and emotional well-being in these very ill and very frightened patients.

2. Problems of Pregnancy

ABORTION

ASSESSMENT

I. Abortion—the termination of pregnancy before the fetus becomes viable
II. Classifications
  A. Threatened abortions
    1. vaginal discharge or frank vaginal bleeding during the first 20 weeks of pregnancy

      2. occasional mild, menstrual-like cramps or backache
  B. Imminent abortion
      1. increasing hemorrhage
      2. continuous pain which has persisted unabated for at least 6 hours or more
  C. Inevitable abortion
      1. rupture of membranes
      2. pain
      3. bleeding
  D. Incomplete abortion
      1. hemorrhage
      2. increasing contractions of uterus
      3. cervix dilated
      4. rupture of membranes
      5. placenta detached, partially expelled, fragments remain
  E. Complete abortion
      1. increasing hemorrhage
      2. uterus contracting
      3. cervix dilated
      4. entire product of conception delivered

PATHOPHYSIOLOGY

Threatened Abortion

The occurrence of signs and symptoms of impending loss of the embryo or fetus indicates threatened abortion. Blood makes its way from ruptured paraplacental blood vessels and eroded epithelium into the uterine cavity. Additional causative factors include inflammatory lesions of the external os, polyps, certain abnormalities of the developing fetus which are inconsistent with life and fibroid uterus. It may follow acute infectious diseases, toxemias of pregnancy, emotional disturbances, and endocrine dysfunctions.

Imminent Abortion

Imminent abortion is characterized by severe bleeding. This bleeding into the layers of the decidual basalis causes separation of the ovum from the decidua, along with opening of the venous sinuses.

Inevitable Abortion

Inevitable abortion is one that has advanced to a stage where termination of the pregnancy can no longer be prevented. If the membranes rupture and this is followed by bleeding or pain, or if rupture follows after bleeding or pain, abortion is inevitable.

Incomplete Abortion
This is an abortion in which a part of the products of conception is retained in the uterus and bleeding persists. Uterine contractions, together with the expulsion of the fetus and amniotic fluid, cause a partial separation of the placenta. If partial separation occurs, muscle fibers are unable to clamp down and hemorrhage occurs.

Complete Abortion
Complete abortion occurs when all of the products of conception are expelled from the uterus. Uterine contractions, together with the expulsion of the fetus and amniotic fluid, cause a complete separation of the placenta.

MANAGEMENT

  I. Threatened abortion
    A. Bed rest
    B. Sedation
    C. Cessation of coitus for at least 2 weeks after bleeding ceases
 II. Imminent and inevitable abortion
    A. Hospitalize patient
    B. Type and crossmatch blood
    C. Large bore IV with administration of lactated Ringer's solution
    D. Oxytocin 0/5 ml every ½ hour for 6 doses, IV, or 10 units per liter of 5 percent D/S
    E. Sedation
III. Incomplete abortion
    A. Hospitalization
    B. Type and crossmatch blood
    C. Oxytocin drip (10 units/liter of 5 percent D/S)
    D. Sedation
    E. Save tissue to ascertain if abortion is complete
    F. Dilatation and curettage
 VI. Complete abortion
    A. Monitor vital signs
    B. Check fundus
    C. Oxytocin drip 10 units/liter of 5 percent D/S
    D. Dilatation and curettage may be indicated

RATIONALE

Threatened Abortion
During the early course of pregnancy, many women experience painless vaginal bleeding which subsides spontaneously. Others who have pain tend to progress to imminent abortion despite all efforts to avert it. Treatment is then directed toward

delaying or averting the abortion through use of bed rest, sedation, and the cessation of coitus.

Imminent and Inevitable Abortion

Because the possibility of continuing hemorrhage is usually inevitable, it is wise to prepare for blood replacement. Abortion, at this point is imminent and is encouraged to completion. Oxytocin is administered to aid uterine contractions to expel the fetus. Because the oxytocin increases pain, mild sedation is ordered.

Incomplete Abortion

If the patient does not respond to an oxytocin drip, dilatation and curettage may be necessary. Sodium thiopental (Pentothal) is the preferred anesthetic agent as it is short acting. Hemorrhage from incomplete abortion is rarely fatal, because as the blood pressure drops, bleeding stops and replacement therapy can be instituted while the dilatation and curettage are in progress.

Complete Abortion

When abortion is complete, the uterine wall contracts to control hemorrhage. Oxytocin may be administered to aid uterine contractions and dilatation and curettage may be indicated for retained products of conception.

PREECLAMPSIA/ECLAMPSIA

ASSESSMENT

A. Increased bp (greater than 140/90 mm Hg)
B. Hyperreflexia
C. Rapid respirations
D. Proteinuria, oliguria, hemoglobinuria
E. Diffuse peripheral edema
F. Visual disturbances
G. Convulsions
H. Coma

PATHOPHYSIOLOGY

This disease primarily involves women in their first pregnancy, usually during the last 3 months up to the 20th week of gestation. Because the vast majority of patients with mild to moderate eclampsia are asymptomatic, attempts to recognize mild preeclampsia before it progresses to eclampsia necessitates frequent prenatal visits during the last trimester of pregnancy. Progression of symptoms may occur in weeks or may occur in several days. Symptomatology is associated with poor tissue perfusion to a number of vital organs including the liver, kidneys, brain, and most importantly the uterus. Cardiac output is unchanged, therefore the increased blood pressure and visual disturbances are due to increased total peripheral resistance. Clinical studies show that the poor perfusion may be the result of a vasospasm. There is a dramatic decrease in the renal glomerular filtration rate due to changes in renal blood flow. There is impaired glomerular filtration with depletion of serum albumin and globulin by proteinuria. There is also a decreased delivery of sodium to the tubules that continue to reabsorb sodium at a normal rate. The imbalance between glomerular and tubular function results in sodium retention which leads to diffuse peripheral edema.

MANAGEMENT

Eclampsia is one of the gravest obstetric emergencies and is preventable by vigorously managing preeclampsia at the onset of presenting symptoms.
  I. Preeclampsia
      A. Complete bed rest
      B. Moderate sedation
      C. Serial urinalysis—monitor proteinuria and hemoglobinuria
      D. Low salt diet
      E. Diuretics, if indicated
 II. Eclampsia
      A. Immediate hospitalization
      B. Baseline laboratory studies—urinalysis, coagulation studies, renal and hepatic function tests, type and crossmatch blood
      C. Central venous line
      D. Monitor vital signs and peripheral reflexes—CVP, bp, temperature, pulse, respirations
      E. Nasal oxygen at 6 liters/minute
      F. Light restraints to prevent injuries
      G. Padded tongue blade at bedside
      H. Minimize outside stimuli
      I. Foley catheter to gravity drainage
      J. Strict monitoring of intake and output
      K. Magnesium sulfate drip 20 g/liter of D5.33. This drip is titrated to run at 2 g/hour. Postpartum, the drip dose is gradually reduced over a 12-hour period of time providing the blood pressure is stable. If peripheral reflexes are hypoactive, it is best to withhold this drug because hyporeflexia is an early sign of magnesium intoxication and always precedes respiratory depression. If respiratory depression develops, discontinue magnesium sulfate and administer calcium gluconate, 20 ml of a 10 percent solution IV slowly several times a day up to 160 ml/24 hours
      L. Phenobarbital 60 mg IM for 4 to 6 hours postpartum
      M. Antihypertensive medication, perferably hydralazine IV in 5 mg bolus and repeat every 20 minutes to lower diastolic blood pressure to between 90 to 95 mm Hg and improve renal flow

N. As soon as the patient has been stabilized for 24 to 36 hours, delivery should be considered. Induction of labor is the preferable procedure. However, if induction is not successful, cesarean section should be performed

RATIONALE

Baseline laboratory data are essential to monitor electrolyte balance and to correct hemoconcentration. Constant and expert nursing care is of paramount importance to prevent injury and to evaluate and report any changes in the patient's condition. A padded tongue blade should be available in the event the patient bites her tongue during a convulsion. The intracranial pressure is frequently raised in patients with eclampsia causing irritability which could trigger a convulsion. It has been suggested that patients with eclampsia might profit from sedation before initiating emergency measures in order to minimize outside stimuli. Because the vasospasm of the arterioles causes hypoxia, oxygen is indicated. Magnesium sulfate is used as a central depressant in circumstances characterized by seizures associated with eclampsia of pregnancy. Whenever magnesium therapy is employed, a preparation of a calcium salt should be readily available to counteract the potential hazard of magnesium intoxication. Calcium counteracts the effects of magnesium sulfate on the muscle tissue. Magnesium sulfate is the central nervous system depressant of choice as it has the least affect on the fetus. Magnesium has additional favorable properties that lower blood pressure and promote diuresis. Magnesium is excreted solely by the kidneys, therefore it is most important to monitor urinary output. Hydralazine is a direct acting vasodilator, reduces peripheral vascular resistance, and tends to cause a reflex increase in cardiac output and renal blood flow. Central venous lines aid in fluid replacement therapy and serve as an indicator of cardiac function. The cessation of symptoms occurs only after the uterus has been emptied, therefore delivery is indicated.

PLACENTA PREVIA

ASSESSMENT

A. Patient presents with painless vaginal bleeding which usually does not appear until after the seventh month of pregnancy
B. Bleeding may be continuous or intermittent

PATHOPHYSIOLOGY

Placenta previa involves the abnormal implantation of the placenta in the lower uterine segment. The extent to which the placenta grows over the internal os of the cervix determines the degree of placenta previa. Although the etiology is unknown, two factors appear to favor its occurrence: multiparity and age. When the placenta is inserted over the external os, it is evident that, as the formation of the lower uterine segment and the dilatation of the internal os progresses, its attachments must inevitably be torn through. The rupture is then followed by hemorrhage from the maternal vessels. Furthermore, the bleeding is augmented by the inability of the stretched fibers of the lower uterine segment to compress the torn vessel as occurs when the normally implanted placenta separates during the third stage of labor.

MANAGEMENT

A. Type and crossmatch blood
B. Central venous line
C. Monitor vital signs—CVP, bp, temperature, pulse, respirations
D. Postpone delivery until 36 weeks gestation, if possible
E. Ultrasound B-scan
F. If bleeding persists, delivery should be contemplated either vaginally or by cesarean section. This is decided under double setup in the operating room
G. Amniotomy
H. Oxytocin drip

RATIONALE

Blood should always be available to correct blood loss and stabilize the patient should hemorrhage occur. If the blood loss is minimal and the patient is not in labor, hospitalize the patient with bed rest and sedation. This is particularly important prior to 36 weeks of gestation in order to give the infant the advantage of further development in utero. A central venous line should always be available should massive hemorrhage occur and to monitor fluid resuscitation. Ultrasound may aid in placental localization. This examination clarifies fetal presentation, possibility of multiple gestation, and provides an estimate of gestational age by measurement of the biparietal diameter. Vaginal examination is extremely hazardous as it can provoke massive hemorrhage if the extremely vascular placenta is penetrated either with a speculum or the examining finger. If the fetus is mature or if the initial hemorrhage persists or recurs, a double setup is performed as soon as blood for replacement is available, in order to determine the optimal route for delivery. A double setup is a vaginal exam performed in an operating room, the patient and the medical team being prepared for immediate cesarean section in case this becomes necessary. Cesarean section is indicated in all cases of partial or total placenta previa, whenever bleeding is profuse, fetal distress is present, fetal presentation is abnormal, or progress of labor is abnormal. Vaginal delivery is indicated when the placenta is marginal to the cervical os and does not occupy any area of cervical dilatation, bleeding is minimal, presentation is cephalic, there is no fetal distress, and rapid labor is anticipated. Under these circumstances, amniotomy and IV oxytocin may be administered as long as uterine contractions and fetal heart rate can be monitored carefully. Rupturing the membranes (amniotomy) aids engagement and provides a tamponade effect on the bleeding portion of the placenta.

Complications for the mother can include (a) hemorrhage and hypovolemic shock, (b) operative trauma, including cervical laceration and rupture of the uterus, and (c) postpartum vascular thrombosis and embolization.

PLACENTA ABRUPTIO

ASSESSMENT

A. Dark red vaginal bleeding (approximately 20 percent of patients have internal hemorrhage, thus bleeding is not apparent)
B. Boardlike, tightly contracted uterus
C. Uterine tenderness
D. Absent fetal heart sounds, depending on the severity of separation
E. Shock

PATHOPHYSIOLOGY

Premature separation of the placenta is a complication of pregnancy involving separation of the placenta from its uterine attachment after the 20th week of pregnancy. Although there are many theories regarding the etiology, the primary cause of abruptio placentae is unknown. In abruptio placentae, there is an effusion of blood into the decidua basalis. The decidua then splits, with a thin layer remaining in contact with the maternal surface, while the thicker layer goes on to form a hematoma. This leads to separation, compression, and destruction of function of the portion of the placenta directly adjacent to it. When bleeding is profuse, the placenta may separate to its margin, and the blood may appear externally by escaping between the membranes and uterine wall. Concealed hemorrhage may occur when the infant's head compresses the pelvic floor, thereby inhibiting the flow of blood. Central separation of the placenta, with blood trapped behind the placenta, may also lead to internal bleeding. Generally, with external bleeding, the separation of the placenta is incomplete, whereas with internal bleeding, the separation is more likely to be complete.

MANAGEMENT

A. Plasma until fresh whole blood is available, cryoprecipitate and platelet packs
B. Nasal oxygen at 6 liters/minute
C. Central venous line

D. Monitor vital signs—CVP, temperature, pulse, respirations, bp
E. Electronic fetal monitoring
F. Fluid resuscitation
G. Rupture membranes
H. Cesarean section if labor does not proceed rapidly or if bleeding is profuse

RATIONALE

The primary emphasis is directed toward preventing and controlling shock. Therefore, it is imperative that blood be available immediately. In abruptio placentae, plasminogen is converted to plasmin, and secondary fibrinolysis occurs. The secondary fibrinolysis digests fibrinogen to small molecules that exert a heparinlike anticoagulant action. The bleeding time will be prolonged and shock often develops. Fresh-frozen plasma is administered to treat clotting factor deficiency. Cryoprecipitate contains fibrinogen, factor VIII, and factor XIII, and may be used to correct the deficiencies encountered in hypofibrinogenemia. Fresh whole blood eliminates the need for combining components because it contains red blood cells, clotting factors, and platelets. Oxygen assists in preventing fetal distress. Two separate intravenous lines are preferable, one to monitor central venous pressure and maintain electrolyte balance, and the second for the rapid administration of blood or blood products. Electronic fetal monitoring assists in evaluating placental insufficiency and fetal hypoxia. With moderate placental separation, the fetus may show fetal heart rate changes suggestive of placental insufficiency. With severe placental separation, the fetus dies or is in severe distress. Uterine contractions are often tetanic in nature with no relaxation between contractions. Rupture of the membranes may help to control bleeding and also hastens labor and delivery. If spontaneous delivery is not rapid enough or if bleeding is profuse, cesarean section is indicated.

ECTOPIC PREGNANCY

ASSESSMENT

Ruptured ectopic pregnancy accounts for up to 11 percent of maternal deaths in the United States and presents a major diagnostic challenge for emergency department personnel. The symptomatology is dependent upon the amount and extent of intraperitoneal bleeding, the site of implantation, and the duration of the pregnancy. For purposes of clarity, the assessment focuses on the acute ectopic pregnancy and the chronic ectopic pregnancy.
 I. Acute ectopic pregnancy
    A. Obtain careful menstrual history—amenorrhea 85 to 90 percent of cases
    B. Abdominal pain (sudden onset)
    C. Irregular vaginal bleeding

    D. Adnexal mass on pelvic exam with cervical tenderness on palpation
    E. Additional signs of pregnancy—breast engorgement, morning nausea
    F. Postural hypotension
    G. Pallor and diaphoresis
    H. Positive culdocentesis (evidence of unclotted blood)
II. Chronic ectopic pregnancy
    A. Amenorrhea
    B. Gradual onset of lower abdominal pain
    C. Irregular vaginal bleeding
    D. Alterations of laboratory data
        1. CBC—anemia out of proportion to bleeding history
        2. elevated white blood cell count
    E. Positive pregnancy test using reliable assay techniques to detect low levels of hCG (human chorionic gonadotropin)
        1. radioreceptor assay (RRA)—results available in 1 hour
        2. radioimmune assays β-specific hCG—results available in 1 to 5 hours
    F. Sonography is particularly helpful in the patient with a positive pregnancy test in excluding ectopic pregnancy by identifying a normal intrauterine gestation
    G. Culdocentesis
        1. negative tap—nondiagnostic as it excludes a ruptured versus a nonruptured ectopic pregnancy.
        2. bright red, grossly bloody—peritoneal hemorrhage from a fresh ectopic pregnancy or an abdominal injury to the spleen, liver, or ruptured aneurysm
        3. old blood, brownish colored, nonclotting—ectopic pregnancy with intraperitoneal bleeding over several days or weeks or a delayed splenic rupture

PATHOPHYSIOLOGY

The primary etiologic factor in tubal pregnancies is healed salpingitis secondary to an infection by *Neisseria gonorrhea*. Partial tubal obstruction after tubal infection is one of the most important known causes of ectopic pregnancy. Antibiotics and antimicrobials used to treat salpingitis have been successful in eliminating the infection but have interfered with the tubal epithilium leading to an open but not fully patent lumen. Perhaps the most important factor in the etiology of ectopic pregnancy is that of a previous pelvic infection which results in the formation of adhesions both in and around the tubes. In most instances the etiology of ectopic pregnancy is linked to mechanical interference with the passage of the fertilized ovum. There are several additional risk factors associated with ectopic pregnancy: advancing age, black race, urban resident, low socioeconomic status, and increasing gravidity. It has been speculated that the incidence of ectopic pregnancy in non-white women is higher because sexually transmitted diseases are reported more frequently and hospitalization for pelvic inflammatory disease is more common in non-white than white women. Differences in health care availability for non-white women could also account for their higher mortality rates from ectopic pregnancy.

An increasing cause of ectopic pregnancy is surgical scarring from salpingo-plasty for infertility and previous ectopic pregnancy. PID affects both tubes so that patients with a history of prior ectopic pregnancy are at risk for recurrence.

The extent to which an ectopic gestation will progress within the tube depends in part on the location and the ability of the tubal mucosa to sustain the pregnancy. The impregnated ovum may implant anywhere along the course of the tube but the majority attach in the outer or ampullary portions of the tube near the narrow isthmus section (Fig. 11). The tubal mucosa lacks the elements to nourish and sustain the fetus. This produces a ruptured embryonic sac and its subsequent symptoms as the respective thin walls are eroded. The tubal pregnancy is destroyed and separated from the original site of implantation. Several sequelae may follow:

1. As blood flows around the chorionic sac, the tube becomes overdistended and the sac ruptures into the lumen of the tube.
2. If the separation occurs early enough or the tubal bleeding is not too excessive, the products of conception may be wholly or partially resorbed with only mild to moderate lower abdominal pain for several days with slight vaginal bleeding.
3. A tubal "abortion" may occur where the ovum is extruded through the fimbriated end of the tube either partially or completely.
4. The fallopian tube itself may rupture directly into the abdominal cavity or develop a slow hemorrhagic leak rather than extrude blood into the tubal lumen. This usually occurs if the ectopic implant occurs in the interstitial or isthmic portion of the tube because there is less opportunity for the tube to expand.

When a patient ruptures an interstitial or cornual pregnancy, the hemorrhage is immediate and excessive. There is little to restrict the development of the ovum and rupture may not occur until the fourth month of gestation.

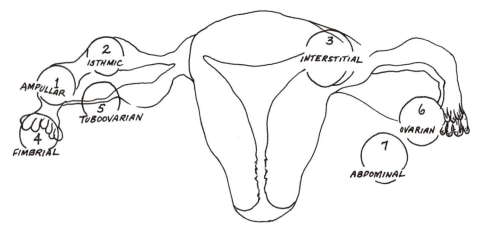

Figure 11. Common sites of ectopic pregnancy.

MANAGEMENT

A. O$_2$ via nasal cannula
B. Blood type and Rh determination
C. Two large bore IV lines with lactated Ringer's solution
D. Monitor vital signs—CVP, temperature, pulse, respirations
E. Insert nasogastric tube
F. Foley catheter to gravity drainage
G. Maintain and/or apply MAST trousers if bp below 80 mm Hg
H. Prepare for operative intervention if culdocentesis is positive

RATIONALE

Although ectopic pregnancy is one of the leading causes of maternal death, it is almost totally preventable. The use of RAI and RAA plus culdocentesis should provide invaluable indications in the early diagnosis of ectopic pregnancy. Oxygen is administered initially to overcome cerebral hypoxia associated with shock states. Rapid volume replacement with blood and crystolloids is necessary to stabilize the patient for anticipated surgery. MAST trousers are a relatively new concept in the treatment of peritonial hemorrhage. The application of a MAST suit may be lifesaving for patients in shock. It increases the central circulating blood volume and total peripheral resistance, particularly in the lower extremities. If the patient arrives in the emergency department with the suit in place it should not be removed until intravenous lines are in place and blood and fluid volumes are restored. A nasogastric tube is inserted with aspiration of stomach contents and as a prophylaxis to postoperative ileus which may occur as a result of blood in the peritoneum. Careful monitoring of vital signs and urinary output ensures the efficacy of volume expanders and fluid replacement. If the culdocentesis is positive or the patient is exhibiting signs of shock, immediate emergency surgery is indicated.

RUPTURED UTERUS

ASSESSMENT

A. Sudden intense abdominal pain and tenderness
B. Cessation of uterine contractions
C. Pale, thready pulse
D. Circumoral pallor
E. Increasing diaphoresis
F. Disturbances of vision
G. Air hunger
H. Copious vaginal hemorrhage
 I. Occasional hematuria
 J. Unconsciousness

PATHOPHYSIOLOGY

Rupture of the uterus is a serious obstetric emergency in which there is a separation of the edges of the uterus with extrusion of all or part of the uterine contents into the peritoneal cavity. Ruptures are classified etiologically as rupture of a previous uterine scar, spontaneous rupture of the intact uterus, and traumatic rupture of intact uterus. Patients who have had a prior cesarean section are potential candidates for a ruptured uterus, particularly those with prior fundal incisions. In this instance, rupture occurs as a result of a weakened wall. Although spontaneous rupture of the uterus is a rare occurrence, several predisposing factors have been identified. It is known that the multiparous aging uterus is more prone to rupture. Cephalopelvic disproportion, in which there may be a long period of obstructed labor, further weakens the uterine wall. Although the uterus is surprisingly resistant to external trauma, occasionally some force causes rupture. Traumatic rupture during delivery is most commonly produced by version breech extraction. Oxytocin in the first and second stage of labor and overly strong fundal pressure have been known to cause rupture. When the uterus ruptures, supporting structures of the bladder are torn, causing hematuria.

MANAGEMENT

A. Type and crossmatch 4 to 6 units of blood
B. Establish a central venous line
C. Monitor vital signs—CVP, bp, temperature, pulse, respirations
D. Ringer's lactate (until blood is available)
E. Nasal oxygen 4 to 6 liters/minute
F. Foley catheter to gravity drainage
G. If rupture is imminent, immediate laparotomy is imperative
H. After the infant is removed, a hysterectomy is performed. On occasion the laceration in the uterus is sutured
I. Systemic antibiotics

RATIONALE

The primary emphasis is directed toward preventing and controlling shock. Therefore, it is imperative that blood be immediately available. Because it is known that certain high-risk groups are more prone to rupture of the uterus, these patients should be carefully monitored during the course of labor. A central venous line facilitates the rapid administration of blood and fluids and the ability to monitor the effectiveness of circulating blood volume. The decision to repair or remove the ruptured uterus is based on the rupture site, nature of tear, extent of bleeding, cause of rupture, presence of a uterine scar, stage of gestation, patient's general condition, and future childbearing concerns. Antibiotics are useful to protect against infection to which the traumatized pelvic tissues are very susceptible.

Genitourinary Emergencies References

ACUTE RENAL FAILURE

Brenner, B. M., & Stein, J. H. (Eds.). *Acute renal failure.* Edinburgh: Churchill Livingstone, 1980.

Bergstein, J. M. Acute renal failure in children. *Critical Care Quarterly,* 1978, **1**, 41–51.

Eknoyan, G. Axioms on acute oliguria. *Hospital Medicine,* 1977, **13**, 32–33.

Fay, F. C. Pulling a patient through acute renal failure. *R.N.,* 1978, **11**, 61.

Flamenbaum, W. Pathophysiology of acute renal failure. *Archives of Internal Medicine,* 1973, **131**, 911.

Freedman P., & Smith, E. Acute renal failure. *Heart Lung,* 1975, **4**, 873.

Kennedy, A. C., Burton, J. A., & Luke, R. G. Factors affecting the prognosis in acute care. *British Medical Journal,* 1973, **42**, 73.

Lancour, J. ADH and aldosterone: How to recognize their effects. *Nursing '78,* 1978, **9**, 36.

Lazarus, J. M. Uremia: A clinical guide. *Hospital Medicine,* 1979, **15** (1), 52–73.

Leste, G. W. Nondialytic treatment of established acute renal failure. *Critical Care Quarterly,* 1978, **1**, 11–24.

McMurray, S. D., Luft, F. C., & Kleit, S. A. Iatrogenic factors in acute renal failure. *Postgraduate Medicine,* 1978, **73**, 523.

Mitchell, J. C. Axioms on uremia. *Hospital Medicine,* 1978, **14** (7), 6–23.

Roberts, S. L. Renal assessment: A nursing point of view. *Heart Lung,* 1979, **8** (1), 105–113.

Robinson, R. L. Laboratory findings in the differential diagnosis of renal failure. *Critical Care Quarterly,* 1979, **1**, 87–89.

Thomson, G. E. Acute renal failure. *Medical Clinics of North America,* 1973, **57**, 6.

Schrier, R. W. Acute renal failure: Pathogenesis, diagnosis and management. *Hospital Practice,* 1981, **16** (3), 93–112.

Stark, J. L. BUN/creatinine: Your keys to kidney function. *Nursing '80,* 1980, **10** (5), 33–38.

Szwed, J. J. Pathophysiology of acute renal failure: Rationale for signs and symptoms. *Critical Care Quarterly,* 1978, **1**, 1–9.

PROBLEMS OF PREGNANCY

Baker, D. A., Catalano, P., Makowski, P., & Gibson, M. Value of computed tomography (CT) in an obstetrical emergency. *Diagnostic Gynecology and Obstetrics,* 1982, **4** (1), 53–55.

Berek, J. S., & Stubblefield, P. G. Anatomic and clinical correlates of uterine perforation. *American Journal of Obstetrics and Gynecology,* 1979, **135** (2), 181–184.

Cederquist, L. L., & Birnbaum, S. J. Rupture of the uterus after midtrimester prostaglandin abortion. *Journal of Reproductive Medicine,* 1980, **25** (3), 136–138.

Cunanan, R. G., Courey, N. G., & Lippes, J. Laparoscopic findings in patients with pelvic pain. *American Journal of Obstetrics and Gynecology,* 1983, **146**, 589.

Farrell, R. G., et al. Incomplete and inevitable abortion: Treatment by suction curretage in the emergency department. *Annals of Emergency Medicine,* 1982, **11**, 655.

Gallagher, J. C. Ovarian pregnancy: A series of 24 cases. *Obstetrics and Gynecology,* 1983, **61** (2), 174–180.

Hibbard, B. M. Preeclampsia–eclampsia. *Practitioner,* 1978, **221** (1326), 847.

Hollatt, J. G. Repeat ectopic pregnancy—A study of 123 consecutive cases. *American Journal of Obstetrics and Gynecology,* 1975, 520–24.

Novak, E. R. *Textbook of gynecology* (10th Ed.). Baltimore: Williams & Wilkins, 1981.

Parsons, L., & Sommers, S. C. *Gynecology.* Philadelphia: W. B. Saunders, 1978.

Patrick, J. D. Ectopic pregnancy—A brief review. *Annals of Emergency Medicine,* 1982, **11,** 576–581.

Pedersen, J. F. Ultrasound in suspected ectopic pregnancy. *British Journal of Radiology,* 1980, **53,** 1.

Pritchard, J. A. The use of magnesium sulfate in preeclampsia–eclampsia. *Journal of Reproductive Medicine,* 1979, **23** (3), 107.

Pritchard, J. A., & McDonald, P. C. *Williams obstetrics* (16th Ed.). New York: Appleton-Century-Crofts, 1980.

Purdie, F. R., Nieto, J. M., Summerson, D. J., & Lauermore, W. E. Rupture of the uterus with DIC. *Annals of Emergency Medicine,* 1983, **12,** 174.

Roberts, J. M. Preeclampsia and eclampsia. San Francisco Medical Staff Conference Univ. of California. *Western Journal of Medicine,* 1981, **135,** 34–43.

Roberts, M. R., Jackimczyk, K., Mark, J., & Rosen, P. Diagnosis of ruptured ectopic pregnancy with peritoneal lavage. *Annals of Emergency Medicine,* 1982, **11** (10), 556–558.

Rosen, P., et al. *Emergency medicine* (Vol. II). St. Louis: C. V. Mosby, 1983.

Royko, M. A. An obstetric emergency: Abruptio placentae vs. ruptured uterus. *Journal of Emergency Nursing,* **8** (1), 4–5.

Schwartz, R. D., & Di Pietro, D. L B-hCG as a diagnostic aid for suspected ectopic pregnancy. *Obstetrics and Gynecology,* 1980, **56** (2), 197–202.

Webster, H. D., Barclay, D. L., & Fischer, C. K. Ectopic pregnancy. *American Journal of Obstetrics and Gynecology,* 1965, 23–24.

F. INTEGUMENTARY SYSTEM EMERGENCIES

1. Burns

First Degree
First degree burns, also known as superficial burns, are tissue injuries limited to the outer layer of the epidermis, such as a sunburn.

Second Degree
Second degree burns, also known as partial-thickness burns, are tissue injuries extending to the dermis. These injuries are complicated by vesicles, blebs, or bullae (Fig. 12). Examples include scalds or results from exposure to flash.

Third Degree
Third degree burns, also known as full-thickness burns, are tissue injuries involving the epidermis and dermis, extending to the subcutaneous fat and possibly muscle tissue with destruction of nerve endings. The surface area may appear coagulated, charred, or white (Fig. 13).

ASSESSMENT

    I. Initial data
        A. Patient's age and weight
        B. Where and how burn occurred
        C. Nature of burning agent
        D. Presenting conditions
            1. cardiac
            2. respiratory
            3. renal

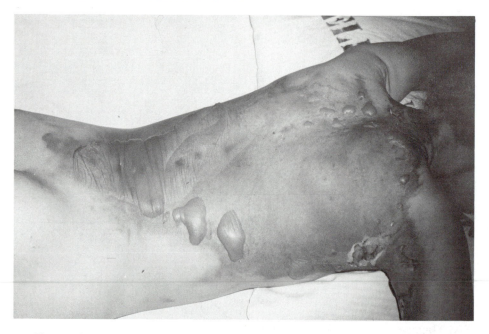

Figure 12. Primarily second degree burn. Note the blister formation. (*Courtesy of New York University Hospital and Bellevue Hospital Center, New York.*)

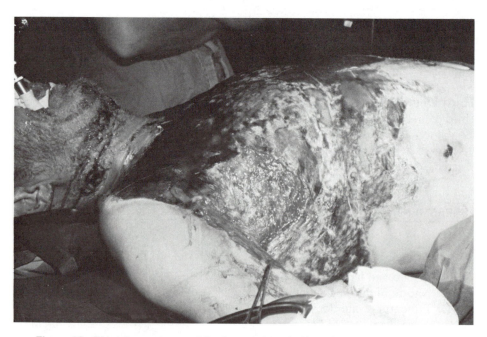

Figure 13. Third degree burns of the face and trunk. Note the pearly white, charred appearance of skin with eschar. Complication: respiratory burns. (*Courtesy of New York University Hospital and Bellevue Hospital Center, New York.*)

4. metabolic
5. vascular
6. hypertension
7. chronic alcoholism
II. Remove all clothing to determine
  A. Degree of burn
  B. Extent of burn
  C. Particular parts of body burned
  D. Damage or injury to deeper structures
III. Evaluate
  A. Respiratory tract for
    1. singed nasal hair; blackened rim of nares
    2. carbon deposits on tongue or oropharynx
    3. rapid noisy respirations
    4. blood-tinged sputum
  B. Electrolyte and/or acid–base imbalances
    1. hyponatremia—muscle weakness/cramps, apathy, tremors, anorexia, increased pulse, decreased pulse pressure, orthostatic hypotension
    2. hypokalemia—nausea and vomiting, anorexia, abdominal distention, paralytic ileus, muscle weakness, absent or weak deep tendon reflexes
    3. metabolic acidosis—headache, malaise, nausea and vomiting, abdominal pain, decreased P_{CO_2}, decreased pH of blood
  C. Urinary output
    1. character (e.g., myoglobinuria)
    2. amount
  D. Edema (in and around burn site)
  E. Hypovolemic shock (see Section on Shock)
  F. Pain (presence or absence of)
  G. Hydration status
  H. Monitor peripheral circulation for
    1. cyanosis
    2. impaired capillary refilling
    3. neurologic signs
      a. deep tendon pain
      b. paresthesias
    4. changes in pulsatile flow
      a. distal vessels of palmar arch
      b. posterior tibial vessels
  I. Other associated injuries
IV. Obtain blood for
  A. Hemoglobin
  B. Hematocrit
  C. Prothrombin time
  D. Serum protein
  E. Electrolytes
  F. Arterial gases including pH and serum bicarbonate

    G. Sputum for culture and sensitivity

    H. Blood cultures

  V. Chest films postintubation

PATHOPHYSIOLOGY

In treating burns in the emergency department, it is important to remember and understand that burns are long-term injuries, and that emergency management is just beginning therapy. For the purpose of this chapter, emphasis is placed on the first critical hours.

An observational priority is an evaluation of the respiratory tract because injury to the tract is one of the major causes of death in patients with burns. Extensive flame burns on the body, and any type of burns on the face and neck including those parameters listed, should be considered suspicious of inhalation injury and respiratory damage. Any airway obstruction noted is usually due to inflammation or edema of the vocal cords, epiglottis, and upper trachea.

The type and classification of burn must be evaluated to establish a tentative diagnosis, and to help influence a prognosis. Following the removal of all clothing, an estimate is made of the extent of burn, depth of burn, and areas burned. The extent of burn is usually determined by the rule of nines. This information is generally transferred to a burn summary chart (Fig. 14) which indicates the various areas burned, the estimate of the depth of burn, and other information related to the patient. As with any kind of trauma, the effect of preexisting conditions and/or associated injuries can definitely alter the patient's progress and therapy, and for this reason it is very important to establish an adequate history in the early moments of admission to an emergency area.

Following a burn, the body floods the injured areas with fluid containing valuable proteins and electrolytes. With this pooling of fluids in the tissues comes a rapid decrease in the blood volume. As heat injures the cells, injured cells lose potassium as well as magnesium and phosphates, and take on sodium. The end result of this process is edema caused by increased capillary permeability, plasma oncotic pressure, and vasodilitation. Although the tissues are filled with fluid, the fluid is not available for general use by the body, and the patient may exhibit signs of dehydration, such as thirst. The unsupervised patient may at this time develop hyponatremia from free water ingestion in trying to overcome this dehydration.

Metabolic acidosis may result from many sources, but it is known that following tissue destruction, lactic acid and other acids that accumulate during intervals of impaired circulation and tissue anoxia, pass into the blood. They cause a metabolic acidotic state characterized by a reduction in plasma bicarbonate.

The burned patient may exhibit both hypovolemic and neurogenic shock (see Section on Shock). Regardless of the kind of shock, the common denominator is a decrease in effective blood volume. The shock state is characterized by a drop in blood pressure, poor perfusion of tissues caused by microcirculatory stasis, and decreased blood volume as a result of a shift of fluid from the extracellular to the in-

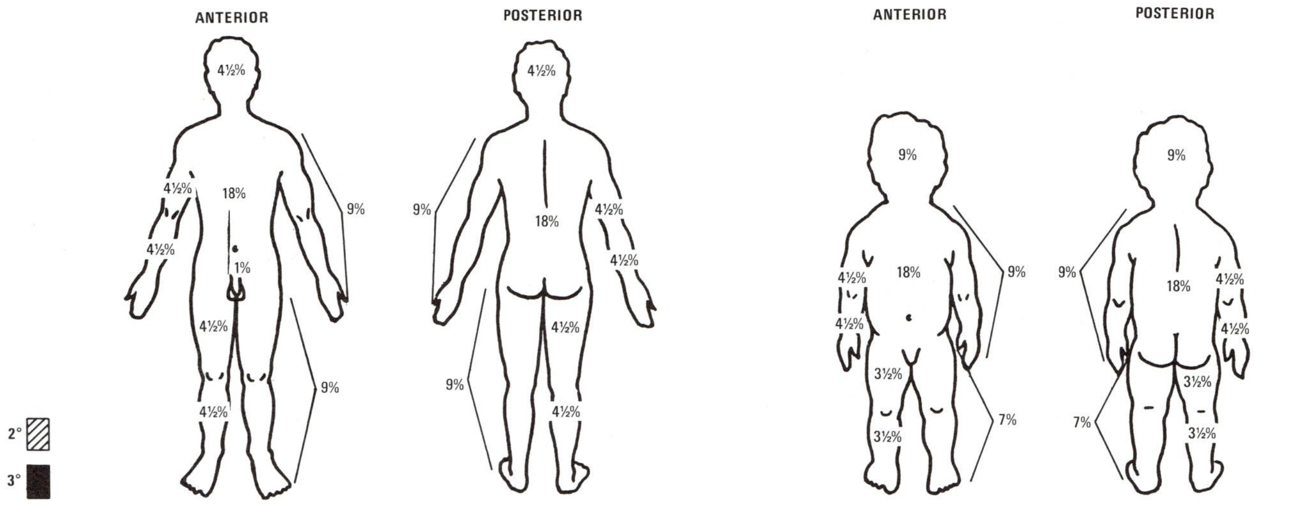

NAME: ______________ AGE: ______________ WEIGHT: ______________

AREA(S) BURNED		HEAD	FACE	ANTERIOR TRUNK	POSTERIOR TRUNK	ARMS (R)	ARMS (L)	LEGS (R)	LEGS (L)	HANDS (R)	HANDS (L)	FEET (R)	FEET (L)	GENITALS
(√)	2°													
	3°													

PERCENT 2° BURN: ______________ PERCENT 3° BURN: ______________ TOTAL PERCENT B.S.A. BURNED: ______________

NATURE OF BURNING AGENT: FLAME ______ CHEMICAL ______ ELECTRICAL ______ SCALD ______ OTHER ______

PREEXISTING CONDITIONS: CARDIAC ______ RESPIRATORY ______ RENAL ______ METABOLIC ______ VASCULAR ______

HYPERTENSION ______ CHRONIC ALCOHOLISM ______ OTHER ______

ALLERGIES: ______________ IMMUNIZATION STATUS: ______________

PREEXISTING DRUG THERAPY: ______________

Figure 14. Burn summary chart.

tracellular compartments. An immediate threat to the electrically burned patient, in addition to acidosis and hypovolemia, is the precipitation of myoglobin in the renal tubules. This occurs as a result of destruction to muscles, nerves, and blood vessels with a concomitant release of myoglobin, a precursor of acute renal failure.

The amount of pain experienced by the patient varies with the depth and extent of the injury. Third degree, or full-thickness, burns are painless because the nerve endings are destroyed. Pain, however, is felt around the area of third degree burns where there are first and second degree burns.

Second degree burns involving 15 percent of the body surface, third degree burns involving 10 percent of the body surface, burns that involve the respiratory tract or critical anatomical areas, electrical and chemical burns, burns accompanied by other injuries, in individuals over the age of 60, in children less than 1½ years of age, and in those individuals with cardiac, pulmonary, metabolic, or renal diseases are all considered serious and must be hospitalized.

MANAGEMENT

I. Provide adequate airway and oxygen therapy to promote optimal ventilation and relief of hypoxia
   A. Mask or nasal prongs
   B. Oro- or nasopharyngeal tube (edema of pharynx)
   C. Mechanical ventilation
   D. Tracheostomy (noncorrectable airway obstruction)
II. Institute measures to support management modalities by establishing
   A. Intravenous lines
      1. central line
      2. peripheral line
   B. Foley catheter
   C. Chest film (postintubation)
   D. Laboratory tests
      1. CBC and differential
      2. type and crossmatch
      3. serum electrolytes
      4. lactate levels
      5. blood and sputum cultures
      6. BUN and creatinine
      7. prothrombin time
   E. Nasogastric tube, if necessary
III. Monitor continuously for trends and response to management modalities
   A. Temperature, pulse, respiration, bp
   B. Central venous pressure
   C. Level of consciousness
   D. Skin quality and appearance
   E. Arterial pH and arterial gases

F. Bicarbonate levels

G. Hemoglobin, hematocrit, and prothrombin levels

H. Serum electrolytes

I. Hourly urine output, character, quantity, and specific gravity

J. Subjective responses

K. Pain levels

IV. Promote and institute measures aimed at restoring fluid balance

  A. Type of fluid

    1. Ringer's lactate (preferred initial therapy)

    2. normal saline

    3. glucose in water

    4. colloids

  B. Formulae (Table 14)

    1. burn budget of F.D. Moore

    2. Evans

    3. Brooke

    4. Parkland (presently preferred)

    5. hypertonic sodium solution

    6. modified Brooke

TABLE 14. FORMULAE USED FOR ESTIMATING ADULT BURN PATIENT RESUSCITATION FLUID NEEDS (FIRST 24 HOURS)

Formula	Electrolyte	Colloid	Glucose in Water
Burn budget of	Lactated Ringer's	7.5 percent of body weight	1500–5000 ml
F. D. Moore	1000–4000 ml 0.5 normal saline 1200 ml		
Evans	Normal saline	1.0 ml/kg/percent burn	2000 ml
	1.0 ml/kg/percent burn		
Brooke	Lactated Ringer's	0.5 ml/kg/percent burn	2000 ml
	1.5 ml/kg/percent burn		
Parkland	Lactated Ringer's 4 ml/kg/percent burn		
Hypertonic sodium solution	Volume to maintain urine output at 30 ml/hour (fluid contains 250 mEq Na/L)		
Modified Brooke	Lactated Ringer's 2 ml/kg/percent burn		

(*From Pruitt, B. A. Jr. Fluid resuscitation for extensively burned patients. Journal of Trauma, 1981,* **21,** 691.)

    C. Rate
       1. half total estimated volume during first 8 hours
       2. quarter over next 8 hours
       3. quarter over last 8 hours
    D. Fluid needs
       1. children: 3 ml/kg for each percent burned area during first 24 hours
       2. adults: 4 ml/kg for each percent burned area during first 24 hours

V. Restore, maintain, and support urinary output
    A. Hourly readings
       1. children 30 lb or less: 1 ml/kg/hour
       2. adults: 50 ml/hour (minimum)
    B. Treat myoglobinuria, if present
       1. increase fluids
       2. insure output of 75 to 100 ml/hour
       3. mannitol
         a. 25 g bolus stat
         b. 12.5 g to each subsequent liter
         c. reduce dose for children

VI. Promote and initiate measures aimed at restoring acid–base and/or electrolyte imbalances
    A. Possible imbalances
       1. respiratory alkalosis
       2. metabolic acidosis
       3. metabolic alkalosis
       4. electrolyte imbalances (sodium, chloride, potassium, etc.)
    B. Frequent determinations and collections of
       1. blood gases (pH, Po_2, Pco_2)
       2. serum bicarbonate
       3. serum albumin
       4. serum electrolytes

VII. Promote measures designed to combat infection or counteract reduced resistance to infection
    A. Prophylactic antibiotic and/or antiinfective therapy
       1. sodium penicillin G, IV (check allergies)
         a. 600,000 U q 12 hours (adults)
         b. 300,000 U q 12 hours (children)
       2. silver sulfadiazine cream (check allergy)
       3. sulfamyalon acetate cream (check allergy)
    B. Wound care
       1. debridement
       2. dressing changes prn
       3. frequent inspection for infection
       4. evaluate for need to dress or leave exposed
    C. Tetanus prophylaxis
       1. 0.5 ml tetanus toxoid, subcutaneously (if unclear history)

2. 250 U, IM human immune globulin plus 0.5 ml tetanus toxoid subcutaneously at different site (no immunization)

D. Use of sterile sheets

E. Maintain reverse isolation

F. Monitor for initial signs of clinical sepsis
   1. altered sensorium
   2. increased respiratory rate
   3. decreased platelet count
   4. glycosuria

VIII. Institute surgical modalities for continual support of peripheral and deep tissue perfusion and circulation

   A. Escharotomy

   B. Fasciotomy

IX. Initiate measures to control pain and promote comfort

   A. Low doses of narcotics or analgesics
      1. morphine, Demerol, Talwin (narcotics)
      2. Tylenol, acetominophin (analgesics)

   B. Keep patient warm to prevent shivering

   C. Environmental temperature regulation

   D. Methods to reduce anxiety

   E. Proper positioning, proper body alignment, contracture prevention, and range of motion

   F. Measures to reduce hypoxia

RATIONALE

Assurance of an adequate airway is of vital importance and treatment of oxygen deprivation might include any of those modalities listed. Tracheostomy may be considered for noncorrectable upper airway obstruction, but it must be remembered that this procedure carries a high morbidity and mortality rate in burned patients, especially in children. A chest film should be obtained as soon as an airway is established to rule out the possibilities of parenchymal lung injuries, chemical pneumonitis, pulmonary edema, and/or decreasing lung compliance.

A wide variety of measures are instituted to support management. A central venous line is established for continuous fluid replacement and for the monitoring of the central venous pressure—an indicator of fluctuation in hydration and cardiac function. A Foley catheter is inserted and attached to a urimeter so that the character, output, and specific gravity of urine can be monitored on an hourly basis. This management modality is an excellent and reliable measure for adequacy of hydration and, indirectly, of vital organ perfusion. The laboratory blood tests suggested should be drawn several times during the first 24 hours to estimate electrolyte imbalances, kidney function, depletion of the circulating plasma, and for determinations of acid–base balance in relation to impending acidotic or alkalotic states. These results, along with the vital signs and other parameters listed, must be monitored continuously in terms of trends and responses to management modalities and corrective measures employed. If nausea, vomiting, or abdominal distension is present, or if more than 25 percent of the total body surface is burned, a nasogastric tube should be inserted.

Fluid replacement during the first 24 hours is paramount, administered in amounts sufficient to minimize blood and plasma volume changes, and to reduce injurious effects on vital organ function. A variety of formulae are available for estimating adult burn patient resuscitation fluid needs during the first 24 hours. Of these, the Parkland formula appears to be the one most generally agreed upon, although clinical successes have been achieved with any one of these formulae. It must be noted that those individuals for whom resuscitation has been delayed, those with respiratory burn injury, and those who have incurred high voltage injury may require additional amounts of fluids. Conversely, there are those who demonstrate an intolerance to the volume calibrated. In these individuals, the volume must be minimized, with the possible substitution of colloid solutions. The most important statement to be made regarding fluid resuscitation and the use of various formulae, is that they are only to be used as a guide for initial administration, and that the patient's physiologic state be a practical consideration. In addition, if more than 50 percent of the body is burned, the number 50 becomes the constant used in the formulae chosen. Hourly urinary output measurements can serve as a primary guide in evaluating circulating volume. Other indices of optimal resuscitative efforts are clear mentation, absence of shock signs, normal cardiac output within the first 10 hours, and correction of electrolyte and/or acid–base imbalances. In the case of electrical burns when myoglobinuria is present, intravenous fluids have to be increased to produce 75 to 100 ml per hour. If the red pigment does not clear, a bolus of mannitol can be administered immediately, and additional mannitol added to each successive liter of fluid. The reason for use of the osmotic diuretic is to block tubular reabsorption in the kidney.

Interruption in skin integrity is interruption in the first line of defense against invading organisms, therefore, the burned area becomes the most frequent source of infection. Damaged tissue from burns results in intravascular clotting so that the area becomes avascular, thereby preventing the defense mechanisms from functioning. Bacterial growth begins immediately deep in the hair follicles, and does not reach clinical significance for 4 to 5 days. On this basis, antibiotic therapy should begin immediately. Cultures, sensitivity, and colony count must be performed frequently so that appropriate antibiotic therapy may be instituted, and a history of specific drug allergies must be elicited from the patient or from significant others. Devitalized tissue, an ideal growth medium for the anaerobic tetanus organism, necessitates tetanus immunization.

It is obvious that severe burns have important systemic consequences and the treatment of such is urgent, but, the primarily injured organ is the skin. For this reason, treatment of the wound is of ultimate concern. The wound care should be performed under as sterile a setup as possible. Gentle cleansing and removal of devitalized tissue is followed by the application of a topical antibacterial agent. Dressings are to be changed as necessary with frequent inspection of the wound site for infections. If dressings are used, hands, face, and small areas should remain un-bandaged. Reverse isolation must be maintained, and the patient closely monitored for impending signs of clinical sepsis. Circumferentially burned limbs or encircling trunkal burns may require escharotomy to relieve compromised distal circulation or chest wall motion. For those individuals suffering high voltage injury or skeletal trauma, a fasciatomy may be necessary to restore effective circulation to the affected area(s).

Pain varies with the extent and depth of the burned area, and also with the patient's state of consciousness. The kind and dose of analgesic or narcotic depends on the individual. Sedatives may be used to allay anxiety and restlessness. Caution must be exercised before administration of any of these preparations to determine whether or not the anxiety or restlessness is due to hypoxia or hypovolemia rather than due to the pain. If so, additional oxygen and/or fluids may be used in the management. Another consideration of primary importance is to provide as much comfort as is possible to the patient. This may be accomplished by interventions such as keeping the patient warm to prevent shivering, environmental temperature regulation, proper positioning, and body alignment. The latter is valuable in preventing contractures. As much as possible, an appropriate range of motion program should be established. Another important area of responsibility for the nurse is to find methods to reduce anxiety and to help develop coping mechanisms within the patient, which will help the patient deal with the psychologic impact of the injury and the possible alteration to the body image.

2. Hypothermia (Accidental)

ASSESSMENT

There are three stages of hypothermia, and biologic changes will occur in accordance with temperature coefficients:

- Stage I—32 to 35 °C (89.8 to 95 °F) (minor)
- Stage II—30 to 32 °C (86.6 to 89.8 °F) (moderate)
- Stage III—temperatures less than 30 °C (86.6 °F) (severe)

I. Abnormal physiologic effects of hypothermia on body systems
   A. Central nervous system—clumsiness, slowed response to noxious stimuli, ataxia, dysarthria, delirium, stupor, coma
   B. Heart—cardiogram may demonstrate atrial fibrillation, atrial flutter, conduction defects, premature contractions and junctional rhythms. Of note is the Osbourn or J point distortion of the QRS complex (Fig. 15). Asystole occurs at core temperatures of less than 15 °C (59 °F)
   C. Lungs—initial hyperventilation followed by hypoventilation as hypothermic state progresses

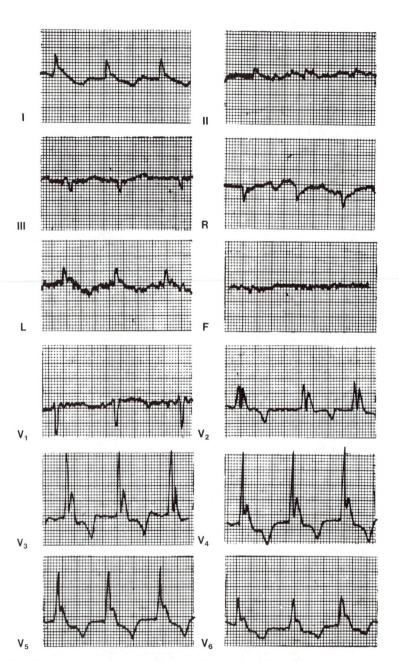

Figure 15. Typical ECG seen in hypothermia. This patient was a 69-year-old man with a core temperature of 24 °C (75.2 °F). Note the typical J wave abnormalities (Osbourn waves) in the terminal phase of the QRS complex. This patient's ECG returned to premorbid state upon rewarming. (*From Goldfrank, L. R. Toxicologic Emergencies: A Comprehensive Handbook in Problem Solving (2d ed.). New York: Appleton-Century-Crofts, 1982, p. 191.*)

    D. Kidneys—oliguric

    E. Hematologic—increased blood viscosity secondary to cryofibrinogen and/or cryoglobulin activation, thromboemboli, decreased blood volume, leukopenia, thrombocytopenia, left shift of oxygen hemoglobin dissociation curve, increased oxygen affinity of red blood cells

    F. Metabolic—metabolic acidosis, hyperglycemia, elevated serum enzymes and free fatty acids, decreased basal metabolic rate

    G. GI tract—decreased motility leading to possible ileus. Depressed hepatic metabolism, increased serum amylase

PATHOPHYSIOLOGY

For a person to remain in thermal equilibrium, the body must gain as much heat as it loses. Therefore, it is important to understand the mechanisms for heat loss.

1. Radiation—when body heat is greater than the environment, this heat is transferred to solid objects and surrounding air. The amount of heat lost by radiation depends on the area of skin exposed and is proportional to the thermal gradient

2. Conduction—is the direct transfer of heat to cooler objects by direct contact. As with radiation, heat loss is proportional to the thermal gradient

3. Convection—heat transfer is dependent upon the wind velocity and ambient temperature. Moving air carries away heat faster than radiation into still air

4. Evaporation—at least 20 percent of total body heat lost is the result of evaporation, about two thirds from the skin surface and about one third from the respiratory tract

Environmental factors such as ambient temperature, relative humidity, and the movement of air (wind–chill factor) affect heat loss. The amount of body surface exposed and the insulating quality of the patient's clothing also affect heat loss. Severe hypothermia depresses the central nervous system, the medullary respiratory center, and the cardiovascular system. The profoundly hypothermic patient is comatose and hyperreflexive. When there is a need for conservation of heat, adrenergic autonomic stimuli cause a sharp reduction in the blood flow to the surface. This causes vasoconstriction and transforms the skin and subcutaneous tissue into layers of insulation. The control of body temperature is a function of cerebral centers located in the hypothalamus. In normal individuals the compensatory mechanism of shivering results in greater heat production. Many of the cases of hypothermia reported in the literature note an absence of shivering ascribed to deficient heat producing capability rather than to heat loss. There is an inherent inability to produce adequate heat as the core temperature drops below a certain point, further aggravated by poor metabolic output. Many alcoholics present with hypothermia because alcohol ingestion causes peripheral vasodilitation that may increase heat loss and also may retard shivering. As cooling occurs, bradycardia develops due to vagal response as well as to some hypothermic effect on the sinoatrial node. There is a shift of potassium across the cell membrane, causing a lowering of the T wave on the electrocardio-gram, and ventricular irritability is evident. Delayed ventricular emptying may be reflected on the electrocardiogram by the presence of the J wave described by Os-bourn. The body's physiologic response to stress leads to a breakdown of tissue and the production of aldosterone and antidiuretic hormone. Both of these mechanisms lead to excretion of potassium and nitrogen and the retention of sodium and water. The presence of edema signifies that hyponatremia is due to the presence of water in excess of sodium. Blood pressure falls because of deleterious effects of anoxia on the capillaries, with a consequent increase in their permeability and loss of blood pro-teins. Urinary output is decreased due to lowered blood pressure, with subsequent decreased glomerular filtration. Antidiuretic hormone secretion leads to water re-tention and subsequent lowered urinary output as evidenced by oliguria. Most of the symptomatology in mild to moderate hypothermia disappears with restoration of normal body temperature. However, at temperatures below 30 °C (86 °F), the myo-cardium becomes irritable and ventricular fibrillation ensues. If this arrhythmia is not corrected, death occurs (usually associated with a core temperature below 30 °C.)

MANAGEMENT

I. Mild to moderate hypothermia
   A. Ensure adequate airway
   B. Remove wet clothing
   C. Arterial IV line (5 percent D/S or Ringer's lactate)
   D. Cardiac monitoring
   E. Monitor vital signs—CVP, bp, temperature, pulse, respiration
   F. Monitor temperature via electronic thermometer with rectal probe
   G. CBC, BUN, electrolytes, toxicology screen, arterial blood gas, urinalysis
   H. Chest x-ray
   I. Foley catheter to gravity drainage
   J. 100 ml 50 percent dextrose in water
   K. 5 ml (2 mg) naloxone hydrochloride (Narcan), IV
   L. 100 mg thiamine IM
   M. Passive rewarming blankets
II. Severe hypothermia with ventricular fibrillation
   A. Monitor ABC (airway, breathing, circulation)
   B. Mechanical cardiopulmonary resuscitation, if indicated, utilizing oxygen powered thumper
   C. Intubation, if apneic
   D. Vasopressors, if warranted
   E. Core rewarming
      1. peritoneal dialysis with warm dialysate
      2. hemodialysis with blood warmed to 110 °F
      3. cardiopulmonary bypass to warm blood

RATIONALE

Initial efforts should be directed toward basic life support techniques. After blood specimens are obtained, an IV line is inserted with the administration of saline or Ringer's lactate to expand intravascular volume. Fifty percent glucose is given to the comatose hypothermic patient to combat hypoglycemia secondary to alcoholism, exogenous insulin, possible overdose of oral hypoglycemic agents and cachexia. The elderly with underlying medical disorders, individuals with psychiatric backgrounds, and alcoholics are at risk of becoming hypothermic, not always associated with low external temperatures. Shock associated with myocardial infarction of sepsis may cause hypothermia. Leukopenia is frequently associated with hypothermia making it difficult to rule out infections. Organic central nervous system lesions or cord transections may affect the hypothalamus and thermal regulators. Toxic inhalations or ingestions may also interfere with thermoregulation; included are carbon monoxide, alcohol, narcotics, chloral hydrate, barbiturates, phenothiazines, general anesthetics, tetracycline, and tricyclic antidepressants. In patients with mild to moderate hypothermia, passive rewarming is usually enough to restore normal body temperature. In our emergency department, the method of choice is a slow passive rewarming at room temperature using warm blankets. The goal is to achieve rewarming at a rate of 0.5 to 0.8 °C per hour.

The patient with severe hypothermia who is in ventricular fibrillation must have core rewarming, because defibrillation cannot be accomplished until normal body temperature is restored. Because it may take several hours to restore normal temperatures, a mechanical oxygen powered thumper is recommended for continuous cardiopulmonary resuscitation. Resuscitation efforts should not be discontinued until normal temperature is reached. The use of peritoneal dialysis or warm lavage or gavage techniques should be employed initially as they are easily accessible to the emergency department. Hemodialysis, if readily available, should also be considered. A recent approach in the management of hypothermia is a portable cardiopulmonary bypass with a heat exchanger, which has been used to warm the blood outside the body. During the rewarming process ventricular fibrillation is common, because of the local temperature gradients that exist as a result of the varying temperatures in adjacent muscle fibers. Atrial dysrrhythmias are also commonly seen. Therefore, careful monitoring, both during the hypothermic episode and the rewarming process is vital.

3. Heat Stroke

ASSESSMENT

A. Tachycardia
B. Tachypnea

C. Headache, lethargy—progressing to coma
D. Hot dry skin (anhydrotic, particularly in elderly)
E. Hyperpyrexia (T 104 °F) (40 °C)
F. Metabolic acidosis
G. Cardiac arrhythmias
H. Initial hypertension followed by hypotension
 I. Leukocytosis
 J. Coagulation abnormalities (prolonged PT and PTT)
K. Decreased platelets and fibrinogen
L. Elevated muscle enzymes (CPK, LDH, SGOT)
M. Myoglobinuria
N. Hematuria
O. Elevated BUN and creatinine

PATHOPHYSIOLOGY

Thermoregulation is a function of the hypothalamus, which is located at the base of the cerebrum. This area responds to increases in temperature of the brain's blood supply as well as to thermoreceptors located in the skin. Heat is a by-product of cellular metabolism and as the body temperature rises, the rate of metabolism increases producing more heat. Under normal conditions heat is dissipated by several mechanisms: radiation, convection and conduction, and by evaporation through the skin and lungs. When environmental temperatures exceed body temperatures, heat loss by radiation, convection, and conduction ceases and heat absorption occurs. As the ambient temperature rises, the major means of heat loss is by the evaporation of sweat. If the environmental humidity is high and the air is already saturated with vapor, evaporation decreases. Sweating is the most effective natural means of combating heat stress with little or no change in the normal body temperature. As long as sweating continues, humans can withstand remarkably high temperatures. The cardiovascular system is responsible for the dissipation of heat. The circulating blood is shifted from the host inner core to the cooler skin vessels with subsequent dilatation of the cutaneous tissues. To maintain this vascular dilatation, cardiac output increases. In addition, there is a compensatory splanchnic vasoconstriction leading to decreased renal blood flow. Hematuria, hemoglobinuria, and myoglobinuria are seen as a result of increased tubular permeability. Abnormal coagulation studies result when the liver is damaged to the point where it ceases to manufacture several clotting factors. Hyperpyrexia and endothelial damage also deplete clotting factors. All of these findings are transient and disappear with rest. The basic problem in heat stroke is one of heat imbalance: heat production occurs in the body without heat dissipation. There is a breakdown of the thermoregulating capability in the hypothalamus leading to cessation of sweating. There are several groups of individuals who are at risk for heat stroke: the inactive aged with underlying cardiovascular disease, overexercised young adults unable to dissipate heat, neonates and young infants, and patients taking certain medications (Table 15).
    As thermal stress continues and the body's defense mechanisms break down, the

body temperature rises precipitously. The accompanying hyperpyrexia causes damage to cells and organs throughout the body. Kidney damage is common due to acute tubular necrosis. Skeletal muscles show widespread degeneration of fibers, and rhabdomyolysis is evidenced by an elevated CPK level and myoglobinuria. Coagulopathy can progress to full blown DIC. Cardiac output doubles and oxygen consumption increases. If blood flow is unable to meet tissue needs, tissue hypoxia develops with resultant metabolic acidosis. The patient becomes progressively comatose as a result of thermal damage to neurons, cerebral hypoxia, and electrolyte imbalance. Anhydrosis usually occurs in the aged and is generally insidious occurring during several days of elevated temperature humidity index. The acute onset of hyperpyrexia in the young may or may not present with anhydrosis. The progress of hyperpyrexia occurs over several hours and is usually due to overexertion and the inability to dissipate heat. If heat stroke is not treated immediately, cardiovascular collapse and death soon occurs.

MANAGEMENT

I. Initial management modalities
 A. Intubation, if apneic
 B. 100 percent O_2
 C. IV arterial line
 D. Serial blood gases
 E. CBC, BUN, glucose, electrolytes, PT, PTT
 F. Urinalysis
 G. Rectal probe to monitor temperature
 H. Place patient in ice bath until temperature is lowered to 38.8°C (102°F)
II. Secondary management modalities
 A. Monitor fluid volume
 B. Monitor vital signs, including temperature, pulse, and CVP
 C. Mannitol, 12.5 g bolus
 D. Furosemide (Lasix), 12.5 g bolus
 E. Intravenous with 12.5 g mannitol in each liter of IV fluid
 F. Monitor urinary output via Foley catheter
 G. Cardiac monitor

RATIONALE

Heat stroke is a medical emergency which if left untreated may lead to death. Cellular death may occur with prolonged elevated temperatures, therefore initial measures should be directed toward rapid cooling. Patients should be undressed and wrapped in cold sheets and ice applied to areas of large superficial vessels such as neck, axilla, and inguinal region while initial assessment takes place. Establish and maintain a patent airway and administer 100 percent oxygen. Because most patients present in coma with the risk of seizures and vomiting, intubation with ventilatory

TABLE 15. DT-LIKE STATES RESPONSIBLE FOR HYPERTHERMIA AND DEATH

Case	Clinical Characteristics	Mechanisms of Action	Suggested Management of Hyperthermia or Agitation
Delirium tremens Ethanol withdrawal	Sympathomimetic effects: tremor, sensorial disturbances, hallucinations, hyperthermia, cardiovascular collapse	Stimulation of the anterior hypothalamus, excessive muscular rigidity, peripheral vasoconstriction	Cooling Glucose Fluid replacement Benzodiazepines Paraldehyde Barbiturates

Sedative–hypnotic withdrawal
  barbiturates
  ethchlorvinyl
  glutethimide
  meprobamate
  benzodiazepines
	Sympathomimetic effects
	Hyperthermia
	Cardiovascular collapse
		Stimulation of the anterior hypothalamus, excessive muscular rigidity, peripheral vasoconstriction	Cooling
			Barbiturates
			Benzodiazepines

Malignant-neuroleptic syndrome (Therapeutic Doses)	Hyperpyrexia Rigidity Dysarthria Stupor Akinesia Mutism Dystonic reaction	Excessive muscular rigidity	Cooling Benztropine Benzodiazepines Diphenhydramine
Lithium and neuroleptics (during manic phase) (Therapeutic Doses)	Extrapyramidal symptoms Rigidity Tremulousness Severe parkinsonism Persistent dyskinesia Hyperthermia No sufficient extrapyramidal effects	Excessive muscular rigidity	Cooling Discontinue therapy Avoid anticholinergics Fluid replacement
Lithium (overdose)	Delirium Seizures Hyperthermia Cardiovascular collapse Tremulousness No significant extrapyramidal effects	Excessive muscular rigidity	Cooling Discontinue therapy Avoid anticholinergics Fluid replacement

Drug/Condition	Clinical Effects	Mechanism	Treatment
Amphetamine methylenedioxy amphetamine	Sympathomimetic effects: diaphoresis, tachycardia hypertachycardia hypertension, hyperhydrosis, dry mouth, hyperactivity, active bowel sounds, reactive mydriasis coma, hyperthermia, seizures, hallucinations, delirium, refractory shock	Stimulation of the anterior hypothalamus	Cooling Benzodiazepines
Cocaine overdose	Tachycardia or bradycardia (initial), hypertension, mydriasis, hyperthermia, hyperactive bowel sounds, verticle and/or horizontal nystagmus, arrhythmias, anorexia, nausea, vomiting, hyperactivity, tonic-clonic seizures, muscle paralysis, oliguric renal failure	Stimulation of the anterior hypothalamus Excessive muscular rigidity Calorigenic activity of liver Peripheral vasoconstriction	Cooling Benzodiazepines
Phencyclidine	Hyperthermia, agitation coma, ventilatory failure, sympathomimetic effects, parasympathomimetic and anticholinergic effects	Stimulation of the anterior hypothalamus Excessive muscular rigidity	Cooling Benzodiazepines
Malignant hyperthermia	Intense muscle rigidity, tachypnea, tachycardia, hypermetabolic state, diaphoresis, cardiac arrhythmias, metabolic acidosis, pulmonary edema, renal failure, shock	Excessive muscular rigidity	Stop anesthesia or muscle relaxant Dantrolene Cooling
Anticholinergic antihistamines belladonna alkaloids tricyclic antidepressants (overdose)	Unreactive mydriasis, hypertension, hyperactivity, hyperexcitability, tachycardia, dry skin and mucous membranes, absent bowel sound, urinary retention, disorientation, seizures, coma	Decreased sweating Excessive muscular rigidity	Cooling Physostigmine

(From Goldfrank, L., Flomenbaum, N., Lewin, N., & Weisman, R. S. Toxicologic emergencies: Nonseasonal heatstroke. *Hospital Physician*, 1982, **6**, 63.)

assistance may be required. An intravenous line is started to provide fluid replacement, promote urine flow, and to administer any necessary medication. Baseline laboratory studies are vital to assess electrolyte imbalance and to determine a course of appropriate replacement therapy. Serial electrolytes are used to determine cardiovascular response to therapy and to demonstrate any possible untoward effects of hyperperexia. A rectal probe is then inserted in the rectum and the patient is put into an ice bath. The goal is to lower the temperature quickly until it reaches 102°F (38.8°C). If the temperature falls below 102°F, it may then plummet beyond control. (The temperature should be carefully monitored as rebound hyperthermia may occur within 3 to 6 hours.) A large volume of ice should be available to the emergency department particularly during high-risk periods of sustained heat and humidity. Hyperthermic patients may have seizures, arrhythmias, and metabolic acidosis which remain uncorrected until hyperthermia is reversed. Hyperthermic patients are not suffering from volume depletion, therefore replacement with a normal electrolyte solution should not exceed 2½ liters in the first 24 hours. A CVP line is established to monitor wedge pressures and prevent fluid overload. In severely hypotensive patients, a Swanz–Ganz catheter may be required. Hypotension in heat stroke does not reflect dehydration but rather fluid shunting through dilated skin vessels. This high output failure is usually reversible after cooling and cutaneous vasoconstriction. Urine output and osmolality should be monitored due to the possibility of acute tubular necrosis. Patients with myoglobinuria or with shock should be given an osmotic diuretic, such as mannitol and furosimide (Lasix) to increase renal blood flow.

Heat stroke is preventable and efforts should be directed toward the high-risk population. The young active population should be cautioned regarding acclimatization, especially during period of high temperature humidity index. Acclimatization is an adaptive process to high temperatures. With slow, repeated exposure to heat, cardiovascular and metabolic efficiency increase. There is a smaller rise in body temperature, less tacchycardia, and an increase in sweating with less sodium and chloride loss. Young and old, overweight and underconditioned individuals should be advised to avoid exertion during sunlight hours and the hottest period of the day. Light clothing should be worn and fluid intake encouraged. Professional staff in supervised facilities such as nursing homes and psychiatric facilities should be aware of the increased risk for the elderly with chronic associated illness and those medications which may produce or potentiate heat stroke.

Integumentary System Emergencies References

BURNS

Baxter, C. R. Guidelines for fluid resuscitation. *Journal of Trauma*, 1981, **21** (8), (Suppl.) 687–689.

Bjornson, A. B., Altemeier, W. A., & Bjornson, H. S. Host defense against opportunist microorganisms following trauma. *Annals of Surgery*, 1978, **188**, 83.

Caldwell, F. T., & Bowser, B. H. Critical evaluation of hypertonic and hypotonic solutions to resuscitate severely burned children: A prospective study. *Annals of Surgery*, 1979, **189**, 546.

Curreri, P. W. Overview of recent progress in the treatment of burn wound. *Journal of Trauma*, 1981, **21** (8), (Suppl.), 674–676.

Edlick, R. F., Larkham, N., O'Hanlan, J. T., et al. Modification of the American Burn Association's injury severity grading system. *Journal of the American College of Emergency Physicians*, 1978, **7** (6), 226–228.

Holleman, J. H., Gabel, J. C., & Hardy, J. D. Pulmonary effects of intravenous therapy in burn resuscitation. *Surgery of Gynecology and Obstetrics*, 1978, **147**, 161–166.

Mason, A. D., Jr. The mathematics of resuscitation, 1980 Presidential address, American Burn Association. *Journal of Trauma*, 1980, **20**, 1015–1020.

Pruitt, B. A., Jr. Fluid resuscitation. *Journal of Trauma*, 1981, **21** (8), (Suppl.), 690–692.

Pruitt, B. A. Jr. Initial care of the burn patient. In M. Ravitch (Ed.), *Current problems in surgery*. Chicago: Year Book Medical, Vol. XVI, No. 4, April, 1979.

Pruitt, B. A., Jr. The effectiveness of fluid resuscitation. *Journal of Trauma*, 1979, **19** (8), 868–870.

Wolfe, R. R. Caloric requirements of the burned patient. *Journal of Trauma*, 1981, **21** (8), (Suppl.), 712–713.

HYPOTHERMIA

Barman, M. R. Hypothermia—In summer? *R.N.*, 1982, **45** (6), 42.

Collins, K. J., Dore, C., & Exton-Smith, A. N. Accidental hypothermia and impaired temperature homeostasis in the elderly. *British Medical Journal*, 1977, **2**, 353.

Eggleton, R. C. *Non-invasive temperature determination for the hypothermia victim under field conditions*. Paper presented at the First International Hypothermia Conference, Kingston, Jan 23–27, 1980.

Goodfrank, L. R. *Toxicologic Emergencies—A comprehensive handbook in problem solving* (2nd Ed.). New York: Appleton-Century-Crofts, 1982.

Jessen, K., & Hagelsten, J. O. Peritoneal dialysis in the treatment of profound accidental hypothermia. *Aviation Space and Environmental Medicine*, 1978, **49**, 426.

MacClean, D., & Emslie-Smith, D. *Accidental hypothermia*. Philadelphia: J. B. Lippincott, 1977.

Miller, J. W., et al. Urban accidental hypothermia, 135 cases. *Annals of Emergency Medicine*, 1980, **9**, 456.

O'Keefe, K. M. Accidental hypothermia: A review of 62 cases. *Journal of the American College of Emergency Physicians*, 1977, **6**, 491–496.

Rango, N. A. Action needed to prevent deaths from hypothermia in the elderly. *J. A. M. A.* (Medical News), 1980, **243**, 407.

Reuler, J. B. Hypothermia: Pathophysiology, clinical settings, and management. *Annals of Internal Medicine*, 1978, **89**, 519–527.

Rich, J. Hypothermia. *Journal of Emergency Nursing*, 1983, **9** (1), 8–10.

Smith, D. S. *The cold water connection*. Presented at the First International Hypothermia Conference, Kingston, Jan 23–27, 1980.

Weyman, A. E., Greenbaum, D. M., & Grace, W. J. Accidental hypothermia in an alcoholic population. *American Journal of Medicine*, 1974, **56**, 13–20.

HEAT STROKE

Allexenberg, R. S. Combatting the heat wave of 1980. *Urban Health,* 1981, 26–30.

Burch, G. E., Knochel, J. P., & Murphy, R. J. Stay on guard against heat syndromes. *Patient Care,* 1979, 67–80.

Clowes, G. H. A., Jr., & O'Donnell, T. F. Current concepts: Heat stroke. *New England Journal of Medicine,* 1974, **291,** 557.

Costrini, A. M., Pitt, M. A., & Gustafson, A. B. Cardiovascular and metabolic manifestations of heat stroke and severe exhaustion. *American Journal of Medicine,* 1979, **66,** 296–302.

Goldfrank, L. R. *Toxicologic emergencies—A comprehensive handbook in problem solving* (2nd Ed.). New York: Appleton-Century-Crofts, 1982.

Goldfrank, L., & Osborn, H. Heat stroke. *Hospital Physician,* 1977, **8,** 14–18.

Knochel, J. P. Environmental heat illness. *Archives of Internal Medicine,* 1974, **133,** 841.

Larkin, J. T. Treatment of heat related illness. *J. A. M. A.,* 1981, **245,** (6), 570–571.

Levine, J. A. Heat stroke in the aged. *American Journal of Medicine,* 1969, **47,** 251–258.

Pickard, C. G., Jr. Summertime emergencies. *Nurse Practitioner,* 1978, **3** (3), 15–16.

Sprung, C. L. Hemodynamic alterations of heat stroke in the elderly. *Chest,* 1979, **75** (3), 362–366.

Wheeler, M. Heat stroke in the elderly. *Medical Clinics of North America,* 1976, **60,** 1289–1296.

G. METABOLIC EMERGENCIES

1. Disorders of Glucose Metabolism

Refer to Table 16, on the following pages.

Maintenance of a Normal Blood Glucose Level

In light of man's feeding–fasting cycles, it is quite remarkable that the blood glucose concentration remains fairly constant. This concentration is a function of the inter-relationship between food intake, absorption, energy needs, storage of energy, and excretion rates. It represents the results of many control systems intracellularly and in a variety of organs and tissues.

The metabolism of food molecules converts the energy in the carbon–hydrogen bonds of food molecules into cellular and stored energy. Once glucose enters a cell it is immediately phosphorylated to glucose-6-phosphate. This reaction is not revers-ible and the glucose is trapped inside the cell. Glucose can be converted to glycogen and stored. It can take part in the synthesis of mucopolysaccharides or it could be oxidized to yield ribose phosphate, a substance necessary for the synthesis of ribo-nucleic acid.

Glucose is most commonly oxidized to provide cellular energy in the form of adenosine triphosphate (ATP), pyruvic acid, and hydrogen ions. The splitting of glucose into two molecules of pyruvic acid is called glycolysis. Pyruvic acid is also oxidized and decarboxylated which produces acetic acid. Acetic acid is activated by combining with coenzyme A to produce acetylcoenzyme A. In this activated form it enters the citric acid cycle (Krebs cycle) where it eventually will be oxidized to car-bon dioxide and water. The key event in the Krebs cycle is the combining of acetyl-coenzyme A with oxaloacetic acid to produce citric acid. In a series of many oxidative steps of this cycle, hydrogen is removed from the food molecule and passed to coenzyme, nicotinamide adenine dinucleotide (NAD), producing reduced coenzyme, $NADH_2$. Most of the energy now is tied up in $NADH_2$. The hydrogen or

TABLE 16. COMMON BLOOD GLUCOSE IMBALANCES: ASSESSMENT FINDINGS

Parameter	Hypoglycemic Reaction	Ketoacidosis	Hyperosmolar Syndrome
History			
Age of patient	All age groups, especially those on insulin or hypoglycemic agents	Usually younger age group "Brittle diabetics"	More common in 60-to- 70-year old group and those with mild or undiagnosed diabetes
Onset	Rapid, in minutes	Gradual, 12 hours or more	Slowly, days and weeks
Precipitating events	1. Diabetes related: too high a dose of insulin or hypoglycemic medication insufficient food intake sudden strenuous exercise without extra food	1. Diabetes related: too little insulin or missed dose too much food mild or severe infection injury stress of any kind	1. Diabetes related: enough insulin to depress excessive lipolysis but not to allow utilization of glucose
	2. Nondiabetic problems: patients with partial gastrectomy pancreatic islet cell tumors liver disease alcohol induced other endocrine problems medications	2. Nondiabetic problems: hepatocellular disease malnutrition and starvation stress secondary to CVA, MI, surgery, febrile illness chronic renal disease and uremia Other endocrine problems medications	2. Nondiabetic problems: CVA, cardiovascular disease Renal disease Sepsis, stress Medications
Physical findings			
General appearance	A well person who has fainted: may be excited	Very ill, lethargy, confused, drowsy person	Confused, stuporous, comatosed
Skin and tissue turgor	Diaphoretic, normal turgor	Dry, flushed, dehydrated	Very dry, dehydrated
Temperature	Normal or below	Elevated	Could be elevated
Breathing	Normal, no air hunger	Acetone odor, rapid, deep (Kussmaul) air hunger present	Rapid, no air hunger, no acetone odor
Blood pressure	Normal or may be elevated	Subnormal	Subnormal, postural hypotension common
Pulse	Full, rapid	Weak, rapid	Weak, rapid
Palpitations	Frequent	Absent	Absent
Eyes	Staring, pupil dilated	Sunken, soft	Sunken, soft

Vision	Diplopia, difficult to focus	Haziness	Absent
Headache	Common	Absent	
Muscle twitching	Common	Absent	Focal seizures common
Reflexes	Babinski may be present	Normal or decreased	Unilateral hyperreflexia
Hunger	Great	Present early followed by anorexia	Present early followed by anorexia
Tongue	Moist	Dry	Dry
Thirst	None	Great	Great
Vomiting	Rare	Along with nausea, common	Seen in some cases
Abdominal pain	Absent	Common along with distention	May be present
Laboratory findings			
Glucose (60–100 mg)	Below 40 mg	Severely elevated (400–800 mg)	Extremely elevated (over 900 mg)
Ketones (2–4 mg)	Normal	Elevated	Normal to mildly elevated
Osmolarity (280–300 mOsL)	Normal	Moderate increase	Severely increased over 350 mOs/L
pH (7.35–7.45)	Normal	Falls below 7.25	Falls, averages 7.26
P_{CO_2} (35–45 mm Hg)	Normal	Decreased	Decreased
Cations			
Sodium (135–145 mEq/L)	Normal	Decreased	Usually high but may be normal or low
Potassium (3.5–5.5 mEq/L)	Normal	Normal or high / Total body amount low	Low, normal or high / Total body amount low
Magnesium (1.5–2.5 mEq/L)	Normal	Decreased	Decreased
Calcium (4.5–5.5 mEq/L)	Normal	Decreased	Decreased
Anions			
Chloride (95–105 mEq/L)	Normal	Decreased	Decreased
Bicarbonate (24–28 mEq/L)	Normal	Decreased	Decreased, but higher than keto-acidosis
Phosphorus (1.7–2.6 mEq/L)	Normal	Decreased	Decreased
Blood urea nitrogen	Normal	Increased	Increased
WBC (5–10,000)	Normal	Increased	Increased
Hematocrit (35–45)	Normal	Increased	Increased
Urine results			
Sugar	Usually negative	Highly positive	Positive
Ketones	Negative	Moderate to strong	Minimal or negative

its electron is passed along a chain of hydrogen acceptors via the hydrogen (electron) transport system resulting in the gradual release of energy, the formation of ATP and water. This aerobic process yields 36 moles of ATP. The ATP produced diffuses out of the mitochondria into the cytoplasm and cell nucleus where energy is used to energize all cellular functions. This pathway is a common pathway for the oxidation of proteins and fats after they have been converted to one of the compounds that lies on the pathway.

The operation of the Krebs cycle and hydrogen transport system are totally dependent upon a continuous supply of oxygen. In the absence of oxygen the hydrogen acceptors of this system cannot accept hydrogen. In addition, the small amounts of cellular coenzyme NAD is quickly depleted. Without free NAD to act as a hydrogen acceptor, the entire Krebs cycle and hydrogen transport system ceases.

Glycolysis can continue in the absence of oxygen in some tissues, especially in skeletal muscle. The end product of this metabolism is not pyruvic acid, but rather lactic acid. Anaerobic metabolism is inefficient because only 2 moles of ATP are formed instead of the 36 moles formed by the aerobic process.

The uses of the end products of nutrient digestion are regulated to meet the changing conditions of the body. During the absorptive state the levels of glucose, fatty acids, and amino acids are high. Most body cells remove the glucose and fatty acids and oxidize them to supply their energy needs in addition to taking in amino acids for protein synthesis. The liver and muscle cells convert glucose to its storage form, glycogen. Excess glucose and amino acids are metabolized to fatty acids and stored as neutral fat in the liver and adipose tissue.

Glucose molecules do not simply cross a cell's membrane. Rather, their passage is facilitated by a carrier molecule, namely insulin. Insulin therefore lowers blood sugar because it promotes the entry of glucose into select cells and increases the anabolism of large molecules. The major stimulus for insulin's secretion from the beta cells of the pancreas is a high blood glucose level which is normally found in the absorptive state.

During the absorptive state other hormones play vital roles. Anterior pituitary growth hormone and somatostatin synthesize proteins from amino acids, whereas circulating estrogens act to antagonize insulin's activity. In addition, thyroxine increases the absorption of carbohydrates from the intestinal tract. The absorptive state is a time of energy storage and essentially all of its events are stimulated by insulin.

In the postabsorptive or fasting state, the body's cells still require glucose as a source of energy. The liver plays a major role at this time. It converts its stored glycogen into glucose (glycogenolysis) which it releases into the blood. The amount of stored liver glycogen has its limits and is insufficient to meet prolonged deprivation of food. Under these conditions, the body metabolizes its fat and protein stores (gluconeogenesis).

The end products of fat digestion are fatty acids and glycerol. Glycerol can be converted to glyceraldehyde and undergo transformation that eventuates in glucose. The fatty acids undergo oxidation which eventuates in the production of three ketones: acetoacetic acid, β-hydroxybutyric acid, and acetone. Normally, these strong acids are rapidly catabolized and do not accumulate in the blood. However, when the metabolism of carbohydrate is abnormally low, fatty acids are used to satisfy energy needs and ketones build up in the blood.

Amino acids, the end product of protein metabolism, are stored in the liver and muscle tissue. When carbohydrates are not available to meet energy needs, the liver deaminates its amino acids to produce ammonia, which is converted to urea and excreted, and keto acids. Most of the keto acids thus formed enter the Krebs cycle in the form of α-ketoglutaric acid and liberate energy. A gram of protein produces about as much ATP as does a gram of glucose. However, prolonged use of protein as an energy source leads to a negative nitrogen balance and severe consequences.

There are four hormones that stimulate the various metabolic processes in the postabsorptive state to maintain a fairly constant blood glucose level. Glucagon, secreted by the alpha cells of the pancreas, opposes the glucose lowering effects of insulin. A low blood glucose concentration stimulates its release. Glucagon stimulates the breakdown of glycogen, fats, and proteins and is considered the hormone of energy release. Epinephrine, one of the catecholamines secreted by the adrenal medulla, augments the effects of glucagon in stimulating the breakdown of glycogen to glucose and fats to free fatty acids. Cortisol from the adrenal cortex acts with glucagon and stimulates the breakdown of body proteins to amino acids and their subsequent conversion to glucose. In the fasting state, somatostatin acts to minimize the breakdown of amino acids. It inhibits the use of glucose by most of the body's cells except nerve cells. Along with glucagon, somatostatin stimulates the breakdown of fats to fatty acids and ketone bodies. The postabsorptive state is considered a time of energy release.

It is well to remember that not all body cells require insulin for glucose to enter. Nerve tissue, erythrocytes, liver cells, intestinal mucosal cells, kidney tubule cells do not need insulin. As such they are most sensitive to fluctuations in blood glucose levels. It is estimated that the brain and nerve cells require 6 grams of glucose per hour to function properly.

HYPOGLYCEMIA

PATHOPHYSIOLOGY

Hypoglycemic reaction is a symptomatic state occurring in the presence of blood glucose levels below 50 mg/100 ml. In the majority of cases, it produces a radical change in the body's energy supply and triggers a series of regulatory events to restore the blood glucose to normal or near normal. Hypoglycemia can occur in the fasting, postabsorptive state, or in the postprandial, absorptive state.

The most common cause of fasting hypoglycemia is an excess of insulin. The diabetic who gives him or herself insulin and who, for any reason, lowers the food intake experiences hypoglycemia. In addition, if he or she performs sudden, strenuous exercise, hypoglycemia occurs because it is believed that exercise increases receptor site affinity for insulin and thus lowers the blood sugar.

The elderly patient who has type II diabetes, in addition to other medical problems associated with aging, is at risk of fasting hypoglycemia. Although all of the sulfonylurea drugs can induce hypoglycemia in the absence of food, chlorpropramide (Diabinese) is the drug most frequently implicated. Perhaps this is because it is the longest acting oral agent and its duration time may overlap in some individuals. In addition, alcohol and other medications these patients may be taking could lead to hypoglycemia. Examples of drugs that augment the action of sulfonylurea drugs are: anticoagulants, allopurinol, chloromycetin, phenylbutazone, MAO inhibitors, phenytoin, probenecid, salicylates, and sulfonamides.

Excessive alcohol ingestion over a long period of time leads to hypoglycemia. Typically, the intake of alcohol occurs in the absence of food. Alcohol in the body competes for the metabolic cofactors which are required for gluconeogenesis during a fasting state. This competition results in hypoglycemia.

Hypoglycemia can be seen in patients with endocrine problems other than pancreatic problems and in patients with liver problems. Conditions such as Addison disease (decrease in cortisol) and hypopituitarism (decrease in growth hormone) cause hypoglycemia by not producing enough substances that antagonize insulin's blood lowering activity. Severe hepatitis, cirrhosis, or cholangitis, which produce hepatic necrosis, cause hypoglycemia because of the loss of hepatic glycogenolysis and gluconeogenesis. Glycogen storing disease such as Von Gierke type I (deficiency of glucose-6-phosphatase) could lead to severe hypoglycemia in children.

Hypoglycemia may be caused by ectopic production of insulin or by the secretion of antigluconeogenic or antiglycogenolytic agents. Carcinoid tumors arising from the enterochromaffin cells produce many substances, one of which is almost identical to insulin. This production is not under any feedback controls and thus hypoglycemic reactions occur. Hepatomas and large fibrosarcomas are not usually associated with excessive insulin production but do cause hypoglycemia. The mechanism is not clearly understood. Gastrointestinal tumors and adrenocortical tumors may produce hypoglycemia by producing substances that inhibit gluconeogenesis or glycogenolysis. Islet cell tumors or islet cell hyperplasia is a rare cause of hypoglycemia but should be suspected in cases of fasting hypoglycemia when no other apparent cause is found.

Postabsorptive (postprandial) hypoglycemia does occur in some situations. Alimentary hypoglycemia is seen in patients who have had gastric surgery, increased gastric motility, and hyperthyroidism. This type of hypoglycemia peaks at 1½ to 2 hours after the ingestion of a meal. In these cases, the duodenum is flooded with carbohydrate which, when absorbed, causes an excessive amount of insulin to be secreted which lowers the blood glucose dramatically. Hypoglycemia can occur 3 to 4 hours after a meal. The exact mechanisms are not clear but faulty cholinergic control of insulin secretion or deficient glucagon secretion have been proposed as causative reactions.

The clinical manifestations of hypoglycemia result from the metabolic changes in the brain and nerve tissues which are quite vulnerable to inadequate supplies of glucose. There may be some slowing of mental responses with disorientation, confusion, diplopia, and emotional instability (inappropriate laughter or tears). The immediate and primary response is the release of epinephrine from the adrenal medulla which produces widespread activation of the sympathetic nervous system.

The early clinical features of hyperepinephremia are weakness, diaphoresis, tingling in fingers and around the mouth, tachycardia, palpitations, high blood pressure, anxiety, nervousness, and tremors. In some adults and children sudden irritability, anger, belligerence, giddiness, or other mood swings are seen. These are considered premonitory signs but all patients do not experience them.

The later clinical manifestations of hypoglycemia are indicative of central nervous system involvement and occur when the hypoglycemia is of extreme degree or prolonged. These signs include: headache, blurred vision, faintness, lightheadedness, mental confusion, clumsiness, hypotonia, staggering gait, hypothermia, twitching, seizures, and deep coma.

The symptoms of hypoglycemia tend to appear rapidly and the patient may be easily misdiagnosed. Frequently, patients are labeled drunk, epileptic, hysterical, psychotic, or as having a CVA before the appropriate cause is discovered. Because many patients do not exhibit the early manifestations, it is not uncommon to see them in a comatosed state. Why this happens is not clear but it appears to be related to the rate of glucose level decline and differences in nerve cell metabolism. In any event, repeated severe attacks of hypoglycemia can lead to permanent brain death. Prompt diagnosis and treatment prevents this occurrence.

MANAGEMENT

I. Identify the possible cause of the presenting symptoms
  A. Inquire as to the events that preceded the onset of the symptoms
  B. Ascertain a history of diabetes mellitus
    1. ask accompanying person, family, friends, co-workers, attendant
    2. check personal items for diabetic identification card
    3. note any jewelry that would alert staff to a medical condition
  C. Establish the prior management regimen of the diabetes
    1. insulin: type taking, amount, when last dose was taken, any recent changes in dose or type of insulin
    2. oral agents: type taking, amount, last dose, any recent changes
    3. diet: total calories allowed, time of last meal, what meal consisted of
    4. exercise: usual activity level, any change in activity pattern
    5. urine testing: materials used, recent test results
    6. complications: note any awareness of neuropathy, retinopathy, nephropathy, angiopathy
  D. Consider the presence of medical problems and/or substance abuse that could contribute to the problem
    1. note any known cardiovascular, pulmonary, neurologic, gastrointestinal, or renal problems and their treatment
    2. obtain a complete list of prescribed and over-the-counter drugs patient is taking

3. identify the use and/or abuse of ethanol
4. note any allergic conditions patient may have

II. Detect and characterize the signs of the presenting and/or other problems
   A. If patient is unconscious, rapidly assess airway patency, breathing and circulation. Initiate measures to relieve airway obstruction, maintain breathing and support circulation, if necessary
   B. Rapidly perform a systems analysis
      1. cardiovascular: take bp, pulse, temperature, note heart sounds and rhythm, note any palpitations
      2. pulmonary: note rate of respirations, breathing pattern, odor to breath, presence of air hunger, breath sounds
      3. state of hydration: note skin turgor, diaphoresis, appearance of tongue, presence of thirst, intraocular tension
      4. neurosensory–motor functioning: note any visual disturbances, pupillary changes, headache, muscle twitching, tremor, type of gait, paresthesias, seizures, responses to motor and sensory testing
      5. gastrointestinal: note any nausea, vomiting, hunger, diarrhea, constipation, palpate for abdominal or retroperitoneal masses
      6. renal functioning: note the usual voiding pattern, quantity of urine

III. Perform diagnostic studies that contribute to the diagnosis
   A. Do a fingerstick blood glucose determination
   B. Obtain a second urine specimen for sugar and acetone levels
   C. Send samples of blood to the laboratory for glucose, ketones, osmolality, BUN, electrolytes, CBC, WBC, Hct, Hgb
   D. Obtain heparinized blood samples for insulin and cortisol assay
   E. Obtain a urine specimen for urinalysis

IV. Restore the serum glucose levels to normal
   A. Administer rapid-acting carbohydrate
      1. for the conscious patient who can swallow, offer 10 g of carbohydrate in the form of 4 ounces of a soft drink or 4 ounces of orange juice. It is not necessary to add sugar to these solutions. Wait 15 minutes. If patient does not feel better, repeat the dose every 15 minutes until the symptoms abate
      2. if the patient cannot swallow, administer glucagon 1 mg subcutaneously or intramuscularly. Wait 5 to 10 minutes for the patient to react. Glucagon is now available sublingually. In this case, wait 10 minutes for it to be effective. Once patient arouses and can swallow, offer a meal or 10 g of glucose in the manner described above
      3. if patient is unconscious, give a bolus of 50 percent dextrose IV which is equivalent to 50 g of glucose. In some situations, start an intravenous of 50 percent D/W. The patient should respond immediately and dramatically to this dose
      4. if there is a history of ethanol abuse, thiamine 50 to 100 mg IV or IM should be administered *before* the dextrose is given
   B. Observe patient for a rebound hypoglycemic effect in 2 to 3 hours

  V. Prevent subsequent hypoglycemic episodes
   A. Treat the cause of the hypoglycemia, if nondiabetic related
   B. If diabetic-related, teach the patient about the need for adequate food intake, the relationship of insulin peak times and hypoglycemia and the role that exercise plays in initiating hypoglycemia
   C. Refer patient to diabetic clinic or private physician for follow-up care

RATIONALE

The purpose of the initial history is to identify what the patient is currently experiencing and to elicit anything in the background that could relate to the current problem. Because the most common cause of hypoglycemia is an excess of insulin, it is prudent to detect the presence of diabetes mellitus, how this patient is managing it and what, if anything, i.e., missed meal, sudden exercise, could have contributed to the problem. If the hypoglycemia is not related to diabetes mellitus, the acute problem can be dealt with in the emergency department, and a search for its cause can be done at a later date.

The rapid physical examination of the patient is aimed at discovering abnormalities and establishing the observable rather than reported signs of the problem. If the patient presents in an unconscious state, other abnormalities which can cause coma must be eliminated quickly. The hypoglycemic reaction differs greatly from other diabetic comas (see preceding Assessment section) and the diagnosis of hypoglycemia can usually be tentatively made after the history and physical are performed.

Laboratory tests contribute to the diagnosis and in most cases confirm the impression of hypoglycemia. It is not wise to wait for laboratory results of serum glucose level. The fingerstick glucose test provides a fairly accurate estimation of the glucose level in only 60 seconds with just one drop of venous or capillary blood. One would expect that the fingerstick test and blood sample results to be below 50 mg/100 ml.

Glucosuria and ketonuria are not expected in hypoglycemic reactions. However, patients with hypotonic bladders or those who have not recently voided have glucosuria from antecedent hyperglycemia. Therefore, a second specimen should be collected. It is unwise to catheterize patients for these specimens but in some cases it is unavoidable. Ketones may be found in the urine of a hypoglycemic patient who has been unconscious for a long period of time and has not ingested any food. Thus, ketonuria is not a clue either to the presence or absence of hypoglycemia.

The patient's blood chemistries and hematologic picture should be well within normal limits unless there is a concomitant medical condition. Insulin levels, if they can be obtained, are usually high. Cortisol may or may not be elevated.

Once the diagnosis is confirmed, the treatment goal is to restore the serum glucose levels to normal. If the patient is conscious and is able to swallow, administer fast-acting oral carbohydrate (4 ounces of orange juice, soda, 2 lumps of sugar). This dose of 10 grams of carbohydrate will reverse the progression of the symptoms and raise the blood glucose level. There is no need to add rapid-acting table sugar to the solutions because such a high oral dose of glucose leads to nausea and vomiting. The patient may require repeat doses of the 10 grams every 15 minutes until improvement is seen. Under no circumstances should fluids be forced on the patient who cannot swallow for fear of aspiration.

If the patient is unable to swallow and the cause of the hypoglycemia is not related to a glycogen storage problem or severe liver disease, glucagon may be administered parenterally. Glucagon activates phosphorylase with the resultant increase in gluconeogenesis. The liver normally stores 100 to 150 grams of glucose as glycogen for emergency use. A single injection usually produces a favorable response in 10 minutes. If not, a second injection may be given. If the patient is at home and no response is seen in 30 minutes, he or she should be hospitalized immediately. Once the patient is alert, oral glucose containing solutions and/or food should be offered.

Even when the patient is known to be a diabetic, but as yet the diagnosis is uncertain, glucose may be administered. A bolus of 25 ml of 50 percent dextrose or an intravenous injection of a 50 percent dextrose in water solution will promptly reverse the symptoms of hypoglycemia. It is believed that even if the patient is in a state of ketosis or hyperosmolarity, the amount given is so small compared to the total glucose pool, that it is essentially harmless.

If the hypoglycemia is related to ethanol abuse, the patient should receive a parenteral dose of thiamine before giving glucose. If glucose is given to the thiamine deficient patient, it may precipitate Wernicke encephalopathy. Thus, the cerebral deficits can be avoided.

After the glucose level has been raised and the patient is out of immediate danger, it is wise to observe for 3 to 4 hours. It is possible that the interventions aimed at raising the blood glucose level to normal do, in fact, overshoot the mark producing hyperglycemia. Insulin secretion is stimulated and hypoglycemia could again occur.

When the cause of the hypoglycemic reaction is not related to diabetic control measures, the patient should be admitted for further workup. If the hypoglycemia is related to diabetes, the patient should be taught to recognize the early signs: the need for adequate food intake, the relationship of insulin peak times and hypoglycemic reactions, and the role of sudden strenuous exercise plays in initiating hypoglycemia. In any case, the patient must be given a clinic appointment for follow-up care or referred to a private physician.

DIABETIC KETOACIDOSIS

PATHOPHYSIOLOGY

Diabetic ketoacidosis (DKA) is a state that develops over a period of time and is characterized by hyperglycemia, fluid loss, electrolyte derangements, and acid–base imbalances. Although DKA is more common in the type I insulin-dependent diabetic who is usually young, it can occur in the 80-year-old patient who is lean and presents with polyuria, weight loss, and dehydration. There are reported cases that substantiate ketoacidosis as the initial event in a patient with undiagnosed diabetes mellitus. DKA is an acute, life-threatening state which demands prompt diagnosis and treatment.

Severe ketoacidosis can be precipitated by many factors and a combination of events. Insulin deficiency can occur in the diabetic patient who omits to take insulin or fails to take the prescribed dose, in a patient who is building up resistance to insulin, or in one who is noncompliant with the dietary plan and increases food intake. It can also occur in diabetics who have an increased demand for insulin as it occurs during a period of infection, inflammation, surgery, stress, trauma, pregnancy, or periods of growth. Insulin deficiency and the resultant hyperglycemia leads to a number of homeostatic mechanisms in an attempt to restore balances.

The lack of insulin results in the body's inability to use available glucose to meet its energy needs with the result that massive lipolysis occurs and some proteolysis to meet the energy requirements. DKA is interpreted by the body as a state of prolonged fasting and triggers the release of hormones to raise the blood glucose level, namely, glucagon, epinepherine, cortisol, and growth hormone. It also triggers glycogenolysis but within hours glycogen stores are depleted.

Unrestrained lipolysis results in the liberation of free fatty acids. Many of these fatty acids are degraded to acetylcoenzyme A (ACoA) and are channeled into the common metabolic pathway to produce carbon dioxide, water, and ATP. However, in a state of extreme lipolysis, the Krebs cycle cannot handle the excess ACoA being produced and it tends to accumulate in the liver. The liver converts this excess ACoA to ketone bodies: acetoacetate, β-hydroxybutyrate, and acetone. (Acetoacetate can be decarboxylated to acetone or it can be reduced to form β-hydroxybutyrate.) When the rate of production of ketones exceeds the liver's ability to oxidize them, they are released into the circulation resulting in ketonemia and when the kidney excretes them, ketonuria.

Ketones are acids and as such are buffered by the bicarbonate buffer system and excreted mainly as sodium salts resulting in a loss of the blood alkali, or base reserves of the body, which contributes to a low serum pH, acidosis. Acidosis triggers a number of compensatory mechanisms. The low pH stimulates the respiratory center and results in rapid, deep (Kussmaul) breathing. Hyperventilation produces a compensatory respiratory alkalosis in an attempt to restore pH to near normal by blowing off carbon dioxide thereby reducing acidity. The absence of Kussmaul breathing does not rule out DKA because, as the pH falls below 7.1, the patient may lose the respiratory drive and this normal compensatory mechanism. If one were to smell the breath of a patient with DKA, it would smell like decaying apples or Juicy fruit gum. Acetone is responsible for this sign. It may not be detectable in patients whose ketone production has shifted more to β-hydroxybutyrate than acetoacetate. A second compensatory mechanism in acidosis occurs in the kidney which increases its excretion of hydrogen ions by combining them with ammonia ions to form ammonium which is readily excreted as ammonium chloride. Acidosis depresses all neuronal cellular activity.

The fluid imbalance, which occurs with severe DKA, is caused by several events and results in intracellular and extracellular fluid deficits. Hyperglycemia increases plasma osmolality and draws intracellular fluid into the extracellular spaces resulting in cellular dehydration. Usually, when the hyperglycemia rises above 175 mg/100 ml, it exceeds the nephron's tubular reabsorption capacity resulting in glucosuria. Glucosuria leads to polyuria because it takes approximately 15 ml of water to excrete 1 gram of glucose. Many calories are lost in the urine, resulting in the patient experiencing hunger (polyphagia). In addition, the accelerated lipolysis and proteolysis, which occur with DKA, produce an excess of ketones and urea which are excreted in the urine. Excessive amounts of these molecules in the urine accentuates the solute diuresis because they also exert an osmotic pull. As much as 14 percent (or 7 liters) of the total body water can be lost during severe DKA. Dehydration initiates the thirst mechanism in an attempt to reduce osmolality and the patient drinks more. However, some patients have a disturbance in the thirst mechanism and do not exhibit polydipsia.

The cation electrolyte derangements associated with DKA are manifested by total body deficits of sodium and potassium. Sodium ions are lost in the urine because of the osmotic diuresis which is secondary to the glucosuria. Sodium ions also combine with ketones, in an attempt to neutralize them, and are excreted in the urine which results in a significant loss of body sodium. It has been estimated that patients in DKA have a 15 percent (or 350 mEq) loss of body sodium. The serum sodium levels of the patient are usually low but they can be normal or high, if dehydration is severe, and it occurs in association with vomiting and hypotonic urine.

Total body potassium is depleted, even in the face of a normal serum level, for the following reasons. In the absence of insulin, potassium ions move from the intracellular space to the extracellular space and then to the plasma where they are rapidly excreted by the kidney. Potassium ions, like sodium ions, combine with ketones, in an attempt to neutralize them, and are excreted as potassium salts. If vomiting, which commonly accompanies DKA, or diarrhea occurs, the potassium loss is even greater. Concomitantly, a secondary hyperaldosteronism exists which is caused by the sodium depletion and/or extracellular fluid volume depletion. Hyperaldosteronism favors the reabsorption of sodium ions and the secretion of potassium and some hydrogen ions. A total potassium body deficit as high as 9 percent (or 500 mEq) could occur. Cellular hypokalemia leads to weakness, flaccidity, hypotonia, ECG changes, nausea, vomiting, and mental depression.

The anion electrolyte losses associated with DKA appear as chloride, bicarbonate, and phosphate deficits. The chloride is lost in the urine along with sodium during the osmotic diuresis secondary to glucosuria. The bicarbonate ions are given up to neutralize the acidic ketones with the resultant formation of carbonic acid which dissociates to form carbon dioxide and water. Severe phosphaturia accompanies DKA which can lead to a decrease in the red blood cell's ability to release oxygen to the tissues. In total, there is a substantial loss of anions in DKA which contributes to the acidosis.

The dehydration associated with DKA has severe consequences. The lowered blood volume results in a lower blood pressure and diminished blood flow to the vital organs. Hypoperfusion of the body's tissues produces an oxygen deficit which favors anaerobic metabolism resulting in the build up of lactic acid and only adds to the acidosis. Circulatory and renal failure is soon followed by coma.

The neurologic status of patients in DKA varies widely. Approximately 10 percent are comatosed on admission. Most present lethargic and sometimes confused. However, their level of consciousness does not correlate with the extent of the metabolic derangements found and is not a clue to the severity and/or improvement in their condition. It is wise to remember that vascular thrombosis could provoke ketoacidosis.

Patients in DKA commonly complain of abdominal problems such as nausea, vomiting, and pain, and may appear distended. These signs and symptoms are probably the result of electrolyte depletion and high levels of glucagon which both result in altered gastrointestinal motility. However, it is prudent to keep in mind that although these signs could be secondary to ketoacidosis, they might also be the provoking cause of the ketoacidosis.

Most patients with DKA have an elevated white blood cell count. The leukocytosis is probably due to the presence of the severe acidosis. Although a majority of the patients do not have demonstrable infection, pneumonia, MI, pancreatitis, peritonitis, urinary tract infection, skin infections, or meningitis should be considered and ruled out as the provoking cause of the ketosis. Frequently, the temperature is normal even in the presence of an infection.

MANAGEMENT

I. Determine the status of the airway, breathing, and circulation
   A. Visually assess the patency of the airway
      1. suction, if not clear; assist with intubation, if needed; support ventilation, if needed
   B. Record the respiratory rate and pattern
      1. chart respiratory rate, pattern, and use of accessory muscles; chart skin color; assess odor of breath for acetone or ETOH
   C. Record temperature, pulse, and bp
      1. report hypotension and/or signs of cardiac dysrhythmias; note the presence of tachycardia
   D. Assess the neurologic status
      1. chart the level of consciousness; record motor and sensory deficits; note any seizures or history of seizures
II. Complete the systems survey and collect a history
   A. Detect changes in the level of hydration
      1. note skin turgor, condition of mucous membranes, intraocular pressure; note the presence of thirst and approximate fluid intake; note the presence of polyuria
   B. Identify the presence of gastrointestinal symptoms
      1. chart the presence or history of nausea, vomiting, diarrhea; note the

time of the last meal and what it consisted of; palpate the abdomen to detect pain or tenderness; pass a nasogastric tube and attach to intermittent low suctioning, if abdomen is distended or if vomiting is present

C. Detect any changes in the urinary system
  1. assess for flank pain and note time of last micturition; chart any complaints of urgency, frequency, dysuria; collect a urine specimen; if unable to void, insert a catheter

III. Search for a history of diabetes mellitus or other conditions
  A. Inquire of the events that led up to current situation
    1. ask patient, family, co-workers; note any recent injuries, infections, pain, or stress
  B. Search personal belongings and body for any medical identification that would indicate current condition
  C. If patient is a diabetic, note the following
    1. time and amount of insulin or oral hypoglycemic agent taken
    2. time and amount of last food intake
    3. time and level of recent activity
    4. other prescribed or over-the-counter medications taken
  D. Perform a fingerstick blood glucose determination and test for sugar and acetone in the urine

IV. Verify the hypothesis of DKA and screen for concurrent problems
  A. Draw bloods for the following tests: glucose, electrolytes, BUN, creatinine, acetone, osmolarity, phosphate, RBC, ESR, WBC, and arterial blood gases. If patient is unconscious and febrile add: serum enzymes, amylase, blood, throat, urine and stool cultures, toxicology screen, type and cross-match
  B. Do a stat ECG and chest x-ray
  C. Estimate the anion gap and serum osmolality
  D. Initiate a flow-sheet which includes vital signs, I&O, laboratory data and therapy initiated

V. Correct the fluid imbalance
  A. Administer IV solutions as ordered, usually 5 to 8 L/24 hours; 1000 ml may be given the first 30 to 60 minutes then 500 ml/hour
  B. Check the vital signs q 15 to 30 minutes; record all I&O and report deficits and excesses
  C. Observe for overhydration: note any distension of neck veins, bounding pulse, loud heart sounds, gallop rhythm, pulmonary edema, cerebral edema, and CHF
  D. Insert a CVP line
  E. Be prepared to administer plasma or whole blood, if patient is in shock

VI. Correct the electrolyte imbalances
  A. Replace the sodium and chloride ions
    1. initial fluid replacement is usually in the form of 0.9 percent saline solution

2. monitor serum sodium levels q 1 to 2 hours; if sodium rises above 155 mEq/L, IV should be changed to 0.45 percent saline

B. Replace the potassium ions
1. administer KCL 20 to 40 mEq/L in the IV, only if patient has a urinary output of 30 ml/hour
2. potassium may be started early if serum potassium is low but it may also be delayed for 1 to 4 hours after therapy is begun
3. monitor serum potassium levels q 1 to 2 hours
4. chart any signs of hypokalemia: muscle weakness, decreased peristalsis, lowered bp, weak pulse, ECG changes such as a prolonged QT interval, depressed T wave, prominent U wave
5. chart any signs of hyperkalemia such as bradycardia, peaked T wave, no P wave, and a wide QRS interval
6. continuous cardiac monitoring is needed
7. when patient is able to swallow and retain fluids, offer solutions high in potassium

C. Replace phosphate ions
1. usually 40 to 60 mEq/L as a potassium salt is prescribed early in the course of treatment
2. it is alternated with KCl in the IV and given as a potassium salt
3. monitor phosphate levels, may *not* be given if patient is hyperphosphatemic or if possibility of uremia exists

VII. Correct the glucose imbalance
A. Administer regular insulin on an intermittent dose basis
1. a large bolus IV (1.5 U/kg or 50 to 200 U) followed by subcutaneous or IM doses. This is repeated q 1 to 2 hours depending on the serum glucose levels
2. check serum glucose levels, potassium levels, and watch for precipitous falls

B. Administer regular insulin on a continuous low dose basis
1. a bolus of 0.33 U/kg body weight is given followed by 4 to 7 units per hour continuously
2. if added to IV, calculate the binding factor or coat bottle, tubing and filters with albumin
3. if given "piggy back," an infusion pump will insure proper flow rate

C. Be prepared to administer hydrocortisone (100 to 200 mg), if insulin resistance develops

D. Monitor serum glucose levels q 1 to 2 hours
1. report a drop in the serum glucose at 250 to 300 mg levels
2. closely observe for signs of hypoglycemia
3. if hypoglycemia occurs, insulin may be discontinued and a 5 percent dextrose in saline solution started

E. Never mix regular insulin with sodium bicarbonate solution

F. Monitor urine samples every hour for glucose and ketones
1. collect a fresh second specimen or aspirate catheter with a needle

      2. use the 2-drop Clinitest method, if testing level with the 5-drop method is 2 percent (4+)

VIII. Correct the base deficit

    A. Sodium bicarbonate replacement is only necessary if the arterial pH is below 7.1 or if the patient is in shock or has a cardiac problem

    B. 80 to 100 mEq or 2 ampules may be prescribed to be placed in the first liter of saline.

    C. Do not mix insulin with bicarbonate solutions, precipitation results

    D. Monitor the pertinent laboratory data to assess the status of the acidotic state: pH, P_{CO_2}, bicarbonate levels and/or carbon dioxide combining power

    E. Calculate the anion gap: $(Na + K) - [(Cl) + (HCO_3) + 17] = 3$ or less

    F. Monitor lactate levels

RATIONALE

The priorities of the nursing assessment upon initial contact with the patient is to assess the respiratory and cardiovascular systems. The primary evaluation will detect any airway obstruction, respiratory distress, and presence of cardiovascular collapse. The patient in DKA does present as an acutely ill patient and at times, basic life support measures may be required. The rapid initial assessment may also provide clues to the precipitating factors or concomitant problems the patient may have (i.e., cardiac dysrhythmias, fever, hypotension, Kussmaul respirations, acetone breath). These patients do not always present as comatosed but do appear rather lethargic and confused. The level of consciousness on admission and during treatment gives clues to cerebral perfusion. Quite commonly the tendon reflexes are depressed.

    Once the primary considerations have been assured, a general systems survey is completed and historic data collection is begun, if possible, to form a working hypothesis of the presenting problem and establish the urgency of the condition. The nurse notes a significant degree of dehydration as clinically manifested by flushed, dry skin with poor turgor, soft eyeballs, dry mucous membranes, low blood pressure, thirst, and tachycardia. A reliable measure of hydration is urinary output.

    Patients who present with abdominal distension and/or vomiting should have a nasogastric tube passed. This relieves the distension by decompressing the stomach. It also eliminates the threat of aspiration.

    The presence of conditions that might have led to DKA should be identified. Urinary retention and cystitis are seen with DKA. An indwelling catheter might be prescribed for the patient who is unable to void or who presents in coma. An accurate record of output is vital to the successful management of this patient.

    Although ketoacidosis is not restricted to diabetics, it most commonly occurs to them. Thus the nurse should search for a history of diabetes; how it has been managed and what events could have evoked the state of ketoacidosis. The time of onset is significant because ketoacidosis develops over a period of time whereas hypoglycemic reactions occur suddenly. Ketoacidosis can be evoked by respiratory, gastrointestinal, or urinary tract infections as well as by stress, trauma, and vascular thrombosis, but most commonly it is caused by ignorance and/or neglect of insulin or dietary regimens. A fingerstick glucose determination quickly establishes the presence or absence of hyperglycemia.

The laboratory data verifies the clinical impression of DKA and identifies concurrent medical problems. The most immediate tests are serum glucose, acetone dilutions, electrolytes, BUN, creatinine, RBC, ESR, WBC, arterial blood gases, ECG, and chest x-ray. Depending upon the patient's condition and history, other tests might be ordered such as serum amylase, toxicology screen, pyruvate levels, and type and crossmatch. If the patient is febrile or comatosed, its cause must be detected and the blood, urine, throat, and stool samples must be cultured. At times a lumbar puncture is indicated.

The initial test results indicate a severe hyperglycemia when they are in the range of 400 to 800 mg. Sodium and potassium concentrations may be low but usually appear normal, however, a total body deficit of these ions does exist. The serum phosphate may be normal on admission but it generally falls during treatment. The hematocrit is elevated because of hemoconcentration. A leukocytosis is commonly seen. Arterial blood gases reveal a low pH indicating acidosis, an unremarkable P_{O_2}, a low P_{CO_2}, and HCO_3. The carbon dioxide combining power, arterial carbon dioxide and bicarbonate levels are low because of the hyperventilation that occurs as a compensatory mechanism and they reflect the decrease in the body's alkali. The ketone determinations of the blood and urine may appear as though very little ketones are present.

Ketosis is associated with the accumulation of ketone bodies: acetoacetate (AcAc), β-hydroxybutyrate (BOHB), and acetone. Clinically it is important to roughly estimate the contribution of ketones to the acidosis. Normally, the ratio of BOHB:AcAc is 3:1 but can rise to 6 to 12:1 in DKA. As a rule of thumb it is at least 6:1 when the pH is below 7.1. In many facilities quantitative plasma ketone levels may not be routinely available or their results delayed, therefore the emergency department staff relies on the qualitative tests using the nitroprusside reaction.

The nitroprusside reaction using the Acetest tablet can be very misleading. It primarily reacts with AcAc and very weakly with acetone. It does not react with BOHB. Thus, in patients with DKA, a negative trace or weakly positive reaction may lead one to underestimate the severity of the ketosis present. Likewise, during therapy as the BOHB is reoxidized to AcAc, strongly positive results could lead one to believe the condition is worsening. In addition, the build up of lactic acid blocks the conversion of BOHB to AcAc.

There is a technique for measuring ketones at the bedside which does use the nitroprusside tablet. The Acetest tablet must be crushed into a powder because it is intended to be used with urine and has a water-permeable coating that is impermeable to fluid containing protein such as plasma. A drop of the patient's serum is placed on the powder. If a positive reaction occurs, the serum must be diluted. First with an equal volume of water (i.e., 5 drops of water to 5 drops of serum) to produce a 1:2 dilution. Further dilutions are obtained by taking samples of this 1:2 serum dilution and adding equal volumes of water. At each dilution, test for a reaction. The process continues until a negative reaction occurs.

To estimate the AcAc concentration, multiply the highest positive dilution by 0.1 mM. Because the normal BOHB:AcAc ratio is 3:1, multiply the results obtained by 3 to get an estimate of the BOHB. For example, in a patient whose pH is not below 7.1

1. Reaction last positive at a dilution of 1:32
2. $32 \times 0.1 = 3.2 =$ estimate of AcAc
3. $3.2 \times 3 = 9.6 =$ estimate of BOHB
4. Conclusions
   Ratio of BOHB:AcAc = 9.6:1
   Total ketones present is = 12.8

Two hourly serial dilutions are a reasonable index of progress in clearing the ketoacidosis. But remember that as the ketoacidosis clears, the BOHB:AcAc ratio changes because of an increase in AcAc which occurs from the loss of the hydrogen ion from the BOHB and its conversion to AcAc. The test may appear more positive. But in the face of a lowered serum glucose and an improved clinical picture, treatment should be continued.

If the total quantified ketones arrived at in this manner is equal to the anion gap, most of the acidosis is due to ketosis. If the anion gap is greater than the quantified ketones, an additional source should be considered to be contributing to the acidosis.

The anion gap provides an estimate of the unmeasured anions in the serum (i.e., phosphates, sulfates, proteinates). In the following formula used to calculate the anion gap, the number 17 approximates their contribution.

$$(Na + K) - [(Cl) + (HCO_3) + 17] = 3 \text{ or less}$$

The anion gap is clinically significant and is a useful tool to follow during treatment because it reflects biochemical recovery.

The serum osmolality is elevated in ketoacidosis and results from the loss of more water than electrolytes. It can be estimated by the following formula:

$$2(Na + K) + \frac{Glucose}{18} + \frac{BUN}{2.8} = mOsm \text{ (norm is 280 to 300 mOsm)}$$

A comprehensive flowsheet for careful record keeping is essential for managing this patient. The sequential recording of vital signs, fluids, laboratory values, and replacement therapy assists the staff in assessing the patient's responses to therapy and in making adjustments to the therapy.

Immediate fluid replacement is of primary concern once the diagnosis is confirmed to correct hypovolemia, hemoconcentration, and dehydration. Rapid rehydration of 1000 to 2000 ml might be prescribed the first 2 hours of therapy and then 500 ml/hour until the deficits are corrected. The initial fluid is usually isotonic saline (0.9 percent) solution or some physicians prefer one half saline (0.45 percent) because of its hypotonicity. If the serum sodium is above 155 mEq, a 0.45 percent solution should be used. When the serum glucose levels are reduced to a range between 250 and 300 mg, a 5 percent dextrose in saline solution is prescribed to avoid hypoglycemia and possible cerebral edema. The nurse should monitor the CVP (normal 6 to 12 cm water), intake and output, and blood pressure. The expected outcomes are a rise in CVP, systolic blood pressure, and an increase in urinary output.

The two dangers associated with rapid rehydration are fluid overload and cerebral edema. Clinical signs of overhydration are distended neck veins, bounding pulse, loud heart sounds, gallop rhythm, pulmonary edema, and CHF (especially in the elderly). Cerebral edema can (but rarely) result from the liberal use of fluids and insulin. The patient will be doing well and then suddenly lapse back into coma. The postulated cause of this event is related to sorbitol accumulations in the cerebral cells resulting in cellular hyperosmolality and subsequent drawing of fluid into the brain's cells. The edematous brainstem then herniates into the foramen magnum resulting in coma and death.

Replacement of lost electrolytes is another significant aspect of managing the patient in ketoacidosis. The sodium and chloride ions are replaced by the early administration of saline solutions. Hyper- and hyponatremia are avoided by the frequent monitoring of the serum levels.

Potassium replacement deserves special consideration and is carried out cautiously to avoid the hazard of either hypo- or hyperkalemia. If the potassium level is normal or elevated on admission, some physicians wait until it falls before treating. If the potassium level is low on admission, potassium is administered immediately, usually 20 to 40 mEq/L. Some physicians give 20 mEq/L until the laboratory reports of the serum levels are back and if there is a urine output of at least 30 ml/hour. Potassium levels fall during therapy. As the patient is rehydrated, given insulin, and the acidosis clears, potassium shifts from the extracellular space back into the intracellular space. Frequent serum potassium determinations (every 1 to 2 hours) are the best guide to prescribing the amount of replacement. A 12-lead electrocardiogram will pick up subtle clues of hypo- or hyperkalemia. Potassium is given intravenously as potassium chloride and added to the saline solution. As the patient recovers, it may be given orally.

During the treatment of DKA, the phosphate ion also shifts back to the intracellular space resulting in a deficit (level below 1 mEq/L) in the blood. In order for the red blood cell to accept and release oxygen, it requires the substance 2,3 diphosphoglycerate (2,3 DPG). If the red blood cell levels of 2,3 DPG are low, the hemoglobin preferentially binds to whatever is present and markedly lowers its own affinity for oxygen. The blood delivered to the body tissues therefore does not release its oxygen readily and the stage is set for anaerobic metabolism which results in the production of lactic acid and a superimposed lactic acidosis. The phosphate ion is usually replaced as potassium phosphate, 40 to 60 mEq/L and is alternated with potassium chloride in the intravenous fluid. It may also be given orally. But it needs to be replaced early in the course of management.

The goal of insulin administration is to reduce the serum glucose and inhibit ketogenesis. The exact amount of insulin is determined by the clinical picture, serum glucose level, and the method of administration.

One method is to deliver a large dose of insulin by intravenous bolus (usually no more than 50 U/minute) followed by intermittent subcutaneous or intramuscular injections every 1 to 2 hours. This system has been questioned because the subcutaneous or intramuscular absorption rate is quite variable and unpredictable especially in a dehydrated acidotic patient. The danger exists that large depots of insulin will collect in poorly perfused tissue only to be suddenly released when perfusion improves resulting in precipitous falls in glucose levels and potassium. However, it is a time honored approach to insulin administration for ketoacidosis.

Another method of insulin delivery is to administer continuous low doses intravenously. Advocates of this system feel that this method is more physiologic and negates the absorption variables. Because insulin has a biological half-life of 10 minutes, the blood glucose changes can be estimated fairly accurately and thus avoid precipitous hypoglycemia and cerebral edema. One of the problems associated with continuous infusions of insulin is its tendency to bind to the delivery system (bag, bottle, filters, tubing). Almost 20 to 30 percent of the insulin dose can be lost this way. Some physicians coat the entire delivery system with 3 to 5 ml of a 25 percent albumin solution, others prime the delivery system to saturate it with insulin, and still others calculate for this loss when prescribing dosage. When giving insulin intravenously, the nurse must be certain that the prescribed rate of flow is accurate to insure that the amount of insulin prescribed is, in fact, delivered. Infusion pumps are needed and a piggy-back system is used. Although this approach of continuous intravenous low doses of insulin is gaining wide acceptance, it does not appear to be effective for the insulin resistant patient.

Insulin resistance develops because of circulating antibodies that counteract the effects of insulin. These patients require thousands of units of insulin before the desired effects are seen. At these doses, the antibodies are thoroughly saturated and the remaining insulin can perform its functions. Hydrocortisone (100 to 200 mg), intravenously, has been used to decrease the antibody response in some patients.

Regardless of the method of administration, serum glucose monitoring every 30 to 60 minutes and urine testing for glucosuria is required of all patients receiving insulin. The nurse would use the 2-drop Clinitest tablet, if the urine glucose is 4^+ (2 percent) when the usual 5-drop Clinitest tablet is used. The urine testing for glucose is not always a reliable indicator of the serum level and has come under some dispute as a valid test. It is commonly recognized that the renal threshold varies widely in individuals thus a patient may have a 400 mg blood glucose but be negative for sugar in the urine.

Hypoglycemia is a potential problem with all patients receiving insulin. The nurse should be aware of the epinephrine response that hypoglycemia induces (see Chapter on Hypoglycemia) and report these findings to the physician. It is common to see a rebound hypoglycemia approximately 4 hours after recovery.

The replacement of the body's alkali reserve is of immediate concern only if the patient is in shock, has a cardiac problem, or the serum pH is below 7.1. In these cases, two ampules of sodium bicarbonate (80 to 100 mEq) are added to the first liter of saline. Overtreatment with bicarbonate can lead to deactivation of insulin, hypokalemia, cerebrospinal fluid acidosis, and an impaired oxygen–hemoglobin dissociation. The nurse would closely monitor the blood gases, serum pH, bicarbonate level, and/or carbon dioxide combining power. The acidosis corrects itself after the patient has been rehydrated and received insulin.

If the patient has been treated fairly early in the ketoacidotic state and is fairly healthy, an uneventful recovery should be seen in 8 to 24 hours. It is the duty of the staff to educate the patient about diabetes and follow-up care must be planned for. However, if complications such as a myocardial infarction, CVA, or sepsis have occurred, further hospitalization is needed.

HYPEROSMOLAR HYPERGLYCEMIC NONKETOTIC SYNDROME

PATHOPHYSIOLOGY

Hyperosmolar syndrome is a sympton complex that occurs more often to people in their middle to later years of life. The patient may be a mild, type II noninsulin dependent diabetic or may not be a known diabetic. The syndrome occurs over a period of time and in most patients a prodromal phase of polyuria, polydipsia, and polyphagia is present for several days or weeks prior to emergency care. On arrival, the patient is commonly quite stuporous or unconscious.

The distinguishing features of hyperosmolar syndrome are profound hyperglycemia, severe hyperosmolarity of the intravascular fluid, and a striking dehydration in the face of minimal lactate or ketone elevations. In addition, these patients typically have underlying renal, cardiovascular, and cerebral impairments which may have precipitated the crisis and must be considered in the management of this problem. Reported mortality rates range from 40 to 70 percent during the first 24 hours of care, thus, prompt diagnosis and treatment are crucial to survival.

The profound hyperglycemia associated with hyperosmolar syndrome ranges between 600 and 1000 mg/100 ml but can rise as high as 2000 mg. It is caused by a relative lack of insulin or a defect in insulin's activity. The type II noninsulin dependent diabetic has some insulin but its release and activity are disturbed. Although the exact cause or causes for this deficit remain obscure, the following theories have been postulated. Some researchers believe that a primary problem exists in the pancreatic glucoreceptors resulting in a decreased or an abnormal amount of insulin released in response to a glucose load. Others believe that the relative insulin deficiency, especially in the genetically susceptible, obese patient, is probably related to excessive secretory demands made upon the pancreas leading to the eventual inability of the β cells to respond to a glucose load. Still others attribute the hyperglycemia to a cellular insulin resistance because they found the levels of circulating insulin to be adequate but the number of cellular insulin binding sites decreased in the obese patient.

The results of this basal lack of insulin or its inefficiency are exaggerated under conditions in which the body requires more energy. Thus, it is common for hyperosmolar syndrome to accompany or be precipitated by acute illnesses such as pneumonia, MI, CVA, pyelonephritis, and trauma. In addition, it may be iatrogenically induced by medical procedures that involve the use of hyperosmolar glucose or protein solutions such as those used during peritoneal dialysis, total parenteral nutrition, and nasogastric tube feedings. Furthermore, the administration of drugs that inhibit the peripheral activity of insulin (i.e., corticosteroids), or drugs that impair insulin's response (i.e., thiazide diuretics, diphenylhydantoin, furosemide, propanolol, alcohol) could be implicated as contributing to the hyperglycemia. Thus, it is apparent that these patients cannot produce enough biologically active insulin in the face of increased demands.

Without enough insulin, glucose cannot be transported into the body's cells in sufficient quantities, and it accumulates in the blood. The liver responds as if the body were fasting and it increases its rate of glycogenolysis, which only adds to the hyperglycemia. However, secretions of the other glucogenic hormones (i.e., cortisol and growth hormone) are not as pronounced in this syndrome as they are in diabetic ketoacidosis. The patient does experience hunger in the early phase of this syndrome and eats more, polyphagia, if possible.

The severe hyperglycemia creates a hyperosmolar state in the vascular fluid compartment. In the normal state, sodium, as the primary extracellular ion, is the chief determinant of the extracellular fluid osmolarity. An exception occurs in hyperosmolar syndrome because glucose molecules and not sodium ions make up a greater portion of the serum solute load. The hyperosmolarity created by the glucose (and in some cases, sodium) favors the movement of water from the intracellular and interstitial spaces into the intravascular space in an attempt to equalize osmotic pressure. However, more water is lost in the urine than solute, resulting in the retention of glucose and other nitrogenous substances. In addition, glomerular filtration rate decreases as hyperosmolarity increases resulting in severe dehydration.

Dehydration and hyperosmolarity lead to central nervous system disturbances. At osmolarity levels above 310 mOsm/L, the patient manifests signs of confusion and stupor. At levels above 350 mOm/L, coma is likely to occur. Other central nervous system symptoms seen in these patients include hallucinations, vestibular disturbances, hemiparesis, unilateral hyperreflexia, and focal motor seizures. The patient in hyperosmolar coma is most commonly misdiagnosed as a CVA.

Hyperglycemia causes an osmotic diuresis and leads to dehydration from such tremendous fluid losses. Because the blood concentration of glucose exceeds the kidney's tubular reabsorptive capacity, glucose spills over into the urine. Glucosuria usually occurs at a blood glucose of 170 to 180 mg/100 ml but in some patients with a high renal threshold, the blood sugar must be higher before sugar is detected in the urine. The excretion of glucose results in an obligatory water loss.

The body usually responds to this fluid loss by initiating the thirst mechanism.

If possible, the patient drinks more, polydipsia. However, this response is not as acute in the elderly and if the patient has physical and/or cerebral impairments, the ability to increase fluid intake is limited. Hypovolemic shock can result.

Polyuria, a response to the osmolar load, results in the excretion of an isotonic urine and loss of electrolytes. Sodium, potassium, chloride, and other ions are washed out as they are diluted in the tubular filtrate. Hyperglycemia can produce an artificial hyponatremia because for every 100 mg/100 ml rise in the serum glucose above the normal, there is a decrease of 1.6 mEq/L in the serum sodium levels. Thus, although the reported serum electrolyte values vary from low to normal to high, patients in hyperosmolar syndrome have some total body loss of these ions.

A certain amount of renal impairment exists in patients who present with hyperosmolar syndrome. Nearly all patients have an elevated BUN (60 to 90 mg range) but are not in uremia. This azotemia can be related to prerenal conditions such as dehydration or existing renal pathology. As part of the normal aging process, the kidney looses some of its functioning nephrons and its ability to concentrate the urine. In addition, the kidney tubule is less sensitive to the action of ADH. Thus, the resulting renal impairments exaggerate the hyperglycemia and hyperosmolar conditions seen in these patients.

Hyperosmolar syndrome patients are generally only mildly acidotic. The absence of ketosis distinguishes this syndrome from diabetic ketoacidosis. The precise explanation for this lack of ketosis waits further study but the following hypotheses have been offered. Ketosis does not occur because adipose tissue needs less insulin to inhibit fatty acid release than it requires for glucose uptake. The small amount of insulin present appears to be sufficient to inhibit ketogenesis. Others theorize that the profound hyperglycemia may cause some glucose to enter cells by a mass action type of mechanism and thereby eliminate the need for fatty acid release. Others propose that the lack of ketosis is related to the lower levels of lipolytic factors (i.e., cortisol, growth hormone) found in these patients or that the severe dehydration might act as an antiketogenic force.

If a greater degree of acidosis is present, the possibility of lactic acidosis or ketoacidosis should be ruled out because it is possible for diabetic ketoacidosis and/or lactic acidosis to overlap hyperosmolar syndrome. Once these processes are excluded, other common causes of acidosis such as excessive intake of salicylates, methanol, paraldehyde, chloral hydrate, and ethylene glycol should be considered.

The reader is directed to review the materials in this chapter on normal glucose metabolism and diabetic ketoacidosis because the principles of physiology and pathophysiology are valid for hyperosmolar syndrome and should help to amplify understanding.

MANAGEMENT

I. Determine the status of the airway, breathing, and circulation
   A. Visually assess the patency of the airway; if necessary, suction, assist with intubation and support ventilation

    B. Record the respiratory rate and pattern
        1. chart the rate, pattern and use of accessory muscles
        2. note any odor to the breath
    C. Record the temperature, pulse and bp
        1. report pyrexia, tachycardia, hypotension and/or signs of cardiac arrhythmias
    D. Evaluate neurologic status
        1. chart the level of consciousness; pupillary responses; motor and sensory responses
        2. note any hemiparesis, hyperreflexia and/or seizure activity
II. Complete the systems survey and collect a history
    A. Estimate changes in hydration
        1. note the skin turgor, condition of the mucous membranes, eyeball pressure; history of thirst and/or polyuria
    B. Detect changes in gastrointestinal functioning
        1. chart the presence or history of vomiting, diarrhea
        2. palpate the abdomen; note any tenderness or distention
        3. auscultate for bowel sounds; note their presence or absence. If abdomen is distended, pass a nasogastric tube
    C. Identify changes in the excretory system
        1. palpate the urinary bladder; if distended, pass a catheter
        2. chart any complaints of urgency, frequency or polyuria
        3. collect a urine specimen for analysis. If patient is unconscious, pass an indwelling catheter
III. Consider conditions that could have precipitated this crisis
    A. Establish the events leading up to the current situation
        1. note treatment for recent or chronic medical–surgical problems
        2. note any unusual medical–surgical therapies patient has received
        3. interview family, nursing home personnel, if patient unconscious
    B. Determine the presence of diabetes mellitus
        1. if patient unable to respond, search personal belongings for medical identification; check with family, friends
        2. if patient is diabetic, how is it managed and does patient comply with regimen?
IV. Verify the hypothesis of hyperosmolar syndrome and screen for concurrent illnesses
    A. Draw bloods for the following
        1. glucose
        2. electrolytes
        3. BUN
        4. creatinine
        5. ketones
        6. osmolarity
        7. RBC, Hct, Hgb
        8. WBC and differential

9. Blood gases
    a. pH
    b. P_{CO_2}
    c. P_{O_2}
B. If patient is unconscious and/or febrile: culture blood, sputum, throat, urine and stool. Perform a toxicology screen
C. Obtain a stat ECG and chest x-ray
D. Estimate serum osmolarity, if patient appears dehydrated

$$2(Na^+ + K^+) + \frac{Glucose}{18} + \frac{BUN}{2.8}$$

E. Insert a CVP line
F. Initiate a flowsheet wherein the following data is recorded: time, LOC, VS, I&O, laboratory data, therapy given

V. Restore the intravascular fluid losses
A. Administer IV solutions as ordered (6 to 16 liters in 24 hours)
    1. initial solution may be 0.9 percent saline (approximately 2 to 3 liters) until hypotension is abolished
    2. 0.45 percent saline may follow or may be used instead of the above
    3. exact volume and rate of administration is determined by the clinical state of the patient
B. Take the vital signs q 15 to 30 minutes; report all changes
C. Record all I&O; report deficits and excesses
D. Record CVP q 1 hour; report readings outside the normal of 6 to 12 cm
E. Chart the specific gravity of the urine
F. Observe for overhydration: distended neck veins, bounding pulse, pulmonary friction rub or rales, galloping rhythm
G. Observe for cerebral edema: patient awakens from coma and then slips back into coma
H. Be prepared to administer volume expanders, if hypovolemic shock is present

VI. Correct the hyperglycemia gradually
A. Administer regular crystalline insulin as prescribed
    1. may be ordered IV, subcutaneously or IM
    2. initial doses may be small for the patient who has never taken insulin (10 to 30 units) or somewhat higher in those dependent on insulin (25 to 50 units)
B. If insulin is prescribed intravenously
    1. give no more than 50 U over 1 minute via bolus technique
    2. be aware that insulin binds to bottles, bags, tubing, filters and this loss must be corrected
    3. check pumps to insure proper delivery rate
    4. do not mix insulin with sodium bicarbonate solution
C. Monitor serum glucose levels q 30 to 60 minutes
    1. report readings that fall below 300 mg

   D. Monitor urine levels of glucose and acetone q 30 to 60 minutes
      1. use only fresh specimens
      2. use the 2-drop Clinitest method, if a 4^+(2 percent) level is read using the 5-drop method
      3. notify physician of any changes
   E. Observe patient for hypoglycemia: excitability, palpitations, tremors, dilated pupils, tachycardia
   F. Observe patient for cerebral edema
VII. Correct the electrolyte losses
   A. Sodium: sodium and chloride ions are replaced immediately via the IV solutions of normal saline
      1. monitor serum sodium levels frequently
      2. report any increase or dramatic drop in levels
      3. assess the patient for signs of hyponatremia: abdominal cramps, diarrhea, diaphoresis, tachycardia, apprehension, cyanosis, seizures
   B. Potassium: replacement not as urgent and considered after hydration has abolished the hypotension and adequate renal functioning is present
      1. KCl (10 to 20 mEq/L) IV may be prescribed (or potassium phosphate)
      2. monitor serum potassium levels—continuous cardiac monitoring
      3. recognize signs of hypokalemia: muscle weakness, decreased peristalsis, hypotension, weak pulse, ECG changes (prolonged QT interval, depressed T wave and U wave), respiratory arrest
      4. recognize the signs of hyperkalemia: ECG changes (heart block, ventricular fibrillation, cardiac arrest, peaked T wave, no P wave and a wide QRS interval)
      5. once patient is alert and bowel sounds are heard, fluids high in potassium may be offered orally
VIII. Observe the responses of other body systems to treatment
   A. Monitor the pulmonary status
      1. auscultate lungs frequently, suction prn, note results of chest x-ray
      2. check the results of blood gases determination; administer oxygen, if needed
   B. Monitor neurologic status
      1. chart neurologic vital signs every 30 to 60 minutes
      2. report changes in level of consciousness, cranial nerve responses, and motor/sensory responses
   C. Monitor body defense systems
      1. observe for signs of infection, take temperature q 2 hours, note the integrity of the skin
      2. be prepared to administer antibiotics, if needed
   D. Monitor gastrointestinal functioning
      1. auscultate bowel sounds q 2 hours; chart I&O hourly
      2. offer mouth care, frequently
   E. Monitor urinary functioning
      1. give catheter care q 4 hours, if catheter used

2. note the color, consistency, and amount of output
3. check urinalysis report

RATIONALE

Any delay in the diagnosis of hyperosmolar syndrome can prove fatal and yet the syndrome is frequently overlooked or misdiagnosed. Often these patients are brought into the emergency department because they cannot be aroused and appear to have suffered a CVA. Because many do arrive unconscious, airway, breathing, circulation, and neurologic status must be rapidly assessed and life support measures initiated, if necessary.

The patient's vital signs are important indicators and changes in body functioning are reflected as deviations from the normal. The patient with hyperosmolar syndrome is hypovolemic because of the water losses associated with this condition. These losses are reflected as hypotension and a compensatory tachycardia which is the heart's response to a lowered intravascular volume. Tachypnea may happen but a Kussmaul breathing pattern occurs only if overlapping diabetic ketoacidosis and/or lactic acidosis is present. The breath does not smell of acetone, because ketoacidosis is usually not a part of this problem. The patient's temperature could be elevated.

The most apparent physical findings are those related to the dehydrated state: dry skin, parched tongue and mucous membranes, soft eyeball pressure, and cerebral changes. Gastrointestinal signs are probably related to the fluid and electrolyte losses. Symptoms range from vomiting, diarrhea, abdominal tenderness, to an absence of bowel sounds. Passing a nasogastric tube and attaching it to low intermittent suctioning relieves distention, prevents vomiting, and possible aspiration.

Clinical observations of dehydration should be supplemented by accurate measurements of urine output and venous pressure. The volume of urine output is a reliable indicator of tissue perfusion and an output below 40 to 60 ml/hour is evidence of inadequate renal perfusion. The patient should exhibit a high urine output resulting from the glucosuria induced diuresis unless in hypovolemic shock. Blood and urine specimens need to be tested frequently for sugar and acetone. The nurse would expect 4^+(2 percent) glucosuria, but negative to mild ketone readings are also seen. An unconscious patient may experience urinary retention which can be detected by palpation. Permanent damage to the urinary bladder can result from overdistension and it is wise to pass a urinary catheter in these cases with gradual emptying of the urinary bladder, 500 to 750 ml at a time. The central venous pressure reading is a relatively simple procedure to perform and it yields important data about the amount of fluid entering the right heart and the ability of the right heart to pump this fluid to the lungs. The normal CVP is 6 to 12 cm water. The measurements of urine output and CVP are continued throughout the management of this patient and serve as useful indicators of recovery.

There are so many acute or chronic conditions, medical therapies, and drugs that can precipitate or accompany hyperosmolar syndrome that a good history and laboratory data are vital to support the diagnosis. The nurse plays an important role in not only eliciting the past health history from persons who accompany the patient to the emergency department but also in identifying the events leading up to this crisis. Generally, the patient is somewhat elderly and has been ill for a period of time. He or she most likely has a history of diabetes which has been controlled with diet or hypoglycemic agents but this may also be the first time that a diabetic condition appears. It is also important for the nurse to ascertain the presence of current stressful situations in the patient's life that may have precipitated the problem. If the patient is unconscious, a fingerstick glucose determination rules out coma due to a hypoglycemic reaction.

The laboratory data verifies the hypothesis of a hyperosmolar syndrome. A severely elevated serum glucose without an elevation in serum ketones plus a high degree of glucosuria should lead the staff to consider hyperosmolar syndrome. However, the severity of the osmolarity awaits the laboratory glucose, electrolytes, and BUN results. A serum osmolarity above 350 mOsm/L is not uncommon. The patient with pure hyperosmolar syndrome is not acidotic but may exhibit a slight fall in pH to around 7.26 and a likewise fall in serum bicarbonate. The anion gap will be relatively normal.

The serum electrolyte picture may vary widely. Cations and anions are lost in the osmotic diuresis, but the water imbalance may cause the serum levels to be low, normal, or high. The serum sodium may appear unusually high but this may be a factitious event due to the hyperglycemia. As a general rule, there is some loss of total body stores of sodium and potassium. The 12-lead ECG may reflect hypokalemic changes.

Other laboratory tests are helpful in assessing the total picture of this patient. BUN is generally elevated indicating some degree of azotemia. Hematocrit is elevated due to hemoconcentration and a leukocytosis will be evident. In the face of pyrexia and leukocytosis, body fluids and excreta need to be cultured to identify the offending organism.

The restoration of fluid balance is of prime importance in managing hyperosmolar syndrome because these patients can lose as much as 20 percent of their total body water. Although a controversy exists as to the relative merits of hypotonic versus isotonic fluid replacement, the nurse should expect to administer either a 0.9 percent or 0.45 percent saline solution. The administration of 1 to 2 liters of a 0.9 percent saline solution restores the blood volume and pressure and the 0.45 percent saline solution restores the free water thereby correcting the osmolarity. The exact amount of fluid volume given and its rate of administration are determined by the patient's clinical condition. It is not uncommon to see large volumes prescribed during the first few hours of therapy. If the patient exhibits hypovolemic shock or vascular collapse, plasma expanders may be administered before the saline solution.

The administration of large volumes of fluid to an elderly patient with cardiovascular and/or renal impairments must be done judiciously to avoid fluid overload. Thus, the patient's responses must be monitored very frequently which means that serum osmolarity, blood pressure, urine output, CVP, and urine specific gravity results must be done every 15 to 30 minutes, charted and reported. The nurse should further observe the patient for signs of overhydration which include noting any distension of the neck veins, bounding pulse, pulmonary edema, and galloping heart rhythm.

Rapid rehydration can lead to cerebral edema. In diabetics, abnormal amounts of glucose are converted to sorbitol by the action of an enzyme, aldose reductase. Sorbitol, it is believed, moves into vulnerable cells of the central nervous system and accumulate. Sorbitol remains in these cells despite rehydration because it does not easily cross the cell's membrane. It exerts an osmotic pull and draws water into these cells resulting in cerebral edema.

Most patients in hyperosmolar syndrome require insulin to reduce their hyperglycemia and thus restore normal energy metabolism. However, because ketosis is not usually present, large insulin doses are not required. Rather, small doses are ordered, especially if the patient has never received insulin before. These patients exhibit a sensitivity to exogenous insulin. Falling blood glucose levels have been observed with rehydration alone, thus obviating the need for insulin.

If prescribed, insulin can be administered by any parenteral route. The intravenous route is most common because the response is immediate. Because the biological half-life of intravenous insulin is 10 minutes and glucose levels fall at 70 to 100 mg/hour, accurate predictions in blood glucose levels can be made. The insulin may be prescribed to be given by bolus or continuous low-dose infusion. The nurse should remember that insulin binds to bags, bottles, tubing, and filters used in intravenous apparatus and that this loss must be calculated in the prescribing dose. The nurse should frequently test the urine and blood for glucose levels to monitor the patient's response to rehydration and insulin administration.

Hypoglycemia can result from rehydration and insulin administration. The nurse should report when the blood glucose levels fall below 300 mg and observe the patient for signs of hypoglycemia: excitability, perspiration, tremors, tachycardia, dilated pupils, and fall in blood pressure. However, these sympathetic nervous system responses may be diminished in the patient who has had diabetes for a long time. If hypoglycemia does occur, a 5 percent intravenous glucose solution should be ordered to reverse the process.

Electrolyte losses are replaced to restore a normal serum concentration and thus promote proper ionic functioning. Sodium and chloride ions are replaced by way of the saline solutions administered early in the management of these patients. The nurse should be monitoring the serum sodium and chloride levels frequently and observing the patient for signs of hyponatremia. Potassium replacement is usually delayed until the rehydration and insulin maneuvers have shifted potassium back into the cells and only if adequate renal functioning is present. Potassium chloride and phosphate can be added to the infusions. The nurse should observe the patient for signs of hypokalemia: muscle weakness, weak pulse, ileus, or distention. ECG monitoring indicates a prolonged QT interval, a depressed T wave and U wave, if the patient is hypokalemic. On the other hand, hyperkalemia is manifested by these ECG changes: peaked T waves, absence of a P wave, and a wide QRS interval.

Many patients with hyperosmolar syndrome have a secondary underlying disorder that precipitates and accompanies this syndrome. The nurse is in a unique position to assist the physician in identifying these secondary factors by closely monitoring the patient's responses to therapy as well as detecting clues of disruptions in other body systems. Thus, the proper treatment of hyperosmolar syndrome includes not only rectifying the primary disorder but also correcting secondary disruptions that contributed to the problem.

2. Disorders of Thyroid Metabolism

ASSESSMENT

Refer to Table 17, on the following pages.

Maintaining Normal Thyroxine Levels

The biosynthesis and secretion of thyroid hormones usually follows a sequential pattern and involves enzymatic regulation throughout the process. The quantity of thyroid hormones produced is dependent upon an adequate supply of iodine which is found in foods such as enriched cereals, milk, seafood, iodized salt, eggs, and bread. It is also found in our water supplies and many medications such as lozenges, cough syrups, gargles, suntan lotions, vitamin–mineral preparations, amebiacides, vaginal and anal suppositories, and x-ray contrast preparations. There are some inland areas of the world where the soil is iodine deficient resulting in an increased incidence of goiter in these regions.

Ingested iodine is converted to iodide in the upper portions of the gastrointestinal tract and absorbed there. The thyroid clears the blood of this iodide very rapidly. The usual thyroid to plasma iodide concentration is 25:1. The thyroid apparently has a "trapping" mechanism for iodide and because iodide is transported into the thyroid against an electrical gradient, an "iodide pump" is believed to exist. Anions, such as perchlorate and thiocyanate, which are found in many foods, inhibit this pump resulting in the thyroid's inability to concentrate iodide. Other tissues, such as the salivary glands, lining of the stomach, mammary glands, and placenta are also capable of concentrating iodide. The kidney passively removes iodide from the blood whereas thyrotrophic stimulating hormone (TSH) actively increases the iodide pump.

In the thyroid gland, iodide is converted to free iodine which is able to enter into organic combination. The conversion of iodide to iodine is accelerated by various oxidizing enzymes such as perioxidase found in thyroid colloid. Thiouracil drugs depress the activity of perioxidase. Oxidized iodine spontaneously reacts with tyrosyl radicals in the thyroglobulin molecule and through a series of reactions, monoiodotyrosine and diodotyrosine are produced. Pituitary TSH enhances the iodination of tyrosine whereas propylthiouracil, methimazole, goitrogens (such as cabbage, ru-

TABLE 17. THYROID IMBALANCES: ASSESSMENT FINDINGS

Parameter	Hypothyroidism and Myxedema Coma	Hyperthyroidism and Thyrotoxicosis
Age	Old to elderly	Young to middle age
LOC	Extreme lethargy to unconsciousness	Very alert, but could be disoriented and become comatose as condition progresses
Blood pressure	Hypotension	Systolic hypertension Wide pulse pressure initially Hypotension follows as condition worsens
Temperature	Below normal (75–90°F)	Above normal (100–103°F)
Pulse	Bradycardia	Tachycardia
Respirations	Very slow Dyspnea on exertion	Rapid with shortness of breath
Cardiogram	Wide, depressed or inverted T wave; prolonged QT interval	Sinus or tachyarrhythmias AV heart block
Psychologic status	Placid, apathetic but could exhibit signs of "myxedema madness"	Agitated, restless, nervous, labile moods

Systems Survey—Past and Present

Parameter	Hypothyroidism and Myxedema Coma	Hyperthyroidism and Thyrotoxicosis
Neuromuscular	Slowed mentation, forgetfulness Excessive fatigue, no energy Speech is slow, guttural Intolerance to cold Prolonged relaxation of deep tendon reflexes (Achilles tendon)	Overactive, excessive energy followed by fatigue Tremors present Speech is rapid, hoarse Intolerance to heat Increase in sweating Decreased relaxation of deep tendon reflexes (Achilles tendon)
Cardiovascular	Cardiac function depressed Myocardium weak and flabby Decreased output and rate Increased capillary fragility and anemias	Cardiac function increased Palpitations and hyperdynamic precordium Increase output and rate
Gastrointestinal	Weight gain, yet decrease in appetite Constipation, possibly ileus, abdominal distension Decreased bowel sounds Liver functioning may be depressed; carotemia and ascites do occur	Weight loss, yet increased appetite Frequent stools, diarrhea, abdominal pains Some nausea and vomiting Increased bowel sounds Liver frequently enlarged; at times mild jaundice
Eyes	Periorbital edema	Retraction of upper or lower lid, decreased blinking; exophthalmos

(continued)

TABLE 17. (Continued)

Parameter	Hypothyroidism and Myxedema Coma	Hyperthyroidism and Thyrotoxicosis
Skin	Dry, thick, boggy skin Swollen hands. Yellow discoloration. Bruises easily	Velvety smooth skin Cutaneous vasodilatation Palmar erythema, warm and moist
	Loss of total body hair Hair is coarse and brittle	Hair is thin, will not curl
Endocrine	Goiter possible	Goiter probable
	Menstrual irregularity	Menstrual irregularity
Laboratory Findings		
RAIU Norms 2 hours 5–10% 6 hours 10–20% 24 hours 20–40%	Low or normal	Usually increased but may vary with etiology Rate of uptake fast and peak is early
Serum T4 Norm 4–12 μg/dl	Below normal. Could be 1 μg/dl	Above normal. Could be as high as 15–25 μg/dl
Serum T3 Norm 110–200 ng/dl	Below normal	Above normal
TBG saturation (resin T3 uptake) Norm 25–35%	Low saturation Resin uptake low	High saturation Resin uptake high
TSH Levels Norm up to 10 mIU/ml	High in primary causes Low in secondary causes	Low except when pituitary tumor implicated
Serum chemistries Sodium	Low, could be below 120 mEq/L	No change
Cholesterol	Usually increased	Low to no change
Phospholipids	Usually increased	Low to no change
Triglycerides	Usually increased	Low to no change
Glucose	Usually low	No change
Enzymes	May be elevated	No change

tabagas, and white turnip), cobalt, phenylbutazone, and soybean-based infant formulas block this process. After a number of oxidative and coupling processes, thyroglobulin-bound triiodotyrosine (T3) and tetraiodotyrosine (T4, thyroxine) are formed.

The two thyroid hormones are stored as thyroglobulins until acted upon by proteases that free the hormones allowing them to diffuse out into the plasma. TSH accelerates this rate of proteolysis and release of thyroid hormone whereas the lithium ion blocks this release. Most of the hormone released is in the form of T4 and only a small quantity of T3 is released.

In the plasma, most of the T4 binds to thyroxine-binding globulin (TBG) and only a minute amount binds to albumin and prealbumin. There normally is only a very small quantity unbound or free in the plasma. There are many factors that alter the ability of thyroxine to bind to TBG. Illnesses and medications that decrease the binding of thyroxine to TBG include cirrhosis, nephrotic syndrome, corticosteroids, testosterone, salicylates, and dilantin. These situations increase the percentage of active free thyroid. Conversely, conditions that raise plasma protein levels increase the binding of thyroid to TBG and decrease the free levels of the hormone. Illnesses and drugs capable of this include infection, hepatitis in its early stage, acute porphyria, pregnancy, patients taking oral contraceptives, and estrogens.

Whereas freely circulating T4 determines the metabolic rate, T3 is much more active at the cellular level. In the liver, T4 can be converted to T3 and in fact, 80 percent of T3 production occurs in this manner. It has been found that large doses of steroids block the conversion of T4 to T3. Thyroxine can also be converted to inactive T3, which is then called reverse T3, under conditions of stress and/or starvation which probably functions to reduce the catabolic effects of thyroid hormone during these critically ill periods.

Thyroid hormones are chemically changed before excretion. The liver is an important site for the distribution as well as the metabolism of thyroid hormone. In the liver, thyroid hormones may be deiodinated, deaminated, decarboxylated, or conjugated with glucuronic acid or sulfate. Much of the biodegraded iodine is recycled and reused to synthesize new hormone. The remainder is excreted in the urine, bile, and feces.

The previous material has pointed out the many roles of TSH in the synthesis and release of thyroid hormones. In addition to these roles, TSH can increase the number, size, and secretory activity of thyroid cells. The level of TSH is controlled by a hypothalamic-releasing hormone called thyrotrophic-releasing hormone (TRH). In the normal individual, the amount of circulating T4 influences the hypothalamic center to release TRH which, in turn, directs the anterior pituitary to release TSH via a negative feedback mechanism. Thus, a fall in T4 levels leads to an increase in TRH and TSH release. The pituitary is very sensitive to increases in circulating thyroid hormones. In fact, the administration of exogenous thyroid preparations can completely block TSH release, even if TRH is administered.

Other psychophysiologic factors effect the release of thyroid hormones. Exposure to hypothermic conditions for a period of days, trauma, and emotional stress precipitate an increase in thyroxine output. Conversely, when a state of iodine excess exists, thyroid activity is reduced due to a decrease in the gland's vascularity. There appears to be an autoregulatory mechanism to maintain a constant store of the hormone.

Freely circulating thyroid hormones must enter the body's cells to perform their function. It is now accepted that thyroid is a polypeptide hormone and as such, reacts with receptor sites on the cell membrane. Here, this hormone-receptor molecule activates cell membrane-bound adenylcyclase which, in turn, catalyzes the conversion of adenosine triphosphate (ATP) to cyclic adenosine monophosphate (cAMP). cAMP in turn activates a protein enzyme which converts the inactive enzyme formed into an active enzyme. It is this active enzyme that carries out the primary functions of the thyroid hormone.

Thyroid hormones exert their physiologic action on all body tissues. The earliest discoveries focused on their ability to increase oxygen consumption and produce heat (calorigenic effect). The basic metabolic rate of all cells is accelerated under their influence, and as a result, the fetus matures normally. The bones and muscles of the child grow, the rate and utilization of carbohydrates and fat is accelerated, proteins are synthesized and catabolized at a faster rate, electrolytes are mobilized, pulmonary ventilation and cardiac output increase, plasma volume and bone marrow activity increase, gastrointestinal motility and glomerular filtration rate are accelerated, the liver becomes more active and the central nervous system matures and responds to stimuli.

MYXEDEMA COMA

PATHOPHYSIOLOGY

Hypothyroidism is a systemic disease resulting from the effects of too little thyroid hormone delivered to the body's tissues. It can range from a mild, chronic condition to an acute, florid state of coma and death. Myxedema coma is an extreme form of hypothyroidism which is most commonly seen in the elderly hypothyroid female during the winter months following some stressful event.

This condition can arise from primary or secondary causes. Primary hypothyroidism occurs when pathologic processes interfere with thyroxine synthesis and destroy thyroid tissue. The most common causes of hypothyroidism are iatrogenic. For example, it is relatively common to encounter this problem after radioactive iodine therapy or surgery to treat hyperthyroidism. Iodine excesses or deficiencies, antithyroid medications (i.e., propylthiouracil, methimazol), and lithium are substances that can lead to hypothyroidism. The administration of opiates, sedation, and tranquilizers have been known to precipitate a crisis state. The second most common cause is chronic lymphocytic (Hashimoto) thyroiditis and then sequentially, congenital thyroid hypoplasia or aplasia, inborn defects in the biosynthesis or action of thyroid hormone, and endemic cretinism. Secondary hypothyroidism is caused by a pituitary and/or hypothalamus disorder which results in insufficient amounts of TSH or TRH. Tumors of the pituitary region have been associated with this cause of hypothyroidism.

The clinical manifestations of the disease are related to the degree of pathology and are reflected as an overall diminution of metabolic processes. In the early stages, the diagnosis is difficult because of the vagueness and variability of the signs and symptoms but as the condition worsens, the diagnosis is usually more obvious. It must be noted however, that in the advanced stage of hypothyroidism, the patient rarely complains. Rather it is friends and family who become upset over the patient's deterioration.

Myxedema coma may occur gradually or spontaneously. It can be precipitated by exposure to cold, infection, water intoxication, trauma, CVA, severe angina, upper respiratory infection, and the administration of a narcotic or analgesic agent.

In the myxedematous state, progressive respiratory depression occurs and is a reflection of hypoventilation, the build-up of carbon dioxide and respiratory acidosis. Obesity and respiratory muscle myopathy contribute to the condition as do the pleural effusions that are commonly associated with this disease. A respiratory infection aggravates the situation and an upper airway obstruction must be searched for in the unconscious patient. The situation of alveolar hypoventilation, decreased maximum ventilatory volume and decreased vital capacity in myxedema coma necessitates prompt action on the part of the emergency department staff.

The cardiovascular effects of deficient thyroid hormone have far-reaching implications. The lack of thyroid hormone is reflected in a decreased rate and force of myocardial contractility resulting in bradycardia and a decreased stroke volume. On x-ray, the cardiac silhouette is enlarged and on echocardiogram, a pericardial effusion is observed in a significant number of patients. However, cardiac tamponade is rare, probably because of the slowed rate and force of myocardial contractions. The combination of decreased circulating blood volume and increased peripheral resistance leads to a noticeable reduction in cerebral, cutaneous, and renal blood flow. There is a high incidence of atherosclerosis and coronary artery disease associated with myxedema coma, and a history of angina is common. The major manifestations of cardiac problems in myxedema coma are severe bradycardia, distant heart sounds, and an ECG reading that depicts very low voltage, prolong QT intervals and a wide, depressed or inverted T wave. The slowed rate of the heart beat, the decrease in its output, and disturbances in its conduction play a major role in the development of hypotension, CHF, and general tissue hypoxia associated with myxedema.

The fluid, electrolyte, and nutritional imbalances associated with myxedema coma are related to a combination of gastrointestinal, endocrine, and urinary system changes. These patients have ascites and peripheral edema which is due to a collection of protein-rich mucinous material in the interstitial spaces that draws water to it. In addition hyponatremia and hypoglycemia are present. The origins of the hyponatremia and its accompanying water intoxication is not clear. It is most likely due to a dilutional situation but some believe that it could be due to inappropriate secretion of ADH, a change in the "set" of the osmoreceptors or perhaps a result of adrenal insufficiency. The hypoglycemia is clearly suggestive of adrenal insufficiency.

The gastrointestinal changes could result in acute processes. Decreased gastric emptying and motility of the bowel could result in nausea, vomiting, and abdominal distension. Constipation frequently accompanies this illness and paralytic ileus could occur to the patient in coma. The history reveals a reduction in appetite but a 10 to 20 pound or more weight gain. The tongue is enlarged which makes swallowing and talking somewhat difficult. There is an increase in the incidence of cholelithiasis which is a reflection of the poor lipid metabolism that exists with this disorder. Histologically, the bowel shows mucosal atrophy and infiltration with lymphocytes and protein-like mucinous material.

The hemopoietic symptoms are related to the reduced peripheral oxygen consumption. The body's bone marrow adapts by decreasing its production of red blood cells resulting in an overall anemia. A problem with vitamin B_{12} absorption in the stomach and intrinsic factor in the ileum would account for the B_{12} anemias seen in some patients. The decrease in tissue synthesis results in capillary fragility with easy bruising. These patients are extremely sensitive to normal doses of opiates, sedation, and tranquilizer and have very little resistance to infections which suggests depressed liver functioning. Infection is difficult to recognize because the typical symptoms of fever, tachycardia, sweating, and leukocytosis often do not develop.

The effects of thyroid deficiency on the skin and appendages are quite obvious. The accumulation of mucinous material in the interstitial space and tissues results in facial, periorbital, peripheral edema (usually nonpitting), and ascites. The skin pallor is a reflection of a thickened dermis, decreased blood flow, and anemia. A yellowish color suggests carotenemia wherein the depressed liver is not converting carotene to vitamin A. The decrease in sebaceous and sweat gland activity adds to the skin's dry, scaly appearance. There is a decrease in overall body hair growth, especially if a pituitary problem coexists.

The severely depressed metabolic state and inadequate production of thermal energy results in a very low core body temperature. These patients suffer from a long-standing intolerance to cold. Although the body temperature is far below the normal, shivering is not observed.

The neuromuscular symptoms of myxedema are most characteristic and are caused by the hypoglycemia and the cerebral hypoxia which follows a reduction of oxygenated blood flow to the brain. Early clinical signs are complacency, sluggishness, and inattentiveness, and these proceed to memory losses and the inability to maintain normal physical and mental activity. Sensory changes include hearing loss, paresthesias, and polyneuropathies. Motor changes include delayed Achilles tendon reflex time and a slowed, hesitant speech pattern. The voice is very hoarse and almost guttural. Grand mal seizures and/or cerebellar symptoms such as ataxic gait and hand clumsiness precede myxedema coma in 25 percent of all cases. At this stage of the illness, somnolence advances to coma.

The psychologic response to hypothyroidism is usually apathy and depression. However, there is a rare form of excitement called myxedema madness that may precede unconsciousness. In this state, the patient appears anxious and agitated. Paranoia, disorientation, and hallucinations may also be part of this picture. It can be appreciated that the appearance of these symptoms causes considerable confusion for the diagnostician.

Laboratory studies support and confirm the clinical impression of severe hypothyroidism, however, supportive therapy is usually begun before all of the test results are returned because the patient's condition is critical.

The best screening tests for hypothyroidism are the serum T4 and the free T4 index. The total concentration of T4 is precisely measured by radioimmunoassay techniques and is a good indicator of thyroid function. The results in this situation would be lower than the normal (4.5 to 11 g/100 ml). However, T4 is bound to a serum globulin (TBG) and anything that would alter TBG effects this test. Factors that do effect TBG levels are described in the opening remarks of this chapter.

Because current practices hold that the unbound or free fraction of T4 exerts the metabolic effect, it should be measured. This test does require special techniques. However, an index of free T4 can readily be obtained by measuring the relative saturation of the serum binding proteins with T4. In this test, it is necessary to measure the relative saturation of T4 binding proteins. To do this, it is more convenient to use radioactive T3 as an indicator of this saturation which has been attached to a resin (resin T3 uptake). The mean normal value for the resin T3 uptake is 32 percent, which would be lower in hypothyroid conditions. By itself, this value does not give a precise estimate of thyroid function but calculating the products of T4 and T3 uptake gives an acceptable estimate.

$$\text{Free thyroxine index} = \text{T4} \times \frac{\text{Patient's resin T3 uptake}}{\text{Control resin T3 uptake or 32}}$$

Primary hypothyroidism is also confirmed by an elevation in TSH levels because this hormone should rise even with mild reductions in thyroid hormone secretion. A low result in a hypothyroid patient indicates secondary hypothyroidism. This is another radioimmunoassay test and the average level does not go beyond 10 U/ml.

Serum T3 concentrations are frequently normal in mild hypothyroidism but are noticeably lower in the severe myxedema patient. However, systemic diseases also lower T3 levels thus rendering this test less useful than T4.

There are no accurate, sensitive tests of the metabolic effects of thyroid hormone and the following tests are very nonspecific. The Achilles tendon reflex time is slower in hypothyroid patients. The BMR is no longer clinically used because of the many artifacts that effect this test. The PBI has been superseded by direct measurements of T4 and T3. However, the hypothyroid patient will probably have anemia, hypercholesterolemia, elevated serum enzymes, and hypoglycemia. The hypercholesterolemia is most likely a primary disorder. The elevation in serum enzymes could be a reflection of skeletal muscle breakdown.

MANAGEMENT

   I. Obtain a history
      A. Interview the patient, family, and friends
      B. Search for previous events that could have precipitated the problem: exposure to cold, thyroid surgery, thyroid radiation, ingestion of antithyroid medications, lithium, opiates, sedatives or tranquilizers. Inquire if patient has undergone diagnostic tests in recent past
      C. Identify behaviors that immediately preceded hospitalization: presence of seizure activity, presence of unusual clumsiness or staggered gait, a change in mood from lethargy to anxiety
      D. Search for the presence of possible coexisting problems: MI, CHF, CVA, URI, trauma, hemorrhage
  II. Determine the status of the airway, breathing, and circulation
      A. Visually assess the patency of the airway
         Suction upper airway, if necessary

Assist with endotracheal intubation *or* prepare for tracheostomy

Support ventilation with mechanical devices and oxygen

   B. Record temperature, pulse and respirations

Take temperature with mechanical thermometer

Count pulse for 1 full minute

Chart the rate, depth and pattern of respirations

   C. Take bp

   D. Assess neurologic status

Note the level of consciousness, motor and sensory responses, and mental status, if possible

III. Perform a rapid systems survey in addition to above

   A. Cardiovascular: obtain a stat ECG; note any rhythm disturbance

Auscultate heart sounds: note any history of angina, dyspnea and/or edema

   B. Pulmonary: obtain a chest x-ray; auscultate the lungs, note the presence of rales or congestion

   C. Gastrointestinal: note any history of nausea, vomiting and/or constipation. Note if abdomen is distended. Auscultate the bowel sounds: note their presence or absence. Note past and current weight, time of last meal and last bowel movement

   D. Integumentary: inspect skin. Note color, temperature, turgor, periorbital edema, peripheral edema

   E. Endocrine: note the presence of a goiter

IV. Assist with diagnostic studies

   A. Obtain blood samples

     1. RBC: Hgb, Hct

     2. WBC and differential

     3. Serum electrolytes

     4. BUN, creatinine

     5. Serum lipids

     6. Serum enzymes

     7. Serum T4 levels

     8. Serum TSH levels

     9. Resin T3 uptake

     10. Cortisol levels

     11. Arterial blood gases

   B. Assist with stat ECG, chest x-ray, and possibly skull x-rays

   C. Collect a specimen of urine for analysis

V. Correct fluid and electrolyte imbalances

   A. If hypotension and hypovolemia are severe: start IV fluids and run very slowly, usually dextrose–saline solution

Monitor blood pressure response to fluids; measure I&O

If vasopressors are prescribed, doses are unusually small and they must be administered very, very slowly with frequent bp monitoring

   B. A very low serum sodium may be corrected by restricting fluids *or* IV of 3 percent saline

Monitor serum sodium levels frequently

IV may be stopped when sodium level rises to 120 mEq/L

C. Observe for fluid overload and/or signs of CHF

D. Correct any hypoglycemia

Oral or IV glucose fluids may be prescribed

Check the serum glucose levels frequently

E. I&O must be charted

Anticipate diuresis after thyroxine replacement has begun

VI. Prevent acute adrenal insufficiency

A. Administer hydrocortisone, as prescribed, usually, 300 mg IV in divided doses; then daily doses and eventually tapering of dosage

B. Observe for the side effects of steroid therapy

VII. Replace the missing thyroid hormone

A. Administer sodium levothyroxine (T4) as prescribed

Route: usually IV

Dosage: 300 to 500 μg

B. Observe patient closely for: tachycardia, palpitations, restlessness, tremor, sweating

C. Monitor pulse every 30 minutes and take frequent ECG

D. Monitor serum TSH and T4 levels

VIII. Observe for any adverse effects of thyroxine replacement

A. Cardiovascular: report any signs of myocardial ischemia, tachyarrhythmias, or CHF

Monitor TPR, bp q 4 hours, pulse rate should not rise above 100

B. Nervous system: chart the neurologic vital signs q 4 hours

Observe for and report any increasing anxiety, headache, sweating or tremor

C. Excretory systems: monitor I&O and bowel sounds

Expect an increase in intestinal motility and diuresis

IX. Prevent further heat loss

A. Adequately cover patient; monitor body temperature q 1 to 2 hours

B. Do not use mechanical warming devices

C. Once replacement therapy has begun, check skin for rash

RATIONALE

The coma associated with severe hypothyroidism in the adult is generally insidious and progressive. The delay of onset is a reflection of substantial stores of thyroxine or a decrease in its degradation. The previous medical picture, the search for recent precipitating events, and the systems survey suggest the etiology of this presenting picture. Laboratory studies confirm the hypothesis of myxedema coma and help identify coexisting problems, if any.

The respiratory depression in myxedema is marked and respiratory failure is always a threat. To combat hypoxia and hypercapnea, airway and ventilatory assistance must be provided. Tracheostomy is preferred to endotracheal intubation because these patients do not fair well postextubation. Monitoring the arterial blood gases and periodic chest x-rays give an indication of the patient's response to therapy. The cardiac and pleural effusions commonly associated with this condition tend to disappear once therapy is begun.

The hypothermic state is a reflection of the very severe decrease in basal metabolism and inadequate production of thermal energy. The prognosis is poor, if the body temperature remains below 90°F. It is more accurate to take body temperature with an electrical thermometer because, if the commonly used mercury thermometer is not shaken all the way down, an inaccurate reading is obtained. The patient requires adequate covering but mechanical rewarming techniques are not employed because they lead to peripheral vasodilatation, depletion of blood to the vital organs and thus, possibly precipitate shock.

Correcting fluid and electrolyte imbalances is done cautiously and slowly. Until thyroid levels are restored, this patient is not able to properly excrete a water load and heart failure follows. In addition, it must be recalled that there is a decrease in the insensible fluid losses from the skin and respiratory tract thus the total calculated fluid replacement is much lower than usual. However, if hypovolemia and hypotension persist, intravenous fluids are required. If vasopressors are prescribed to support blood pressure, they are given in much smaller doses because once thyroid replacement is begun, the thyroid acts synergistically with the vasopressor. This combination, in an already sensitive patient, could lead to severe reactions. The nurse must monitor the intake and output, blood pressure, and electrocardiogram during fluid replacement.

It is widely accepted that the adrenal gland in this condition responds sluggishly to stress and that the state of hypoglycemia is related to this insufficiency. To prevent further adrenal problems, cortisol is administered daily in divided doses and then tapered off around the second week of hospitalization. The nurse should observe the patient's responses to this therapy by monitoring serum electrolytes, glucose levels, and counteracting gastric hyperacidity with antacids. Broad spectrum antibiotics may be prescribed because cortisol therapy depresses the immune and inflammatory responses.

Thyroid hormone replacement is the cornerstone in managing this patient. Levothyroxine is most commonly prescribed, and it is administered intravenously because of poor gastrointestinal absorption and poor circulation. The large initial dose of 0.4 to 0.5 mg should rapidly restore levels to normal. This dosage is followed by 0.05 to 0.1 mg daily. The nurse should observe the patient for an increase in pulse, blood pressure, temperature, and improvement in mental status. All should occur within 24 hours. If the level of consciousness does not improve in this time, the prognosis is poor. The patient's urinary output should increase as will the motility of the bowel. Accurate intake and output, neurologic vital signs, and cardiac monitoring must be done while the hormone is being replaced.

Replacing the missing hormone is fraught with many dangers. It could precipitate cardiac arrhythmias, angina, myocardial infarction, and/or congestive heart failure. The patient's heart activity must be monitored continuously and any signs of ischemia or tachyarrhythmias be reported immediately so dosage adjustments of T4 can be made. Any symptoms of headache, tremor, sweating, and/or increasing anxiety indicate that the central nervous system is adversely responding to the increased levels of T4 and adjustments need to be made.

This patient requires admission to a critical care unit and further supportive care. Measures to avoid skin breakdown, aspiration, and urinary retention begun in the emergency department are all continued.

HYPERTHYROIDISM AND THYROTOXICOSIS

PATHOPHYSIOLOGY

Hyperthyroidism is a metabolic state resulting from the effects of excessive amounts of circulating thyroid hormone delivered to the body tissues. The onset may be so gradual that its manifestations may go unnoticed by the patient. However, toxic or crisis states exist when the patient can no longer tolerate the multisystem strain of this excess thyroid hormone.

There are a variety of conditions that can stimulate an overproduction of thyroid hormones. The most common cause is Graves disease which occurs to adults in their thirties and forties. These patients produce and release an immunoglobulin G, which is referred to by many names, long-acting thyroid stimulator (LATS), human thyroid stimulator, and thyrotropin-displacing substance. This immunoglobulin is capable of stimulating adenylcyclase activity in human thyroid tissue thus producing an excess of thyroid hormone. These patients tend to have hyperplasia of the gland with depletion of thyroid colloid. At times lymphocytic infiltration of the gland is found. The thyroid is large and commonly palpable. The increased blood flow to the enlarged gland causes a bruit to be heard. In severe cases, it may be possible to detect a thrill over the upper lobes.

Hyperfunctioning autonomous or multinodular goiters are two common causes of hyperthyroidism. A nodule larger than 3 cm can produce excessive thyroid hormone which would be evident on the radioactive iodine uptake scan. Uptake concentration would be greatest in the nodule whereas the rest of the gland takes up little. Multinodular goiters give a picture of diffuse hyperactivity of the tissue between the nodules. Nodular goiters are more common in the elderly but one should note that the clinical picture presented by the hyperthyroid elderly is quite misleading. Thyroid nodules may be inactive or active. Multiple nodules are usually benign but solitary "cold" nodules have an increased chance of being malignant.

Inflammatory conditions of the thyroid could result in hyperthyroidism, if thyroid hormones leak from the inflamed gland. Hashimoto thyroiditis is an autoimmune process resulting in the inflammatory process. The patient may be euthyroid, hypo- or hyperthyroid. Clinically, the thyroid is very large and may cover the isthmus of the gland but it is nontender to touch. The laboratory will report high titers of antithyroglobulin antibodies as well as marked lymphocytic infiltration of the gland. Subacute granulomatous thyroiditis is associated with viral conditions such as sore throats and mumps. Clinically, the patient has fever, malaise, pain, and tenderness in the neck around the thyroid which may radiate up to the angle of the mandible. Histologically, the thyroid cells appear disorganized, fibrotic, and infiltrated with multinucleated giant cells. Subacute granulomatous thyroiditis may also present as hypothyroidism or euthyroidism.

Less common causes of hyperthyroidism exist. Ingestion, iatrogenically or surreptitiously, of excessive thyroid hormone (thyrotoxicosis medicamentosa) is seen frequently in persons who wish to lose weight and medical personnel who feel they need a boost of energy. Hydatidiform mole and choriocarcinoma can secrete enough human chorionic gonadotropin which would stimulate the production of thyroid hormones. A rare form of ovarian teratoma (struma ovarii) can produce an excessive amount of thyroid hormone. Pituitary adenomas, which secrete excessive TSH, could also cause hyperthyroidism.

Hyperthyroid states have been associated with psychologic and physiologic stressors. It has long been observed that during periods of psychologic stress, such as emotional shock, worry, loss of esteem, loss of job, the symptoms of hyperthyroidism appear, and worsen. It is not clear which came first, the emotional problem or the hyperthyroid condition. It has been suggested that the catabolic processes associated with the hyperthyroid state produces and releases tissue breakdown products which have a detrimental effect on the central nervous system. Physical stressors such as infection, trauma, pregnancy, and surgery do increase the rate of TSH secretion and could lead to a hyperthyroid state. In the past, thyrotoxicosis commonly followed thyroidectomy but today with better medical management this is rare. Thyroid crisis can occur in undiagnosed, inadequately treated, or untreated patients. It can be precipitated by concomitant conditions such as ketoacidosis, CVA, pulmonary embolism, vigorous palpitation of the gland, x-rays using contrast media, ether anesthesia, and postirradiation of the thyroid.

Because there are no criteria that clearly differentiate a patient with severe hyperthyroidism from one who is thyroid-toxic, an explanation of the major manifestations of this metabolic problem follows. The manifestations discussed are seen in the young and middle-aged patient. The elderly may only manifest hyperthyroidism by an arrhythmia or CHF of unknown etiology. There is an extreme form of hyperthyroidism in the elderly called apathetic hyperthyroidism wherein the patient fails to exhibit any of the typical signs of hyperthyroidism.

At the cellular level, in vitro, excess thyroid hormone increases mitochondrial protein synthesis. And in high doses, in vitro, the by-product is heat instead of the energy of ATP. Thyroid hormone appears to activate the sodium pump in the cell membrane causing a great expenditure of energy. Fever is most prominent in thyrotoxicosis and is considered the sina qua non. It usually ranges from 100° to 103°F.

The integument of the hyperthyroid patient is the organ that dissipates the heat produced at the cellular level. There is a decrease in peripheral vascular resistance resulting in greater blood flow to the tissues and cutaneous vasodilatation. Some patients compensate by perspiring even under very cool conditions and, in fact, have a heat intolerance. The palms are warm, moist, and reddened. Another dermopathy of Graves disease is a benign condition called pretibial myxedema wherein the skin on the legs and feet appears raised and thickened. Some patients experience excessive melanin pigmentation, which results from an accelerated cortisol metabolism. The severe vasodilatation that accompanies thyrotoxicosis is manifested by hypotension and profuse diaphoresis.

Hyperthyroidism has a profound effect on the cardiovascular system. An increase in β-adrenergic activity occurs with this condition and thyroid hormones, themselves, exert a direct chronotropic and ionotropic effect on the myocardium. The results are a tremendous increase in stroke volume and heart rate associated with a decrease in peripheral vascular resistance. Clinically, tachycardia is observed and the increased force of cardiac contractions causes palpitations. Eventually, cardiac enlargement and mild edema are observed. Atrial dysrhythmias are another cardiac manifestation of hyperthyroidism and atrioventricular heart block can occur in severe cases. A systolic heart murmur can be heard and pulse pressure will be wide due to the rise in systolic pressure and a decrease in diastolic pressure. In thyrotoxicosis, the patient may go into high output cardiac failure or suffer from AV heart block accompanied by pulmonary edema.

The hyperthyroid patient needs more oxygen to keep up with the metabolic demands. The increased utilization of oxygen causes more carbon dioxide to be formed which stimulates the respiratory center and the patient increases the rate and depth of respirations. Some patients complain of shortness of breath. In the toxic state, the patient needs an additional supply of oxygen to meet the accelerated demands.

The gastrointestinal system and nutritional state are effected by excess thyroid hormones. The patient has an increase in appetite but commonly complains of weight loss. The nausea, vomiting, abdominal pains, and diarrhea associated with this condition are attributed to the increase in gastric and intestinal motility. As the condition worsens, the patient can no longer take in enough calories to meet the metabolic needs. A state of negative nitrogen balance occurs leading to weight loss, muscle wasting, and hypoalbuminemia. In some cases, the parathyroid gland becomes overactive causing an imbalance in calcium. Hypercalcemia and hypercalciuria result in demineralization of bone which could possibly lead to pathologic fractures. The hypermetabolic state could also result in a deficiency of vitamin B complex which could, but rarely does, result in neuropathy. The thyrotoxic patient manifests hepatomegaly, mild jaundice, complains of nausea and abdominal pains. Vomiting and diarrhea plus dehydration are also significant in this stage of the disease process.

Neuropsychiatric symptoms associated with hyperthyroidism could lead the examiner towards a diagnosis of anxiety neurosis. Frequently, the patient is restless, agitated, anxious, has outbursts of uncontrolled behavior, has problems with interpersonal relationships, becomes suspicious, paranoid, and depressed. Individuals complain of chronic fatigue as well as insomnia. Others have fleeting thoughts and their ideas run together so swiftly that they become disoriented. Others experience delusions, hallucinations, and believe they are going mad. This tense, hyperkinetic individual has brisk reflexes and a tremor. The tremor may be so severe that it becomes impossible to drink from a cup. Choreiform movements have been reported in some cases. Men more than women complain of muscle weakness and myopathy of the quadriceps. Myasthenia gravis is occasionally associated with hyperthyroidism. In thyrotoxicosis, the neuromuscular–psychiatric effects of excess thyroid hormone are most prominent and the patient's condition progresses to extreme weakness, disorientation, and possibly coma and death.

There are two ophthalmopathies associated with hyperthyroidism. First, the commonly called "stare of thyrotoxicosis" which is caused by the increased sympathetic tone and results in retraction of the upper eyelid and infrequent blinking. The second is true exophthalmos wherein there is an accumulation of mucopolysaccharides and lymphocytes behind the eye causing varying degrees of protrusion. Exophthalmos may be unilateral or bilateral. It may precede, run concurrent with, or follow a hyperthyroid state.

Laboratory studies confirm the clinical impression of thyrotoxicosis, however, therapy is usually begun before the results are known because the patient's condition is critical and test results may take too long to complete. It is beyond the scope of this text to describe each test in detail and only the highlights of the most common tests are discussed.

Because the body metabolizes all the isotopes of iodine in the same manner and because iodine is the building block for thyroid hormonal synthesis, studying radioactive iodine uptake provides a fairly accurate picture of the speed at which the thyroid traps iodine. Radioactive tracer doses of ^{131}Iodine (25 to 50 μc) can be administered orally or intravenously. The radioactivity over the thyroid gland can be measured within 10 minutes, if the dose was given intravenously or in 60 minutes, if given orally. The normal uptake in a euthyroid patient is 10 to 30 percent in 24 hours. The hyperthyroid patient exhibits a rapid uptake and therefore, 1-hour, 2-hour, and 6-hour scannings are done to catch the peak activity and to determine the percentage of uptake before thyroidal radioactivity declines. The results can only be assumed accurate if the patient's total iodine pool is normal. If the iodine pool is expanded, then the administered dose occupies only a small proportion and only a small uptake is depicted. Similarly, if the total pool of iodine is small, the dose given occupies a larger proportion of the total supply and uptake is faster. Factors that increase or decrease the iodine pool were described in the opening comments of this section.

Directly measuring T4 levels bypasses the problem of iodine contamination. The methods that can be used involve competitive thyroid-binding globulin assay or radioimmunoassay. Normal values range from 4 to 12 μg/dl. The hyperthyroid patient has a much higher level. Anything that effects the level of TBG in the serum effects the results of this test. Factors that do effect TBG levels were described in the opening remarks of this section.

Measuring circulating T3 is more difficult because it is present in far lower concentrations than T4 and also because it is biologically much more active and has a shorter serum half-life. Radioimmunoassay is the only effective technique. The normal range is 110 to 200 ng/dl. Serum T3 measurements are frequently increased in hyperthyroidism. If thyroxine levels are normal and T3 levels are high, a clinical state known as T3 toxicosis exists.

Measuring the degree of saturation of TBG indirectly depicts the level of circulating hormone. If a large quantity of endogenous hormone is present, practically all the thyroid-binding sites are occupied and only a few sites are free to bind to a test dose of radioactive labeled hormone which is administered along with a secondary binding substance, usually a resin. The test is called the resin T3 uptake. In hyperthyroid conditions, the resin uptake is high because the TBG is saturated. This test is most useful for those patients who give a history of taking iodine containing substances because iodine does not affect the results. However, any factor that increases or decreases the level of TBG affects these test results. Factors that do effect TBG levels were discussed earlier in this section.

In an effort to distinguish variations from the normal due to hormone binding from hormone concentration and because so many factors can affect the level of T3, the free thyroxine index can be calculated.

$$\text{Free thyroxine index} = \text{T4} \times \frac{\text{Patient's resin T3 uptake}}{\text{Control's resin T3 uptake}}$$

However, this is a more elaborate test and may not be in general clinical use.

The level of pituitary TSH can be directly measured by radioimmunoassay techniques. One would expect low levels of TSH in the hyperthyroid patient and one with toxic nodular goiter because the information that high levels of thyroxine is circulating is fed back to the pituitary and there is no need to produce TSH which would only stimulate more hormone to be produced.

MANAGEMENT

I. Obtain a history to identify the causes of the presenting picture
   A. Interview the patient, family, personal physician, and others
   B. Chart the events that immediately preceded the current episode
   C. Identify thyroid or other endocrine problems present in the patient or family
   D. Note the presence of recent physical stressors (i.e., x-ray studies, uncontrolled diabetes, surgery of any kind, pregnancy, upper respiratory infection)
   E. Note the presence of recent psychologic stressors (i.e., prolonged worry, loss of a loved one, changes in employment, family problems, loss of esteem)
   F. List all the medications, prescribed and over-the-counter, that patient is using (i.e., cough medicine, vitamin–mineral preparations, suppositories, losenges, salicylates, synthetic hormones, steroids, oral contraceptives). Note, if patient has abruptly stopped taking antithyroid medication
   G. Note any allergies patient may have
   H. Search for the presence of concomitant problems (i.e., sore throat, viral infection, trauma, slight CVA, ketoacidosis)
II. Detect and characterize the signs of the presenting picture
   A. If patient is unconscious, assess airway patency, breathing and circulation.

Initiate measures to relieve airway obstruction, maintain breathing and support circulation

B. Rapidly perform a systems analysis
   1. cardiovascular: obtain the temperature, pulse, respirations, and a stat ECG; chart any complaints of palpitations, orthopnea, or edema. Auscultate the heart and note the presence of a systolic murmur, tachycardia and gallop rhythm. Determine the degree of hypotension, and/or pulse pressure
   2. pulmonary: determine the rate, depth and regularity of respirations. Observe for signs of cyanosis. Chart any complaints of dyspnea or shortness of breath. Obtain a stat chest x-ray
   3. endocrine: observe for goiter. Note the size and symmetry of the thyroid. Report any tenderness of the gland, difficulty in swallowing or complaints of pain in the jaw. Listen for bruit over the thyroid and thrill over thyroid arteries. Note the distribution and texture of the hair. Obtain a menstrual history
   4. neurologic: evaluate the level of consciousness and general behavior. Note the degree of emotional lability, anxiety, agitation, insomnia and presence of psychotic symptoms. Assess muscle tone, strength and reflexes. Chart complaints of fatigue, evidence of twitching, tremor and/or involuntary movements. Note the presence of "thyroid stare" or exophthalmos. Record any intolerance to heat and the characteristics of the voice, report hoarseness
   5. gastrointestinal: chart a history of nausea, vomiting, or diarrhea. Auscultate abdomen to detect hyperactive bowel sounds. Check for hepatomegaly. Assess the skin's turgor, texture, and color. Note any palmar erythema and/or tibial myxedema. Chart the hydration of the tongue and level of thirst. Assess for changes in appetite, weight, taste and difficulties in swallowing. Note any flushing and diaphoresis

III. Assist with diagnostic studies that contribute to the diagnosis
   A. Obtain blood samples for
   RBC hemoglobin, hematocrit: WBC and differential electrolytes, BUN, glucose, cholesterol, triglycerides, enzymes, serum T4, T3 resin uptake, thyroid antibodies, blood gases
   B. Chest x-ray and ECG
   C. Radioactive iodine uptake studies

IV. Reduce the increased β-adrenergic activity of hyperthyroidism
   A. Propranolol (Inderal) is usually prescribed
      1. dosages may range from 20 to 120 mg/24 hours, if oral or 2 to 10 mg diluted in 5 percent D/W and infused slowly IV
      2. before giving report any existing contraindications to this drug: asthma, COPD, AV block, CHF, pregnancy. If any are present, the physician may choose to give metoprolol (Lopressor)
      3. before, during, and after giving this medication, record the bp, pulse, respirations and cardiac rhythm
      4. assess for adverse effects of this drug: sudden bradycardia, sudden hy-

potension, syncope, CHF, respiratory wheezing, dyspnea. Be prepared to give atropine, vasopressor, and bronchodilators if these symptoms arise

    5. assess for therapeutic effects of this drug: reduction in pulse rate, sweating, tremor, agitation, palpitations, and psychomotor activity

V. Inhibit the biosynthesis of thyroid hormones

  A. Propylthiouracil (PTU) may be prescribed

    1. dosage: 300 to 600 mg/24 hours; divided into q 4- to 6-hour doses has to be given orally or via NG tube, or

    2. Methimazole (Tapazole) may be prescribed
dose: 30 to 60 mg/24 hours which may be given in divided doses has to be given orally or via NG tube

  B. Observe for side effects: skin rash, pruritus, epigastric distress, paresthesias, arthalgia, myalgia. Hepatitis has been reported in patients receiving this drug

VI. Inhibit the release of thyroid hormones

  A. Iodine preparations may be prescribed

    1. drugs and dosages: sodium iodide injectable, 1 to 2 g infused over 8 hours
potassium iodide, 300 to 650 mg q 4 to 6 hours orally
Lugol's solution 10 to 20 gtts, tid, po

    2. precautions: do not administer before giving PTU or methimazole, wait one or more hours, if these drugs will be given

    3. observe for signs of iodinism (metallic taste, stomatitis, sneezing, vomiting, parotitis), pulmonary edema, and skin rash

  B. Lithium carbonate may be prescribed

    1. dose: 900 to 1200 mg daily to achieve blood levels of l mEq/L

    2. observe for nausea, vomiting, diarrhea, and lessening of the manic symptoms. Draw serum lithium levels periodically to avoid toxic levels of the drug

VII. Inhibit the peripheral conversion of T4 to T3

  A. Glucocorticoids may be prescribed

    1. drugs and dosages: hydrocortisone, 100 to 200 mg/24 hours
prednisone, 40 mg/24 hours
dexamethazone, 8 mg/24 hours

    2. observe for esophagitis, peptic ulcer, sodium and water retention, potassium loss

VIII. Remove excessive circulating hormone from blood (rare)

  A. Prepare for an exchange transfusion

  B. Prepare for peritoneal dialysis

IX. Counteract the harmful hypermetabolic state

  A. Reduce body temperature

    1. nurse patient on a hypothermia mattress or place ice packs around patient

    2. offer frequent sponge baths and provide good skin care

      3. reduce the amount of clothing and bed covers on patient

      4. lower temperature of room via air conditioning, if possible

      5. avoid using aspirin because it increases thyroxine levels

  B. Rehydrate and restore nutritional balance

      1. start an IV of 10 percent dextrose

      2. offer supplemental parenteral vitamins and electrolytes

      3. offer high protein, high caloric feedings, if patient can swallow

      4. monitor I&O, daily weight, serum electrolytes, and serum albumin levels

      5. assess for signs of fluid overload: dyspnea, abdominal pains, nausea, vomiting, diarrhea

      6. monitor bowel sounds

  X. Reduce the neuropsychiatric effects of excess thyroid hormones

    A. Modify environment so that extraneous stimuli are absent

      1. provide a cool, darkened, single room

      2. limit visitors to supportive relative or friend

      3. orient patient to person, place, and time

      4. provide a clock and a calendar

      5. provide simple explanations of events

    B. Avoid restraints; administer a mild sedative

    C. Obtain the neurologic vital signs q 4 hours and report any worsening of responses and/or deterioration in mental status

  XI. Monitor for cardiac decompensation or increased cardiac output

    A. Provide for continuous cardiac monitoring. Report any episodes of atrial fibrillation, aberrant beats or patterns of heart block

    B. Check bp, pulse, and respirations q 1 to 2 hours. Report widening of the pulse pressure or falling of bp

    C. Digitalis preparations may be prescribed or other drugs to treat the atrial dysrhythmias

    D. Obtain periodic chest x-rays to detect further cardiac enlargement

  XII. Provide for adequate oxygenation

    A. Place patient on complete bed rest. Nurse in semi-Fowler position. Limit involvement of patient in daily care

    B. Initiate oxygen therapy via nasal cannula

    C. Monitor pulmonary status: assess rate, depth, rhythm of respirations. Check blood gases and auscultate lungs. Report any lung congestion

RATIONALE

Because hyperthyroidism is a multisystem disease of unknown etiology and because the neuropsychiatric parameters predominate in most cases, it is quite possible to misdiagnose the gravity of the situation. The initial history identifies what the patient has experienced in the recent past and what presently has occurred to make him or her seek medical help. History taking may prove difficult, if the patient cannot concentrate or is constantly moving. In these cases, data must be collected from significant others who are familiar with the patient.

The systems analysis is performed rapidly and systematically. It will uncover overt, as well as covert, signs of disease. In many instances, the diagnosis is made on the basis of history and clinical findings because very few rapid thyroid tests are available. The young and middle-aged patient with true hyperthyroidism exhibit a fairly classic picture but the elderly patient's symptoms may be masked. It is imperative that the emergency department nurse maintain a high index of suspicion of hyperthyroidism and possible thyrotoxicosis in patients who present with unexplained fever, agitation, atrial dysrhythmias, and cardiac decompensation. If the patient is unconscious when first seen, other causes must be quickly eliminated.

The β-adrenergic blocking drug propranolol's principal advantage in this life-threatening situation is its ability to bring the symptoms rapidly under control. It reduces the tachycardia, tremor, sweating, and nervousness. The effects are due to its ability to inhibit the peripheral conversion of T3 to T4 and its competitive blocking action at all β-adrenergic receptor sites resulting in a negative inotropic and chronotropic effect on the heart. It slows AV conduction, decrease plasma renin levels, constricts the bronchioles, dilates peripheral blood vessels, and reduces sympathetic outflow from the vasomotor center in the brain. Because of these effects on the heart and circulation, the patient requires close monitoring.

The antithyroid drugs, propylthiouracil (PTU) and methimazole, most likely block the peroxidase enzyme system in the thyroid and thus inhibit biosynthesis of new hormone. Because they do not interfere with previously formed hormone or exogenously administered hormone, their clinical effects take longer. PTU, but not methimazole, blocks the conversion of T4 to T3. PTU has a short serum half-life and duration necessitating its administration several times a day. Methimazole is more potent than PTU and has a longer duration of action. Both these drugs must be taken orally because the parenteral solution is not yet available. These drugs cross the placental barrier and may produce cretinism and goiter in the developing fetus. A possible state of pregnancy must be ascertained when taking the history to prevent this occurrence. Antithyroid drugs can harmfully interact with other drugs such as with anticoagulants wherein hypoprothrombinemia can result. Along with many other drugs, they could lead to agranulocytosis, but this is rare.

Excessive iodine causes a marked reduction in the thyroid's activity and at one time, stable iodine preparations were the only available treatment for hyperthyroidism. Iodine preparations suppress the release of hormone from the thyroglobulin and interfere with the synthesis of new hormone probably by blocking the peroxidase system. The effects are seen within 24 hours but are short lived. The size of the gland shrinks as does its vascularity. Iodine preparations are best given after antithyroid medications to prevent some of the iodine from being made into new thyroid hormone. The nurse must observe for the acute signs of iodinism when the intravenous preparation of sodium iodide is used.

Lithium has an effect similar to iodine in that it blocks the release of thyroid hormone from the gland. Its benefits are rapid in onset and reduce the manic symptoms that accompany the disease. Its toxic levels are very close to its therapeutic levels, which necessitates that serum lithium levels be performed periodically.

Large doses of glucocorticoids have proven beneficial in treating thyrotoxicosis. The adrenal gland is close to a state of exhaustion in this state of hyperthyroidism and replacement therapy is warranted. Furthermore, glucocorticoids have been shown to reduce serum TSH levels probably by suppressing TRH release from the hypothalamus. Glucocorticoids are also capable of blocking the conversion of T4 to T3. Because they are given in therapeutic doses, the nurse should closely observe for gastrointestinal ulcer formation. Antacids may be prescribed prophylactically to combat this occurrence.

In extreme life-threatening situations of thyrotoxicosis, the excess hormone can be removed by mechanical rather than chemical means. Exchange blood transfusions and peritoneal dialysis have been performed but these techniques are rarely required.

General supportive measures are directed at reducing the complications of thyrotoxicosis: dehydration, hypovolemic shock, CHF, exhaustion, coma, and death. Parenteral fluids restore fluid volume and combat hypotension in addition to providing the needed route for additional calories. The 10 percent dextrose solution not only provides carbohydrate but it spares the liver's need to convert glycogen to glucose. Extra vitamins and minerals are given parenterally to make up the deficits. Needed protein can usually be supplied orally via diet or with supplemental high protein drinks. Monitoring the effects of this therapy are aimed at avoiding fluid overload, especially if the heart is decompensating. The nausea, vomiting, and/or diarrhea usually subside with treatment.

Hyperpyrexia and diaphoresis accelerate fluid losses and must be combated. Cooling measures, which include sponge baths, ice packs, hypothermia blanket, and air conditioning, all increase the rate of evaporation from the skin thereby lowering body temperature. The nurse must exert special efforts to preserve the integrity of the patient's skin during such treatments. Aspirin, as an antipyretic medication, is not used in this condition because it can increase thyroxine levels. Other nonsalicylate antipyretics may be prescribed.

High output cardiac failure or heart block are serious complications of thyrotoxicosis. Continuous cardiac monitoring, assessment of the vital signs, digitalization, and reduction of the β-adrenergic activity are all measures aimed at treating these cardiovascular changes. Periodic chest x-rays depict any changes in heart size.

The neuropsychiatric symptoms of thyrotoxicosis are most often the cardinal features of this syndrome. The administration of the β-adrenergic blocker drugs helps control the autonomic nervous system manifestations until more definitive therapy is begun. The nurse should initiate measures to prevent exhaustion and decrease the level of agitation and/or confusion. Although the patient needs meaningful sensory information, sensory overload has a deleterious effect and must be avoided. Thus a quiet, nonstimulating, cool room is preferred placement for this patient. It is important for the patient to understand that the symptoms are disease-related and that they will subside with time and treatment. Soft tone of voice and gentle handling promotes calmness. Visitors should be limited. Confusion is corrected by pointing out reality and orienting the patient as needed. Monitoring neurologic responses and mental status at frequent intervals detects improvement or deterioration in the patient's condition. A mild sedative may be needed during the acute phase but then the medication may blunt responses.

In the hypermetabolic state, the body cells need a large and constant supply of oxygen. Depending upon the severity of the patient's condition, oxygen may be prescribed to relieve shortness of breath and dyspnea. Keeping the patient on complete bed rest, if possible, lessens the need for oxygen. The nurse must be alert for signs of pulmonary edema because atrial dysrhythmias and cardiac failure frequently accompany thyrotoxicosis.

3. Disorders of Adrenal Hormone Functioning

ADRENALCORTICAL INSUFFICIENCY

ASSESSMENT

  I. Presenting clinical picture (depends upon the extent of adrenal destruction)
     A. Cardiovascular system alterations
        1. severe hypotension; history of postural hypotensive episodes
        2. hypovolemia progressing to hypovolemic shock
        3. rapid, thready pulse (in adrenal crisis)
        4. decreased heart size
        5. ECG changes consistent with hyperkalemia
           a. widening QRS complex, spiked T waves
     B. Respiratory system alterations
        1. rapid, shallow respirations (in adrenal crisis)
     C. Urinary system alterations
        1. oliguria progressing to anuria (in adrenal crisis)
     D. Integumentary system alterations
        1. increased pigmentation of areolar, elbows, knees, knuckles, palmar creases, moles, freckles; "bronze" appearance; blotches in buccal mucosa, conjunctiva (only primary disease)
        2. vitiligo (depigmented skin patches) or pallor in some
        3. scanty body hair
        4. cool, clammy skin (in adrenal crisis)
     E. Gastrointestinal system alterations
        1. anorexia; weight loss
        2. fasting hypoglycemic episodes
        3. vague abdominal pain (could mimic peritonitis or ulcerations)
        4. nausea, vomiting, diarrhea (in adrenal crisis)

    F. Neuromuscular system alterations
        1. lethargy, weakness, easy fatiguability, progresses to exhaustion
        2. muscle flaccidity
        3. increased sensitivity to noise, odors, tastes
        4. could be restless, irritable
        5. confusion and decreased LOC progressing to coma (in adrenal crisis)
II. Possible precipitating and/or contributing causes
    A. Primary adrenalcortical insufficiency
        1. autoimmune pathology: search history for diagnosis of other autoimmune disorders such as Graves disease, Hashimoto thyroiditis, hypoparathyroidism
        2. history of acute or chronic infectious disease
           a. acute: septicemia, usually due to bacterial meningococcus
           b. chronic: fungal (histoplasmosis) or bacterial (tuberculosis)
        3. presence of other problems: amyloidosis, metastatic carcinoma, hemochromatosis, adrenal vein thrombosis, bilateral adrenalectomy
        4. presence of acute and/or prolonged stress
    B. Secondary adrenocortical unsufficiency
        1. hypothalamic problems: tumor, encephalitis, vascular lesions, basal skull fractures
        2. pituitary problems: chromophobe adenomas, postpartum necrosis, hypophysectomy
        3. medications: high-dose glucocorticoid therapy, abrupt cessation of glucocorticoid therapy, and long-term heparinization
III. Pertinent laboratory and radiologic findings
    A. Hematologic studies reveal
        1. decrease in the number of RBC; increased hematocrit; increased WBC count, if infection present; increased eosinophils
    B. Blood chemistries and electrolytes reveal
        1. decreased serum sodium, chloride, and bicarbonate
        2. increased potassium, calcium, and magnesium
        3. elevations in BUN and creatinine
        4. decreased serum glucose
    C. Blood gases reveal a mild metabolic acidosis
        1. pH, P_{CO_2} and bicarbonate levels decreased somewhat
    D. Chest x-ray reveals a small heart size
    E. ECG changes are consistent with hyperkalemia
        Widened QRS wave and spiked T wave
    F. Hormonal studies
        1. plasma or serum cortisol levels
           a. fluorescence method: normal 5 to 30 μg/dl. This value varies with the time of day drawn. It is normally higher in the morning and lowest after 8 PM
           b. Peterson method: normal 6 to 27 μg/dl
           The cortisol levels are usually lower in adrenal insufficiency

2. Plasma or serum aldosterone levels. Normal up to 20 ng/dl
   This value varies with the time of day drawn
3. 60-minute ACTH test
   An inadequate response of cortisone and aldosterone to ACTH is specific
   to diagnose adrenal insufficiency
4. 11-deoxycortisol levels in the serum or plasma. Normal is less than 1
   μg/dl
5. urine studies: a 24-hour urine specimen is required
   Creatinine levels in the urine are also done on these specimens to determine the completeness of specimen collection
   a. 17-hydroxycorticosteroids: normal, 3 to 12 mg/24 hours
   b. 17-ketosteroids
      men: normal 9 to 18 mg/24 hours
      women: normal 6 to 13 mg/24 hours
      Both studies would reveal low values in this illness

PATHOPHYSIOLOGY

The two roughly triangular shaped glands that lie retroperitoneally at the apex of
the kidney are the adrenal glands. Anatomically each gland has an outer portion
(cortex) and an inner portion (medulla). Each portion produces distinctly different
hormones that have diverse physiologic functions. Adrenal insufficiency is a problem
of the adrenal cortex and should correctly be called adrenocortical insufficiency.

There are three histologic zones in the adrenal cortex. First, a thin outer portion called the zona glomerulosa, where the mineralocorticoid, aldosterone, is produced. Second, a fair-sized middle zone called the zona fasciculata where the
glucocorticoid, cortisol, is produced. Third, a small inner zone which abuts the medulla of the gland called the zona reticularis where it is believed that the sex hormones or androgens are produced.

Mechanisms which control the synthesis and release of adrenocortical hormones are subject to a number of influences. Glucocorticoids, and to a degree
adrenal androgens and aldosterone, are regulated by the hypothalamus–pituitary–adrenal axis by way of a negative feedback mechanism. Low levels of cortisol
stimulate the hypothalamus to secrete corticotropin-releasing hormone (CRH),
which stimulates the pituitary to secrete adrenocorticotropic hormone (ACTH).
ACTH controls the synthesis and release of glucocorticoids by regulating the
amount of free cholesterol available to the cell's mitochondria where it is converted
to pregnenolone and then the various steroid hormones. The adrenal cortex responds
maximally to a small increment of ACTH. Increased serum cortisol levels inhibits
ACTH and CRH secretion.

ACTH release follows a circadian (24-hour) pattern and there is considerable
diurnal variation in its secretion. The highest levels of plasma cortisol, approximately 20 μg/dl, are normally found between 6 AM and 8 AM and the lowest levels of
less than 5 μg/dl found around midnight. This rhythm of ACTH release can be in-

fluenced and altered by environmental synchronizers such as the daily light–darkness cycle. In addition, ACTH secretion is regulated by neural inputs from higher centers. The circadian pattern, negative feedback system, and neural influences can be overcome by such stressful events as mass infections, shock, hypoglycemia, and surgery. Stressors tend to increase the secretion of ACTH and after several days of stress, the adrenal can secrete as much as 300 mg of cortisol in 24 hours.

ACTH is structurally similar to hormones released from the intermediate lobe of the pituitary, MSH (melanocyte-stimulating hormones). MSH occurs in two forms, the alpha amino acid and the beta amino acid. In humans, β-MSH which may be an artifactual fragment of another pituitary hormone accounts for promoting pigmentation. However, ACTH has some MSH-like biological activities and some researchers believe it to be the single pigmentary hormone.

ACTH has only an acute, unsustained ability to effect the release of aldosterone. The major regulator of aldosterone secretion is the renin–angiotensin system. The juxtaglomerular cells of the afferent arterioles of the glomeruli secrete renin, a proteolytic enzyme, in response to a lowered renal perfusion. Renin acts on angiotensinogen, a circulating α-2-globulin made in the liver, to form angiotensin I, a decapeptide. Angiotensin I is converted by enzymes in the blood to an octapeptide, angiotensin II. Angiotensin II is a powerful vasoconstrictor plus a potent, direct stimulus in the production of aldosterone. The serum potassium levels may also have a direct stimulatory effect in aldosterone's release. In vitro studies have shown that high levels of potassium injected directly into the adrenal artery produce an immediate increase in serum aldosterone levels.

The metabolic functions and effects of the adrenocortical hormones are multiple. Cortisol's most predominant effects are concerned with the intermediary metabolism of carbohydrates, proteins, and fats to maintain the blood sugar at acceptable levels. Thus, it is commonly referred to as the glucocorticoid. It does enhance gluconeogenesis from protein catabolism and it antagonizes the activity of insulin. It participates in water metabolism by increasing the clearance of free water, promoting the shift of water into the cells, and helps to maintain extracellular fluid volume and thus blood pressure. It acts directly on the arterioles of the cardiovascular system by sensitizing them to the actions of epinephrine thereby playing some role in maintaining blood pressure. Cortisol has a catabolic effect on skeletal tissue and cartilage growth. All components of the inflammatory response are depressed by cortisol and immunologic competence is inhibited. A decrease in the number of eosinophils and an increase in neutrophils, platelets, and red blood cells is an effect of cortisol. Cortisol affects the gastrointestinal tract by increasing gastric acid and pepsin secretion and decreasing gastric mucous secretion. Excessive amounts of cortisol decrease the absorption of calcium by apparently antagonizing the effects of vitamin D. The neuromuscular system's threshold for electrical excitation is depressed in the presence of cortisol and deficiencies or excesses of cortisol may lead to psychiatric disturbances and muscle weakness.

Aldosterone's primary functions are the regulation of sodium and potassium metabolism and thus, it is commonly referred to as the mineralocorticoid. Aldosterone enhances the reabsorption of sodium, the secretion of potassium and to a lesser extent, secretion of the hydrogen ion in the distal renal tubule. Although aldosterone acts mainly in the renal tubule, it helps the salivary ducts, sweat glands, and intestinal glands to reabsorb sodium in exchange for potassium. Despite this potent sodium-retaining property, the body has a protective "escape" mechanism to guard against overretention of sodium. There probably is a natriuretic or "third factor" involved in this escape phenomenon.

The role of the adrenal androgens is not totally clear. They appear to play an anabolic role particularly in women. In addition, they appear to enhance virilization and feminization.

The functions of the adrenalcortical hormones are essential to life. They play a major role in the body's physiologic adaptation to stress. Within a short period of time of any stress, the quantity of these hormones released into the bloodstream is increased many fold. The adrenal cortex hypertrophies in the presence of prolonged stress but its reserve capacity is not limitless. Prolonged stress results in lipid depletion of the zona fasciculata and in some cases hemorrhagic changes. Death can follow the loss of functioning and/or surgical removal unless replacement hormone therapy is rapidly reinstituted.

Adrenalcortical insufficiency is usually a chronic condition which can exacerbate into an acute, life-threatening disorder. Although it occurs more commonly in adults between the ages of 30 and 50, it has been reported in children and the elderly. Destructive lesions within the adrenal cortex result in primary adrenal insufficiency or Addison disease, so named after Thomas Addison (1855) who first wrote the classical description of this illness. Secondary adrenocortical insufficiency results from dysfunctions of the hypothalamus or pituitary gland.

Primary adrenocortical insufficiency can result from a number of situations that destroy the cortical cells. The majority of cases in the United States today are due to idiopathic atrophy of the glands resulting in fibrous replacement of the cortex with mononuclear inflammatory cells. The process is believed to be due to an autoimmune disorder because circulating adrenal antibodies have been found in these patients and this condition is associated with other immune disorders such as Graves disease, Hashimoto thyroiditis, and idiopathic hypoparathyroidism.

The most common chronic infectious causes of primary insufficiency are due to fungal and bacterial organisms. Histoplasmosis, and less commonly Cryptococcus and Coccidioides, are the most commonly implicated fungi. Tubercular destruction was once the most prevalent bacterial cause but is now considered an uncommon etiology in the United States. Both fungal and tubercular etiologies lead to destructive caseating granulomatous inflammatory reactions in the gland.

Acute bacterial infections of an overwhelming nature could lead to hemorrhagic destruction of the adrenal glands (Waterhouse–Friderichsen syndrome). The offending organism is commonly the meningococcus but can be others which lead to an overwhelming septicemia.

There are other less common causes of primary adrenal insufficiency. Amyloidosis could result in adrenal deposits which cause total pressure atrophy of the adrenals and destroy them. Metastatic carcinoma of the breast or bronchi has been known to cause the disease, as have adrenal vein thrombosis, hemochromatosis, and, understandably, a bilateral adrenalectomy. In addition, acute or chronic stress could lead to lipid depletion of the zona fasciculata and decrease cortisol production. Primary adrenocortical insufficiency results in deficiencies of both cortisol and aldosterone and to some extent androgens.

Secondary adrenocortical insufficiency originates in the hypothalamus and/or pituitary gland and results in a reduction primarily of cortisol. Hypofunctioning of the anterior pituitary and hypothalamus result in a deficiency of ACTH production and eventual adrenal atrophy producing secondary adrenal insufficiency. The hypothalamus could be injured by metastatic tumors of the breast and lung, inflammatory conditions of the brain, vascular lesions, and basal skull fractures. Craniopharyngioma, the most common pituitary tumor found in children, is located usually in the suprasellar area and may cause hypothalamic dysfunctioning. Hypothalamic disorders lead to hypofunctioning of secondary glands stimulated by the pituitary's trophic hormones because of the failure to produce and secrete releasing hormones.

The most frequently implicated anterior pituitary problems which could result in secondary adrenocortical insufficiency are chromophobe adenomas, postpartum necrosis, and surgery. Chromophobe adenomas could lead to hypo- or hyperproduction of ACTH. The tumor causes compression and destruction of the normal surrounding tissue and could lead to severe panhypopituitarism. Shock and excessive bleeding at the time of delivery could result in thrombosis and infarction of the pituitary (Sheehan syndrome), and could also result in hypoadrenalism depending upon which cells of the pituitary are destroyed. Pituitary ablation or surgery, hypophysectomy, used in the treatment of diabetic retinopathy, metastatic breast and lung cancer, or pituitary tumors result in adrenal insufficiency as well as other trophic hormone deficiencies.

Medications have the ability to suppress the adrenal cortex. The administration of high-dose glucocorticoids suppresses the hypothalamic–pituitary–adrenal axis and results in varying degrees of adrenal insufficiency. Within only a few days after a high dose of glucocorticoids is taken, a decrease in adrenal weight can be observed. After more prolonged therapy, a decrease in the response to ACTH is seen as well as suppression of CRH. The adrenal gland suppression is reversible, if therapy is of short duration. However, hypothalamic–pituitary recovery could take up to 6 to 12 months. Therefore, patients with a history of glucocorticoid therapy of greater than 1 month and/or patients who abruptly stop taking their glucocorticoids, should be considered to be in a state of relative adrenocortical insufficiency. In some cases, this state lasts up to 1 year following therapy. It has also been reported that patients on long-term anticoagulation therapy using heparin could have adrenal insufficiency. Structural abnormalities in the zona glomerulosa have been found in these patients.

Secondary adrenocortical insufficiency should alert the examiner to the possibility of other pituitary trophic deficiencies and/or lesions that could endanger neural structures. Deficiencies in gonadotropin, somatostatin, and thyrotropin have accompanied secondary adrenocortical insufficiency.

The clinical course of primary adrenal insufficiency is usually insidious with the signs and symptoms developing over a period of time. The earliest and most conspicuous sign noticed by the patient or the family is hyperpigmentation. The increased pigmentation or "bronzing" may be diffuse and is similar to tanning on exposure to sunlight. More commonly, it appears where the skin is subject to pressure, in scars of past injuries and on exposed surfaces. There is a predilection for pigmentation to accumulate on the elbows, knees, knuckles, palm creases, freckles, and areas that are normally richer in pigment: areolar, perianal, perivulvar, and scrotal skin. In some cases buccal, vaginal, and conjunctival blotches can be observed. However, pigmentation is not a universal sign and in some cases patients have vitiligo, depigmented skin patches. None of the pigmentary changes are helpful in examining dark-skinned patients. The cause of these integumentary changes is believed to be related to the lack of cortisol's inhibitory feedback on ACTH and MSH secretion. Hyperpigmentation is not found in secondary adrenal insufficiency because ACTH and MSH levels are low.

The major and constant cardiovascular finding of primary adrenocortical insufficiency is hypotension. In the early stages of this illness, the systolic pressure ranges from 80 to 100 mm Hg whereas the systolic pressure ranges between 50 and 65 mm Hg. Postural hypotension with the systolic and diastolic dropping 20 mm Hg or more is frequently noted in chronic forms of this disease. Attacks of severe hypotension can be triggered by even relatively minor stressors. The basic mechanism for the hypotension is a hypovolemia caused by a lack of aldosterone. Without aldosterone, the kidney excretes sodium, chloride, and water but retains potassium and the hydrogen ion. The serum electrolytes reflect this sodium loss (hyponatremia) and potassium retention (hyperkalemia). The mild acidosis is reflected in the lowered serum pH and bicarbonate.

Although dyspnea and palpitations do occur on exertion because of low cardiac reserve, cardiac failure is not a common finding. On x-ray, the heart does appear smaller and this is probably due to the decrease in blood volume the heart receives. As the condition worsens, the electrocardiogram reflects the hyperkalemia by a widened QRS wave and spiked T wave.

Gastrointestinal dysfunctions occur in over 75 percent of patients with primary adrenocortical insufficiency. Anorexia is the initial symptom to appear. A weight loss averaging 30 pounds or more is another consistent finding and is reflective of the severe anorexia and dehydration that accompanies the loss of aldosterone. The lack of glucocorticoids is responsible for the fasting hypoglycemia seen in these patients as well as their vague gastrointestinal complaints. Many give a history of episodic abdominal pains. There is usually a hypochlorhydria probably due to the loss of chloride which is caused by the aldosterone deficiency. Nausea and vomiting are harbingers of impending adrenal crisis. In some attacks of vomiting, the abdominal picture may be confused with peritonitis.

Asthenia which may vary from easy fatiguability to extreme exhaustion is another constant finding in untreated adrenocortical insufficiency. In the later stages of this disease, the patient may only be able to sit up with assistance and even talking becomes too much of an effort. Asthenia and extreme muscle weakness is associated with creatinuria and results from a lack of both cortisol and aldosterone.

The neuropsychiatric disturbances associated with this illness do not occupy a prominent part of the clinical picture. Mood changes are consistent with a picture of a chronic disease. Psychoses have been observed in some cases. The EEG does depict slower than normal oscillations of the alpha rhythm and an absence or decreased number of beta waves. The flaccid muscle tone is reflective of electrolyte imbalances. The changes in the sensitivity to noise, odors, and tastes are unexplainable at this time. In the acute stage of crisis, the decrease in level of consciousness is a reflection of the low serum glucose, electrolyte losses, fluid losses, and acidosis.

At any time, the patient may lapse into a shock-like condition, referred to as Addisonian crisis. This crisis could occur in the undiagnosed or undertreated patient. Any situation which creates a demand for cortical hormones could trigger a crisis despite the adequacy of previous treatment because the patient cannot respond to stress. Stimuli that produce a crisis situation are varied and nonspecific. A slight upper respiratory infection, exposure to the sun, and emotional upsets could be enough to trigger a crisis. It usually happens in patients with chronic insufficiency in the setting of severe infection, trauma, or surgery. Crisis may develop rapidly, within a few hours or gradually, with the patient deteriorating over a period of time.

Addisonian crisis is characterized by severe hypotension, hypovolemia, nausea, vomiting, and possibly high fever. Fever may be reflective of the infectious process or dehydration. However, subnormal temperatures may occur in shock despite the presence of infection. When aldosterone deficiency exists severe hyponatremia and hyperkalemia are found. Poor renal perfusion leads to retention of urea and an elevated BUN is seen.

While the emergency department team focuses their efforts upon stabilizing the patient's condition, diagnostic tests can be performed to assess the status of the adrenals and distinguish primary from secondary insufficiency.

A practical, reliable, and fairly rapid test of adrenal functioning is the 1-hour ACTH test. A baseline cortisol and aldosterone level is drawn. Synthetic 1-24 ACTH (cosyntropin), 250 μg is given intramuscularly. In 60 minutes, blood is drawn for cortisol and aldosterone levels. Normally, cortisol levels would rise in increments greater than 7 μg/100 ml over the baseline or an absolute level greater than 18 μg/100 ml is seen. An inadequate cortisol response to this test is specific for adrenal insufficiency. The aldosterone response to this test helps differentiate primary from secondary insufficiency. If the problem is in the adrenal gland, primary insufficiency, the aldosterone response is minimal. On the other hand, if the problem is secondary insufficiency, the mean increment in aldosterone levels over the baseline is two to threefold in 60 minutes after ACTH administration.

Several other adrenal diagnostic tests are available but they take longer to complete and although they may be started in the emergency department (i.e., 24-

hour urine collections), their results take longer to return. The emergency department team should begin searching for the underlying cause of the crisis and this is the basis for culture and sensitivity of urine and blood.

MANAGEMENT

I. Detect and characterize the signs of the presenting picture
   A. If patient is unconscious, assess airway patency, breathing, and circulation. Institute measures to relieve airway obstruction, maintain breathing, and support respirations
   B. Rapidly perform a systems survey
      1. cardiovascular: obtain temperature, respiration, pulse, bp, stat ECG auscultate the heart: note rate and rhythm
         evaluate the extent of dehydration: chart skin turgor, status or mucous membranes, presence of thirst, eyeball tone, urinary output
      2. respiratory: determine the rate, depth and regularity of respirations. Note any signs of dyspnea, at rest or on exertion. Note any cyanosis. Obtain a stat chest x-ray
      3. gastrointestinal: chart any history or presence of nausea, vomiting, diarrhea, abdominal pains. Palpate and auscultate the abdomen. Note bowel activity. Obtain a weight, if possible. Note a history of weight loss
      4. neuromuscular: note the LOC and general behavior. Assess muscle strength, tone and reflexes. Chart complaints of weakness, fatigue, exhaustion
      5. integumentary: note the overall skin color, temperature and turgor as well as distribution of body hair. Note operative scars that might suggest adrenal, breast, lung or renal surgery
II. Assist with the collection of specimens and diagnostic tests
   A. Obtain blood samples for: RBC, hemoglobin, hematocrit; WBC, and differential: serum electrolytes, glucose, BUN, creatinine: serum hormone studies, cortisol, aldosterone and ACTH
   B. Collect sample of body fluids for culture
   C. Collect urine sample for analysis
   D. Obtain stat chest x-ray, ECG, and possible flat plate of abdomen
III. Obtain a history to identify the cause of the presenting picture
   A. Interview patient, family, friends or others. Note the circumstances leading up to and accompanying the onset of the problem
   B. Search the patient for identification that would alert staff to a chronic medical condition
   C. Obtain a complete inventory of all the medications the patient has taken the past 6 to 12 months. The reasons for taking them and the dosages. Consult with patient's personal physician, if possible

D. Note a history of diabetes mellitus, tuberculosis, carcinoma, thyroid problems, past surgical procedures, recent exposure to infections, head trauma, postpartum status

E. Note the presence of physical and/or psychologic stressors in the patient's life

IV. Correct the severe dehydration and hypovolemia

   A. Establish an IV line; cut down may be required, if circulatory collapse is present

   B. A CVP line or pulmonary artery catheter may be inserted

   C. Insert an indwelling urinary catheter. Save all urine

   D. For severe dehydration, the following may be prescribed: 250 ml of glucose in physiologic saline given within 30 minutes, followed by 300 to 500 ml of this solution every hour; up to 3 liters of fluid may be required the first few hours. Subsequent fluid therapy: 5 percent dextrose in saline, 1000 ml q 4 to 6 hours/24 hours

   E. Monitor the patient's responses to this high fluid volume:

     1. check the bp q 30 minutes

     2. check the CVP or PWP q 1 to 3 hours

     3. monitor I&O

     4. monitor serum electrolytes, BUN, creatinine

     5. check the urine specific gravity q 1 hour

   F. If hypotension is not corrected with rapid hydration and corticoid replacement, a pressor agent such as Neo-synephrine 0.25 to 0.5 mg IV bolus may be prescribed (rarely needed)

V. Replace the missing glucocorticoid

   A. Administer an IV bolus of hydrocortisone, 100 mg; follow with hydrocortisone, 100 mg in a liter of 5 percent dextrose/saline and administer at a rate of 100 ml/hour. The total dose of hydrocortisone in the first 24 hours may range from 300 to 400 mg

   B. Monitor patient's responses to therapy

     1. note improvement in muscle strength, tone

     2. observe for increasing awareness, orientation and less confusion

     3. note an increase in systolic and diastolic bp

     4. note an increase in serum sodium and decrease in potassium

VI. Assess effects of hyperkalemia on cardiac muscle

   A. Place patient on continuous cardiac monitoring

     Initially heart rate will be slow, QRS wave wide and T wave spiked; these should disappear with treatment

   B. Monitor serum potassium levels frequently. If potassium levels remain above 6.5 mEq/L, and if cardiac dysrhythmias occur, IV sodium bicarbonate may be prescribed

VII. Institute measures to relieve pyrexia

   A. Take a rectal temperature every hour during acute crisis

   B. Fever may be controlled with tepid sponges or a cooling mattress

   C. If fever is due to an infectious problem, antibiotics may be prescribed

VIII. Institute measures to reduce physiologic and psychologic stress
  A. Patient is on complete bed rest and is not allowed to do anything during the acute phase of this illness
  B. Provide a quiet, nonstimulating environment
  C. Give short explanations concerning nursing and medical activities
  D. Keep family informed about patient's condition

RATIONALE

Because adrenocortical insufficiency is not a common occurrence and because the laboratory picture could be confused with chronic renal failure, it is imperative that the emergency department staff pay special attention to the data gathered from the history and systems survey. Adrenal crisis should be suspected in patients in shock and where hypotension cannot be explained. Once the diagnosis is established, the goals of management are to correct the dehydration and electrolyte imbalances, restore the cortisol levels to their maximum, and search for an underlying precipitating or contributing cause of the problem.

Dehydration and hypovolemia are best corrected by the rapid administration of intravenous fluids. The fluid of choice is a solution of 5 percent dextrose in normal saline which will yield per liter 50 grams of glucose and 154 mEq of both sodium and chloride. This solution helps restore the blood glucose level as well as the sodium and chloride levels. The rate of repletion is determined by the degree of dehydration. In many cases, large volumes of fluids are required. This necessitates close and careful monitoring of the patient's responses to this fluid load. Therefore, a catheter is inserted into the urinary bladder for accurate output measurement; a CVP line or PWP line may be inserted and serum and urine electrolytes must be obtained frequently.

This patient requires maximal replacement doses of glucocorticoids. Hydrocortisone is the steroid of choice because it has a rapid onset of action, is short-acting, and produces less side effects and hypothalamic–pituitary–adrenal axis suppression. After an intravenous bolus of the drug is given, the patient is maintained on an intravenous drip until oral therapy can be started. The large initial dose precludes the need to replace mineralocorticoids. However, once oral therapy begins, the patient requires mineralocorticoid replacement. As the patient recovers from the acute episode, glucocorticoid dosages are reduced 20 to 30 percent daily until a maintenance dose can be established for this patient. During the crisis stage, the glucocorticoids, glucose, saline, and water will correct the fluid and electrolyte imbalances as well as the hypotension. Rarely are vasopressor agents required to correct the hypotension.

The rapid hydration and high doses of glucocorticoids should be sufficient to lower the hyperkalemia. To monitor the heart's response to therapy and to observe for untoward effects of the hyperkalemia on the heart, the patient should be placed on a cardiac monitor. If cardiac arrhythmias do develop, in rare conditions, sodium bicarbonate may be prescribed. The mild metabolic acidosis will also correct with the glucocorticoid administration and does not need further therapy.

Hypo- or hyperpyrexia could accompany adrenal crisis. The hourly temperature needs to be recorded to monitor this parameter. Severe hyperpyrexia can be managed by tepid sponges and/or a cooling mattress. Even slight changes in body temperature should be reported to the physician once glucocorticoids are begun because they mask the signs and symptoms of infection.

The asthenic patient cannot and should not be expected to participate in the care. The nurse should perform all aspects of care and allow for as much rest as possible. Likewise, the nurse will do all possible to reduce psychologic stressors that may be affecting the patient.

4. Disorders of Acid–Base Balance

The internal environment of the human body is composed of acids, bases, and salts in solution. Acids are substances that produce hydronium ions (hydrogen) when placed in solution and because the hydrogen ion is a proton, an acid can be described as a substance that yields protons (proton donor). A base is a compound containing one or more hydroxyl groups which are capable of dissociating in solution producing hydroxyl ions which are negatively charged. Because bases combine with protons, they are referred to as proton acceptors.

When acids and bases are mixed together, the hydrogen ions of the acid combine with the hydroxyl to form water and another compound. Salts are also products of the reaction of an acid with a base. These compounds contain the negative ion of an acid combined with the positive ion of a base and result in the formation of (a) a neutral salt, one without replaceable hydrogen or hydroxyl ions, (b) an acid salt, one that contains replaceable hydrogen in its molecule, or (c) a basic salt, one that contains a hydroxyl group in its molecule which it will yield when dissolved in water.

Acids, bases, and salts are known as electrolytes because, as dissolved ions, they conduct an electrical current. Within the body they function in a number of ways to maintain fluid balance and acid–base balance within reasonably normal limits so that the cells of the body can continue to live and function properly.

Acid–base balance in the body is a reflection of hydrogen ion concentration of the blood. Although some of the body's physiologic fluids are very acidic or basic, the body can only tolerate minimal fluctuations in this concentration of hydrogen ions, if cellular enzymatic processes are to proceed at their normal rate. The concentration of hydrogen ions is expressed by the symbol, pH, which is a negative logarithm. pH is a more convenient means for expressing the minute quantity of hydrogen ions in a fluid. Sorenson's pH scale ranges from 0 to 14. A pH of 7 is neutral, meaning that there are as many hydrogen ions in this solution as there are hydroxyl ions. At a pH below 7, a solution is acid. A pH above 7 is alkaline or basic. The pH of the human blood ranges between 7.35 and 7.45 with a normal of 7.4.

Therefore, human blood is slightly basic. Acidosis refers to the process which cause acidemia. Likewise, alkalosis refers to the process which causes alkalemia. Acidosis is present when the blood pH is below 7.35. Alkalosis is present when the blood pH is above 7.45.

It is quite extraordinary that the body's pH is maintained within such narrow limits, because hydrogen ions are constantly being added to and removed from the body by chemical reactions and exchanges with the environment. Endogenously, each day volatile acids are produced as an end product of cellular metabolism. The potential volatile acid is carbonic acid which results from the cellular production of carbon dioxide. Carbon dioxide combines with water to produce carbonic acid. In addition, nonvolatile or fixed acids are produced by metabolic processes such as in the metabolism of amino acids which contain sulfur, which could be a potential source of sulfuric acid; lactic acid is a product of carbohydrate metabolism; aceto-acetic acid arises from fatty acid metabolism. Exogenously, organic acids and bases enter the body by way of the foods we eat and additions to these foods in the processing or preparation.

The body has three well-integrated control systems that help to maintain the constancy of the hydrogen ion: (a) the activities of chemical buffer systems in its body fluids, (b) the ability to alter the activity of the respiratory system, (c) the ability to secrete either an acid or an alkaline urine. The respiratory system regulation of acid–base balance is faster and more powerful than the other two control systems.

Chemical buffers are substances that resist changes in hydrogen ion concentration of a solution when an acid or base is added to that solution. They have the unique ability to keep the pH of a solution fairly constant unless they are overwhelmed. In the body, they usually appear in pairs and consist of a weak acid accompanied by its conjugated base, usually a sodium salt, if extracellular, or a potassium salt, if intracellular. Examples of important chemical buffer pairs in the body are:

1. carbonic acid–sodium bicarbonate (H_2CO_3/$NaHCO_3$)
2. monosodium phosphate–disodium phosphate (NaH_2PO_4/Na_2HPO_4)
3. hydrogen proteinate–sodium proteinate
4. oxyhemoglobin–reduced hemoglobin

The action of chemical buffers is predictable. The conjugated base of a weak acid of a buffer pair reacts with strong acids to produce a weaker acid and salt. Examples would be:

$$NaHCO_3 + HCl \rightarrow H_2CO_3 + NaCl$$
$$Na_2HPO_4 + HCl \rightarrow NaH_2PO_4 + NaCl$$

The weak acid of a buffer pair reacts with strong bases to produce the conjugated base of the weak acid plus water. Some examples are:

$$H_2CO_3 + NaOH \rightarrow NaHCO_3 + H_2O$$
$$NaH_2PO_4 + NaOH \rightarrow Na_2HPO_4 + H_2O$$

The carbonic acid–bicarbonate buffer system is the most important buffer system in the body. Activities of the bicarbonate part of this buffer pair accounts for approximately 50 percent of the buffering potential of the blood. In the normal, healthy person, there exists approximately 1 molecule of carbonic acid for every 20 molecules of bicarbonate ions. Although bicarbonate is found in plasma, red blood cells, and other body fluids, the cells lining the renal tubules are most capable of conserving or excreting this ion as needed. The respiratory system, principally by altering its ventilatory rate, regulates the amount of carbon dioxide in the blood, thus changing carbonic acid levels.

Conditions that increase the level of anions (chloride, sulfate, phosphate, organic acids) in the body reduce the number of sodium ions available to combine with bicarbonate ions because these ions combine with available sodium. The "free" bicarbonate ion combines readily with hydrogen ions to form carbonic acid, which will dissociate in water to form carbon dioxide and water. As the carbon dioxide is increased, the rate and depth of respirations increase resulting in the carbon dioxide being blown off. As the level of carbon dioxide is lowered, more carbonic acid dissociates resulting in a lowering of the bicarbonate and hydrogen ions in the plasma and diminished respirations.

Conversely, when anion concentration is low, especially the anion chloride, it will lead to an increase in the bicarbonate ion concentration of the blood because more sodium is available to combine with bicarbonate. In this situation, the number of free hydrogen ions and thus the amount of carbonic acid is reduced. Changes in the anion concentration are frequently used diagnostically and therapeutically. The physician looks at the results of the base excess values and the anion gap values in many cases to make the proper diagnosis.

The phosphate buffer system acts almost identically to the bicarbonate buffer system. It is found primarily in the cells of the renal tubule and intracellularly. Monobasic and dibasic phosphates can trap hydrogen ions and the processes involved in these chemical reactions accounts for the elimination of approximately 20 mEq of acid per day. The quantity excreted is titratable because it can be quantified by laboratory procedures.

The amino acids in the form of proteinates are very effective buffers because of their ability to neutralize either acids or bases. The amino groups in their radical neutralize acids, whereas their carboxyl groups neutralize bases. Their greatest activity takes place intracellularly and they contribute about 7 percent to the total buffering done in whole blood.

Hemoglobin not only acts to transport oxygen but it also functions as a buffer. In fact approximately 35 percent of the total buffering of the blood is contributed by the oxyhemoglobin–reduced hemoglobin buffer. The hemoglobin molecule contains a number of imidizole groups, each of which can accept or donate hydrogen ions which are bound by reduced (or unoxygenated) hemoglobin. Oxygen transport is a function of the iron-containing groups of the hemoglobin molecule, which is bound to oxyhemoglobin. When oxygen is bound by the iron containing groups, the imidizole groups show less affinity for binding hydrogen ions and vice versa. At the tissue level, oxygen is released and carbon dioxide diffuses into the blood. Carbon dioxide is hydrated to carbonic acid because of the presence of the activator, carbonic anhydrase, found in the red blood cells. Hydrogen ions from the carbonic acid are further buffered by the reduced hemoglobin, to produce bicarbonate. Some of this bicarbonate diffuses out to the plasma in exchange for chloride ions to preserve the electroneutrality of the compartments. When the blood is exposed to alveolar gas, reduced hemoglobin is oxygenated; it dissociates more hydrogen ion which reacts with bicarbonate in the red blood cells to form carbonic acid, which again in the presence of carbonic anhydrase will be dehydrated to carbon dioxide and water. Carbon dioxide escapes in the exchange gas. As the red blood cell bicarbonate is consumed, plasma bicarbonate enters the red blood cells and chloride ions come out.

Although the actions of the body's buffers are described individually, it must be understood that they actually all work together. Thus, any condition that changes the hydrogen ion concentration results in changes in the balance of all the buffer systems. It should also be noted that most of the chemical buffer systems are arranged to neutralize acids. In fact, the body handles an acid load much better than a basic load.

The respiratory system is able to respond to changes in the pH of the body's extracellular fluids in a physiologic manner by either retaining or blowing off carbon dioxide. The hydrogen ion concentration of the body fluids has a direct influence on the medulla's respiratory center. A decrease in pH results in an increase in respiratory rate which could be four to five times the normal. Conversely, an increase in pH results in a decrease of approximately 50 to 75 percent in respiratory rate. The respiratory system's physiologic "buffering" ability is greater than all the chemical buffers in our body.

Approximately 60 mEq of fixed acids are produced daily and they cannot be eliminated by the lungs. The kidney has a number of mechanism that excretes excess hydrogen ions: (a) directly excreting them, (b) excreting them in exchange for sodium ions, (c) excreting them as titratable phosphate acids, and (d) excreting them as nonacidic ammonium ions. When the body excretes a large amount of hydrogen ions in any form, the urine becomes acid. Likewise, when the body has an excess of base, the kidney excretes the base causing the urine to become alkaline. The renal response of changing the acidity or alkalinity of the urine takes longer than other mechanisms to maintain acid–base balance.

The direct excretion of hydrogen ions in the urine can continue until an ultimate level, pH 4.5, is reached. At this level, this mechanism stops. The phosphate buffers in the tubular mechanism will efficiently remove excess hydrogen ions, but if the tubular fluids remain highly acidic for a long period, ammonia ions are produced in greater numbers. Ammonia combines with hydrogen to produce ammonium ions. The ammonium ions are excreted in combination with chloride or other tubular anions. The net effect is the removal of hydrogen ions and no change in urinary pH because ammonium chloride is a neutral salt. Ammonium excretion can account for the excretion of more than 50 mEq of acid per day.

METABOLIC ACIDOSIS

ASSESSMENT

Refer to Table 18, following.

PATHOPHYSIOLOGY

Metabolic acidosis can be described as a condition created by (a) an increase in the unspecified fixed acid levels or (b) bicarbonate losses without a change in the unspecified acid levels. The most common causes can be categorized as follows:

I. Accumulation of strong acids (primary base deficit)
   A. Increases in endogenous acid production
      1. lactic acid build up: shock, hemorrhage, cardiac arrest, hypoxia, lactic acidosis
      2. ketoacid build up: starvation, diabetic ketoacidosis, alcoholic ketoacidosis
      3. unspecified anion retention (phosphates, sulfates, creatinates): glomerulonephritis, renal failure
   B. Ingestion of acids or acid precursors
      1. late in salicylate intoxication (salicylic and lactic acids)
      2. ethylene glycol–antifreeze (oxaloacetic acid)
      3. methyl alcohol–wood alcohol (formic acid and lactic acids)
II. Losses of strong base
   A. Intestinal losses: prolonged or severe diarrhea, pancreatic or biliary drainage
   B. Renal tubular acidosis
   C. Medication overtreatment with acetazolamide (Diamox or ammonium chloride)

The most frequent cause of acute metabolic acidosis in the critically ill or injured patient is related to an inadequate supply of oxygen to the body cells. The body cells require oxygen for the cellular metabolism of food molecules. This metabolism proceeds in sequential phases: (a) glycolysis, wherein glucose is converted to pyruvate with the release of small amounts of hydrogen and 2 moles of ATP, (b) pyruvate is converted to acetylcoenzyme A which enters, (c) the Krebs cycle, where the oxidation of the molecule takes place and results in liberated hydrogen ions which combine with an acceptor, nicatinamide adenine dinucleotide to form $NADH_2$ plus 2 moles of ATP, and (d) in the electron transport system, the hydrogen ions of $NADH_2$ are passed along a chain of acceptors (the final one being oxygen) releasing sufficient energy for the synthesis of 32 moles of ATP plus water. Carbon dioxide is also released in these phases.

In the absence of oxygen, all the hydrogen acceptors remain reduced and cannot accept hydrogen ions. With no free NAD, fuel molecules cannot be oxidized and the whole processes of the Krebs cycle and electron transport system cease. The same effect results if the enzymes of the electron transport system are poisoned, for example, with cyanide.

TABLE 18. METABOLIC ACIDOSIS AND METABOLIC ALKALOSIS: ASSESSMENT FINDINGS

Parameter	Metabolic Acidosis		Metabolic Alkalosis	
	Primary	Compensated	Primary	Compensated
pH (7.35–7.45)	Low	Near normal	Increased	Near normal
P$_{CO_2}$ (35–45 mm Hg)	Normal	Decreases	Normal	Rises
H$_{CO_3}$ (22–26 mEq/L)	Below normal	No change	Above normal	No change
Base excess (0, ±2)	Low, deficit	Less of a deficit	High, excess	Less of an excess
Respiratory rate		Hyperpnea		Shallow
		Kussmaul type		Hypoventilation
Urine pH		Acid		Alkaline or paradoxically acid
Serum sodium		Could be decreased	Decreased	
Serum chloride		Could be increased	Decreased	
Serum potassium		Could be increased	Increased	
Serum calcium				
Central nervous system effects	Depressed motor and sensory activity; lethargy, listless, stuporous, coma		Hyperactive motor and sensory responses; increased muscle tone, tetany, seizures	
Level of hydration	Usually hypovolemic		Could be hypo- or hypervolemic depending on the cause	

Glycolysis can continue in a reduced oxygen environment (anaerobic glycolysis) in some body tissues. The small amount of hydrogen produced in this process is passed along to the pyruvate (pyruvic acid) which becomes reduced to lactic acid because pyruvate, itself, cannot enter the Krebs cycle. The circulation of large amounts of lactic acid eventually exceeds the capacity of the buffering systems and results in an imbalance of the lactate–pyruvate ratio of 1:10 to shift to the left. This build up of lactic acid exceeds the liver's capacity to extract it and the kidney's ability to excrete it, furthering regional hypoperfusion and acidemia.

Lactic acidosis is a metabolic acidosis caused by the acccumulation of lactate ions to almost twice the normal (normal is 1 mEq/L) and is associated with an arterial pH below 7.35. Circulatory collapse, hypoxia, and hypoperfusion contribute to type A lactic acidosis. Type B is more commonly associated with hepatic disease, renal disease, the ingestion of alcohol, formerly the ingestion of Phenformin, and with hereditary defects of carbohydrate metabolism.

Lactic acidosis could coexist in patients with diabetic ketoacidosis, hyperglycemic hyperosmolar nonketotic coma, and in alcoholic ketosis. Ketoacidosis contributes to lactate accumulation when the primary ketone, acetoacetate (AcAc), is reduced to form excess quantities of β-hydroxybutyric acid (BOHB) rather than decarboxylating it to form the volatile ketone, acetone. The normal BOHB–AcAc ratio is 3:1. In acidosis, this ratio can rise to 6 or 12:1. When the pH is below 7.1, the BOHB–AcAc ratio is at least 6:1. When BOHB accumulates first, the excess hydrogen ions favor lactic acid formation. Ethanol and formerly Phenformin caused an excess in lactic acid in a similar manner, in addition they are able to elevate the amount of NAD that is reduced.

Lactic acidosis should be suspected in patients who present in shock, particularly if a history reveals diabetes, hepatic or renal disease. The anion gap is greater than the estimated contribution of ketones to the acidosis. Serum glucose and ketone levels may be normal but lactate levels are extremely high in pure lactic acidosis.

Uncontrolled diabetes mellitus, starvation, and excessive alcohol ingestion result in an excess of acidic ketones being produced in the body. These conditions are examples of a "fasting" state wherein low levels of insulin are found, glycogenolysis is depleted, and gluconeogenesis exists. Lipolysis produces the necessary energy required for cellular activity. However, unrestrained lipolysis results in the overproduction of ketones because of the failure to oxidize glucose for energy.

The primary ketone body is acetoacetic acid and from it β-hydroxybutyric acid and acetone are formed. Acetone is a volatile acid and is blown off by the lungs. These ketones are the end result of the breakdown of fatty acids in the liver. Excess ketones must be neutralized by bases and/or excreted with bases. Thus, excess ketone formation, ketosis, exhausts the base buffering ability of the body causing a rise in the serum hydrogen ions to acidotic levels.

The kidney plays a major role in the excretion of body acids and any disease of its parenchyma (i.e., chronic glomerulonephritis) interferes with this capacity. Acid excretion, being a function of the tubules, is most effected by tubular diseases (i.e., pyelonephritis). The basic pathologic mechanism appears to be related to the inability to produce ammonia (NH_3) in normal quantities because of a total loss of the number of functioning nephrons as is seen in acute or chronic renal failure. The impaired ability to excrete hydrogen ions with ammonia results in hydrogen ion retention as well as the retention of sulfates and other organic anions. The body attempts to neutralize these substances by giving up its bases. If overwhelmed, acidemia results.

The ingestion of acids or their precursors could lead to acidemia. The most common causes are the accidental or intentional ingestion of ethylene glycol, methyl alcohol, and aspirin. Ethylene glycol is a complex alcohol and when dissolved in water, it lowers the freezing point. It is commonly called antifreeze and is used in automobile radiators. It is known to be lethal at approximately 100 ml. Once ingested it is metabolized to oxalic acid, which is quite toxic to the kidney, and results in tubular necrosis, the deposit of calcium oxylate crystals in the renal tubules, marked acidosis, hypocalcemia, and other electrolyte disturbances. Ethanol 50 percent has been used to treat this condition but dialysis may be required.

Methyl alcohol, methanol or wood alcohol, may be ingested as a substitute for ethanol. Once ingested, it is oxidized to form formaldehyde. Formaldehyde is a protein precipitant and is highly toxic to protoplasmic proteins. Blindness and death can occur, if as little as 30 ml is ingested. Formaldehyde is further oxidized to produce the fatty acid, formic acid. Formic acid is a weak acid and will not dissociate readily, thus building up the acid load of the body fluids. It is also possible that methyl alcohol enhances the conversion of pyruvate to lactic acid. The antidote used in treating this patient is ethanol 50 percent, however, dialysis may be required.

The accidental ingestion of an excess of salicylates is unfortunately common in children. Once absorbed, aspirin is rapidly hydrolyzed to salicylic acid in the body fluids. The liver has a limited capacity to biotransform salicylic acid to its water soluble form for excretion. A blood salicylate level of 600 to 700 μg/ml is indicative of moderate to severe poisoning. In the early stages, the patient is in a state of respiratory alkalosis because salicylate acts as a respiratory stimulant increasing oxygen consumption and carbon dioxide output. After compensatory mechanisms are depleted, the body gives up its bicarbonate buffer resulting in acidemia. In addition, high levels of salicylic acid induce disturbances in carbohydrate metabolism resulting in the accumulation of lactic acid and ketones.

All the aforementioned causes of metabolic acidosis result from the accumulation of strong acids and anions. Anions such as phosphates, sulfates, proteinates, and other organic anions are left behind to replace the bicarbonate used in the titration of hydrogen ions. Thus an anion gap exists. Normally, the sum of chloride and bicarbonate in the blood is about 10 to 12 mEq/L less than the concentration of sodium. When strong acids accumulate in the body, the sum of chloride plus bicarbonate is less than the sodium minus 10 to 12 mEq.

Metabolic acidosis can be caused by excessive losses of the bicarbonate ion. In comparing the bicarbonate concentration of various gastrointestinal fluids to that of plasma, it is quite evident that the bicarbonate concentration of all these intestinal fluids, with the exception of gastric juice, is higher in bicarbonate ions. Thus, any condition associated with large losses of these fluids such as diarrhea, biliary and/or pancreatic drainage, small intestine drainage, obstruction, would be accompanied by a loss of bicarbonate. Decreasing the level of bicarbonate in the body fluids results in an increase in the dissociation of carbonic acid, because sodium is not available to combine with the bicarbonate. The result is an increase in hydrogen ions free to combine with water to form carbonic acid or to join with anions to make acids.

Another mechanism in which bicarbonate ions are lost from the body is reflective of renal tubular disease. In proximal renal tubular acidosis, the kidney is unable to generate hydrogen ions which results in the distal tubule receiving a large load of filtered bicarbonate. The distal tubule has a decreased ability to secrete hydrogen ions resulting in the bicarbonate being lost in the urine. Thus the urine produced is alkaline. If patients with this problem do develop acidemia, the reduced rate of bicarbonate delivery to the distal segment allows it to excrete some hydrogen ions; thus, the urine could become acidic.

Distal renal tubular acidosis is reflective of the inability to develop normal hydrogen ion gradients resulting in an alkaline urine even when the patient is acidemic. In chronic states of this disease, the patients can achieve a reduced but stable serum bicarbonate level because the mineral salts of the bones provide an additional source of buffer.

Certain medications can iatrogenically result in a loss of body bases. Acetazolamide (Diamox) may be prescribed (a) to alkalinize the urine, (b) in the treatment of glaucoma, and (c) in combination with other anticonvulsant medication in treating seizures. This drug inhibits the formation of the enzyme carbonic anhydrase, and thus promotes the excretion of bicarbonate, sodium, and potassium ions in the urine, while retaining hydrogen ions and titratable acids. Patients receiving moderate amounts of this medication have an acidemia with an accompanying alkaline urine.

Ammonium chloride is another medication that leads to a loss of the body base. It is commonly used as part of cough expectorants, as a means for acidifying the urine, and a part of drugs which decrease the fluid retention associated with menstruation. When ammonium chloride is ingested, the ammonium dissociates to form ammonia and hydrogen chloride. The hydrogen chloride (hydrochloric acid) is buffered by the sodium bicarbonate ions producing sodium chloride and carbonic acid. The ammonia is converted to urea in the liver, which necessitates using carbon dioxide from the plasma. The net result is a loss of the total body base leading to acidemia.

Mild to moderate systemic acidosis accompanies other electrolyte disturbances and is a prominent feature of salt depletion syndromes. Recall that the normal renal mechanism exchanges a sodium ion for each hydrogen and potassium ion in the distal tubule. Impaired bicarbonate reabsorption, which occurs in renal and gastrointestinal problems, leads to losses of sodium as well as bicarbonate ions resulting in the retention of hydrogen and potassium ions. The loss of sodium ions leads to (a) an obligatory water loss, (b) retention of chloride ions to maintain electroneutrality, (c) hyperchloremic acidosis, because the chloride ions combine with the hydrogen ions, (d) hyperchloremic acidosis, which mobilizes calcium from the bones leading to a hypercalcemia and a hypercalcinuria, and (e) the release of intercellular potassium. Excess parathyroid hormone, lack of aldosterone, and lack of glucocorticoids are examples of conditions that cause sodium depletion and are accompanied by metabolic acidosis of varying degrees.

Regardless of its cause, primary acidemia lowers the pH because of the build up of the hydrogen ions. The body's chemical buffer pairs increase their activity to titrate this load. In the process most of the base is consumed and this is reflected in a low serum bicarbonate level and base deficit.

The body will compensate for this disturbance in the carbonic–bicarbonate equilibrium. Compensation means that the abnormal pH is returned to near normal by altering that component of the buffer system not primarily affected. However, it must be understood that compensatory mechanisms are never complete.

Compensation for primary metabolic acidosis is done by the lungs. The increase in hydrogen ions is sensed by chemoreceptors located in the aorta and carotid bodies. They send this signal to the respiratory center in the medulla, which stimulates respirations. The increase in rate and depth of respirations lowers the PCO_2 so that the ratio of carbonic acid–bicarbonate returns to 1:20. Because it is the respiratory system doing the compensating, the process can occur fairly rapidly, within hours. If renal pathology is not present, the kidney eventually secretes a very acid urine.

If the metabolic acidosis is very severe and/or chronic, the lungs may not be able to blow off enough carbon dioxide to compensate fully. In fact, chronic metabolic acidosis is identified by smaller decrements in serum bicarbonate, less of a base deficit, and a less marked reduction of PCO_2. In chronic states, the renal mechanism is capable of secreting more acid ammonium salts.

The diagnosis of metabolic acidosis is based upon the clinical picture, the history, and laboratory data. The patient characteristically appears quite ill. Hypovolemia is suspected in those who appear very dehydrated. The body will try to dilute very strong acids. The serum pH in the acute stage will be low as will the bicarbonate and there will be a base deficit.

The calculation of the base excess value (or buffer base value) is helpful in determining whether the alteration in the concentration of bicarbonate is due to an abnormality in (a) cell metabolism, (b) renal functioning, or (c) if it is due to a compensatory change. The term "base excess" refers principally to bicarbonate in the blood and other blood bases. When bicarbonate levels drop below the normal range, base excess values drop below zero (normal −2, 0, +2) and a base deficit exists.

Because metabolic acidosis can be due to an increased production and/or absorption of acids, it should be differentiated from those conditions that cause it by loosing bicarbonate. This can be accomplished by calculating the anion gap. The anion gap represents the sum of the unmeasured serum anions (i.e., sulfates, phosphates, proteinates, and other organic acids such as lactate). The anion gap is calculated in a number of ways:

1. $(Na + K) - (HCO_3 + Cl) = 12 (\pm 2)$
2. $(Na + K) - (HCO_3 + Cl + 17) = 3$ or less
3. $(Cl + HCO_3) =$ less than $(Na - 12)$

Patients with excessive acid production or absorption have an increase in the anion gap. Whereas patients with metabolic acidosis due to a bicarbonate loss have a relatively normal anion gap. In the first formula, a value above 20 is indicative of metabolic acidosis in azotemic patients.

MANAGEMENT

   I. Obtain a history and review it for possible causes of acidosis
     A. Interview the patient, family, friends, and others
     B. Ascertain for a history of diabetes, starvation, alcoholism, renal failure, heart disease, or circulatory problems
     C. Identify the accidental ingestion of salicylates, antifreeze, methanol
     D. Obtain an accurate list of all medications patient is taking, especially Diamox and ammonium chloride
     E. Search for evidence of losses of intestinal fluids: ostomies, diarrhea, obstruction, pancreatic losses
     F. Note the time of onset of the problem and behaviors that the patient exhibited
  II. Determine the status of airway, breathing, and circulation
     A. Clear upper airway, if necessary, and support ventilation
     B. Establish an intravenous line for fluid administration
     C. Record the temperature, pulse, respiration, and bp
 III. Perform a rapid systems survey
     A. Cardiovascular: obtain a stat ECG; note any rhythm disturbance
     B. Pulmonary: note the rate, depth and pattern of respirations: note any odor to the breath; note the presence of cyanosis
     C. Central nervous system: note the general behavior, level of consciousness, motor responses, sensory responses
     D. Gastrointestinal: note any nausea, vomiting, diarrhea, fistulas, ostomies, abdominal distention and condition of mucous membrane. Establish what patient has eaten or ingested the past 12 hours
     E. Renal: catheterize and insert an indwelling catheter. Measure the output and test it for sugar and acetone. Send specimen to laboratory for analysis
     F. Integumentary: skin color, turgor, temperature
 IV. Assist with diagnostic studies
     A. Obtain blood samples for
       1. RBC: Hgb, Hct
       2. WBC and differential
       3. serum electrolytes
       4. serum glucose, BUN, creatinine
       5. liver profile
       6. blood cultures
       7. arterial blood gases
       8. toxicology screen
       9. blood ammonia level
      10. blood lactate–pyruvate

  B. Collect and send urine samples for analysis, electrolyte, ammonia levels, cultures and sensitivity glucose, acetone, pH
  C. Calculate the anion gap and base excess values
  D. Initiate continuous cardiac monitoring
V. Correct the underlying problem
  A. For lactic acidosis: improve oxygen delivery, improve tissue perfusion, restore fluid balance and electrolyte status
  B. For ketoacidosis: give insulin, carbohydrates, correct fluid and electrolyte imbalances
  C. For ingestion of acids: remove the offender (see Chapter on Toxicology)
  D. Prevent further losses of base: treat diarrhea, fistulas, obstructions
  E. Withdraw medications that enhance base loss
VI. Restore bicarbonate ion levels, if pH is below 7.25
  A. Administer sodium bicarbonate IV (one ampule = 50 ml of 7.5 percent solution = 44.6 mEq of bicarbonate)
    1. calculate dosage required: formulas used are
      a. needed bicarbonate $= \dfrac{\text{base deficit (mEq/L} \times \text{body weight in kg)}}{4}$
      b. needed bicarbonate = (25 mEq − reported bicarbonate) × 0.5 (kg body weight)
      c. needed bicarbonate = kg body weight × (25 mEq − reported bicarbonate) × 0.3
    2. administer at rate prescribed: bolus or in 1000 ml 5 percent D/W
      a. bolus of ½ calculated dose in first 40 to 60 minutes. Reevaluate blood gases
      b. no more than 2 ampules every 10 minutes. Evaluate blood gases frequently
      c. give 1 mEq/kg body weight initially, repeat in 10 minutes. Reevaluate blood gases
    3. observe for signs and symptoms of hypokalemia
      a. check cardiac monitor for signs of rhythm disturbances
      b. check serum potassium levels; report any below 3.5 mEq
      c. note any signs of: weakness, hyporeflexia, paresthesias, flat or inverted T waves, depressed ST segment, prominent U wave
    4. observe for signs of fluid overload
    5. observe for signs of respiratory alkalosis: hypertonic muscles, decreased respirations, hypokalemia, tetany
    6. administer alone to avoid undesirable interaction with other medications
    7. use very cautiously in patients with CHF, kidney disease, hypertension, or arrhythmias
  B. Administer Thromethamine (THAM), IV as prescribed (rare)
    1. this highly alkaline, sodium free organic amine solution is administered as a 0.3M solution in 0.2 percent NaCl
    2. dosage: 3.5 to 6.0 ml/kg body weight; administer slowly

3. check infusion site for inflammation, venospasm, thrombosis, chemical phlebitis. Must be given through large bore needle. Infiltration can result in tissue necrosis and sloughing

4. observe closely for depressed respirations as a result of drug; have ventilatory assistance equipment nearby during and after treatment

5. monitor blood gases frequently during administration. Watch for signs of alkalosis. Monitor serum electrolytes and glucose.

6. monitor urine output; drug has an osmotic effect

VII. Systematically record the patient's responses to therapy

   A. Chart temperature q 1 hour; pulse, respirations, bp q 30 minutes

   B. Accurately record all I&O; weigh patient

   C. Test urine specimens for sugar, acetone, pH

   D. Monitor CVP or pulmonary artery pressures, if lines inserted

   E. Assist with collection of frequent blood samples for electrolytes and blood gases; chart the result

   F. Calculate the anion gap and base excess values

   G. Record the time and dosages of all medications given

   H. Chart the neurologic responses; neurologic vital signs q 1 hour

   I. Follow ECG for subtle changes suggestive of potassium imbalances

RATIONALE

Acute metabolic acidosis is a life-threatening disorder which can depress myocardial function, counteract insulin's activity, inhibit glycolysis and increase gluconeogenesis. Because it could be due to a number of problems, a carefully elicited history is vital, if appropriate treatment is to be initiated. Analysis of the history and systems survey should provide the examiner with many clues as to the basic problem. Results of the laboratory tests quantify the clinical impression and are useful parameters to monitor responses throughout therapy.

All efforts are directed at identifying and treating the underlying problem(s). Once proper treatment for the underlying condition is begun, the acidosis may correct itself. Because severe acidosis is commonly associated with dehydration, intravenous fluids are begun to restore blood volume.

In cases where the pH is markedly depressed, alkali therapy may be a useful therapeutic adjunct to other measures aimed at correcting the underlying problem. Sodium bicarbonate is the drug of choice to raise the serum bicarbonate ion level and lower the hydrogen ion concentration. Even though acetate and lactate ion solutions normally are metabolized to bicarbonate ions, their use is limited because of the possibility that the acidosis is due to an increase in these organic acids and thus, they cannot be further metabolized to generate bicarbonate ions.

Sudden additions of bicarbonate ions into the blood could drive large amounts of potassium into the cells resulting in a hypokalemia and serious cardiac arrhythmias. This is especially serious in patients who have received digitalis. Therefore, continuous cardiac monitoring to detect subtle changes associated with hypokalemia and frequent potassium blood levels are an essential part of this patient's regimen.

Overtreatment with sodium bicarbonate leads to other severe problems that could be lethal. The high sodium load leads to an increase in extracellular osmolarity. Intracellular water shifts extracellularly to maintain osmotic equilibrium, thereby diluting the extracellular fluid and concentrating the intracellular fluid. The nurse should look for signs of edema because water will be retained, again in an effort to keep a normal sodium ion concentration in the extracellular fluid. Frequent serum sodium levels must be taken. In addition to the hypernatremia and hyperosmolarity, excess alkali could result in metabolic alkalosis. Frequent monitoring of the blood gases, respirations and neuromuscular responses will pick up clues of this event.

The complications of bicarbonate administration can be avoided. The dosage should be carefully calculated. It is preferred to administer it as a bolus because dosage delivery is difficult to regulate otherwise. Furthermore, continuous infusions will inactivate other drugs administered simultaneously during a cardiac arrest (i.e., catecholamines, calcium salts). The nurse should also be aware that solutions of sodium bicarbonate are incompatible with a wide variety of other drugs and that nothing should be added to this solution or its delivery set. Serial blood gases, electrolytes, and frequent estimations of the anion gap are useful parameters to guide therapeutic needs of this patient.

Tromethamine (THAM) has been used on occasion to treat metabolic acidosis associated with a cardiac arrest. This medication is a highly alkaline, sodium free, organic amine that acts as a hydrogen acceptor. It may function as an osmotic diuretic resulting in the excretion of fixed acids, carbon dioxide, and other electrolytes. Therefore, it is contraindicated in patients with impaired renal functioning and in those who are anuric or uremic.

THAM has several undesirable effects. It can lead to severe respiratory depression, transient hypoglycemia, metabolic alkalosis, and, if extravasation occurs, tissue necrosis. Parameters such as respirations, blood gases, glucose, electrolytes, and urinary output must be closely and continuously monitored before, during, and after its administration to detect these complications.

METABOLIC ALKALOSIS

ASSESSMENT

Refer to Table 18, on p. 417.

PATHOPHYSIOLOGY

Primary metabolic alkalosis can be described as a condition created by (a) a gain of the bicarbonate ion in the extracellular fluid or (b) a loss of acid from the extracellular fluid. Some causes of this condition can be catagorized as follows:

I. Gain of bicarbonate ion
   A. Ingestion of systemic antacids
   B. Infusions of excessive sodium bicarbonate
   C. Oxidation of organic acid salts: lactate (Ringer's lactate solution), citrate (whole blood transfusions), acetate, phosphates, sulfates
   D. Rapid correction of chronic hypercapnea
   E. Dehydration of moderate degree
II. Loss of acid ions
   A. Loss of hydrochloric acid: vomiting, pyloric stenosis
   B. Depletion of potassium and chloride ions
      1. extrarenal losses: protracted vomiting, prolonged nasogastric tube suctioning
      2. renal losses: diuretic therapy, excess glucocorticoids, excess mineralocorticoids

Metabolic alkalosis can result from the excessive oral or parenteral intake of alkaline drugs. Increasingly in medicine today, large amounts of antacids are prescribed in an effort to raise the pH of the stomach thereby reducing its acidity and decreasing the incidence of stress ulcers. Most of these antacids are not systemic, however, as they remove excess acid by neutralization, they could contribute to the occurrence of metabolic alkalosis. The patient who self medicates with over-the-counter antacids is at higher risk to develop alkalosis because many commercial preparations contain sodium bicarbonate or calcium carbonate, or both. Calcium carbonate antacids are eventually metabolized to sodium bicarbonate. Taking systemic antacids in large amounts over a long period of time results not only in alkalosis but also in rebound hyperacidity and the milk–alkali syndrome. An increase in the intake of bicarbonate raises the blood pH because hydrogen ions are given up to buffer the increase in base.

The intake of organic salts (i.e., lactate, acetate, citrates), whether orally or parenterally, in excessive amounts results also in a gain of base and a loss of acid. When organic acid salts are ingested they alkalinize body fluids because they are oxidized to carbon dioxide, water, and bicarbonate. Whole blood contains large amounts of citrate as an anticoagulant and therefore, could lead to alkalosis, if massive transfusions were given. Likewise, the lactate ions in Ringer's lactate solution, which are not excreted in the urine, can be oxidized to bicarbonate ions.

The rapid correction of chronic hypercapnea results in a temporary metabolic alkalosis. Hypercapnea results in the retention of carbon dioxide and a build up of bicarbonate ions as a compensatory mechanism. When the carbon dioxide levels are rapidly brought down to near normal, the bicarbonate ion change does not occur quickly enough. It may take several days for bicarbonate to reduce. In the meantime, a temporary metabolic alkalosis is present.

If the extracellular fluid volume is contracted, as happens in moderate dehydration that is not severe enough to interfere with tissue perfusion, a contracted metabolic alkalosis could occur. In this situation, water, sodium, and bicarbonate reabsorption increase, resulting in a high level of bicarbonate ions. If the dehydration becomes severe and tissue perfusion is impaired, the tendency toward lactic acidosis is greater than the ability to reabsorb bicarbonate ions.

Vomiting, short-term nasogastric suctioning, and pyloric stenosis lead to excessive losses of hydrochloric acid from the stomach, which leads to an increase in the bicarbonate ion concentration of the extracellular fluids. Two mechanisms contribute to this situation: (a) A loss of pure acid or hydrogen ions is equivalent to a gain in hydroxyl ions. The hydroxyl ions combine with carbonic acid producing bicarbonate and water. (b) A loss of chloride ions is accompanied by increased reabsorption of bicarbonate ions in the kidney.

Protracted vomiting and long-term nasogastric suctioning result, not only in the loss of hydrogen and chloride, but also in losses of sodium and potassium. Hypokalemia and hyponatremia are due to losses in the vomitus, inability to retain food and fluids, and continued urinary losses. Thus, the extracellular fluid delivered to the kidney for filtration is now low in hydrogen, chloride, sodium, and potassium ions yet high in bicarbonate ions. The renal tubule reacts mainly to the tubular deficit of sodium rather than the excess bicarbonate in an attempt to restore volume. Water and sodium are reabsorbed either with bicarbonate or in exchange for hydrogen or potassium ions. This mechanism, while defending the volume of the extracellular fluid compartment, sustains the alkalotic state and potassium depletion.

Other conditions associated with hypokalemia and hypochloremia place patients at risk for metabolic alkalosis. Recall that normally 80 percent of the positive ion, sodium, is reabsorbed along with the negative ion, chloride. The other 20 percent of sodium is reabsorbed in the distal tubule in exchange for hydrogen or potassium ions. This is called the distal cation pump. When hypochloremia exists, the amount of sodium reabsorbed with chloride is reduced and more of the sodium must be exchanged for hydrogen or potassium ions. When sodium is exchanged for potassium ions, there is a net loss of potassium ions resulting in a hypokalemic alkalosis. When sodium is exchanged for hydrogen ions, this represents a loss of acid, resulting in a hypochloremic alkalosis.

Usually the urine of a patient in alkalosis is alkaline which is reflective of the kidney's attempt to lower bicarbonate levels. However, if a deficit of potassium ions exists, more hydrogen ions will be excreted in exchange for sodium ions resulting in a paradoxical aciduria, in the presence of alkalosis.

There are many situations that give rise to states of hypokalemia or hypochloremia. Diuretics, the mainstay of antihypertensive regimens, lower serum potassium levels significantly and thus could induce metabolic alkalosis. Excessive adrenocortical steroids, such as cortisone and prednisone, favor the excretion of potassium. Hyperaldosteronism enhances the activity of the distal cation pump resulting in the loss of both hydrogen and potassium ions and a rise in the bicarbonate ion. The degree of this last alkalosis is not severe.

It should be clear now that conditions that raise the bicarbonate ion concentration or lower the carbonic acid concentration of the extracellular fluid lead to an increase in serum bicarbonate, positive base excess, values of a pH greater than 7.45 which is reflective of the decrease in hydrogen ion concentration. Decreases in carbonic acid and thus low carbon dioxide levels are sensed by the body's chemoreceptors. This information is sent to the respiratory center in the medulla which responds by decreasing the rate and depth of respirations. This pulmonary compensatory mechanism has its limits, because as the P_{CO_2} rises, the P_{O_2} falls. The body's chemoreceptors then stimulate respirations once again. Hypoxia, therefore, limits this mechanism.

Alkalosis also induces changes in calcium ionization. Normally 50 percent of the body's calcium is ionized and 50 percent is bound. This concentration is kept in equilibrium by parathyroid hormone and serum pH. When hydrogen ion concentration falls, as in alkalosis, more calcium is bound and less is ionized. Reduced serum levels of ionized calcium can lead to muscular stiffness, aching, and/or muscle cramps. If alkalosis develops quickly, tetany may be observed. Tetany is exhibited as muscle twitching, carpopedal spasms, and seizures.

MANAGEMENT

  I. Obtain a history and review it for possible causes of alkalosis
     A. Interview the patient, family, friends
     B. Obtain a complete record of medications patient has taken, especially diuretics, steroids, antacids
     C. Ascertain the presence of concomitant illnesses: CHF, liver or renal disease
     D. Note the time or date of the onset of vomiting
 II. Determine the status of airway, breathing, and circulation
     A. Clear upper airway and support ventilations, if necessary
     B. Record the temperature, pulse, respirations, and bp
     C. Establish an intravenous line and begin fluids
III. Perform a rapid systems survey
     A. Cardiovascular: obtain a stat ECG; auscultate the heart; note any rhythm disturbances
     B. Pulmonary: obtain a stat chest x-ray; record the rate, depth and pattern of respirations; note color
     C. Nervous system: chart the general behavior, LOC, motor and sensory responses. Report any complaints of paresthesias, muscle twitching or history of seizures
     D. Gastrointestinal: note the time and amount of last food or fluid intake; note the presence of nausea, vomiting, abdominal distention
     E. Renal: catheterize and insert an indwelling catheter; measure all output; check urine pH and send specimen for analysis
     F. Integumentary: note level of dehydration; skin color, turgor and temperature
IV. Assist with diagnostic studies
     A. Obtain blood samples for:
        1. RBC, Hgb, Hct

    2. WBC and differential

    3. serum electrolytes

    4. arterial blood gases

    5. BUN, creatinine

    6. serum glucose

  B. Collect and send sample of urine to the laboratory for analysis, especially pH, electrolytes

  C. Calculate the anion gap and base excess values

  D. Initiate continuous cardiac monitoring

V. Correct the underlying problem

  A. Institute measures to decrease vomiting or loss of gastric fluids.

  B. Discontinue diuretics, steroids, antacid therapy

  C. Take measures to reduce aldosterone secretion

  D. Restore depleted volume: start IV with 5 percent D/W

VI. Correct an existing hypochloremic alkalosis

  A. Adequately hydrate to restore volume

  B. Replace chloride ions

    1. calculate the chloride deficit using 20 percent figure of extracellular fluid space or 60 percent figure, if patient is severely dehydrated

    2. administer chloride and sodium ions as isotonic saline

    3. correct ½ deficit at one time

    4. monitor serum electrolytes and blood gases frequently

VII. Correct an existing hypochloremic, hypokalemic alkalosis

  A. Replace fluid losses

  B. Administer: ¼ chloride deficit as potassium chloride

                 ¾ chloride deficit as sodium chloride

    1. do not administer potassium chloride faster than 40 mEq/hour

    2. some patients will require greater doses of potassium

    3. monitor cardiac rhythm, serum electrolytes and blood gases frequently

VIII. Administer acidifying salts to neutralize bicarbonate (rare)

  A. Salts that may be used are: ammonium chloride (2.14 percent IV), arginine hydrochloride IV, lysine hydrochloride by mouth, and dilute hydrochloric acid by mouth or hydrochloric acid IV.

  B. Closely observe blood gases, serum pH, and base excess value

  C. Dosage given should only correct ½ of base excess value

IX. Systematically record the patient's responses to therapy

  A. Chart temperature, pulse, respiration and bp q 30 to 60 minutes

  B. Record all I&O

  C. Follow cardiac monitor closely for hypokalemic and hypocalcemic changes

  D. Chart the neurologic vital signs q 30 minutes

  E. Assist with frequent collections of blood and urine samples and chart all results; repeatedly calculate base excess value

  F. Record the time and dosages of all medications given

RATIONALE

Acute primary metabolic alkalosis can be a life-threatening disorder and arises in a variety of ways. A carefully elicited history and systems survey should provide the examiner with many clues as to the basic problem. Laboratory results quantify the clinical impression. However, an erroneous impression can be made because of the pulmonary hypoventilatory compensatory mechanism seen in more chronic states of alkalosis.

Treatment should be directed toward identifying and correcting the underlying problem. Once proper treatment is initiated, the alkalosis may correct itself, if it is not too severe. Fluid depletion frequently accompanies this condition, thus intravenous fluids are begun.

Chloride-responsive alkalosis, which is commonly due to vomiting, excessive nasogastric suctioning, and volume depletion responds to infusions of normal saline. In this situation, the lack of chloride ions leads to a decrease in sodium reabsorption in the proximal tubule. At the distal tubule this sodium exchanges with a hydrogen ion or a potassium ion to be excreted allowing the bicarbonate to be reabsorbed. If adequate chloride ions are administered, more sodium is absorbed in the proximal tubule and less bicarbonate is reabsorbed.

More commonly, the patients in metabolic alkalosis have some degree of hypokalemia as well as a hypochloremia. Hypokalemia results from a number of causes: diuretics, which favor the excretion of potassium and other electrolytes, steroids which enhance the retention of sodium but loss of potassium. In addition, whenever a volume depletion exists, serum aldosterone concentration increases resulting in sodium retention and potassium loss. Correction of the hypokalemia by giving potassium chloride allows for the chloride ion to be reabsorbed with sodium in the proximal tubule and bicarbonate to be excreted with sodium in the distal tubule.

Calculating the amount of potassium to be replaced depends upon a number of parameters. As pH rises 0.10, the serum potassium falls by 0.5 mEq/L. Other parameters are length of time the deficit has occurred, patient stature and muscle mass, ECG changes, and coexisting medical problems. If potassium deficit is acute, the patient may require 40 to 60 mEq/L of potassium to raise the serum level 1.0 mEq/L.

When the alkalosis is severe (i.e., P_{CO_2} 45 or more, tetany present) or if it is resistant to therapy, acidifying salts may be administered to neutralize the excess base. Ammonium chloride, arginine hydrochloride, and lysine hydrochloride all act in a similar manner and require adequate liver functioning. In the liver the nitrogen radical of these salts is converted to urea with a hydrogen ion being released. The free hydrogen ion combines with bicarbonate to form carbonic acid which dissociates to carbon dioxide and water. Thus, bicarbonate levels are reduced and the body fluids become more acid. Hydrochloric acid can be delivered by mouth or through a large bore needle but this is the last of the modalities in the treatment of alkalosis.

During the administration of acidifying salts the patient's responses must be carefully monitored. Initially, the dosage given is only enough to correct one half of the excess base. The patient's condition and laboratory data should be reevaluated frequently before continuation of acidifying therapy.

RESPIRATORY ACIDOSIS

ASSESSMENT

Refer to Table 19, following.

PATHOPHYSIOLOGY

Primary respiratory acidosis is a condition characterized by an accumulation of carbonic acid in the blood and is due to disorders in the exchange of carbon dioxide and oxygen. The most common causes can be categorized as follows:

I. Decreased respiratory center drive, sensitivity or function
   A. Chemically induced: drugs such as barbiturates, morphine, alcohol, tranquilizers, narcotics and anesthetic agents
   B. Cranial problems: trauma, ischemia, hemorrhage, tumor, thrombosis, increased intercranial pressure, meningitis, encephalitis
II. Impairment in the mechanics of respiration
   A. Obstructions
      1. acute: aspiration of foreign objects, swelling or spasms of the pharynx, larynx, trachea, or bronchi as seen in smoke inhalation, allergic manifestations and asthma, collection of secretions from any cause, status asthmaticus
      2. chronic: emphysema, bronchitis, asthma
   B. Restrictive problems
      1. musculoskeletal defects: kyphoscoliosis, ankylosing spondylitis, muscular dystrophy, chest wall trauma
      2. neuromuscular impairments: myasthenia gravis, Guillain–Barré syndrome, drugs that relax skeletal muscles such as succinylcholine, curare.
      3. other problems: obesity, abdominal distention, pleural problems, pneumothorax, hydrothorax, hemothorax, hypoventilation with the mechanical respirator
   C. Surfactant deficiency: infant and adult respiratory distress syndromes

Diffusion of carbon dioxide and oxygen continually takes place across the alveoli capillary membrane. This exchange is dependent on a number of factors being intact: adequate ventilation to maintain normal gas exchange and volumes, a pulmonary capillary blood flow, adequate surface area, relative pressure gradients, and solubility of gases on both sides of the alveolar membrane.

Various conditions can affect the ventilatory or perfusion aspects of this pro-

TABLE 19. RESPIRATORY ACIDOSIS AND RESPIRATORY ALKALOSIS: ASSESSMENT FINDINGS

Parameter	Respiratory Acidosis		Respiratory Alkalosis	
	Primary	*Compensated*	*Primary*	*Compensated*
pH (7.35–7.45)	Decreased	Near normal	Increased	Normal
P$_{CO_2}$ (35–45 mm Hg)	Increased	No change	Decreased	No change
H$_{CO_3}$ (22–26 mEq/L)	Within normal	Increases	Within normal	Decreases
Base excess (0, + 2)	Within normal	Excess	Within normal	Deficit
Urine pH		Acid		Alkaline
Respiratory pattern	Hypoventilating Could be dyspneic		Hyperventilating Rapid rate	
Central nervous system effects	Headache Dizziness Disorientation Weak muscle power Coma		Light headed Hypertonic muscles Paresthesias Tetany Seizures	

cess. Abnormalities in ventilation are reflected in acid–base changes of the blood because the rate of carbon dioxide removal from the alveoli is directly dependent upon the rate of alveolar ventilation. Normal alveolar ventilation is sufficient to maintain the $Paco_2$ at approximately 40 mm Hg. Alveolar hypoventilation results in the retention of carbon dioxide (hypercarbia) and a decrease in available oxygen (hypoxia). Whatever is the cause of this hypoventilation, respiratory acidosis results. It can be an acute process or chronic.

Acute respiratory acidosis is a situation that implies a short time span, minutes to hours, and refers only to blood buffer changes. In acute respiratory acidosis, the following blood gases are commonly seen: Pco_2 rises abruptly above 40 mm Hg, HCO_3 rises, base excess value shows a deficit, and pH decreases.

As the amount of carbon dioxide rises in the extracellular fluid, it becomes hydrated to produce carbonic acid. This reaction occurs faster in the red blood cells than in the plasma or interstitial fluid because of the presence of carbonic anhydrase in the red blood cells.

$$CO_2 + H_2O \rightleftharpoons H_2CO_3$$

The initial body responses to mild hypercarbia are an increase in tidal volume and respiratory rate. Internally, the body responds by producing more bicarbonate ions in the blood to buffer the accumulating carbonic acid. This is specifically done by the interaction reaction process whereby carbonic acid reacts with the conjugate bases of nonbicarbonate buffers to form bicarbonate and the corresponding weak acid of the nonbicarbonate system. The reaction appears as:

$$H_2CO_3 + Buffer \longrightarrow H \, Buffer + HCO_3$$

The bicarbonate thus formed diffuses out of the intravascular space into the interstitial fluid to neutralize the acid accumulating in this compartment. This consumption of buffer results in a net decrease in the total amount of buffer. Thus, in acute respiratory acidosis the base excess value may be negative especially because renal compensatory mechanisms have not started. However, this occurrence of a negative base excess value could mislead emergency department staff into believing that the problem is metabolic acidosis.

Brackett and others have quantified the limits for the expected degree of fall of base excess or the expected degree of rise in plasma bicarbonate concentration in acute respiratory acidosis within 95 percent confidence limits. At times, this tool can be used diagnostically for patients who are experiencing hypercarbia of short duration. When using this tool, if the data falls below the 95 percent confidence limits, the possibility of an independent metabolic acidosis should be suspected.

The increase in carbonic acid production and thus, hydrogen ion increase, is reflected in a lower pH value. As the Pco_2 rises 1 mm Hg above the normal of 40 mm Hg, the pH decreases by 1 point. For example: Pco_2 of 40 mm Hg is at a pH of 7.4. A Pco_2 of 41 mm Hg will have a pH of 7.39. This inverse relationship holds true until a 10 point difference is reached. At that time, the renal compensatory mechanisms should begin to handle the acid load.

It takes from 6 to 18 hours for renal compensation to become apparent and 5 to

7 days for it to reach its maximum. The renal compensatory mechanisms need not be maximal nor complete. In this situation, the mechanisms are directed at reabsorbing bicarbonate as well as excreting hydrogen ions in an effort to restore the 1:20 ratio of carbonic acid–bicarbonate.

Filtered bicarbonate ions are not directly reabsorbed in the kidney. The sodium of filtered sodium bicarbonate is reabsorbed leaving behind the bicarbonate ion in the tubular fluid. Sodium is reabsorbed against an electrochemical gradient and in direct exchange for hydrogen ions. The hydrogen ions are formed in the tubular cells by the catalyzed hydration of carbon dioxide which results in the formation of carbonic acid. Hydrogen ions from this acid (or other acids) leaves the tubule cell and joins up with the bicarbonate ion in the tubular fluid. This reaction forms carbonic acid. This acid dissociates rapidly because of the presence of carbonic anhydrase into carbon dioxide and water. The carbon dioxide diffuses back into the tubule cell where it can form more carbonic acid or bicarbonate ions. Thus, bicarbonate ion concentration is conserved. For each mole of bicarbonate ions removed from the tubular fluid, 1 mole of bicarbonate diffuses from the tubular cell into the peritubular capillaries. This mechanism does not get rid of excess hydrogen ions.

Excess hydrogen ions in the tubular urine fluid reacts with the buffer anions sodium dibasic phosphate to form sodium monobasic phosphate. This occurs in the distal tubule. Sodium monobasic phosphate is a weak acid salt and is excreted as such. Each hydrogen ion that reacts with buffer anions, other than bicarbonate, contributes to the titratable acidity of the urine and returns one bicarbonate ion to the blood.

The renal tubule cells produce another buffer, ammonia. Any free hydrogen ions react with ammonia (NH_3) to produce ammonium (NH_4). Ammonium combines with a salt, usually a chloride and is excreted. The amount of ammonia production increases in acidosis but this takes a few days and seems to depend upon the pH of the tubular urine fluid. For each hydrogen ion that combines with ammonia, there is a net gain in one ion of bicarbonate in the peritubular blood.

The retention of carbon dioxide and its concomitant hypoxia affects many other body systems. The chemoreceptors sense the change in P_{CO_2} and O_2 concentrations of the blood and send impulses to the brain which in turn sends impulses to the heart to increase its rate and force of contractions. The patient experiences tachycardia, increased blood pressure, and palpitations. Hypoxia of the pulmonary vascular bed leads to vasoconstriction and an increase in pulmonary artery pressure. The right heart hypertrophies and eventually fails (cor pulmonale). The build-up of acid ions in the extracellular fluid causes the hydrogen ion to enter the body's cells. Potassium leaves these cells in exchange for hydrogen resulting in a net loss of potassium (hypokalemia), general muscle weakness, cramping, cardiac changes, and arrhythmias. The bone marrow responds to hypoxia by increasing its production and output of red blood cells resulting in polycythemia. Hypercarbia causes cerebral blood vessels to dilate thus increasing cerebral blood flow and cerebrospinal fluid pressure. This could result in cerebral edema and increased intercranial pressure. The patient may experience a throbbing occipital headache, dizziness, periods of disorientation, seizures, and asterixis. As the level of carbon dioxide rises and oxygen decreases, the patient becomes more and more lethargic and eventually stuporous (carbon dioxide narcosis).

The blood picture of the patient in respiratory acidosis reflects the renal compensatory attempts to maintain normal pH. Thus, the blood gases indicate a rise in serum pH to near normal, an elevated bicarbonate level, a base excess value that is now within normal limits and the high P_{CO_2} remaining unchanged. If these buffer systems fail or become exhausted, unconsciousness and death soon follow.

MANAGEMENT

I. Determine the status of airway, breathing, and circulation
   A. If patient appears apneic, perform a jaw thrust or Heimlich maneuver
   B. Institute mouth-to-mouth or mouth-to-nose respirations, if breathing does not spontaneously occur
   C. Suction airway to clear secretion
   D. Establish an IV line for the administration of fluids
II. Establish an artificial airway
   A. Assist with endotracheal tube intubation or tracheostomy tube insertion
   B. Select an airway tube that has a low pressure volume cuff. Inflate the cuff with 1 to 3 ml of air, once in place
   C. Safely secure the artificial airway; have a replacement at the bedside
III. Perform a rapid systems survey
   A. Cardiovascular: obtain temperature, pulse, respiration, bp, stat ECG; note any engorgement of neck veins, clubbing of fingers, signs of cyanosis
   B. Respiratory: note the respiratory rate, depth and pattern; obtain a stat chest x-ray; note the color of the lips and fingernail beds; note any purse lip breathing, flaring of nares, grunting respirations, position patient assumes to breathe; check for a deviated trachea, kyphoscoliosis, barrel or pigeon chest, use of accessory muscles, flail chest. Auscultate breath sounds: report any musical, crepitant, atelectatic, subcrepitant, rhonchi, or rales heard
   C. Nervous system: note any restlessness, headache, delirium, confusion, hallucinations, irrational behavior. Chart the LOC, muscle, and sensory responses; observe eyes for signs of engorged eye veins and/or papilledema
   D. Excretory: note any abdominal distention, or rigidity; note the time of last food or fluid intake. Obtain a urine sample, if not possible, catheterize and insert indwelling catheter
IV. Obtain a history and review it for possible causes of the problem
   A. Interview the patient, if possible, family, friends, others
   B. Identify the accidental or intentional ingestion of chemicals that depress respirations: narcotics, barbiturates, alcohol, tranquilizers.
   C. Obtain an accurate list of all medications patient has taken
   D. Search for evidence of acute or chronic problems that could lead to respi-

ratory depression: central nervous system, neuromuscular, allergies, smoke inhalation, respiratory blockage or restrictive problems
  E. Note the date and time of the onset of the problem
V. Assist with diagnostic studies
  A. Obtain blood samples for blood gas analysis, electrolytes, BUN, creatinine, liver profile, toxicology screen, RBC, Hgb, Hct, WBC and differential
  B. If fever is present: culture blood, urine, sputum, nose and throat
  C. Collect and send urine samples for analysis, electrolytes, glucose, acetone, pH, ammonia
  D. Institute continuous cardiac monitoring
VI. Treat the underlying condition
  A. For cranial injuries: institute measures to decrease cranial pressure, combat infection, offer ventilatory assistance
  B. For drug overdose: use antagonists, remove offender
  C. For acute obstructions: reestablish airway or bypass airway, suctioning
  D. For chest wall trauma: reexpand lung with appropriate therapy
  E. For bronchiole or alveolar collapse: IPPB, PEEP, bronchodilator medications
VII. Improve alveolar ventilation
  A. Place patient on a volume-cycled or pressure-cycled ventilator
    1. Volume-cycled ventilators are used in critically ill, intubated patients who most likely have underlying lung disease and will require long-term ventilatory assistance
    2. Pressure-cycled ventilators are used in critically ill patients, who may or may not be intubated and in whom lung disease is absent as well as insults to the thoracic cavity
  B. Assist the inhalation therapist to initiate the therapy. Note the prescribed setting on all ventilators. Do not change without physician's direction. In general, settings provide
    1. tidal volume of 400 to 800 ml. The amount of needed tidal volume can be estimated by multiplying the patient's weight in pounds by 3
    2. oxygen concentration delivered at 30 to 40 percent, but this could be lower or higher depending upon patient's condition
    3. respiratory rate between 10 and 14 per minute with a longer expiration than inspiration
  C. Check for air leaks around the airway; check the position of the airway; check the airway pressure and oxygen concentration frequently. Be certain water is in the humidifier
  D. Be certain that safety alarm systems are set in case of accidental disconnect or loss of delivered tidal volume
  E. Periodically hyperinflate or "sigh" patient; monitor ABG
VIII. Evaluate patient responses to ventilatory assistance
  A. Chart the actual respiratory rate, minute and tidal volumes, color, breath sounds, amount and characteristics of secretions, bp, heart rate, urine output. Continuously monitor heart rhythm

B. Observe for oxygen toxicity, absorption atelectasis, decreased cardiac output, cardiac dysrhythmias, respiratory alkalosis

C. Suction airway prn; change positions unless contraindicated, monitor blood gases, chest x-rays

RATIONALE

Acute respiratory acidosis is a life-threatening problem resulting from a number of conditions that have lead to hypoventilation. The first priority in caring for this patient is to establish an airway and restore breathing. In the emergency department, an artificial airway will most likely be put in place if the patient has a flail chest, inhaled smoke, is comatose, has ARDS, peritonitis, and so forth. Additional indications are a P_{CO_2} of 45 to 50 mm Hg in a patient with previously normal lung function who is not in metabolic alkalosis or a P_{O_2} of 50 mm Hg on room air or if the P_{O_2} does not improve with 40 percent oxygen delivery.

The physical survey and history should provide the examiner with clues as to the causes and extent of the respiratory problem. Laboratory results quantify the clinical impression. The information obtained from the systems survey and laboratory provide a baseline of data to which future comparisons are made.

Therapy is directed at identifying and treating the underlying cause, treating concomitant disease, and improving ventilations. Pharmacologic approaches cannot be generalized and are directed mainly toward the individual needs of the patient. In most cases, respirations will need to be assisted. Volume ventilators or pressure-limited models are available and the choice is usually based upon the severity of the patient's condition and availability of the ventilator. Because of all the various controls, accessory equipment and features they possess, ventilators are a mystery to staff. Nurses must familiarize themselves with the type of ventilator used, its purpose in this patient and be on the lookout for patient and ventilator problems while on this therapy. This patient requires constant attention and reevaluation to assure the prescribed delivery and removal of gases.

Because mechanical ventilators deliver oxygen and remove carbon dioxide from the patient, they correct respiratory acidosis. However, it is imperative that severe chronic respiratory acidosis *not* be corrected too quickly, especially if a compensatory alkalosis is exhibited. In these patients, the respiratory sensitivity to P_{CO_2} levels is lost and low P_{O_2} tension is the respiratory stimulus. Elevating the P_{O_2} too quickly removes the respiratory drive resulting in decreased rate and depth of respirations, a worsening of the acidosis or could result in a combined respiratory and metabolic alkalosis, cardiac arrhythmias, seizures, and death.

Oxygen toxicity is a hazard associated with ventilator therapy especially if the patient is receiving a high (above 40 percent) inspired oxygen concentration. The patient will complain of substernal pain after 8 to 24 hours of treatment. The arterial blood gases will deteriorate. Tachycardia and blood pressure changes will be seen. High oxygen levels decrease surfactant production and worsen the condition of patients in distress due to this problem. Other changes that may occur with high oxygen delivery are alveolar edema, pulmonary congestion, and intraalveolar hemorrhage.

Absorption atelectasis is another potential hazard of high oxygen delivery. In this situation, nitrogen is washed out of the lungs. The alveoli remain inflated with only oxygen, carbon dioxide, and water vapor. If the oxygen is absorbed from the alveoli faster than it is replaced, the alveoli collapse. A post end expiratory pause or "sigh" is a necessary part of this patient's care to avoid this problem.

Mechanical ventilation by its very nature reverses the normal processes that occur in ventilation and cardiac filling. Normally, on inhalation, the intrathoracic pressure is subatmospheric and air flows into the lungs. A fall in intrathoracic pressure enhances venous return to the heart which, in turn, increases right ventricular pressure, pulmonary artery pressure, and pulmonary capillary pressure. In passive exhalation, the intrathoracic pressure returns to the resting level of subatmospheric (-2 cm H_2O), venous return is reduced but left atrial filling and left ventricular output are increased. When ventilators exert pressure on inhalation, the intrathoracic pressure rises above atmospheric pressure which leads to left atrial filling. The expiratory phase of ventilated respirations returns the intrathoracic pressure to only atmospheric, not to the normal subatmospheric because the machine operates as a closed respiratory circuit. Exhalation results in an increase of venous return and right atrial filling. Subjecting the heart and its blood vessels to increased intrathoracic pressure for more than a very short time impairs venous return and cardiac output. The nurse should observe for any pulse changes, decrease in urine output, and blood pressure decrease. The inspiratory phase of the mechanical ventilator must be kept as short as possible to avoid these effects and the expiratory phase must be prolonged.

RESPIRATORY ALKALOSIS

ASSESSMENT

Refer to Table 19, on p. 432.

PATHOPHYSIOLOGY

Primary respiratory alkalosis is a condition characterized by an increase in alveolar ventilation and a relative decrease in the rate of carbon dioxide production. This physiologic disorder can be caused by disturbances in different locations in the body and involves differing mechanisms. The most common causes can be categorized as:

I. Responses to stressful situations
   A. Physical: shock, trauma, gram-negative sepsis
   B. Psychologic: acute anxiety, hysteria

II. Increased respiratory drive
   A. Direct stimulation of respiratory center
      1. drugs: early salicylate intoxication
      2. brain dysfunction: trauma, infection
      3. others: fever, hyperthyroidism, compensatory to metabolic acidosis
   B. Reflex stimulation of respiratory center
      1. from peripheral chemoreceptors because of hypoxia, severe anemia, CHF, hepatic insufficiency or hypocarbia from mechanical overventilation
      2. from intrathoracic receptors in conditions such as pulmonary embolism, pneumonia, fibrosis

The maintenance of normal blood oxygen and carbon dioxide levels requires the integration of ventilation, blood flow, and diffusion of gases. During ventilation a volume of air (tidal volume) is moved into and out of the lungs with each inspiration and expiration. Only a portion of this tidal volume reaches the alveoli. The remainder stays in the conducting airway.

Hyperventilation results in a greater amount of air reaching the alveoli than is required for metabolic needs. Carbon dioxide is blown off resulting in less CO_2 available to combine with water to produce carbonic acid. A deficit in carbonic acid results in less of it dissociating into hydrogen ions and bicarbonate ions. The reactions appear as this:

$$CO_2 + H_2O \xrightleftharpoons[\text{Carbonic Anhydrase}]{} H_2CO_3 \rightleftharpoons HCO_3^- + H^+$$

The net loss of carbonic acid in respiratory alkalosis is reflected by the blood gases. In acute respiratory alkalosis, the pH rises due to the loss of hydrogen ions; the P_{CO_2} decreases below 40 mm Hg because it is being blown off; the bicarbonate level and base excess value tend to remain within normal limits.

Because acute changes in P_{CO_2} occur much more rapidly than bicarbonate changes, estimated changes in pH caused by P_{CO_2} changes can be clinically useful. A sudden drop of P_{CO_2} by 1 mm Hg will cause a corresponding rise in pH of 0.01 point. For example: At a P_{CO_2} level of 40 mm Hg the pH is 7.4. If the P_{CO_2} falls to 32 mm Hg the pH will be 7.48. This relationship holds true until there is a 10 point difference.

The body's initial reaction to an abrupt elevation of pH is to use all of its buffers to keep the carbonic acid–bicarbonate ratio at 1:20. Within minutes, the hydrogen ion of other buffers reacts with acids weaker than carbonic acid to form a salt and a slightly stronger acid (carbonic acid). For example, in the blood, hemoglobin is a very weak acid (HHb) that occurs as a potassium salt (KHb). Potassium bicarbonate ($KHCO_3$) in the blood reacts with hemoglobin to produce carbonic acid as in this reaction:

$$KHCO_3 + HHb \rightleftharpoons KHb + H_2CO_3$$

Thus, the initial response, within minutes, to a decrease in carbonic acid is for the body to give up its base and convert it to carbonic acid by various interaction–reaction processes. However, the blood picture is not reflective of this loss because as the bicarbonate buffer is used other buffers enter the picture on a one-for-one basis and in addition, there may be an increase in the rate of acid addition to the extracellular fluid.

The systemic effects of hypocarbia are widespread. The alkalotic state causes the oxyhemoglobin curve to shift to the "left" thus causing the hemoglobin to hold on to its oxygen molecule and resisting its release at the tissue level. Reduced amounts of CO_2 in the extracellular fluid leads to vasoconstriction of the body's arterioles. If the P_{CO_2} falls below 30 mm Hg, cerebral blood flow is reduced. Widespread vasoconstriction and increased intrathoracic pressure from hyperventilation result in less blood returning to the heart and eventually reduced cardiac output. The net result of these pathophysiologic responses is tissue hypoxia. Cerebral hypoxia for any duration results in cerebral ischemia, local acidosis and edema which in turn stimulates further hyperventilation.

An alkaline environment of the extracellular fluid affects calcium ionization. Normally 50 percent of calcium is bound to protein and 50 percent is in its ionized form. Protein bound calcium is in equilibrium with hydrogen ions. When there is a decrease in the amount of free hydrogen ions, as occurs in alkalosis, the reaction is driven to the left, thus reducing the amount of ionized calcium in the extracellular fluid.

$$CaPr + H \rightleftharpoons HPr + Ca^{++}$$

Reduced amounts of ionized calcium alter muscle membrane potential and the muscles become increasingly responsive to the slightest stimuli (irritable). Tingling sensations, muscle stiffness, aches and cramps are signs of low ionized calcium levels. These could progress to twitching, carpopedal spasms, tetany, and seizures.

The activities of the kidney to compensate for the alkalotic state can be detected in 6 to 18 hours after the onset of the problem. The kidney enhances its secretion of bicarbonate ions in exchange for hydrogen ions and nonbicarbonate anions. For every bicarbonate ion reabsorbed, a chloride ion is excreted producing a hypochloremia in some cases. It takes several days for the kidney to reach its maximum level of bicarbonate excretion. This is the only acid–base disturbance that can be fully compensated, thus restoring the pH to normal. The bicarbonate level decreases and there is a base excess deficit in compensated alkalosis.

MANAGEMENT

I. Obtain a history and review it for possible causes
   A. Interview the patient, family, friends, or others
   B. Identify the existence of psychologic and/or severe physical stressors
   C. Search for evidence of cerebral, pulmonary, and other coexisting medical problems
   D. Compile a list of all medications patient has taken
   E. Detect the prior existence of neuromuscular abnormalities and/or seizures

II. Perform a rapid systems survey
   A. Cardiovascular: chart temperature, pulse, respirations, bp; obtain a stat ECG auscultate the heart; note any rhythm disturbances
   B. Respiratory: record the rate, depth, and pattern of respirations; note patient's color and degree of respiratory effort; obtain a stat chest x-ray
   C. Nervous system: chart the general behavior, LOC, motor and sensory responses, cranial nerve responses. Report any complaints of paresthesias, muscle cramping
   D. Excretory: note the time of last intake of food or fluid; auscultate for bowel sounds, obtain a specimen of urine, if not possible, insert an indwelling catheter
III. Assist with diagnostic studies
   A. Obtain blood samples for:
      1. RBC, Hgb, Hct
      2. WBC and differential
      3. arterial blood gases
      4. toxicology screen
      5. serum electrolytes
      6. BUN, creatinine
   B. Initiate continuous cardiac monitoring and establish a CVP line to monitor cardiac rhythm and blood volume
   C. Brain scan and lung scan may be required
   D. Collect and send urine samples to the laboratory
IV. Correct and/or treat the underlying problem
   A. Control hysteria: *use sedation cautiously*
   B. Correct cause of fever and/or other conditions that increase metabolic rate
   C. Take measures to correct hypoxia, cerebral dysfunctions and lung conditions contributing to the problem
 V. Add carbon dioxide to inspired air
   A. Rebreathing inspired air: rebreathing mask, paper bag
   B. Deliver an oxygen–carbon dioxide gas mixture to patient (rare)
VI. Correct electrolyte imbalances
   A. Monitor CVP, fluids may be required
   B. Restore chloride and potassium ion concentration
      1. IV solutions of normal saline with KCL added
      2. Do not administer KCL faster than 40 mEq/hour
   C. Monitor cardiac rate and rhythm, serum electrolytes and blood gases
VII. Administer acidifying salts (rare)
   A. Examples: ammonium chloride, arginine hydrochloride, lysine hydrochloride, dilute hydrochloric acid
   B. Dosage used should only correct ½ base excess value
VIII. Systematically record patient's responses to therapy
   A. Chart temperature, pulse, respirations, bp. Neurologic vital signs q 30 to 60 minutes

B. Record CVP readings, I&O hourly
C. Record the results of electrolyte reports, blood gas analysis
D. Note the time and dosage of all medications administered

RATIONALE

Hyperventilation is a commonly observed phenomenon in the emergency department. It could be a response to a physiologic as well as a psychologic disorder and it is important for staff not to assume that all hyperventilation is related to a psychologic cause. A carefully elicited history and system survey provides the examiner with many clues as to the basis of this problem. Laboratory results quantify the clinical impression. Acute respiratory alkalosis could be a life-threatening event, if not recognized and treated.

Once the underlying problem is identified all efforts are initially directed at correcting this situation. Proper treatment for the underlying problem may correct the alkalosis. Concurrent with activities aimed at correcting the basic problem, measures may be taken to reduce the effects of the alkalotic state. These are aimed at promoting the accumulation of carbonic acid, correcting the electrolyte disturbances and oxygen deficit.

Because the basic defect is a loss of carbon dioxide and thus reduced carbonic acid formation, adding carbon dioxide to inspired air by way of a rebreathing mask or paper bag might prove very helpful. An oxygen–carbon dioxide gas mixture is available but is rarely used in emergency departments. When the patient is rebreathing his or her inspired air, the nurse should be in attendance offering calming reassurance.

Electrolyte imbalances do occur with respiratory alkalosis. Chloride ions are lost in the reabsorption of bicarbonate ions. Hypokalemia could occur because potassium tends to remain intracellular in the alkalotic state and yet potassium is lost with bicarbonate ion excretion in the urine. The amount of replacement depends on the serum electrolyte data, the size and muscle mass of the patient, and coexisting underlying medical conditions. Replacement usually takes the form of intravenous normal saline and intravenous potassium chloride. Acidifying salts are rarely used to treat respiratory alkalosis.

Vasoconstriction and low cardiac output should improve on electrolyte and pH correction. However, in some cases low flow oxygen is offered to patients to reduce the hypoxia associated with alkalosis.

Metabolic Emergencies References

DISORDERS OF GLUCOSE METABOLISM

Alberti, K., & Nattrass, M. Severe ketoacidosis. *Medical Clinics of North America*, 1978, **62**, 799.

Bolinger, R. E. Hypoglycemia. *Critical Care Quarterly*, 1980, **3** (2), 99.

Cataland, S. Hypoglycemia: A spectrum of problems. *Heart & Lung*, 1978, **7**, 455.

Cavalier, J. P. Crucial decisions in diabetic emergencies. *R.N.*, 1980, **43** (11), 32.

Craighead, S. Current views on the etiology of insulin dependent diabetes mellitus. *New England Journal of Medicine*, 1978, **299**, 1439.

Flier, J. S. Receptors, antireceptors, antibiotics and mechanisms of insulin resistance. *New England Journal of Medicine*, 1979, **300**, 413.

Kyner, J. L. Diabetic ketoacidosis. *Critical Care Quarterly*, 1980, **3** (2), 65.

Murray, P. Diabetes today: When hyperglycemia goes critical. *R.N.* 1983, **45** (3), 56.

Podolsky, S. Hyperosmolar nonketotic coma in the elderly. *Medical Clinics of North America*, 1978, **68**, 815.

Shade, D., & Eaton, R. Pathogenesis of diabetic ketoacidosis: A reappraisal. *Diabetes Care*, 1979, **2**, 296.

Sneid, D. S. Hyperosmolar hyperglycemia non-ketotic coma. *Critical Care Quarterly*, 1980, **3** (2), 29.

Stock-Barkman, P. Confusing concepts: Is it diabetic shock or diabetic coma. *Nursing '83*, 1983, **13** (6), 32.

Zipf, W., Bacon, G., & Spencer, M. Hypocalcemia, hypomagnesemia and transient hypoparathyroidism during therapy with potassium phosphate in diabetic ketoacidosis. *Diabetes Care*, 1979, **2**, 265.

DISORDERS OF THYROID METABOLISM

Brown, J. Autoimmune thyroid disease: Graves' and Hashimoto's. *Annals of Internal Medicine*, 1978, **88**, 379.

Degroot, L. F., & Neipumniszce, H. Biosynthesis of thyroid hormone: Basic and clinical aspects. *Metabolism*, 1977, **26**, 665.

Evangelisti, J. T., & Thorpe, C. J. Thyroid storm: A nursing crisis. *Heart & Lung*, 1983, **12** (2), 184.

Greer, M. A., & Ingbar, S. H. Short-term antithyroid drug therapy for thyrotoxicosis of Graves' disease. *New England Journal of Medicine*, 1977, **297**, 173.

Hellman, R. The elevation and management of hyperthyroid crisis. *Critical Care Quarterly*, 1980, **3**, 77.

Ingbar, S. H. When to hospitalize the patient with thyrotoxicosis. *Hospital Practice*, 1975, **11**, 45.

Meek, J. Myxedema coma. *Critical Care Quarterly*, 1980, **3** (2), 131.

Oppenheimer, J. H. Thyroid hormone action at the cellular level. *Science*, 1979, **203**, 971.

Urbanic, R. C., & Mazzaferri, E. L. Thyrotoxic crisis and myxedema coma. *Heart & Lung*, 1978, **7**, 435.

Wake, M., & Brenzinger, J. The nurses' role in hypothyroidism. *Nursing Clinics of North America*, 1980, **15**, 453.

DISORDERS OF ADRENAL HORMONE FUNCTIONING

Gotch, P. Teaching patients about adrenal corticosteroids. *American Journal of Nursing*, 1981, **81**, 78.

Sanford, S. Dysfunction of the adrenal gland: Physiological considerations and nursing problems. *Nursing Clinics of North America*, 1980, **15**, 481.

Schimke, N. R. Adrenal insufficiency. *Critical Care Quarterly,* 1980, **3** (2), 19.

Tzagournis, M. Acute adrenal insufficiency. *Heart & Lung,* 1978, **4,** 603.

Williams, G., Dluh, R., & Thorn, G. Diseases of the adrenal cortex. In T. R. Harrison (Ed.), *Principles of internal medicine* (9th Ed.). New York: McGraw Hill, 1980.

DISORDERS OF ACID–BASE BALANCE

Aberman, A. The lessons of lactic acidosis. *Emergency Medicine,* 1982, **14,** 147.

Brackett, N. C., Cohen, J. J., & Schwartz, W. B. Carbon dioxide titration curve of normal man. Effects of increased degrees of acute hypercapnea on acid-base equilibrium. *New England Journal of Medicine,* 1965, **272,** 6.

Done, A. K. The toxic emergency. Acid-base disturbances: Aids to evaluation. *Emergency Medicine,* 1981, **13,** 68.

Elenbaas, R. M. Critical review of forced alkaline diuresis in acute salicylism. *Critical Care Quarterly,* 1982, **5,** 64.

Emmett, M., & Narins, R. G. Clinical use of the anion gap. *Medicine,* 1977, 56, 38.

Flomenbaum, N. Acid-base disturbances. *Emergency Medicine,* 1980, **12,** 24.

Flomenbaum, N. Acid-base disturbances. *Emergency Medicine,* 1984, **16,** 59.

Fulop, M. Ventilatory response in patients with acute lactic acidosis. *Critical Care Medicine.* 1982, **10,** 3.

Masoro, E. J. An overview of hydrogen ion regulation. *Archives of Internal Medicine,* 1982, **100,** 1.

Mays, E. E. An arterial blood gas diagram for clinical use. *Chest,* 1973, **63,** 793.

Miller, W. The ABCs of blood gases. *Emergency Medicine,* 1984, **16,** 37.

Narins, R. G., & Emmett, M. Simple and mixed acid-base disorders: A practical approach. *Medicine,* 1980, **59,** 161.

Narins, R. G., & Emmett, M. Diagnostic strategies in disorders of fluid, electrolyte and acid-base homeostasis. *American Journal of Medicine,* 1982, **72,** 3.

Quintanilla, A. P. Acute acid-base disorders. *Postgraduate Medicine,* 1976, **60,** 68.

Robertson, K. J., & Guzzetta, C. E. Arterial blood-gas interpretations in the respiratory intensive care unit. *Heart & Lung,* 1976, **5,** 256.

Weil, M. H. Iatrogenic alkalosis in CPR. *Emergency Medicine,* 1981, **13,** 55.

H. MULTISYSTEM EMERGENCIES

1. Hematologic Emergencies

SICKLE CELL CRISIS

ASSESSMENT

  I. Repeated episodes of vascular occlusion
   A. Pain
      1. gnawing, increasing in intensity
      2. involves the extremities, joints, abdomen, and chest
      3. lasts hours or days
      4. fever
 II. Chronic hemolytic anemia
   A. Hematocrit level 20 to 30 percent
   B. Hemoglobin 8 g/dl
III. Frequent severe infections
   A. *Salmonella osteomyelitis*
   B. Pneumococcal pneumonia
   C. Pneumococcal meningitis
   D. *Mycoplasma pneumonia*
 IV. Laboratory tests
   A. Presence of sickle cells on a peripheral blood smear
   B. Sodium metabisulfide—an agent to induce sickling

PATHOPHYSIOLOGY

In normal adults, hemoglobin (hemaglobin A) consists of two A and two B chains. In the sickler, a single amino acid substitution of glutamic acid for valine occurs on the B chains, resulting in alterations in the physiochemical properties of the hemoglobin molecule. The erthrocytes from patients with homozygous sickle cell disease assume the sickle shape at a low oxygen tension especially at a low pH. The S (sickle) hemo-globin is less soluble in deoxygenated form which leads to an increase in blood viscosity with eventual stasis and obstruction of blood flow in the capillaries, veins, and terminal arterioles. The cycle continues as more cells sickle causing local blockage and ischemic infarction in any organs and leading clinically to the painful "sickle crisis."

The chronic anemia usually seen in most sickle patients is due to the short survival time of the rigid sickle cells.

The high incidence of infection may be due to functional asplenia, defective phagocytic activity, local stasis, and tissue necrosis. In patients with sickle cell disease occlusive phenomena (i.e., fat emboli), peripheral vein emboli is always a possibility and should be ruled out as early as possible.

Sickle cell anemia is a hereditary disorder, essentially confined to blacks and transmitted as a dominant trait.

MANAGEMENT

Treatment is symptomatic depending on the clinical signs that manifest.
  I. Repeated episodes of vascular occlusion
     A. Analgesics
     B. Hydration
     C. O_2 therapy
     D. Alkalizing agents, questionable value
     E. Vasodilators
 II. Chronic hemolytic anemia
     A. Exchange transfusions—especially useful during crises, strokes, and/or surgery
III. Frequent severe infections
     A. Early intervention with antibiotic therapy
     B. Immunization with pneumovax

RATIONALE

Treatment for patients who are in sickle cell crisis depends on clinical manifestations. The mainstay of all modalities remains analgesics and hydration. The analgesics provide symptomatic relief of the pain due to vascular occlusion and tissue ischemia. Most sicklers are ordinarily prone to dehydration due to chronic hyposthenuria. It is most important to hydrate patients during crisis to decrease the concentration of hemoglobin S which can only increase the possibility of the red blood cells to sickle.

Other modes of therapy remain controversial, administration of oxygen may in fact lead to suppression of red blood cell production. Use of alkalizing agents, i.e., sodium bicarbonate and sodium lactate, may decrease acidosis and thereby decrease sickling.

Transfusion of several units of blood or exchange transfusion to dilute the percentage of sickled cells is especially beneficial for patients in acute crisis, impending cerebral infarction or surgery.

All sickle cell patients are prone to a variety of infections, particularly in the lungs, urinary tract, and bones. Aseptic necrosis of the femoral head, osteomyelitis, pulmonary infections, hematuria, priapism and cerebral infarction are a partial list of complications. Early intervention is mandatory to prevent further debilitation of the "sickler."

ACUTE LEUKEMIC CRISIS

ASSESSMENT

A. Weakness, malaise, anorexia, fever
B. Bone and joint pain
C. Pallor, petechiae, lymph node swelling, splenomegaly
D. Laboratory findings
    1. platelet—100,000/µl
    2. WBC—10,000 to 100,000/µl
    3. blood smear—immature and abnormal cells
    4. presence of myeloblasts or monoblast proliferation of primitive malignant cells in the bone marrow
E. Bleeding tendencies

PATHOPHYSIOLOGY

Leukemia is a disease characterized by proliferation of a specific type of leukocyte within the body in the absence of a demonstrable cause. The two most commonly seen leukemias are acute lymphoblastic and acute myeloblastic. Assessment parameters are similar in both types. Acute lymphoblastic leukemia is manifested by a large number of lymphoblasts whereas acute myeloblastic leukemia is characterized by an increase in myeloblasts. Cellular proliferation of the leukemic cells leads to a reduced number of normal blood cells, thrombocytopenia with resultant hemorrhage, purpura, and petechiae. Anemia with resultant fatigue, malaise, and anorexia are additional concomitant symptoms. Bacterial infections due to neutropenia and/or decreased circulating antibodies are often seen.

Secondly, the leukemia cells usually form masses, i.e., splenomegaly, lymphadenopathy, and meningeal infiltration.

Patients in acute lymphoblastic leukemia present most commonly with bone and joint pain; infiltration of the meninges with resultant increased intracranial pressure. The presence of lymph node enlargement splenomegaly and hepatomegaly are more commonly seen in this type of leukemia.

Patients with acute myeloblastic leukemia present fatigued with a general sense of poor health, hemorrhagic manifestations, and fever. Patients with this type of leukemia are more resistant to therapy and generally have a shorter life span.

MANAGEMENT

I. Provide organ support depending on area of infiltration
   A. Airway maintenance
   B. Volume replacement
   C. Decreased intracranial pressure
      1. positioning
      2. steriods
      3. chemotherapy
   D. Renal enlargement—increased uric acid production; use of allopuinol
II. Reduction in normal hematopoietic cells
   A. Hemorrhage—platelet concentrates to raise count to at least 60,000/μl.
   B. Organ support
III. Fever and infection
   A. Specific antibiotics to the offending organisms
   B. Surgical drainage of area
   C. Reverse isolation techniques

RATIONALE

The majority of treatment modalities for the acute leukemic patient are usually not begun in the emergency department setting. Paramount during this time would be supportive therapy, maintenance of vital functions, decreasing the chance of infection, and specific organ support. Leukemia patients should be placed in reverse isolation until definitive treatments can be outlined. A regimen of multiple drug therapy is instituted as soon as possible to attack leukemic cells in different phases of the mitotic cycle. (See Appendix B for drug modalities.)

ACQUIRED IMMUNE DEFICIENCY SYNDROME
by Pamela D. Brick

The acquired immune deficiency syndrome (AIDS) renders the body incapable of defending itself against foreign invaders, such as bacteria, fungi, parasites, viruses, and tumors which are usually fought off by the cellular immune system. AIDS is characterized by an invasive form of (a) Kaposi sarcoma (KS) in patients less than 60 years old and (b) opportunistic infections, the most common being *Pneumocystic carinii* pneumonia (PCP) in individuals without any previously recognized immune suppression. The groups at highest risk are homosexual men, intravenous drug users, Haitians, hemophiliacs, and recipients of blood transfusions, as well as the sexual partners of individuals in these risk groups. Children of women at risk for or with AIDS seem also to be at risk.

Because no "agent" has been identified and no diagnostic laboratory tests are currently available, a diagnosis of AIDS has to be based on a working definition.

Working Definition
I. Opportunistic infections in patients without previously recognized predisposing factors
   A. A single infection with one of the following
      1. bacteria—*Mycobacterium avium*—intracellular or other, atypical mycobacteria (disseminated)
      2. parasites—*Pneumocystis carinii*, toxoplasmosis (CNS)
      3. viruses—Cytomegalovirus (disseminated), herpes simplex ulcers, persistent for 2 months, progressive multifocal leukoencephalopathy
   B. Infections with two of the following
      1. bacteria—*Legionella* species, *Mycobacterium tuberculosis* (disseminated or severe)
      2. fungi—*Crytococcus, Candida*—oral or esophageal, *Histoplasma capsulatum* (disseminated)
      3. parasites—cryptosporidiosis, 1-month duration
      4. viruses—Herpes zoster (?)
   C. Possibly, other infections which one might anticipate in patients with impaired cell-mediated immunity (e.g., *Listeria, Norcardia*, blastomycosis, *Coccidioides*, disseminated adenovirus, etc.)
II. Kaposi sarcoma in patients less than 60 years old and without previously explained immunosuppression—must be distinguished from "background" cases

Not included in the case definition, but thought to be associated with AIDS are autoimmune phenomena, such as autoimmune thrombocytopenic purpura, and non-Hodgkin lymphomas.

Also not included is the "wasting syndrome" or adenopathy, which many people believe reflects the AIDS prodrome.

ASSESSMENT

I. Fitting into a high-risk group
   A. Homosexual and bisexual males
   B. Intravenous drug users
      1. men
      2. women
   C. Haitians
      1. men
      2. women

  D. Recipients of blood products
    1. hemophiliacs
    2. transfusion recipients
      a. men
      b. women
      c. infants
  E. Sexual contacts of people at risk for AIDS
  F. Children of women at risk for AIDS
II. Symptoms
  A. Lymphadenopathy
  B. Weight loss/wasting syndrome
  C. Diarrhea/vomiting
  D. Cough
  E. Dyspnea
  F. Fatigue
  G. Fevers
  H. Night sweats
  I. CNS findings
    1. confusion
    2. headache
    3. seizures
    4. reduced mental activity
  J. Pigmented cutaneous lesions (Kaposi sarcoma)

Workup for AIDS Patients
  I. Hematology
  A. CBC
  B. LFTs
  C. SMA-6
  D. Hepatitis panel
  E. Immunoglobulins
  F. Total lymphocyte count
  G. Titers
    1. CMV*
    2. toxoplasmosis*
    3. EBV*
    4. herpes I and II*
    5. cryptococcal antigen
  II. Microbiology
  A. Blood cultures
    1. bacterial
    2. fungal

---

*Usually do not give clinically useful information.

    B. CSF cultures
        1. bacterial, AFB (acid fast bacteria)
        2. mycobacterial
    C. Urine
        1. Gram stain
        2. bacterial, AFB, fungal cultures
    D. Sputum
        1. Gram stain, AFB smear
        2. bacterial, AFB, fungal cultures

III. Radiology: CXR-PA/lateral

IV. Others
    A. ABG (arterial blood gas)
    B. Stool for O&P, enteric pathogens, cryptosporidium, and AFB, PPD and anergy panel

V. Special procedures*
    A. Upper and lower endoscopy
    B. Lumbar punctures
        1. cells
        2. protein
        3. glucose
        4. VDRL
        5. cryptococcal antigen
        6. gamma globulin and oliogoclonal bands
    C. Lymph node biopsy

VI. Immunological procedures†
    A. T cell ratios/identification
    B. Lymphocyte proliferation
    C. Antibody levels
    D. Thymosin levels
    E. Interferon levels

VII. Consulations§
    A. Ophthalmology
    B. Neurology
    C. GI
    D. Hematology (bone marrow aspirate; biopsy for cultures and pathology)

PATHOPHYSIOLOGY

There is sparse data on the pathophysiologic mechanisms involved in the infectious processes and malignancies associated with AIDS. In assessing the patient with AIDS the most important criteria are ascertaining that there is an infectious process

---

* Done if indicated by clinical presentation.

† Not emergency procedures.

§ As indicated.

going on, locating the sites of infection, and identifying the organisms responsible for the infection. It is important to keep in mind that the patient with AIDS may have multiple infections and malignancies.

Fever is one of the most common manifestations of infection. All infectious agents (bacteria, viruses) and neoplasms can cause an inflammatory response. The phagocytic cells involved in this response produce endogenous pyrogen, which acts on the thermoregulatory center of the anterior hypothalmus. The net result is an increase in body temperature and a reduction in mechanisms for heat dissipation. Therefore, fever is the most useful clue to the presence of infection in these patients.

Lymphadenopathy can either be localized or generalized, acute or chronic (greater than 1 month), infectious or noninfectious (due to a neoplasm). Some of the major areas associated with lymphadenopathy are the head, the neck, the axilla, and the inguinal regions. Biopsy of the lymph nodes of patients with AIDS reveals several different morphologies ranging from an explosive follicular hyperplasia to "burnout" of the lymph nodes. The significance of these findings are not known; nor is it known if all lymph nodes progress through these morphologic stages. Individuals presenting with fevers and lymphadenopathy and who fit into one of the high risk groups for AIDS must be evaluated for multiple infections and neoplasms, including those not associated with AIDS.

Pneumocystis carinii (PCP), a ubiquitious parasite, generally causes a focal or diffuse pneumonia. The patient may present with a nonproductive cough, dyspnea, and possibly weight loss. The chest x-ray may or may not show alveolar infiltrates, and the arterial blood gases show varying degrees of hypoxia even before the appearance of respiratory insufficiencies and radiologic findings. Chest x-ray findings are not sufficient to make a diagnosis of PCP; transbronchial or open lung biopsy should be obtained early.

Mycobacterium tuberculosis may cause disease ranging from isolated plural effusions to nonspecific alveolar infiltrates in the superior segments of the lower lobes, or a typical apical posterior fibronodular infiltrate (with or without cavitation) or occult miliary distribution. The clinical picture may include cough, hemoptysis, fever, night sweats, and weight loss. The diagnosis is made by identification of the tubercle bacillus, in sputum, bone marrow, or liver biopsy.

Mycobacterium avium intracellulare has been cultured from the lungs, bone marrow, liver, spleen, and intestinal tract of patients with AIDS. There is a weak inflammatory response with poorly formed granulomas. The role of *M. avium intracellulare* in causing weight loss, fever, fatigue, bone marrow suppression, and other organ dysfunctions is uncertain, but is probably similar to that of miliary tuberculosis.

Legionella is an aerobic bacteria that stains with Dieterele silver impregnation and Giemsa. The clinical picture may include pleuritic chest pain, tachpnea and hypoxemia, malaise, diarrhea, fever, chills, headache, anorexia, athralgias, myalgias, nonproductive cough, and mental confusion. It may cause a unilateral or bilateral pneumonia that rarely cavitates. Some x-ray findings may show poorly marginated, round opacities or a profusion of infiltrates from patchy and localized to multilobar consolidations.

CMV is a DNA herpes virus which can cause intestitial pneumonia typical of most viral pneumonias. A biopsy of lung tissue reveals CMV inclusion bodies in the endothelial cells and in alveolar macrophages. CMV may also be recovered, by viral culture techniques, from peripheral blood mononuclear and polymorphonuclear cells. In addition to pneumonia, CMV causes CNS disease, GI and skin lesions. CMV has also been shown to suppress the cellular immune response in non-AIDS patients, often resulting in superinfection and death. The role of CMV in the suppression of the immune response in patients with AIDS is not known at present, but is not felt to be the primary etiology of the syndrome.

Central nervous system toxoplasmosis may present with a headache, confusion, reduced mental activity, seizures, and possible loss of sight and hearing. CNS findings include diffuse encephalitis, brain abscesses, and areas of cerebritis. Single or multiple lesions which enhance or contrast may or may not be found on CAT scan. Diagnosis is made by identifying the organism from a tissue specimen. In the normal host toxoplasmosis causes a usually mild and self-limited syndrome. In patients with AIDS, toxoplasmosis such as CMV, *M. avium* and *M. tuberculosis* have been found disseminated to multiple organ systems.

Cryptosporidiosis has been described in several patients with AIDS and cannot be overlooked in the patient with chronic profuse watery stools. It has been diagnosed as a cause of self-limited diarrheal syndromes in immunologically competent individuals, but in the immunocompromised host it causes a chronic syndrome to which no therapy is currently available. The cryptosporidia, a protozoan, is found extracellularly on the epithelial lining of the small and large bowel. It can often be diagnosed by the sucrose flotation technique, but a biopsy of the bowel may be required for diagnosis. On biopsy the jejunal tissue reveals distortions of the microvilli, mononuclear inflammatory cells, and 2 to 4 μm spherical parasites on the mucosal surface.

Cryptococcus is a yeast-like fungus characterized by a large polysaccharide capsule. The fungus is acquired via inhalation and is subsequently disseminated hematogenously to the central nervous system, the skin, and the bones. The patients with CNS lesions may present with headaches, nausea, dementia, staggering gait, blurred vision, photophobia, or coma. The clinical signs and symptoms may be mild in relationship to the extent of the disease. Diagnosis is made by lumbar puncture, and identification of capsular antigen in the spinal fluid or the serum using the latex agglutination method or by detection of the cryptococci by the India ink technique. Pulmonary symptoms include chest pain and cough. X-ray findings may include dense granulomatous infiltrates with cavitation and hilar adenopathy. Diagnosis is made by staining biopsied tissues with methenamine silver or periodic acid-schiff.

The lesions associated with Kaposi sarcoma can be found disseminated throughout the body, skin, gingiva, tongue, esophagus, stomach, duodenum, colon, spleen, and lymph nodes. Lymphadenopathy may be associated with this aggressive form of KS and can either be discrete or matted. The most common initial presentation is cutaneous plaques, pink/red, blue/purple or red/brown, flat or raised. These nodules range from a few millimeters to about 2.5 cm in size. KS should be diagnosed by biopsy.

RATIONALE

In the clinical evaluation of the patient with AIDS the first priorities are to stabilize the patient, to locate the life-threatening infection and identify the organisms, to treat with the appropriate antimicrobial or antiviral agent, and to institute the appropriate isolation precautions, e.g., stool precautions for patient with diarrhea.

I. O_2—indicated for the patient with hypoxemia
Po_2—less than 60 mm Hg requires O_2 therapy
Po_2 should be maintained between 60 and 70 mm Hg

II. Fluid replacement—the patient with profuse diarrhea or chronic malnutrition will need fluid replacement (saline, D_5 saline, or D_5 ½ saline) to prevent dehydration.

III. Antidiarrheal therapy—for patients with cryptosporidosis or CMV there are no therapies, therefore the symptoms have to be treated. For the control of diarrhea, antiperistaltics (Kaopectate, Lomotil, or tincture of opium) may be effective. Other etiologies of diarrhea such as Salmonella, Shigella, and amebiasis must be ruled out before antiperistaltic therapy is instituted. Thus therapy of diarrhea is not an emergency issue.

IV. Antimicrobial therapy

PCP	Trimethoprim/	20 mg/kg orally q 6 hours
	Sulfamethoxazole,	100 mg/kg orally q 6 hours
	or Pentamidine*	4 mg/kg IM daily
M. tuberculosis	Isonizid plus	300 mg orally every day
	Rifampin	600 mg orally every day
M. avium	Ansamysin* plus	150 mg daily
intracellulare	Clofazimine*	100 mg daily
Cryptococcus	Amphotericin B	0.5 mg/kg IV daily
neoformans	plus 5 Fluocytosine†	(total of 2 g)
		150 mg/kg orally q 6 hours
Legionella pneumonia	Erythromycin	1 g IV q 6 hours
Herpes, persistent or disseminated only	Acyclovir (reduces viral shedding) topical for ulcers. IV for disseminated Adenine—Arabinoside decreases viral shedding and dissemination	

V. Chemotherapy or immunotherapy for KS
    A. Immunotherapy
    B. Chemotherapy
        1. VP-16 (etoposide)
        2. vinblastine

---

* Optional—may cause leukopenia.
† Investigational—obtained through the Centers for Disease Control, Atlanta, Ga.

3. combination
   a. doxorubicin
   b. bleomycin
   c. vinblastine
VI. Isolation procedures and precautions for health care workers

There is no evidence of AIDS transmission from patients to hospital personnel. But, because of concern over a "transmittable agent" being responsible for AIDS the CDC has made interim suggestions based on what is known about AIDS and other blood-borne viral diseases.

1. Care should be taken to avoid accidental wounds from sharp instruments contaminated with potentially infectious material and to avoid contact of open skin lesions with materials from AIDS patients.
2. Gloves should be worn when handling blood specimens, blood soiled items, body fluids, excretions, and secretions as well as surface materials and objects exposed to them.
3. Gowns should be worn when clothing may be soiled with the blood, excretions, or secretions.
4. Hands should be washed after removing gowns and gloves and before leaving the room of known or suspected AIDS patients. Hands should be washed immediately if they become contaminated with blood.
5. Blood and other specimens should be labeled with a special warning, such as "blood precautions." If the outside of a container becomes contaminated, it should be cleaned with a disinfectant (bleach). Containers should be checked for leaks.
6. Articles soiled with blood should be placed in an impervious bag and labeled "blood precautions" before being sent for reprocessing or disposal. Infectious waste should be labeled as such and incinerated or disposed of in accord with hospital policies for disposal of infectious wastes. Reusable items should be reprocessed in accord with hospital policies for Hepatitis B contaminated items. Lensed instruments should be sterilized after being used.
7. Blood spills should be cleaned up immediately with a disinfectant (household bleach, sodium hypochloride, at a 1:10 dilution is adequate).
8. Needles should not be bent or replaced into their protective shields, because this is a cause of puncture wounds. They should be promptly placed in a puncture resistant container used solely for such disposal.
9. Use only disposable syringes and needles. Only needle-locking syringes or one-piece units should be used to aspirate fluids from patients, so that fluids can be discharged safely through the needle.
10. A private room is indicated for patients who are too ill to use good hygiene, such as those with profuse diarrhea, fecal incontinence, or altered behavior secondary to CNS infection.
11. Precautions appropriate for particular infections that occur in AIDS patients should be taken. Respiratory isolation is being followed in many institutions for patients with PCP or TB or any other infection spread via airborne agents.

From all the epidemiologic evidence, AIDS itself is not spread via an airborne agent or via casual contact. It is inappropriate to avoid contact with AIDS patients. Care should be taken when dealing with blood, blood products, fecal material, and secretions. In addition, because there is no test to determine who has AIDS, care should be taken when dealing with blood and secretions from *all* patients.

Acknowledgment
I would like to thank Dr. Shelley Gordon for her excellent guidance in writing this chapter.

2. Toxicologic Emergencies

DRUGS

Poisonings
The poisoned patient, whether it is a suicide attempt or accidental or whether it is a drug, food, or alcohol-induced poisoning, remains one of the most difficult to assess and manage in the emergency department.

There is no doubt that a problem exists

- 100 million persons drink alcohol
- 8 million persons are poisoned
- 7.5 million persons are taking sedatives and hypnotics
- 400,000 persons are narcotic addicts
- 600,000 persons attempt suicide and about one fifth are successful
- 80 percent of all poisoning victims are children
- 20 percent of all poisonings occur in adults as intentional, accidental drug abuse, and industrial events

The above statistics are given on an annual basis for the United States.

Paramount to the initial treatment of the poisoned patient must be general support of the patient's vital functions. Specific identification and/or antidote administration should not be sought prior to stabilizing. The majority of problems evolve from not dealing with the poisoned patient on a timely basis. Second, after the patient has been stabilized, psychiatric evaluation whenever possible should be done prior to the patient leaving the emergency department.

ASSESSMENT

I. Adequacy of airway
   A. 24 percent or 28 percent ventilation, if breathing; Ambu with 100 percent and intubate if inadequate

    II. Pulse rate
        A. 12 lead EKG
        B. Continuous monitoring
    III. Bp
        A. Hypotensive—lactated Ringer's
        B. Normotensive or hypertensive—D5W K/O
    IV. Level of consciousness—comatose
        A. Administer 100 ml D50W; 100 mg thiamine; 2 mg naloxone (Narcan)
    V. Blood samples for glucose, electrolytes, BUN, CBC, and toxicologic screening
    VI. Blood gases—arterial
    VII. Temperature
    VIII. Urine, gastric samples

PATHOPHYSIOLOGY

A large number of toxic substances taken by patients cause either central nervous system depression or stimulation (Table 20). These substances effect the patient's vital functions, and stabilization should be begun as soon as the patient enters the emergency department. If the patient's level of consciousness is depressed, D50W, thiamine, and naloxone should be given intravenously. Dextrose 50 percent is given to eliminate the chance of the patient being hypoglycemic, because ingestion of certain toxins will increase utilization of glucose. Thiamine is administered with dextrose 50 percent; a carbohydrate load may precipitate Wernicke encephalopathy in a thiamine deficit patient (i.e., alcoholics). Narcan is a narcotic antagonist and in recommended dosage range has no morphine-like activity and will not further depress respirations. A slightly larger dose is necessary to achieve an antagonistic effect on such substances as Darvon, Talwin, and iodine.

Fluids should be administered depending on volume requirements. Initially, a fluid challenge of 150 to 200 ml should be given. If there is no response, one must consider the possibility of an ingested toxin which acts as a myocardial depressant, an extremely potent vasodilator, or there is concomitant trauma.

If there is no response to treatment, more invasive techniques should be considered. Central venous and/or Swan–Ganz catheter should be inserted prior to starting the patient on vasopressors.

MANAGEMENT

    I. Decrease absorption of toxic substance
        A. Conscious patient
            1. ipecac—15 ml po 1 to 5 years old
                30 ml po older children
                30 to 60 ml po adults
            2. apomorphine—1 mg/kg adults

TABLE 20. TOXICOLOGIC SYNDROME

Drugs or Poison	Signs and Symptoms	
Amphetamines	Track marks Toxic psychosis Hyperthermia Dilated pupils (reactive)	"Heat stroke" Flushing, diaphoresis Increased bp Active bowel sounds
Antifreeze	Metabolic acidosis Renal failure	Hypocalcemia
Arsenic	Garlicky breath Profuse diarrhea Polyneuropathy	Abnormal KUB Vomiting, abdominal pain Arrhythmias, cutaneous abnormalities
Barbiturates	Tense vesicular skin lesions Slightly constricted pupils	Coma
Boric acid	Lobster red skin Severe acidosis Coma	Blue-green diarrhea Convulsions
Botulism	Epidemic Vertigo Ptosis Muscle weakness	Sore throat Dilated pupils Ophthalmoplegia Dysphagia
Brominism	Acne	Dementia/psychosis Hyperchloremia "Cation gap"
Carbon monoxide	Epidemic—family illness Charcoal burning—high altitude	Coal gas odor Headache, nausea, vomiting
Cocaine	Perforated nasal septum Psychosis Skin tracks	Dilated pupils (reactive) Hyperthermia
Cyanide	Bitter almond odor Coma	Convulsions Abnormal ECG
Digitalis	Visual disturbances Abnormal ECG	Delirium Nausea
Disulfiram	Flushing Circulatory collapse	Pulsating headache
Ethychlorynol	Deep coma Lowered pulse and bp	Pungent aromatic odor Pink gastric aspirate
Phenothiazines	Postural hypotension Miosis Abnormal KUB	Hypothermia Tremor Increased OT
Salicylates	Hyperventilation Fever	Vomiting Bleeding
Strychnine	Stiff neck Suicide note–track marks	Status epilepticus
Thallium	Alopecia Personality change	Leg weakness Retrobulbar neuritis
Tricyclic antidepressants	Vasodilation ileus Response to physostigmine (Lilliputian)	Dilated pupils (unreactive) Supraventricular arrhythmia

TABLE 20. TOXICOLOGIC SYNDROME (Continued)

Drugs or Poison	Signs and Symptoms
	Convulsions, agitation
Hallucinations	Dry mucosa, axilla

(Adapted from the works of Arena, J., Becker, C., Done, A., Goldfrank, L., and Rumack, B.)

    B. Unconscious patient
        1. lavage 30 to 40 French catheter;
           150 to 200 ml aliquots of water
  II. Decrease absorption of toxic substance
    A. Activated charcoal—20 to 50 g of charcoal mixed in a slurry with 100 to 200
       ml of water po or through lavage tube
 III. Increase elimination of toxic substance
    A. Ionic cathartic
       magnesium sulfate ($MgSO_4$) or sodium sulfate (Na_2SO_4) given
       30 g po adult, 250 mg/kg child
       1. forced diuresis, IV fluids 200 to 400 ml/hour in adults or 5 ml/kg
    B. Diuresis
       1. acid diuresis—ammonium chloride (NH_4Cl), 75 mg/kg/day IV or po;
         urinary pH 5.5
       2. alkaline diuresis—sodium bicarbonate ($NaHCO_3$) 1 to 2 meg/kg IV with
         KCl supplements
    C. Dialysis
       1. hemodialysis
       2. peritoneal dialysis
 IV. Use of specific antibiotics (Table 21)
  V. Use of the toxicology laboratory

RATIONALE

Once the patient has been stabilized, the next step is to eliminate drugs or toxins not yet absorbed.

To decrease the absorption of the drug, a forced emesis (vomiting) should be induced in an *alert, cooperative patient* with a *present gag reflex*. Ipecac is the most commonly used emetic. It should be given with several glasses of water and will usually induce vomiting within 15 to 30 minutes. Other contraindications to emesis other than decreased level of consciousness include:

- ingestion with hemorrhagic diatheses
- patients with hemorrhagic diatheses
- ingestion of petroleum distillates

Apomorphine is another emetic that can be used. It causes emesis by stimulation of the chemoreceptor trigger zone. It acts within 3 to 5 minutes and may have a

TABLE 21. LIST OF ANTIDOTES TO RELATED TOXINS

Antidote	Medication (toxin)
Activated charcoal	General
Ammonium chloride	Phencyclidine, amphetamines, strychinine
Antivenin (Crotalidae)	Crotalid snake
Polyvalent (Wyeth)	Bites
Antivenin (Lactrodectus)	Black widow spider
Mactans (MSD)	Bites
Atropine	Chlolines & Enase inhibitors
Bentonite (7 percent) (Fuller earth)	Paraquat (herbicide)
Botulin antitoxin (ABE-trivalent)	Available from local health department (or Centers for Disease Control)
Calcium chloride	Oxalates, fluoride, ethylene, glycol
Chlorpromazin (thorazine)	General, amphetamines
Corn starch	Iodine
Cyanide kit (amyl nitrite, sodium nitrite, sodium thiosulfate)	Cyanide
Deferoxamine mesylate (Desferal)	Iron
Dextrose in water (50 percent)	Hypoglycemic agents
Diazepam (Valium)	General
Dimercaprol (Bal, British anti-Lewisite)	Arsenic, mercury, gold
Diphenylhydramine (Benadryl)	Phenothiazines
Dopamine HCl	Hypotension
Edrophonium chloride (Tensilon)	Anticholinergic agents
Ethylenediaminetetraacetic acid, CA (calcium EDTA)	Lead, zinc, and other heavy metals
Ethyl alcohol (100 percent)	Methyl alcohol, ethylene glycol
Hyloperidol (Haldol)	General
Ipecac, syrup of	General
Magnesium sulfate (Epsom salts)	General
Methylene blue (1 percent solution)	Methemoglobinemia
N-Acetylcysteine (Mucomyst)	Acetaminophen
Naloxone hydrochloride (Narcan)	Opium alkaloids, Pentazocine, propoxyphene
Nitroprusside	Hypertensive management
Oxygen	Carbon monoxide, cyanide
D-Penicillamine	Copper, lead, mercury, arsenic
Phenobarbital	General
Phospho-soda (Fleets)	General
Physostigmine salicylate (Antilirium)	Anticholinergic agents, antihistamine, atropine, tricyclic antidepressants
Pralidoxime chloride (2-Pam chloride)	Cholinesterae Inhibitors
Protamine sulfate	Heparin
Pyridoxine hydrochloride	Ethylene glycol, isoniazid, monomenthyl hydrazine containing mushrooms
Sodium bicarbonate (5 percent solution)	Iron, general
Thiamine hydrochloride	Thiamine deficiency
Vitamin K (aquamephyton)	Oral anticoagulants

(*From Goldfrank, L. R. Toxicologic Emergencies: A Comprehensive Handbook in Problem Solving (2d ed.)* New York: Appleton-Century-Crofts, 1982, p. 15.)

significant respiratory depressant effect. The major disadvantage of apomorphine is occasional severe and protracted vomiting.

In an unconscious patient gastric lavage should be performed to decrease the absorption of the toxin. Endotracheal or nasotracheal intubation should be done prior to attempting a lavage. A saline solution should be used in 200 ml aliquotes and should be continued for at least several liters. The patient should be placed in the left lateral decubitus position. The major contraindications for lavage are acid or alkali ingestions and significant hemorrhagic diathesis.

Activated charcoal should be used after the stomach has been emptied by either emesis or lavage. It absorbs most chemical ingestants, both organic and inorganic with the exception of small ions (i.e., magnesium, iron, and lithium). Activated charcoal has a small particle size with an enormously large surface area that can absorb 5 to 10 molecules of toxin per molecule of charcoal.

An ionic cathartic should be given following the activated charcoal. It is wise to stay away from oil-based cathartics which in case of aspiration would cause a lipoid pneumonia. An ionic cathartic will also not be absorbed by the charcoal. Administration of the cathartic should decrease transit time of the toxin in the intestine. The contraindications to cathartics include:

- adynamic ileus
- severe diarrhea
- abdominal trauma
- intestinal obstruction
- renal failure (magnesium cathartic)
- congestive heart failure (sodium sulfate)
- ethylene glycol (Phosphosoda)

Some drugs may be removed by increasing urinary excretion (Table 22). Forced diuresis is useful only with water soluble, weakly protein-bound drugs such as phenobarbital, meprobamate, amphetamines, and lithium salts. It is contraindicated in patients with congestive heart failure, shock, and/or renal failure.

Alkalinization or acidification can further increase elimination by acting on those drugs that remain ionized in the renal tubule at a specific pH (Table 22).

Dialysis is indicated when the clinical picture of the patient illustrates extreme toxicity with hypotension and renal compromise, and the patient has, by history and blood levels, taken a lethal dose. The ingested toxin must be water soluble and poorly protein bound (i.e., acetaminophen, amphetamines, ethanol, ethylene glycol,

TABLE 22. DRUGS THAT RESPOND TO ACID AND ALKALINE DIURESING

Acid Diuresis	Alkaline Diuresis
Phencyclidine	Salicylates
Amphetamines	Phenobarbitol
Strychnine	Isoniazid
Quinine	

methanol, phenobarbital and salicylates). Peritoneal dialysis is only about 10 to 25 percent as effective as hemodialysis but does not require the sophisticated equipment and staffing.

Supportive management of the poisoned patient yields dramatic results. At times, laboratory data is vital to the patients survival. Toxicologic screening should be available and used in adjunct with clinical management.

ALCOHOL ABUSE

Alcoholism is often referred to as the country's third most serious public health hazard. There are approximately one million alcoholics in the United States; more men are affected than women and it has been shown that the average age of the alcoholic has been decreasing over the past 10 years. In the emergency department, one is faced with problems related to alcohol abuse. The patient who is acutely intoxicated and the patient who is in acute withdrawal.

ASSESSMENT

I. Intoxication
  A. Vital signs
    1. temperature—normal or decreased
    2. pulse—elevated
    3. bp—normal
    4. respiratory rate—decreased
  B. Incoordinated
  C. Impaired sensory function
    1. ataxia, dysarthria, nystagmus
    2. nausea and vomiting
  D. Laboratory values
    1. blood alcohol level (Table 23)
    2. hypocalemia
  E. ECG
    1. sinus arrhythmias
    2. sinus tachycardia
    3. ventricular arrhythmias in chronic alcoholics
  F. Severe intoxication—respiratory depression and coma

PATHOPHYSIOLOGY

Alcohol acts in the body as a central nervous system depressant. Initially, it may appear as a stimulant, manifesting itself by garrulousness, aggressiveness, excessive activity, and increased electrical excitability of the cerebral cortex. The above is probably due to the depressive action on certain subcortical structures that ordinar-

TABLE 23. CLINICAL SIGNIFICANCE OF VARYING BLOOD ALCOHOL LEVELS

Blood Alcohol Level	Symptoms
50 mg%	Limited muscular incoordination Driving not seriously impaired
50–100 mg%	Incoordination Impaired sensory function Driving increasingly dangerous
100–150 mg%	Mood, personality, and behavioral changes Marked mental impairment, incoordination, ataxia Driving is dangerous (legally drunk in most states)
150 mg%	Prolonged reaction time Driving is very dangerous (legally drunk in all states)
200–300 mg%	Nausea, vomiting, diplopia, marked ataxia
300–400 mg%	Hypothermia, dysarthria, amnesia
400–700 mg%	Coma, respiratory failure, death

ily modulate or inhibit cerebral cortical activity. As the level of alcohol increases, the depressant action spreads to involve the cerebral cortical neurons as well as other cerebral and spinal neurons.

Motor performance, from simply standing to control of speech, eye movements, and complex motor skills are adversely affected. The movements are slower, more inaccurate, and random in character.

Alcohol impairs the efficiency of mental function by interfering with the learning process. The individual is not able to form associations, has a decreased power of attention and concentration, and a marked inability to judge and discriminate.

Alcohol's effect on organs other than the central nervous system is not as dramatic. It has a direct action on the excitability and contractibility of the heart muscle, and results in a rise in cardiac rate and output, and cutaneous vasodilatation. Increased sweating and vasodilatation cause a loss of body heat and may cause the body temperature to drop.

The exact pathophysiology behind the nausea and vomiting is somewhat debatable. It may be caused by a superficial gastritis or it may represent the mildest manifestations of the withdrawal syndrome.

The symptoms of *intoxication* are caused by the depressant action of alcohol on nerve cells acting in some manner as general anesthetics. Unlike general anesthetics, however, the margin between the dose of alcohol that produces surgical anesthesia and that which dangerously depresses respiration is very narrow.

MANAGEMENT

I. Initial therapy
   A. Dextrose 50 percent (50 g), 100 ml
   B. Thiamine, 100 mg IM
II. Complete body assessment

III. Supportive therapy
   A. IV fluids
   B. Vitamins
IV. Avoid sedatives—hypnotics
V. Disulfiram (antabuse) 500 mg od × 7 to 10 days; 125 mg to 250 mg/day as a maintenance
VI. Psychologic support

RATIONALE

Most patients who come to the emergency department intoxicated will improve as ethanol metabolization at the rate of approximately 15 mg percent/hour progresses. Unless vital functions are compromised, therapy should be supportive and conservative. Initial therapy of dextrose and thiamine should be instituted as quickly as possible. It is very difficult to distinguish between acute intoxication and hypoglycemia. Avoid jumping to any conclusions and being liable for your mistakes. A head-to-toe physical assessment should be carried out to rule out concomitant conditions such as trauma, infection, and multiple drug use.

Supportive therapy of intravenous fluids, electrolyte replacement, and vitamin supplements should be given, especially in those patients who are vomiting.

Avoid the use of sedatives and hypnotics because at this point it only tends to confuse the issue.

Disulfiram (Antabuse) can be started when the patient has achieved abstinence and the serum ethanol level is zero. The drug should never be given surreptitiously or as the only component of therapy. The maximum dose is 500 mg once a day for 7 to 10 days followed by maintenance doses of 125 to 250 mg daily. When alcohol is taken by a patient who has a serum level of disulfiram the following symptoms occur: flushing, hypotension, vertigo, headache, diaphoresis, nausea, vomiting, and abdominal pain. Chest pain and occasionally shock may ensue. There is no effective antidote to disulfiram and the patient should be treated supportively.

The most important aspect of management is some type of psychologic and/or behavioral therapy. Involvement of the spouse or other members of the family in treatment is always beneficial. Encourage the patient to join Alcoholics Anonymous (AA) and the family to join Al-Anon. Use other social agencies, religious counseling, and group therapy. Some physicians advocate the use of aversion therapy, the patient is given a shot of whiskey and then a shot of apomorphine. Most people do not retain learned aversion responses.

ALCOHOL WITHDRAWAL

ASSESSMENT

I. Minor (8 to 36 hours of abstinence)
   A. Tremor

B. Mild diaphoresis
C. Irritability
D. Restlessness
E. Gastrointestinal distress
F. Transient hallucinations
G. "Rum fits"
H. Insomnia
I. Mild tachycardia, tachypnea, low-grade fever, elevated bp
II. Major
A. Profuse diaphoresis
B. Marked disorientation
C. Persistent hallucinations
D. Extreme agitation, tremor, restlessness
E. Febrile, tachycardia, tachypnea
F. Orthostatic hypotension
III. Laboratory values
A. Arterial blood gases—may show metabolic acidosis, respiratory alkalosis and metabolic alkalosis
B. Serum ethanol—0 percent in late withdrawal
C. Increased BUN
D. Decreased K, Ca^{++}, Na, PO_4
E. ECG
F. Sinus tachycardia
G. Premature ventricular contractions
1. ventricular tachycardia
2. ventricular fibrillation

PATHOPHYSIOLOGY

The severity of the withdrawal syndrome depends on many factors, such as the age of the individual, the general physical and psychologic condition of the patient, amount of alcohol consumed, how rapidly the alcohol was consumed, the height and duration of the blood alcohol level, and finally the degree of tissue tolerance to alcohol. Tissue tolerance is a biochemical adaptation of the habituated individual to long-continued exposure to alcohol. The precise nature of the adaptation is unknown but it allows the individual to function more effectively at a given alcohol level and is probably the cause of withdrawal symptoms. The nervous tissue is still responding as if there was a high alcohol concentration and it takes the body weeks to further adapt to a lower alcohol level. Another theory is that of a psychologic adaption. The chronic alcoholic learns to compensate for the lack of coordination and the removal of inhibitions in a manner that would be impossible for the nonalcoholic.

The assessment parameters stated for the minor withdrawal syndrome usually occur within 36 hours. Patient is usually alert, startles easily, has a deeply flushed face, and is mildly disoriented. Accompanying symptoms are nausea, vomiting, and tachycardia. Tremors are generalized, more severe in the agitated patient and may be so violent that the patient cannot speak, stand up, or feed him or herself. Most of the above symptoms disappear within a few days.

Symptoms of disorder perception occur in about 25 percent of all tremulous patients. Patient may complain of bad dreams, familiar objects may become distorted. Hallucinations may be purely visual, auditory, olfactory, and/or tactile. They are more commonly animated than inanimate, and occur singly or in groups, may be shrunken or enlarged, and may take distorted and hideous forms.

"Rum fits" usually occur 12 to 48 hours after the last drink. The seizures are grand mal in type, occur in short bursts of two to six or even more, and disappear within several hours or a day or two.

Delirium tremors is the most dramatic and grave complication of alcohol withdrawal. It is characterized by profound confusion, delusions, vivid hallucinations, tremors, agitation, and sleeplessness. A state of increased activity of the autonomic nervous system exists, i.e., dilated pupils, fever, tachycardia, and profuse diaphoresis. The majority of patients are over the delirium tremors in 72 hours. About 15 percent end fatally and the cause is usually underlying infection, illness, or injury.

MANAGEMENT

I. Fluid and electrolyte replacement
  A. Based on osmolarity and electrolyte values
  B. May require 6 to 10 liters of fluid
  C. May require diuretics
II. Reduction of fever
  A. Aspirin
  B. Cooling blankets
  C. Sponge baths
III. Vitamin supplement
  A. Thiamine 100 mg IM stat and thiamine 100 mg bid
  B. Other vitamin supplements—pyridoxine 100 mg/od, folic acid 5 mg tid; ascorbic acid 100 mg bid
IV. Use of sedative/hypnotics
  A. Librium 50 mg or greater IM q 3 to 4 hours until an absence of withdrawal symptoms occur
V. Use of anticonvulsants
  A. Only if status epilepticus occurs

RATIONALE

The overall result of alcohol in fluid and electrolyte balance is an accumulation of water and electrolytes in all fluid compartments and particularly throughout the intracellular spaces of the central nervous system.

A state of dehydration associated with hyponatremia, hypokalemia, and hypochloremia exists when the patient has excessive vomiting, diarrhea, and malnutrition. Low serum potassium may be due to hyperventilation; respiratory alkalosis causes the shift of potassium from the extracellular space to the intracellular space.

If the patient is overhydrated, a dose of Lasix 40 to 80 mg will effect a safe, rapid diuresis.

Use of magnesium, usually as magnesium sulfate remains controversial. There is evidence which suggests that excessive alcohol ingestion causes a decrease in total exchangeable magnesium, and a replacement of such reduces the hyperirritability of neural tissue.

Hypoglycemia has been associated with those individuals who are malnourished, with inadequate glycogen stores in the liver. Intravenous dextrose and water is usually effective.

A reduction in temperature is necessary to decrease fluid loss, central nervous system irritability, and blood coagulation abnormalities. Use of external methods to decrease temperature is preferred over the use of aspirins.

Vitamin supplements are usually necessary because most alcoholics are undernourished. Thiamine should be given immediately because a carbohydrate load in a malnourished individual may precipitate a Wernicke encephalopathy.

Anticonvulsant medications are usually not required for the simple withdrawal seizures. The seizures are usually self-limiting and medications should only be given to those patients in status epilepticus. Valium, 10 to 20 mg IV, may be given every 2 to 4 hours as needed.

Sedatives/hypnotics should be given very carefully and dosage should be determined by clinical responses rather than standing orders. The objective of sedation is to decrease the patient's agitation, restlessness, tremors, and disorientation and not place him or her in a stupor or coma.

Multisystem Emergencies References

HEMATOLOGIC

Clene, M. J. Acute leukemia: Biology and treatment. *Annals of Internal Medicine*, 1979, **91**, 758.

Sheehy, T. W., & Plumbo, V. J. Treatment of sickle cell disease. *Archives of Internal Medicine*, 1977, **137**, 779.

Weinstein, H. T.: Treatment of acute myclogenous leukemia in children and adults. *New England Journal of Medicine*, 1980, **303**, 473.

TOXICOLOGIC

1. Chambers, C. D. Barbiturate use, misuse, and abuse. *Journal of Drug Issues*, 1972, **4** (2), 15.

2. Cohen, A. S. *Medical emergencies: Diagnostic and management procedures from the Boston City Hospital.* Int Editor.
3. Davis, J. M., Bartlett, E., & Termim, B. Overdosage of psychotropic drugs, a review. I. Major and minor tranquilizers. *Diseases of the Nervous System,* 1968, **29,** 157.
4. Ellenwood, E. H., Eibergen, R. D., Kelbey, M. M. Stimulants: Interactions with clinically relevant drugs. *Annals of the New York Academy of Science,* 1976, **281,** 393.
5. Goldfrank, L. R., & Kirstein, R. *Toxicologic emergencies: Handbook in problem solving.* New York: Appleton-Century-Crofts, 1978.
6. Goldfrank, L., Kirstein, R., & Bresnitz, E. Gasoline and other hydrocarbons. *Hospital Physician,* 1979, **50,** 32.
7. Goldfrank, L., & Osborn, H. The barbiturate overdose. *Hospital Physician,* 1977, **9,** 30.
8. Goodman, G. A., Goodman, L., & Gilman, A. (Eds.). *The pharmacological basis of therapeutics* (6th Ed.). New York: MacMillan, 1980.
9. Hollister, L. E. Tricyclic antidepressants. *New England Journal of Medicine,* 1978, **299,** 1106.
10. Jaffe, J. Drug addiction and drug abuse. In L. S. Goodman, & A. Gilman (Eds.). *The pharmacological basis of therapeutics.* New York: MacMillan, 1975.
11. Johnson, R. B., & Lukasa, W. M. Medical complications of alcohol abuse. *Committee on alcoholism and drug dependence.* American Medical Association Publication, 1–48, 1974.
12. Rapport, R. T., Gay, G. R., & Farris, R. D. Emergency management of acute phenocyclidine intoxication. *Journal of the American College of Emergency Physicians,* 1979, **8,** 68.
13. Rosen, P., et al. *Emergency medicine concepts and clinical practice* (Vols. I & II). St. Louis, C. V. Mosby, 1983.
14. Rumack, B. H., & Peterson, R. G. Acetaminophen overdose: Incidence, diagnosis, and management in 416 patients. *Pediatrics,* 1978, **62,** 898.
15. Schuckit, M. A. The disease alcoholism. *Journal of Post Graduate Medicine,* 1978, **64,** 78.
16. Ullman, K., & Groh, R. Identification and treatment of acute psychotic states secondary to the usage of over-the-counter sleeping preparations. *American Journal of Psychiatry,* 1972, **128** (10), 64.

SECTION FOUR

MEDICOLEGAL ASPECTS OF EMERGENCY CARE

MEDICOLEGAL ISSUES

This chapter is intended to provide basic information to emergency medical personnel relative to medicolegal issues in the delivery of emergency services. Individual practitioners should be aware of the variations of statutory provisions.

Emergency departments are chaotic in nature, necessitating rapid decision making with little time to develop any professional relationships. Patients and families expect immediate treatment although the waiting room may already be crowded with more urgent cases. The triage nurse and clerical registration staff must convey a sense of concern and outline realistic time frames for the intake process and treatment according to a prioritized system of care. Many lawsuits arise from the patient's discontent with the attitude and/or behavioral response of the staff and not necessarily any specific act of omission or commission. Patients are also more sophisticated and knowledgeable about health care and expect to be an active participant in plans for care and follow-up. A few minutes invested initially on arrival may improve patient compliance and decrease stress for the rest of the staff.

TYPES OF LAW (Common Law)

The American judicial system is based on a combination of English common law and statutory law. Common law, also referred to as case law, is an interpretation made by judicial discussion rather than legislature enacted. Common law serves two purposes: settles or resolves a dispute as well as setting precedent for future resolution of similar situations.

Statutory law is law enacted by the legislative branch of government and usually declares, commands, or prohibits some activity. Included under statutory laws are state laws that govern and regulate the practice of nursing and medicine.

REGULATORY AGENCIES AND POLICIES

All hospitals have internal mechanisms for operational policy formulated by municipal, governmental, or voluntary agencies. These guidelines are based on judicial and administrative review and are designed to protect the institution, its clinical professionals, and the patient from liability. Federal and state regulatory agencies mandate certain criteria be met for participation in health programs such as Medicaid and Medicare. JCAH standards, although not statutory, may be compulsive if a particular state requires it for licensing. Noncompliance might also result in nonreimbursement penalties. The law as it applies to emergency care is a new era of specialization for lawyers, and in 1973, the ABA recognized the specialty of Health Care and Hospital Law. Additionally, EMSS has developed and expanded with concomitant expansion of prehospital care and emergency department specialization. Standards were originally meant to reflect and compare community standards and professional practice was intended to reflect these standards. The courts have abandoned this custom and expect that emergency practitioners with similar training and expertise must conform to standards regardless of locale. In New York City the EMSS, in cooperation with medical, nursing, and administrative personnel have developed standards applicable to staffing, education, facilities, and resources.

These standards have been used to categorize existing emergency resources in New York City and will eventually be used to designate specialty referral centers.

GENERAL LEGAL PRINCIPLES

Negligence

Most simply defined, negligence is a deviation from an accepted standard of care. Emergency personnel are liable for negligence or malpractice if the standard is not adhered to which results in damage to the patient. There are four basic elements that must be proven in negligence cases: duty, breach of duty, damages, and proximate cause.

A duty is established when the person enters the emergency department, and the staff voluntarily assumes a relationship when they accept responsibility for providing care. Inherent in this responsibility is an obligation to provide care that is reasonably prudent and meets accepted standards. Breach of duty occurs when emergency personnel do not provide the care according to accepted standards. Damage must have occurred to the complainant in order to sue for negligence. There may have been a breach of duty but if there were no untoward effects on the patient the court will not pursue a claim of negligence. Proximate cause requires that there be some evidence of a cause and effect relationship between the damages sustained and the breach of duty.

Res ipsa loquitur is a latin phrase that means the thing speaks for itself. It is meant to assist plaintiffs in situations where it would be impossible to prove all of the elements of negligence. In order to prove this doctrine plaintiffs need to establish (a) that the injury or harm does not ordinarily occur in the absence of somebody's negligence, (b) that the injury occurred under the sole control of the defendant, and (c) that the patient did not contribute to the injury. The effect of this doctrine was to shift the burden of proof from the plaintiff to the defendant.

Statutes of Limitations

Statutes of limitations limit the length of time a lawsuit may be filed. Most statutes of limitations for negligence are 2 to 3 years. In New York, voluntary hospital limits are 2 years and 6 months and municipal hospitals, 1 year and 3 months. Minors are not generally affected by statutes of limitations until they are emancipated or reach the age of maturity.

If the complainant does not file legal action within the allowable period, he or she will then be prohibited from filing suit. Some states apply the statutes of limitations from the time the negligent act occurred, while other states apply the statutes from the time the negligent act has been discovered. It is important to know when the limiting time period begins.

Respondent Superior

Respondent superior is a phrase used to express the area of the employer's liability for the employees arising out of the cause of employment. However, it does not render the employees immune from suit as professionals are always independently liable for their own negligent behavior. The employer is not liable for the torts of independent contractors if the employer has no significant control over the actions of the independent contractors, i.e., physician groups not employed by the hospital and agency nurses who provide services to the emergency department.

ASSAULT AND BATTERY

Assault

Assault is an intentional act designed to place an individual in apprehension of bodily harm without his consent (i.e., threat to apply restraints to uncooperative patient).

Battery

Battery is the unlawful touching of another individual without his consent (i.e., the actual application of restraints without assessment by physician and written orders).

Abandonment

Anyone who presents to the emergency department is entitled to appraisal and initial treatment of any illness or injury. This establishes a physician–patient relationship whereby the physician is responsible for the continued care of the patient until that responsibility is assumed by another physician. This would include appropriate instructions for follow-up care, i.e., instruction sheets with receipt signatures signed by the patient. If continued care is required the patient should be referred to an OPD or other resources until there is full resolution of the presenting problem. In all instances patients should be encouraged to return to the emergency department if symptoms do not improve or complications ensue. Abandonment can also occur when patients are transferred from one emergency department to another. The responsibility for safe transport rests with the sending facility. No patient should be transported unless stable and accompanied by a nurse or physician, if indicated. If the patient leaves "against medical advice," he should sign a witnessed release. If he leaves without signing, this fact should be so noted on the emergency department records.

CONSENT

Implied Consent

When a patient voluntarily presents himself to the emergency department and requests assistance without evidence of duress, written consent is not mandatory. A written consent should be obtained as an added precaution to cover routine emergency department care (i.e., x-rays, laboratory tests, medications). Invasive procedures should involve special consent forms (minor surgery, procedures where anesthesia is used, and risk procedures).

Informed Consent

Every patient has a legal right to be treated only with his consent. This consent should be authorized only after a thorough explanation of the risk involved to the patient and alternatives to the proposed medical treatment.

Emergency Doctrine

If consent is unable to be obtained from the patient or an authorized representative and the patient's life or health is jeopardized, emergency treatment is then valid. Emergency staff must balance the treatment risk of battery vis-a-vis the nontreatment risk which could result in death or disability. It is more preferable to render treatment despite the legal risk. Emergency staff should document the nature of the injury and any/all efforts to contact a next of kin.

Minors

In most states the age of majority is 18 years. Minors lack the legal ability to consent to treatment except in situations where immediate action is required to preserve life or prevent bodily harm. In this instance the rule of implied parental consent is indicated. Another exception is the case of an emancipated minor who is self-supporting, married, or can understand the full significance of contemplated treatment. Additionally, all states have a statutory exception allowing minors to consent to treatment for venereal disease, pregnancy, alcoholism, and drug abuse. School authorities frequently bring minors to the emergency department for treatment. Written consent may be on file in the student's health record, however, efforts should be made to contact one of the parents, either at home or at work. Telephone consent should be verified by having someone listen on an extension and validate this in writing on the chart. In the case of Jehovah Witnesses, the courts act in favor of dependent children.

Refusal of Consent

A competent, conscious patient has the right to refuse treatment if he understands the nature of the consequences of such refusal. This precludes patients who are under the influence of drugs and/or alcohol where sensorium is impaired. Efforts should then be made to contact a family member for consent to treat. Competent, conscious adults who refuse treatment should be encouraged to sign out of the emergency department against medical advise. In instances where refusal may result in serious harm or death, every legal effort should be pursued. The patient should be seen by a psychiatrist where possible, to evaluate the patient's ability to refuse treatment and such consultation be recorded on the medical record. Hospital administration should then petition the courts to institute the prescribed treatment plan. In most instances the courts protect minor children while allowing consenting, terminally ill patients to die with dignity.

Triage

Most contemporary emergency departments have experienced a dramatic increase in use in the last several decades. In order to categorize patients according to the severity of illness–injury triage sorting has evolved. This evolving function has served to broaden emergency department nurses' responsibilities for prioritizing emergency care. Although triage may influence the order of treatment, it may not be used to refuse. Nurses must be aware that they are responsible for their own acts of negligence. For a more comprehensive review of triage see the section on Triage.

EMERGENCY DEPARTMENT RECORD

JCAH standards of 1979 outline the following record keeping requirements:

> A medical record shall be maintained on every patient seeking care and shall be incorporated into the patients' permanent hospital record. Included items—patient identification (when not obtainable, the reason must be entered on the medical record), time and means of arrival, pertinent history of the illness or injury and physical findings including vital signs, care given prior to arrival, diagnostic and therapeutic orders, clinical observations, including results of treatment, reports or procedures, tests and their results, diagnostic impression, conclusion at the termination of evaluation and treatment including final disposition, the patient's condition on discharge or transfer, and any instructions given to the patient or his family, or both for follow-up care and the patient's leaving against medical advice.

Good Samaritan Laws

There is a great variation from state to state regarding good samaritan laws. These laws are meant to protect individuals from civil liability when providing emergency assistance to ill or injured individuals. Some states have laws that only protect professionals (M.D.'s, R.N.'s), therefore emergency personnel should be aware of the law in effect in a particular area.

EMERGENCY PERSONNEL AND THE POLICE DEPARTMENT

Most emergency departments are a microcosm of the communities they service. Most large urban hospitals reflect the rise in criminal activity either from a perpetrator or victim point of view with increased involvement with law enforcement agencies. Several points should be considered:

1. Emergency department staff are not required to report *suspected* criminal activity but *actual* criminal activity must be reported, i.e., victims of gunshot or stab wounds. Additionally, all concealed weapons should be reported.
2. Any clothing or property taken by the police department should be duly recorded on the emergency department record.
3. The obtaining of evidence (blood alcohol or drugs) should not be done forcibly as it violates the fourth amendment, which protects the individual against unreasonable search and/or seizure. Emergency personnel should be aware of the potential civil liability in cooperating with law enforcement agencies particularly when the patient does not consent to treatment. They are liable to be sued for assault, battery, and invasion of privacy. All staff should be aware of institutional malpractice insurance and the existing administrative operative guidelines.
4. Child abuse—Most states have enacted child abuse reporting laws, most of which are mandatory in nature and require the individual to report suspected cases under penalty of fine, imprisonment, or both for not reporting. Reporting statutes usually provide some measure of immunity from civil or criminal liability for good faith reporting of suspected battered children.
5. Rape is classified as a medical emergency in order to minimize or avoid complications of pregnancy, venereal disease, and psychologic damage. The emergency department record should be accurate, complete, and detailed. Exam should include consent, observations, history, physical exam, laboratory tests, preservation of evidence, diagnosis, disposition with regard to possible pregnancy, venereal disease, psychic trauma, and reporting of the alleged incident to the appropriate authorities. There are many evidence collection kits on the market that will assist emergency personnel in obtaining and securing evidence which might be used in future litigation.

PSYCHIATRIC EMERGENCIES

Prehospital personnel (EMT/paramedics) should exercise caution when evaluating a potential psychiatric patient. The patient can sue for assault and battery and/or false imprisonment if physical restraint is applied. Mitigating circumstances require necessary force if by virtue of medical illness or injury the patient is not mentally competent. The overriding concern should be whether the patient is a danger to himself or to the person or property of others. This is sometimes called the common law test of insanity. As soon as the patient enters the emergency department and verbalizes suicidal or homicidal ideation, the emergency staff are responsible for safeguarding the patient or others from harm. Close observation should be maintained until a decision regarding disposition is made.

INVOLUNTARY HOSPITALIZATION OR COMMITMENT

Under its police power, the state has the right to involuntary admit a patient to a psychiatric facility to protect its citizens and personal property.

Categories of Involuntary Hospitalization

1. *Emergency*—temporary measure to suppress and prevent conduct likely to create a clear and present danger to persons or property.
2. *Judicial*—procedure in which a judge or jury had discretion to determine whether hospitalization is required under the law.
3. *Medical*—one or more physicians may involuntarily hospitalize a patient without his consent and for an indefinite period of time.
4. *Observational*—limited amount of time, i.e., drug or alcohol induced psychosis.

All psychiatric patients should have a complete medical evaluation prior to admission to a psychiatric facility. Physiologic illness or injury can present with psychiatric manifestations; therefore, emergency personnel should act in an advocacy role in determining what is in the best interest of the patient and community.

DISCHARGE AND TRANSFER

The JCAH mandates that all patients receive written instructions on discharge for follow-up care. These instructions should be explained in a clear and concise manner comprehensible to the patients and/or family, with the option to return to the emergency department if there is no improvement. Preprinted instruction sheets are beneficial and the signature of the patient and/or family should be documented on the emergency department record. The signature should attest that not only were written instructions given but that they were understood.

Every emergency department should develop risk management programs to identify risks in order to reduce or prevent malpractice claims while improving the quality of patient care.

Medicolegal References

Cameron, C. T. M. *PR in the emergency department.* Bowie, Md.: Brody, 1980.

Creighton, H. Failure to adequately supervise PA's. *Nurse Manager,* 1982, **13** (12), 44–45.

Danis, D. M. Governmental affairs. Paramedic role in emergency departments and intensive care units in dispute in Pennsylvania. *Journal of Emergency Nursing,* 1983, **9** (3), 180.

Darling v. Charleston Memorial Hospital. 33 Ill. 2nd 326, 211 N.E. 2nd 253, Ill. Supreme Court, Second District, 1965.

Dean, K. A. Legal liability in the emergency department. *Focus on Critical Care,* 1983, **10** (6), 44–46.

Finch, J. Law: Negligent but not liable. *Nurse Mirror,* 1983, **156** (9), 41.

Focal point for risk management (slide-tape presentation). Charlotte, N.C.: McNaery Insurance Consulting Services, 1979.

George, J. E. Illegal drugs—police—and the emergency department. *Journal of Emergency Nursing,* 1982, **8** (5), 267.

George, J. E. *Law and emergency care.* St. Louis: C. V. Mosby, 1980.

George, J. E. Law and the ED nurse. Volunteers in the emergency department. *Journal of Emergency Nursing,* 1983, **9** (1), 57–58.

George, J. E. Law and the emergency nurse. *Journal of Emergency Nursing,* 1979, **5 (1), 38.**

George, J. E. The right to refuse medical treatment. *Journal of Emergency Nursing,* 1983, **9** (4), 234.

Gibson, T. C. Skull x-rays in minor head injury. A review of their use and interpretation by casualty officers. *Scottish Medical Journal,* 1983, **2B** (2), 132–137.

Gonzales v. Nork and Mercy Hospital. No. 225866. Superior Court of Calif., Sacramento County, 1973.

Hospital CEO and Risk Managers Newsletter (Vol. 1, No. 4). Detroit, Mich.: Kitch, Suhrheinrich, Smith, Saurbier and Drutchas, 1981.

Langlow, A. The nurse and the law: Causes in casualty. *Aug. Nurses Journal,* 1982, **12** (1); 23–27.

Mancini, M., & Gale, A. T. *Emergency care and the law.* Rockville, Md.: Aspen Systems Corp., 1981.

Manual for seminar on malpractice liability control in the hospital environment. Chicago: InterQual, 1979.

MHAMIC risk management systems. Lansing, Mich.: Michigan Hospital Association Mutual Insurance, 1979.

Michaels, J. L., & Crouter, M.D. Emergicenters and the need for a competitive regulatory approach. *Law Med Health Care,* 1982, **10** (3), 108–114.

NAIC malpractice claims (Vol. 2, No. 2). Milwaukee: National Association for Insurance Commissioners, 1980.

Rabin, P. L., Folks, D. G., & Hollender, M. H. Optimal care and the law. *Southern Medical Journal,* 1982, **75** (11), 1369–1370.

Regan, W. A. Legal case briefs for nurses. MI: Epileptic injured in ER: No liability. NC: Drug administration: Technique errors. *Regan Rep. Nurse Law,* 1983, **24** (4), 3.

Regan, W. A. Licensure: What is "unprofessional conduct?": Case in point: Lunsford v. Bd. of Nurse Examiners (648 S.W. 2nd 391, TX). *Regan Rep. Nurse Law,* 1983, **24** (1), 2.

Vaccarino, J. Incident reporting: For what it's worth. *Forum* (newsletter) 1980, **1** (3), 2. Published by the Risk Management Foundation of Harvard Medical Institutions, Inc., Boston, Mass.

Wilcox, D. P. Hospital emergency rooms—New legal requirements. *Texas Medicine*, 1983, **79** (11), 73–75.

APPENDIX A

1. Definition of Terms and Abbreviations

ABG	arterial blood gases	DPT	diphtheria, pertussis, tetanus
ACH	acetylcholine	DT	diphtheria, tetanus
ACTH	adenocorticotropic hormone	ECG	electrocardiogram
ADH	antidiuretic hormone	EEG	electroencephalogram
AFB	acid fast bacillus	EME	emergent medical exam
ARF	acute rheumatic fever	EMT	emergency medical techni-
ASO	acute streptozyme O test		cians
AV	atrioventricular	ENT	ear, nose, and throat
AVM	arteriovenous malformation	EOM	extraocular movements
BAL	British antilewisite	EPI	epinephrine
bid	2 times a day	ER	emergency room
BMR	basal metabolic rate	ESR	erythrocyte sedimentation
bp	blood pressure		rate
BUN	blood urea nitrogen	ETOH	ethanol
C&S	cuture and sensitivity	FIO_2	forced inspiratory oxygen
CAT	computerized axial tomography	GC	gonococcus
CBC	complete blood count	GI	gastrointestinal
cc	cubic centimeter(s)	GLU	glucose
CHF	congestive heart failure	g	gram(s)
CO_2	carbon dioxide	GTT	glucose tolerance test
COPD	chronic obstructive pulmo-	GTTS	drops
	nary disease	HAA	hepatitis associated antigen
CPK	creatine phosphokinase	HCO_3	bicarbonate
cu mm	cubic millimeter(s)	H_2CO_3	carbonic acid
CVP	central venous pressure	HCT	hematocrit
CXR	chest x-ray	Hg	mercury
D5W	5 percent dextrose in water	Hgb	hemoglobin
D50W	50 percent dextrose in water	HTN	hypertension
dc	direct current	Hx	history
DI	diabetes insipidus	I&D	incision and drainage
DIC	disseminated intravascular	IgA, etc.	immunoglobulin A, etc.
	coagulopathy	IM	intramuscular(ly)

(continued)

I&Os	inputs and outputs		PN	pneumonia
IPPB	intermittent positive pressure breathing		po	orally
			PPD	purified protein derivative
IU	international unit(s)		prn	as needed
IV	intravenous(ly)		Pso_2	arterial oxygen pressure
IVP	intravenous pyelogram		PT	prothrombin time
kg	kilogram(s)		PTT	partial prothrombin time
K/O	keep open		q 4 hours,	
KUB	kidney, ureter, and bladder x-ray		etc.	every 4 hours, etc.
			qd	every day
L&D	labor and delivery		qid	4 times a day
lb	pound(s)		RA	rheumatoid arthritis
LDH	lactic dehydrogenase		RAIU	radioactive iodine uptake
LFT	liver function test; direct bili, total bilirubin, alkaline phosphatase, LDH, SGOT		RHD	rheumatic heart disease
			RME	routine medical exam
			R/O	rule out
LOC	loss of consciousness		RX	treatment
LP	lumbar puncture		SBE	subacute bacterial endocarditis
LS	lumbosacral			
LVEDP	left ventricular end-diastolic pressure		SC	subcutaneously
			SGOT	serum glutamic oxaloacetic transaminase
mEq	milliequivalent(s)			
mg	milligram(s)		SGPT	serum glutamic pyruvic transaminase
MI	myocardial infarction			
mIU	mili-international unit(s)		SL	sublingual
ml	milliliter(s)		SLE	systemic lupus erythematosus
mm	millimeter(s)			
mOsm	milliosmole(s)		SMA6	Na, K, Cl, CO_2, BUN, creatinine
N & V	nausea and vomiting			
neb	nebulized		SOB	shortness of breath
ng	nanogram (= millimicrogram)		SQ	subcutaneously
NG	nasogastric		stat	at once
nm	nanometer (= millimicron)		SX	signs
nmole	nanomole		TB	tuberculosus
non-urgent	RME; routine medical exam		T&C	type and crossmatch
npo	nothing by mouth		TC	throat culture
NS	normal saline		tid	3 times a day
NVD	nausea, vomiting, diarrhea		TM	tympanic membrane
OD	overdose		TPR	temperature, pulse, respirations
OM	otitis media			
O&P	ova and parasites		u	unit(s)
OPD	outpatient department		U/A	urinalysis
Pco_2	carbon dioxide pressure		UME	urgent medical exam
Po_2	oxygen pressure (or tension)		URI	upper respiratory infection
$Paco_2$	arterial carbon dioxide pressure		UTI	urinary tract infection
			VDRL	venereal disease research lab
PAo_2	alveolar oxygen pressure		VS	vital signs
PBI	protein-bound iodine		WBC	white blood cell
PCN	penicillin		wt	weight
PE	physical exam		W/U	workup
PEEP	positive end-expiratory pressure		/	per
			<	less than
pH	hydrogen-ion concentration		>	more than
PLTS	platelets			

2. Metric and Apothecary Equivalents

Metric Weights or Measures (grams or ml)		Apothecary Weights (grains)		Apothecary Measures (minims of water at 4°C)
0.0648	=	1	=	1.0517
0.130	=	2	=	2.11
0.194	=	3	=	3.15
0.259	=	4	=	4.20
0.324	=	5	=	5.26
0.389	=	6	=	6.31
0.454	=	7	=	7.37
0.5	=	7.72	=	8.12
0.518	=	8	=	8.41
0.583	=	9	=	9.46
0.648	=	10	=	10.52
0.713	=	11	=	11.57
0.778	=	12	=	12.63
0.842	=	13	=	13.67
0.907	=	14	=	14.72
0.972	=	15	=	15.78
1.000	=	15.4324	=	16.23
1.296	=	20	=	21.04
1.944	=	30	=	31.55

Metric Weights (grams)		Apothecary Weights (grains)		Metric Weights (milligrams)
0.0001	=	1/640	=	0.1
0.0002	=	1/320	=	0.2
0.0003	=	1/210	=	0.3
0.000324	=	1/200	=	0.324
0.0004	=	1/160	=	0.4
0.000432	=	1/150	=	0.432
0.0005	=	1/128	=	0.5
0.00054	=	1/120	=	0.54
0.0006	=	1/100	=	0.6
0.0008	=	1/80	=	0.8
0.001	=	1/64	=	1.0
0.0011	=	1/60	=	1.1
0.0013	=	1/50	=	1.3
0.0016	=	1/40	=	1.6
0.0018	=	1/36	=	1.8

(*continued*)

Metric Weights (grams)		Apothecary Weights (grains)		Metric Weights (milligrams)
0.0022	=	1/30	=	2.2
0.0026	=	1/25	=	2.6
0.0032	=	1/20	=	3.2
0.004	=	1/16	=	4.0
0.0065	=	1/10	=	6.5
0.0072	=	1/9	=	7.2
0.0081	=	1/8	=	8.1
0.0092	=	1/7	=	9.2
0.011	=	1/6	=	11.0
0.013	=	1/5	=	13.0
0.0162	=	1/4	=	16.2
0.0217	=	1/3	=	21.7
0.0243	=	3/8	=	24.3
0.0324	=	1/2	=	32.4
0.0432	=	2/3	=	43.2
0.0486	=	3/4	=	48.6
0.065	=	1	=	65.0

3. Weights and Measures

WEIGHTS

Apothecary		Apothecary		Metric
1 scruple	=	20 grains	=	1.296 grams
1 dram	=	60 grains	=	3.88 grams
1 ounce	=	480 grains (8 drams)	=	31.1 grams
1 pound	=	5,760 grains (12 ounces)	=	373.24 grams

Metric		Apothecary		Metric
1 milligram	=	1/65 grain*	=	0.001 gram
1 centigram	=	1/6 grain*	=	0.01 gram
1 decigram	=	1½ grains*	=	0.1 gram
1 gram	=	15.432 grains	=	0.001 kilogram
1 kilogram	=	2.2 pounds avdp*	=	1,000 grams

Avoirdupois		Apothecary		Metric
1 ounce	=	437.5 grains	=	28.35 grams
1 pound	=	7,000 grains	=	453.59 grams
1 ton	=	2,000 pounds avdp	=	907.184 kilograms

* Approximate equivalent.

LIQUID MEASURES

1 fluid dram	=	60 minims	=	3.697 ml
1 fluid ounce	=	8 fluid drams	=	29.573 ml
1 pint	=	16 fluid ounces	=	473.167 ml
1 quart	=	32 fluid ounces	=	946.333 ml
1 gallon	=	128 fluid ounces	=	3,785 ml
1 milliliter	=	0.061 cubic inch	=	1 ml
1 centiliter	=	0.61 cubic inch	=	10 ml
1 deciliter	=	6.1 cubic inches	=	100 ml
1 liter	=	61.0271 cubic inches	=	1,000 ml
1 teaspoonful	=	1 fluid dram	=	5 ml*
1 teacupful	=	4 fluid ounces	=	120 ml*
1 glassful	=	8 fluid ounces	=	240 ml*

* Approximate equivalent.

LINEAR MEASURES

1 inch	=	25.4 millimeters	=	2.54 centimeters
1 foot	=	12 inches	=	30.48 centimeters
1 yard	=	36 inches	=	0.9144 meter
1 rod	=	198 inches (16½ ft.)	=	5.029 meters
1 mile	=	5,280 feet	=	1.609 kilometers
1 millimeter	=	0.03937 inch	=	1,000 microns
1 centimeter	=	0.3937 inch	=	10 millimeters
1 decimeter	=	3.937 inches	=	10 centimeters
1 meter	=	39.37 inches	=	10 decimeters
1 kilometer	=	3,281 feet (0.62 mile)	=	1,000 meters

* Approximate equivalent.

4. Conversion Tables

TEMPERATURE

°F	°C	°C	°F
0	−17.7	0	32.0
95	35.0	35.0	95.0
96	35.5	35.5	95.9
97	36.1	36.0	96.8
98	36.6	36.5	97.7
99	37.2	37.0	98.6
100	37.7	37.5	99.5
101	38.3	38.0	100.4
102	38.8	38.5	101.3
103	39.4	39.0	102.2
104	40.0	39.5	103.1
105	40.5	40.0	104.0
106	41.1	40.5	104.9
107	41.6	41.0	105.8
108	42.2	41.5	106.6
109	42.7	42.0	107.6
110	43.3	100.0	212.0
$°C = (°F − 32) \times 5/9$		$°F = (°C \times 9/5) + 32$	

WEIGHT

lb	kg	kg	lb
1	0.5	1	2.2
2	0.9	2	4.4
4	1.8	3	6.6
6	2.7	4	8.8
8	3.6	5	11.0
10	4.5	6	13.2
20	9.1	8	17.6
30	13.6	10	22
40	18.2	20	44
50	22.7	30	66
60	27.3	40	88
70	31.8	50	110
80	36.4	60	132
90	40.9	70	154
100	45.4	80	176
150	68.2	90	198
200	90.8	100	220
1 lb = 0.454 kg		1 kg = 2.204 lb	

LENGTH

in	cm	cm	in
1	2.5	1	0.4
2	5.1	2	0.8
4	10.2	3	1.2
6	15.2	4	1.6
8	20.3	5	2.0
12	30.5	6	2.4
18	46	8	3.1
24	61	10	3.9
30	76	20	7.9
36	91	30	11.8
42	107	40	15.7
48	122	50	19.7
54	137	60	23.6
60	152	70	27.6
66	168	80	31.5
72	183	90	35.4
78	198	100	39.4
1 inch = 2.54 cm		1 cm = 0.3937 inch	

HOUSEHOLD MEASURES

1 teaspoonful	1 fl dr	4–5 ml
1 dessertspoonful	2 fl dr	8 ml
1 tablespoonful	½ fl oz	15 ml
1 jigger	1½ fl oz	45 ml
1 wineglassful	2 fl oz	60 ml
1 teacupful	4 fl oz	120 ml
1 glassful	8 fl oz	240 ml

5. Normal Blood Values

HEMATOLOGY

Hematocrit	Men: 45% (38–54%)
	Women: 40% (36–47%)
Hemoglobin	Men: 14–18 g%
	Women: 12–16 g%
	Children: 12–14 g%
	Newborn: 14.5–24.5 g%

Blood Counts	Per cu mm	%
Erythrocytes		
Men	$5 \ (4.5–6) \times 10^6$	
Women	$4.5 \ (4.3–5.5) \times 10^6$	
Reticulocytes		0–1
Leukocytes, total	5,000–10,000	100
Myelocytes	0	0
Juvenile neutrophils	0–100	0–1
Band neutrophils	0–500	0–5
Segmented neutrophils	2,500–6,000	40–60
Lymphocytes	1,000–4,000	20–40
Eosinophils	50–300	1–3
Basophils	0–100	0–1
Monocytes	200–800	4–8
Platelets	200,000–500,000	

RBC Measurements

Diameter	5.5–8.8 microns (Newborn: 8.6)
Mean corpuscular volume	80–94 cu microns (Newborn: 106)
Mean corpuscular Hb	27–32 micromicrograms (Newborn: 38)
Mean corpuscular Hb concentration	33–38%
Color, saturation, and volume indexes, each	1

Miscellaneous

Bleeding time	1–3 minutes (Duke)
	2–4 minutes (Ivy)
Circulation time, arm to lung (ether)	4–8 seconds
Circulation time, arm to tongue (sodium dehydrocholate)	9–16 seconds
Clot retraction time	2–4 hours
Coagulation time (venous)	6–10 minutes (Lee and White)
	10–30 minutes (Howell)
Fragility, erythrocyte (hemolysis)	0.44–0.35% NaCl
Prothrombin time	70–110% of control value
Sedimentation rate	
Men	0–9 mm/hour (Wintrobe)
Women	0–20 mm/hour (Wintrobe)

BLOOD CHEMISTRY (Whole Blood, Serum, and Plasma Values)[a]

Acetone, serum	0.3–2 mg/100 ml
Alpha amino nitrogen, plasma	3–5.5 mg/100 ml
Ammonia, blood	40–70 μg/100 ml
Amylase, serum	80–180 Somogyi units/100 ml
Ascorbic acid, blood	0.4–1.5 mg/100 ml
Barbiturates, serum	0
	Coma level: Phenobarbital, approximately 11 mg/100 ml; most other barbiturates, 1.5 mg/100 ml
Base, total, serum	145–160 mEq/L
Bilirubin, serum	
Direct	0.1–0.4 mg/100 ml
Indirect	0.2–0.7 mg/100 ml
	(Total minus direct)
Total	0.3–1.1 mg/100 ml
Bromides, serum	0
	Toxic levels above 17 mEq/L
Calcium, serum	4.5–5.5 mEq/L
	(9–11 mg/100 ml)
	(Slightly higher in children)
	(Varies with protein concentration)
Ionized	2.1–2.6 mEq/L
	(4.25–5.25 mg/100 ml)
Carbon dioxide, serum	
Content	26–28 mEq/L
	(Infants: 20–26 mEq/L)
Combining power	24–29 mEq/L
	(53–64 vol %)
Tension P_{CO_2}	35–45 mm Hg
Carbon monoxide, blood	Symptoms with over 20% saturation
Carotenoids, serum	100–300 IU/100 ml
Chloride, serum	100–106 mEq/L
	(355–376 mg/100 ml as Cl)
	585–620 mg/100 ml as NaCl)
Cholesterol, serum	
Total	150–250 mg/100 ml
Esters	68–76% of total cholesterol
Copper, serum	70–140 μg/100 ml
Creatinine, serum	0.7–1.5 mg/100 ml
Cryoglobulins, serum	0
Dilantin (phenytoin) blood or serum	Therapeutic levels: 1–11 mcg/ml
Ethanol, blood	
Marked intoxication	0.3–0.4%
Alcoholic stupor	0.4–0.5%
Coma	Above 0.5%
Fibrinogen, plasma	200–400 mg/100 ml

(continued)

BLOOD CHEMISTRY (Whole Blood, Serum, and Plasma Values)[a]

Glucose (fasting), blood	
True	60–100 mg/100 ml
Folin	80–120 mg/100 ml
17–hydroxycorticoids, plasma	5–25 **m**g/100 ml
Icterus index, serum	4–7
Iodine, butanol extractable, serum	3.5–6.5 **m**g/100 ml
Iodine, protein-bound, serum	3.5–8 **m**g/100 ml (May be slightly higher in infants)
Iron, serum	75–175 **m**g/100 ml
Iron binding capacity, unsaturated, serum	150–300 **m**g/100 ml
Lactic acid, blood	6–16 mg/100 ml
Lactic dehydrogenase, serum	200–450 units/100 ml
Lead, blood	0–50 **m**g/100 ml
Lipase, serum	Less than 1.5 units (ml of N/20 NaOH)
Lipids, total, serum	450–850 mg/100 ml
Lipid partition, blood	
Cholesterol	150–250 mg/100 ml
Cholesterol esters	68–76% of total cholesterol
Phospholipids	6–12 mg/100 ml as lipid phosphorus
Total fatty acids	190–420 mg/100 ml
Neutral fat	0–150 mg/100 ml
Magnesium, serum	1.5–2.5 mEq/L (1.8–3 mg/100 ml)
Nitrogen, nonprotein, serum	15–35 mg/100 ml
Osmolality, serum	285–295 mOsm/L
Oxygen, blood	
Capacity	16–24 vol % (varies with Hb)
Content	
Arterial	15–23 vol %
Venous	10–16 vol %
Saturation	
Arterial	94–100% of capacity
Venous	60–85% of capacity
Tension, P_{O_2}	
Arterial	95–100 mm. Hg
pH, arterial, plasma	7.35–7.45
Phenylalanine, serum	Less than 3 mg/100 ml
Phosphatase, acid, serum	1–5 units (King-Armstrong) 0.5–2 units (Bodansky) 0.5–2 units (Gutman) 0–1.1 units (Shinowara) 0.1–0.63 units (Bessey-Lowry)
Phosphatase, Alkaline, serum	5–13 units (King-Armstrong) 2–4.5 units (Bodansky) 3–10 units (Gutman) 2.2–8.6 units (Shinowara) 0.8–2.3 units (Bessey-Lowry) (Values are higher in children)

Phosphate, inorganic, serum	3–4.5 mg/100 ml
	(Children: 4–7 mg/100 ml)
Potassium, serum	3.5–5 mEq/L
	(14–20 mg/100 ml as K)
Proteins, serum	
Total	6–8 g/100 ml
Albumin	3.5–5.5 g/100 ml
Globulin	1.5–3 g/100 ml
Paper electrophoresis	
Albumin	45–55% of total
Globulin	
alpha$_1$	5–8% of total
alpha$_2$	8–13% of total
beta	11–17% of total
gamma	15–25% of total
Pyruvic acid, plasma	1–2 mg/100 ml
Salicylate, plasma	0
Therapeutic range	20–25 mg/100 ml
Toxic range	Over 30 mg/100 ml
Serotonin	
Platelet suspension	0.1–0.3 mg/ml blood
Serum	0.1–0.32 mg/ml
Sodium, serum	136–145 mEq/L
	(313–334 mg/100 ml as Na)
Sulfates, inorganic, serum	0.5–1.5 mg/100 ml
Transaminase, serum	
SGOT	5–40 units/ml
SGPT	5–35 units/ml
Urea nitrogen, blood (BUN)	10–20 mg/100 ml
Uric acid, serum	3–6 mg/100 ml
Vitamin A, serum	30–100 units/100 ml

[a] For some procedures, the normal values may vary according to the methods used.

6. Normal Urine Values

Acetone and acetoacetate	0
Addis count	
Erythrocytes	0–130,000/24 hours
Leukocytes	0–650,000/24 hours
Casts (hyaline)	0–2,000/24 hours
Aldosterone	6–16 μg/24 hours
Alpha amino nitrogen	64–199 mg/24 hours
	(Not over 1.5% total nitrogen)
Ammonia	20–70 mEq/L
Amylase (Somogyi)	260–950 Somogyi units/24 hours
Calcium	
Low Ca diet (Bauer-Aub)	Less than 150 mg/24 hours
Usual diet	Less than 250 mg/24 hours
Catecholamines	
Epinephrine	Less than 10 μg/24 hours
Norepinephrine	Less than 100 μg/24 hours
Chorionic gonadotropin	0
Coproporphyrin	50–250 μg/24 hours
Creatine	Less than 100 mg/24 hours
	(Higher in children and during pregnancy)
Creatinine	15–25 mg/kg body wt/24 hours
Cystine or cysteine	0
Estrogens	
Male	4–25 μg/24 hours
Female	4–60 μg/24 hours
	(Increased during pregnancy)
Hemoglobin and myoglobin	0
Homogentisic acid	0
5-Hydroxyindolylacetic acid (5-HIAA)	
Qualitative	0
Quantitative	Less than 16 mg/24 hours
17-Hydroxycorticoids	
Male	5–15 mg/24 hours
Female	4–10 mg/24 hours
	(Varies with method used)
17-Ketosteroids	
Under 8 years	0–2 mg/24 hours
Adolescents	2–20 mg/24 hours
Male	8–25 mg/24 hours
Female	5–15 mg/24 hours
Lead	Less than 0.08 μg/ml or less than 120 μg/24 hours
pH	4.6–8; average, 6 (Depends on diet)
Phenylpyruvic acid	0

Pituitary gonadotropins	5–10 rat units/24 hours
	10–50 mouse units/24 hours
	(Increased after menopause)
Porphobilinogen	0
Protein	0 qualitative
	(less than 30 mg/24 hours)
Specific gravity	1.003–1.030
Solids, total	30–70 g/L; average, 50 g/L (To estimate total solids per liter, multiply last two figures or specific gravity by 2.66, Long's coefficient.)
Sugar	0
Titratable acidity	20–40 mEq/24 hours
Urobilinogen	Up to 1 Ehrlich unit/2 hours
	(1–3 P.M.)
	0–4 mg/24 hours
Vanillylmandelic acid (VMA)	1.8–8.4 mg/24 hours

7. Renal Function Studies

Clearance tests (corrected to 1.73 sq M body surface area)	
Glomerular filtration rate (GFR)	Males: 110–150 ml/minute
Inulin clearance	Females: 105–132 ml/minute
Mannitol clearance	
Endogenous creatinine clearance	
Renal plasma flow (RPF)	Males: 560–830 ml/minute
p-Aminohippurate (PAH)	Females: 490–700 ml/minute
Diodrast	
Filtration fraction (FF)	Males: 17–21%
$$FF = \frac{GFR}{RPF}$$	Females: 17–23%
Urea clearance (C_U)	Standard: 40–65 ml/minute
	Maximum: 60–100 ml/minute
Concentration and dilution	Specific gravity > 1.025 on dry day
	Specific gravity < 1.003 on water day
Maximum Diodrast excretory capacity (Tm_D)	Males: 43–59 mg/minute
	Females: 33–51 mg/minute
Maximum glucose reabsorptive capacity (Tm_G)	Males: 300–450 mg/minute
	Females: 250–350 mg/minute
Maximum PAH excretory capacity (Tm_{PAH})	80–90 mg/minute
Phenolsulfonphthalein	25% or more in 15 minutes
(PSP) excretion	40% or more in 30 minutes
	55% or more in 2 hours
	After injection of 1 ml PSP intravenously

8. Pulmonary Function Studies

MEASUREMENTS OF PRINCIPAL LUNG VOLUMES AND FORMULAS FOR THEIR PREDICTION IN NORMAL SUBJECTS

	Age 15–34		Age 35–49		Age 50–69	
	Women	*Men*	*Women*	*Men*	*Women*	*Men*
Vital capacity, supine (ml)	2,312–4,150	2,792–4,950	2,212–3,435	3,300–5,240	1,570–3,525	2,184–5,429
Maximum breathing capacity, standing (L/minute)	63.6–117.5	82–169	47–114	86–144.5	49–101.5	58–139
Ventilation, resting (L/minute/sq M body surface)	2.55–4.27	3.1–4.5	2.4–3.71	2.6–4	2.53–3.95	3.2–4.9
Oxygen consumption, resting (ml/minute/sq M body surface)	111–149	129–186	109–136	118–156	105–150	107–165
Predicted (calculated) total capacity (supine)	$\dfrac{\text{Vital capacity}}{80} \times 100$		$\dfrac{\text{Vital capacity}}{76.6} \times 100$		$\dfrac{\text{Vital capacity}}{69.2} \times 100$	
Ratio $\dfrac{\text{residual volume}}{\text{total capacity}} \times 100$ (supine)	20		23.4		30.8	
Predicted (calculated) vital capacity, supine (ml)	Women: $(21.78 - [0.101 \times \text{age in yrs}]) \times$ height in cm Men: $(27.63 - [0.112 \times \text{age in yrs}]) \times$ height in cm					
Predicted (calculated) maximum breathing capacity, standing (L/minute)	Women: $(71.3 - [0.474 \times \text{age in yrs}]) \times$ sq M body surface Men: $(86.5 - [0.522 \times \text{age in yrs}]) \times$ sq M body surface					

9. Liver Function Studies

Bromsulfalein (BSP)	Less than 5% remaining in serum 45 minutes after injection of 5 mg/kg body weight
Cephalin cholesterol flocculation	0–2 + in 48 hours
Cholinesterase (pseudocholinesterase), serum	0.5 pH unit or more/hour
Galactose tolerance	Excretion of not more than 3 g galactose in urine 5 hours after ingestion of 40 g
Glycogen storage	Increase of blood glucose 45 mg/100 ml over fasting level 45 minutes after subcutaneous injection of 0.01 mg epinephrine per kg body weight
Hippuric acid	Excretion of 3–3.5 g hippuric acid in urine within 4 hours after ingestion of 6 g sodium benzoate *or* Excretion of 0.7 g hippuric acid in urine within 1 hour after IV injection of 1.77 g sodium benzoate
Thymol turbidity	0–5 units
Zinc turbidity	2–12 units

10. Thyroid Function Studies

Basal Metabolic Rate	Minus 10% to plus 10% of Mean Standard	
Radioactive Iodine (I-131) uptake	20–50% of administered dose in 24 hours	
Radioactive Iodine (I-131) excretion	30–70% of administered dose in 24 hours	
Radioactive Iodine, protein-bound	Less than 0.3% of administered dose per L of plasma at 72 hours	

11. Pancreatic (Islet) Function Studies

Glucose tolerance tests	Patient should be on diet containing 300 g carbohydrate per day for 3 days prior to test. Values given are for true glucose; with Folin method, values are approximately 20 mg/100 ml higher
Oral	After ingestion of 100 g glucose or 1.75 g glucose per kg body weight, blood glucose not more than 160 mg/100 ml after 60 minutes, 140 mg/100 ml after 90 minutes, and 120 mg/100 ml after 120 minutes.
Intravenous	Blood glucose does not exceed 200 mg/100 ml after infusion of 0.5 g glucose per kg body weight over 30 minutes. Glucose concentration falls below initial level at 2 hours and returns to preinfusion levels in 3 or 4 hours.
Cortisone-glucose tolerance test	The patient should be on diet containing 300 g carbohydrate per day for 3 days prior to test. At 8½ and again 2 hours prior to glucose load, patient is given cortisone acetate by mouth (50 mg if patient's ideal weight is less than 160 lb, 62.5 mg if ideal weight is more than 160 lb). An oral dose of glucose, 1.75 g/kg ideal body weight, is given and blood samples are taken at 0, 30, 60, 90, and 120 minutes. Test is considered positive if true blood glucose exceeds 160 mg/100 ml at 60 minutes, 140 mg/100 ml at 90 minutes, and 120 mg/100 ml at 120 minutes.

12. Gastric Analysis

Acidity
  Fasting
    Free acidity   0–30 degrees/100 ml
    Total acidity   10–50 degrees/100 ml
  One hour after histamine
    Free acid   30–85 degrees/100 ml
Diagnex Blue (Squibb)
  Anacidity   0–0.3 mg in 2 hours
  Doubtful   0.3–0.6 mg in 2 hours
  Normal   More than 0.6 mg in 2 hours
Volume, fasting stomach content   50–100 ml
Emptying time   3–6 hours
Color   Opalescent or colorless
Specific gravity   1.006–1.009
pH (adults)   0.9–1.5

13. Stool Tests

Bulk   100–200 g daily
  Water content   Approximately 65%
  Dry matter   23–32 g daily
    Protein content   Minimum
    Fat, total   17.5% of dry matter (Up to 30% of dry weight is normal.)
      Fatty acid combined as soap 4.6% of dry matter
      Free fatty acid   5.6% of dry matter
      Neutral fat   7.3% of dry matter (42% of total fat)
Nitrogen excretion   Less than 1.7 g/day
Urobilinogen   40–280 mg/24 hours

14. Gastrointestinal Absorption Tests

d-Xylose absorption test	After an 8-hour fast, 10 ml of a 5% solution of *d*-xylose per kg body weight are given by mouth. Nothing further by mouth is given until the test has been completed. All urine voided during the following 5 hours is pooled, and blood samples are taken at 0, 60, and 120 minutes. Normally, 26% (range, 16–33%) of ingested xylose is excreted within 5 hours; the serum xylose reaches a level between 25 and 40 mg/100 ml after 1 hour and is maintained at this level for another 60 minutes.
Vitamin A absorption test	A fasting blood specimen is obtained, and 200,000 units of vitamin A in oil are given by mouth. Serum vitamin A level should rise to twice fasting level in 3 to 5 hours.

15. Adrenal–Pituitary Function Studies

Insulin tolerance test	Blood glucose usually falls to 50% of fasting level in 20 to 30 minutes with return to normal levels in 90 to 120 minutes after IV administration of 0.1 unit crystalline insulin per kg body weight
Adrenocortical inhibition test Δ-1, 9, α-fluorocortisone or 16-methyl-α-hydrocortisone	0.5 mg of either drug po q 6 hours reduces excretion of 17-hydroxycorticoids from 4–15 mg/24 hours to a level of less than 2 mg/24 hours
Corticotropin (ACTH) response tests Eosinophil count (Thorn test)	Four hours after 25 USP units of ACTH IM, decrease in eosinophil count should exceed 50% of the initial level
Plasma 17-hydroxycorticoids	After 8 hours infusion of 25 USP units of ACTH, plasma 17-hydroxycorticoids rise from a normal level of 5–25 μg/100 ml to 35–55 μg/100 ml
Urinary steroids	After 8 hours infusion of 25 USP units of ACTH, urinary 17-hydroxycorticoids increase 200 to 400%, and urinary 17-ketosteroids increase 50 to 100%

16. IV Flow Rates and Infusion Times

Flow rate (drops/minute)   = $\dfrac{\text{Drops in 1 ml} \times \text{total ml}}{\text{Total time in minutes}}$

Infusion time (hours)   = $\dfrac{\text{Total vol to be delivered}}{\text{ml being delivered/hour}}$

17. Cardiac Function Studies

Blood volume	8.5–9% of body weight
Cardiac output	3 L/min/sq M body surface area
Cardiac pressures:	
Right atrium	Mean, 0–5 mm Hg
Right ventricle	Systolic, 20–30 mm Hg
	Diastolic, 0–5 mm Hg
Pulmonary artery	Systolic, 20–30 mm Hg
	Diastolic, 7–12 mm Hg
	Mean, 12–17 mm Hg
Circulation time	
Arm to tongue	10–16 seconds
Venous pressure	60–120 mm water

18. Cerebrospinal Fluid Values

Cells	Fewer than 5 per cu mm, all mononuclear
Chloride	120–130 mEq/L (20 mEq/L higher than in serum)
Colloidal gold test	Not more than 1 in any tube
Gamma globulin	1.3–4.7 mg/100 ml 4.3–12.3% of total protein
Glucose	50–75 mg/100 ml (20 mg/100 ml less than in blood)
Pressure	70–180 mm water
Protein	15–45 mg/100 ml

19. Intracardiac and Intra-arterial Pressures

Site	Representative Mmttg	Range
Aorta		
Systolic	120	100–140 mm Hg (13.3–18.7 KPa)
Diastolic	70	60–90 mm Hg (8.0–12.0 KPa)
Atrium		
Left	8	2–12 mm Hg (0.3–1.6 KPa)
Right	3	0–5 mm Hg (0–0.07 KPa)
Pulmonary artery		
Systolic	25	15–30 mm Hg (2.0–4.0 KPa)
Diastolic	10	3–13 mm Hg (0.4–1.7 KPa)
Wedge (mean)	9	5–13 mm Hg (0.7–1.7 KPa)
Ventricle, left		
Systolic	120	100–140 mm Hg (13.3–18.7 KPa)
Diastolic	8	4–12 mm Hg (0.5–1.6 KPa)
Ventricle, right		
Systolic	25	15–30 mm Hg (2.0–4.0 KPa)
Diastolic	3	0–5 mm Hg (0.07 KPa)
Venous antecubital	100	5–14 mm Hg (0.5–1.4 KPa)

(*Based on data in Altman, Dittmer* (Eds.). *Respiration and Circulation. Bethesda, Md., Federation of American Societies for Experimental Biology, 1971.*)

APPENDIX B

1. Anaphylactic Syndrome

THERAPEUTIC CLASSIFICATION

Grade I Symptoms—Large local contiguous reaction (15 cm)
Treatment—Cold compress, symptomatic medication

Grade II Symptoms—Pruritus (urticaria)
Treatment—Epinephrine 0.3 cc of 1:1000 SQ every 15 minutes to 3 dose maximum. Antihistamine (like diphenhydramine) 50 mg po, IV, or IM followed by oral dose tid or qid for 24 to 48 hours or ephedrine 25 mg po qid for 24 to 48 hours

Grade III Symptoms—Dyspnea (mild wheezing), angioedema, nausea, and vomiting
Treatment—Epinephrine 0.3 cc of 1:1000 SQ every 15 minutes to three dose maximum. If no response treat as if Grade IV. Admit for at least 24 hours of observation.

Grade IV (a) Symptoms—Asthma (severe dyspnea), tongue swelling (dysphagia). Respiratory distress/hoarseness (laryngeal edema)

Treatment—Early intubation. If refractory dyspnea, give epinephrine 0.3 cc SQ or IM q 15 minutes and aminophylline 5 to 6 mg/kg IV loading dose slowly IV followed by 0.9 mg/kg per hour maintenance

(b) Symptoms—Cardiovascular hypotension (1 to 2 cc IV of epinephrine 1:10,000 if bp < 70). (This preparation (1:10,000) is the standard intracardiac dose.) It can be prepared by diluting 1 cc of 1:1,000 epinephrine with 9 cc of normal NaCl. Supportive care for Grade IV reactions should include hydrocortisone 200 mg IV and an antihistamine (diphenhydramine) 50 mg IV if urticaria is present. Admit to ICU for observation.

Treatment—Epinephrine 1:1,000 0.3 cc SQ. Rapid volume replacement 500 to 2000 ml normal saline in first hour to bp of 80. If crystalloids are ineffective, use colloids. If pressor agents are needed, dopamine should be tried first.

(c) Symptoms—CNS seizures

Treatment—Usually a self-limiting process but phenobarbital 130 mg IV or IM may be given

CLINICAL CHARACTERISTICS (BY SYSTEM)

System	Symptoms and Signs	Mediator(s)
General (prodromal)	Malaise, weakness, sense of illness	
Dermal	Hives, erythema	Histamine
Mucosal	Periorbital edema, nasal congestion pruritus, angioedema (or) flushing and/or pallor, cyanosis	Histamine
Respiratory	Sneezing, rhinorrhea, dyspnea	
Upper airway	Laryngeal edema, hoarseness, tongue and pharyngeal edema, stridor	Histamine
Lower airway	Dyspnea, acute emphysema Air trapping (asthma, bronchospasm, bronchorrhea)	Probably SRS-A Possibly histamine others
GI	Increased peristalsis, vomiting, dysphagia, nausea, abdominal cramps, diarrhea, occasionally with blood	?
Cardiovascular	Tachycardia, palpitations, hypotension (cardiac arrest) ECG coronary insufficiency with ST-T wave changes	?
CNS	Anxiety, seizures	?

2. Management of Animal Bites

ANIMAL BITES

Cat bites and scratches, even if minute, may cause a benign localized low-grade viral infection, "cat scratch fever," or a bacterial infection, typically *Pasteurella multocida*. Protection against tetanus should be provided, in addition to local cleansing and repair as indicated.

Dog bites vary in extent from slight contusions, superficial abrasions, and fang puncture wounds to deep tearing lacerations if the animal or victim attempts to pull away. Contusions without broken skin usually require no treatment. (Abrasions, puncture wounds and lacerations require local treatment as indicated.) Protection against tetanus should be provided. Rabies is rare in urban centers, but must be kept in mind. Whenever possible, the animal should be detained. The case should be reported immediately to the Health Department for disposition and guidance.

PATHOGENS IN SEPSIS FROM DOG BITES

Commonly Found Species	Animal Bite Wound Treatment
Aeromonas hydrophila	1. Adequate tetanus immunization
Bacteroides	2. Thorough wound irrigation
Eikenella corrodens	3. Extensive debridement
Enterobacter sp	4. Consider rabies
Klebsiella sp	5. Suture all wounds except hand
Pasteurella	6. Acute injuries need not be recultured
Proteus mirabilis	7. Prophylactic antibiotics
Pseudomonas	(penicillin or dicloxacillin)
Staphylococus aureus	
Streptoccus progenes	

(Adapted from Callaham, M. L. Human and animal bites, Topics in Emergency Medicine, 4 (1), April, 1982.)

Rat bites require local treatment and tetanus protection. Rat bite fever is, in fact, two diseases caused by different bacteria, *Streptobacillus moniliformis* and *Spirillum minus.* It has systemic involvement, manifests about 10 days after a rat bite, and should be treated with tetracycline.

3. Spouse Abuse

OBJECTIVE

To recognize symptoms and provide physical, emotional, and psychological care for the victim and family of spouse abuse.

PROCEDURE

A. The *triage nurse* will:
   1. suspect any woman with multiple soft injuries, signs of multiple old injury, pregnant women with injury, and women accompanied by an oversolicitous companion or one who refuses to leave the woman's side
   2. document on triage sheet the patient's statement regarding event (with quotes as appropriate). The note should contain the description of obvious injury pattern and the nurse's suspicion of battering
   3. separate patient from spouse/partner/companion as soon as possible by placing patient in a private place
   4. give report to primary nurse for assigned room
B. The *primary care nurse/doctor* will:
   1. privately approach the patient empathetically. Ask the patient if she would want to press charges; if she needs to leave home. Be sure to give message that

no one deserves to be beaten. Assure patient of the confidentiality of her statements and chart. Respect this confidentiality

2. notify clerical staff and hospital police of patient's status and need for confidentiality
3. obtain urine for analysis since beating is often directed to the abdomen and flank areas
4. refer all patients for consultation to the social worker on duty

The *social worker/nurse/doctor* should determine whether victim has children. If so, ages, present location, and whose charge the children are presently in should be established. If children are considered "at risk" for neglect or abuse, the social worker must be involved.

Documentation of injuries should be as explicit as possible. The patient should be encouraged to permit photographs to document the injuries. A camera should be readily available and consent should be obtained for filing and retrieval in the medical record. Photos must be signed and dated by the person taking the picture, and the patient's name and chart number must be on the back of the photos. If a patient refuses/denies the need for intervention, notation must be made on the chart that the pattern of injury is consistent with the patient's history.

If the patient is afraid to return home, every effort should be made for alternate placement. Give all suspected spouse abuse victims the phone numbers of the hospital social work department, Victims' Service Agency and the New York State Department of Social Services.

SUMMARY PROTOCOL/CHECKLIST: IDENTIFYING AND TREATING ADULT DOMESTIC VIOLENCE VICTIMS

A. It is often difficult for hospital staff to identify adult domestic violence victims because most victims try to disguise the cause of their injuries. Hospital staff should consider domestic violence if any of the following is observed:
   1. Common sites of injury—face, neck, throat, chest, abdomen, genitals
   2. Injuries during pregnancy
   3. Substantial delay between onset of injury and presentation for treatment
   4. Multiple injuries in various stages of healing
   5. Extent or type of injury inconsistent with explanation patient gives
   6. Repeated use of emergency room services and/or psychosomatic or emotional complaints
   7. Evidence of alcohol or drug abuse
B. Convey an attitude of concern, interest, and confidentiality to the patient
C. *Interview the patient alone.* Hospital staff should ask any accompanying spouse, friend, or family member to leave the treatment area. Interview the patient in a place that affords privacy so the patient can speak frankly. Interview the spouse or family member if considered appropriate
D. Take the patient's history, conduct a thorough examination, and provide appro-

priate lab tests and x-rays. Treat physical and emotional injuries. Keep detailed medical records
E. Preserve physical evidence. Place torn or blood stained clothing and/or weapon used in sealed envelope or bag. Mark on envelope the date, patient's name and the name of the person who placed the items in the bag. Keep envelope in a locked drawer until you turn it over to police, prosecutor, or patient's lawyer
F. Offer to photograph the patient's physical injuries. Keep in sealed envelope
G. Encourage the patient to call the toll-free domestic violence hot line: 1-800-942-6906
H. Provide information and referrals for counseling, shelter and legal assistance in your community
 I. In the case of abused elderly persons, refer to local Department of Social Services Protective Services for Adults

4. Child Abuse

REPORTING OF SUSPECTED ABUSED OR NEGLECTED CHILDREN

The following procedure for reporting suspected abuse or maltreatment of children is intended to reflect legislative mandates for child protection.

A. *Introduction*
   In review of the continued increase in the number of cases of child abuse, legislation has been passed by the New York State Legislature to improve the reporting and investigation of abuse cases, and to further improve the degree of protection offered to those children. The following administrative information and procedure statement is intended to provide guidelines for assisting the physician in carrying out his legal responsibilities under the law.
B. *Definitions*
   1. "Abused child" means a child less than 16 years of age whose parent(s) or other person legally responsible for his care:
      a. inflicts or allows to be inflicted upon such child physical injury by other than accidental means which causes or creates a substantial risk of death, or serious or protracted disfigurement, or protracted impairment of physical or emotional health, or protracted loss or impairment of the function of any bodily organ, or
      b. creates, or allows to be created, a substantial risk of physical injury to such child by other than accidental means which would be likely to cause death

---

Reprinted courtesy of Bellevue Hospital Medical Center.

or serious or protracted disfigurement, or protracted impairment of physical or emotional health, or protracted loss or impairment of the function of any bodily organ, or

c. commits, or allows to be committed, a sexual offense against such child as defined in the penal law.

2. "Maltreated child" includes a child under 18 years of age,

a. defined as a neglected child by the Family Court Act:

(1) whose physical, mental or emotional condition has been impaired, or is in imminent danger of becoming impaired, as a result of the failure of his parent, or other person legally responsible for his care, to exercise a minimum degree of care:

(a) in supplying the child with adequate food, clothing, shelter or education, or medical, dental, optometrical or surgical care, although financially able to do so, or offered financial or other means to do so, or,

(b) in providing the child with proper supervision or guardianship, by unreasonably inflicting or allowing to be inflicted harm or a substantial risk thereof, including the infliction of excessive corporal punishment, or by using drugs or a drug, or by using alcoholic beverages to the extent that he loses self-control of his actions, or by other acts of a similarly serious nature requiring the aid of the court, or

(2) who has been abandoned by his parents, or other legally responsible for his care.

(3) who has had serious physical injury inflicted upon him by other than accidental means.

C. *Reporting Responsibilities*

1. Persons Legally Responsible for Reporting

According to the law, the following persons and officials are required to report or cause a report to be made when they have reasonable cause to *suspect* that a child coming before them in their professional capacity is an abused or maltreated child: any physician, surgeon, medical examiner, dentist, osteopath, optometrist, chiropracter, podiatrist, resident, intern, registered nurse, hospital personnel, school officials, social service worker, and mental health workers.

2. Immunity from Prosecution

The physician must bear in mind that he need have only reasonable cause to suspect and that proof is not required. He need make no definitive decision and is not required to make any accusation as to who caused the suspected injuries. It is important to note that the law specifically protects the reporting person against any civil or criminal proceedings when the initial report was made in good faith.

3. Penalties for Failure to Report

Any person, official, or institution required to report child abuse or maltreatment, who willfully fails to do so, shall be guilty of a Class A Misdemeanor and shall be civilly liable for the damages proximately caused by such failure. The state law further indicates that failure to provide required surgical or medical treatment, even when the child's parents refuse such treatment, may be defined as an act of "neglect" on the part of the physician and hospital personnel.

D. *Emergency Remand Procedure*
   1. If the parent or guardian of a child suspected of being abused or maltreated attempts to remove that child from the hospital, the physician should notify the Administrator who may decide to institute an Emergency Remand by contacting Special Services for Children. This procedure allows the Administrator to retain custody of an abused or maltreated child until the next regular week day session of the Family Court when a child protection proceeding may be commenced.
   2. Any child who has been admitted to the hospital as a possible case of abuse or maltreatment may not be discharged until release is authorized by Special Services for Children. If a parent or guardian attempts to remove such a child before release is authorized, an Emergency Remand should be immediately obtained from Special Services for Children.

E. *The Physician's Responsibility*
   1. Every abused child must be admitted to the hospital immediately.
   2. Every maltreated child who the physician judges to be in any imminent danger must be admitted to the hospital immediately.
   3. Any child diagnosed as maltreated but who, in the Pediatric Emergency Service physician's opinion, is not in any imminent danger, may be discharged only if a consultant from the Child Welfare Committee reviews the case and agrees, Special Services for Children is properly notified, and the parent or person legally responsible for the child is informed that the case has been referred and that a worker from Special Services for Children will be coming to their home.
   4. Any child brought to the Pediatric Emergency Service by the police as an *abandoned child* must be examined by the physician on duty. If the child is found to be entirely well, a note stating that the child is medically cleared should be given to the police who will then transport the child to the appropriate shelter. If the child has any medical problems or if a work-up for child abuse is indicated, the child must be admitted to the ward and Special Services for Children should be notified of his presence in the hospital. All charts on abandoned children must include the name, badge number, and precinct of the police officer who brought the child to PES.
   5. "Specific Instructions on How to Detect Child Abuse" is attached for informational purposes. Bellevue Hospital has a designated a Child Welfare Committee composed of doctors, nurses, social service workers and administrators who will serve as consultants for any case of child abuse and who are responsible for maintaining a hospital registry of cases of child abuse and maltreatment.
   6. The physician in the Pediatric Emergency Service is responsible for immedi-

ately notifying the appropriate Administrator of any case of suspected abuse or maltreatment. He should also consult the Hospital's Abuse Registry in the Duty Administrator's Office to ascertain if there has been any previous suspicions of abuse or maltreatment of this child or his siblings by Bellevue physicians. He should fill out a hospital abuse card if none exists. The physicians should avoid confronting or accusing any questions that the parents have. All x-ray and lab slips should use SCAMP (Suspected Child Abuse or Maltreated Patient) as diagnosis.

7. If the patient is admitted, it is the responsibility of the primary physician to obtain a clear history without accusations or value judgments and to follow through with the medical examination and report.

8. Should child abuse or maltreatment be suspected on a child admitted to Bellevue for a diagnosis other than abuse, it is the primary physician's responsibility to notify the Pediatric Area Administrator or Duty Officer, the Pediatric Social Service Supervisor, and to verify that the case is reported to Special Services for Children.

9. The primary physician should interview the parent(s) or guardian(s) legally responsible for the child after the examination has been completed, and should inform them that a referral is being made to the Special Services for Children Program as a possible child abuse case. The physician should also explain in detail what the parent(s) or guardian(s) can expect to happen.

F. *Nurse's Responsibility*

If a nurse or nurse's aide believes a child to be abused or maltreated, she shall immediately inform a doctor of her suspicion. If there is any disagreement about the diagnosis, a consulting member of the Child Welfare Committee will be called to make the final disposition of the case.

G. *The Hospital's Responsibility*

1. House Officers will report any case of suspected child abuse or maltreatment to the Administrator.

2. The Administrator upon receiving the report will immediately proceed to the PES, with the camera and proper forms (checklists and DSS-2221-A).

3. In the PES the administrator will confer with the physician who will then telephone notification to the Special Services for Children.

   a. It should be ascertained from SSC whether there has been a previous report of suspected abuse or maltreatment made on this child. SSC is prepared to supply to any *authorized source*, information within minutes from their computerized Central Registry. The Central Registry contains only substantiated reports. Unsubstantiated reports are expunged from the Registry. Therefore, a lack of information in the Central Registry should not lead the physician to assume that the child does not have a past record with SSC.

   b. Whether there is a previous report on this case or it is not on record, the physician will inform SSC of the presence of a suspected child abuse or maltreatment case at Bellevue Hospital.

   c. The telephone and written reports to SSC should contain the following:

(1) The names and addresses of the child and his parents or other persons responsible for his care, if known.

(2) Child's age, sex, and race.

(3) The nature and extent of the child's injuries or abuse or maltreatment to the child or his sibling(s).

(4) The names of the person or persons responsible for causing the injury, abuse or maltreatment, if known.

(5) Family composition.

(6) The source of the report.

(7) The person making the report and where he can be reached.

(8) The actions taken by the reporting source, including the taking of photographs and x-rays, removal or keeping of the child or notifying the medical examiner.

(9) Any other information which the Commissioner may by regulation require, or the person making the report believes might be helpful.

(*Note:* It would be important to indicate the parents' explanation of the injuries, abuse or maltreatment, and the reporter's assessment, as well as the religion of the child, if known. If the child has been hospitalized, it is important to include the *projected length of hospitalization.* The ages and whereabouts of the other children in the family may also be significant.)

4. Form DSS-2221-A and the Physician's Checklist should be *filled out and signed* by the Admitting Resident immediately. Form DSS-2221-A should be completed in duplicate.

5. The Administrator will send written notification within 48 hours to the Central Registry of Child Abuse and Maltreatment of Form DSS-2221-A.

H. *Examination of the Child*

The examination of an abused or maltreated child, and the resultant medical record is relied on heavily by the Family Court in deciding abuse and maltreatment cases. Therefore, it is important that the following be done:

1. In recording the history, the physician should identify the person giving the history and should quote the person in his own words and in as much detail as possible.

2. *Photographs* of the abused child should be taken in duplicate. One copy must go to the SSC with DSS-2221-A. Photographs may be taken without parental consent.

3. X-rays of the injured area(s) and other appropriate films should be taken, unless medically contraindicated to show evidence for use in court, and an official radiologist's report on the films should be made part of the medical record. X-rays may be taken without parental consent.

4. The Physician should note on the medical record (and on Form DSS-2221-A) an accurate description of the injuries and the explanation given. If there is clinical evidence that the injuries were caused in a manner other than that given in the history, it should be clearly stated. If there is contributory evidence (old injuries, evidence of neglect, failure to thrive, etc.) this should also be stated.

5. Communicable Diseases

	Incubation Period	Communicability Period	Symptoms	Treatment
Amebiasis *Entamoeba histolytica*	3 days to several months	During infection	Vary with severity—diarrhea (sometimes intermittent), blood and mucus in feces, abdominal discomfort	Chemotherapeutics or antibiotics
Ascariasis *Ascaris lumbricoides hominis*	2 months	Until fertilized female worms are killed	Vague unless heavily infected; then may exhibit digestive disturbance, abdominal pain, restlessness, exaggerated nervous reflexes	Anthelmintic
Brucellosis (Undulant Fever) *Brucella melitensis, abortus, or suis*	1 week to several months	Not usually communicable from man to man	Irregular fever, profuse sweating, chills, pain in joints and muscles	Antibiotics
Chancroid (Soft Chancre) *Hemophilus ducreyi*	1 to 12 days	Until etiological organisms are destroyed	Necrotizing ulcerations at site of inoculation; usually venereal	Sulfadiazine
Chickenpox (Varicella) Virus	2 to 3 weeks	1 day before to 6 days after first appearance of vesicles	Chills, slight fever, headache, malaise, successive crops of macules, papules, vesicles, crusts	Symptomatic
Diphtheria *Coryne-bacterium diphtheriae*	2 to 5 days, sometimes longer	Several hours before onset and for about 2 weeks during infection	Sore throat, fever, coryza, malaise, grayish patches (pseudomembranes) on tonsils and mucosa of throat and nose	Antitoxin, antibiotics
Dysentery, Bacillary Species of *Shigella* bacillus	1 to 7 days	During infection	Acute onset, diarrhea, sometimes fever, tenesmus, and frequent defecation, often with blood and mucus; symptoms variable in mild cases	Sulfonamides, antibiotics

Disease / Organism	Incubation period	Period of communicability	Symptoms	Treatment
Enterobiasis (Pinworm or Threadworm Infection) *Enterobius vermicularis*	14 to 21 days	During infection	Variable, frequently absent; anorexia, restlessness, insomnia, and pruritus ani	Anthelmintic, all members of family should be considered infected
Erysipelas Hemolytic streptococci, Group A strains	1 to 2 days	Until clinical recovery	Acute febrile infection of skin, characterized by red, tender, edematous, spreading skin lesion which is sharply delineated; fever, malaise	Antibiotics
Gonorrhea *Neisseria gonorrhoeae*	2 to 9 days or longer	During infection	In the male, acute anterior urethritis with burning on urination; serous discharge, becoming profuse, greenish-yellow, and often blood-tinged. In the female, often asymptomatic	Antibiotics
Hepatitis, Infectious Virus	10 to 40 days	From 2 to 3 weeks before until about 1 month after clinical onset	Acute infection, fever, anorexia, nausea, vomiting, fatigue, lassitude, headache, abdominal discomfort, sometimes followed by jaundice	Symptomatic
Hepatitis, Serum Virus	40 to 160 days	Unknown	Slow onset and little fever except in fatal cases; other symptoms similar to those in infectious hepatitis	Symptomatic
Influenza[a] Virus Type A, Type B, subtypes	24 to 72 hours	Unknown, probably during early and febrile stage	Sudden onset, chills and fever, prostration, aches and pains in back and limbs, coryza, sore throat, bronchitis	Symptomatic; antibiotics for secondary infection
Measles[a] (Rubeola) Virus	7 to 14 days	2 to 4 days before appearance of rash until 2 to 5 days thereafter	Mild fever, malaise, conjunctivitis, coryza, cough, photophobia, Koplik's spots, small reddish-brown or pink macules changing to papules. Rash fades on pressure, begins behind ears (and/or on forehead and cheeks), progresses to extremities in 3 days, lasts about 5 days	Symptomatic; gamma globulin

	Incubation Period	Communicability Period	Symptoms	Treatment
Measles, German[a] (Rubella) Virus	14 to 21 days	From as long as 13 days before onset of rash until 6 days after rash disappears. In the case of newborns infected *in utero*, virus may be recovered from the throat, urine, and/or stool for several months after birth	Malaise, fever, headache, rhinitis, postauricular and postoccipital lymphadenopathy with tender nodes, small pink to pale-red macules fused or closely grouped to give scarlet blush which fades on pressure, disappears within 3 days	Symptomatic
Meningococcus Meningitis (Cerebrospinal Fever) Meningococcus or *Neisseria meningitidis*	2 to 10 days	Indefinite, until meningococci are absent from nose and mouth discharges	Sudden onset, fever, intense headache, stiff neck, nausea, vomiting; frequently petechial rash; delirium and coma	Antibiotics, sulfonamides
Mononucleosis, Infectious (Glandular Fever) Cause unknown	4 to 14 days	Unknown	Acute febrile infection, sore throat, malaise, fatigue, headache, often enlargement of cervical and other lymphatic glands	Symptomatic
Mumps[a] (Infectious Parotitis) Virus	12 to 26 days	From about 7 days before first symptoms appear until swelling subsides	Slight fever, malaise, nausea, irritability; swelling, inflammation, and tenderness of salivary glands	Symptomatic
Pertussis[a] (Whooping Cough) *Bordetella pertussis*	1 to 3 weeks, almost uniformly within 10 days	Greatest in catarrhal stage before onset of paroxysms; organism rarely recovered after fourth week of disease	Coryza, dry tracheal cough which is worse at night; paroxysms of several staccato coughs in one expiration, followed by sudden, rapid, deep inspiration and whoop	Hyperimmune serum; symptomatic; antibiotics may be of value

Disease and Causative Organism	Incubation Period	Period of Communicability	Symptoms	Treatment
Pneumonia (Acute Lobar) Pneumococci	1 to 3 days	Unknown (during infectious discharge)	Acute infection, sudden onset with chills and fever, often pain in chest, usually cough and dyspnea	Antibiotics
Pneumonia, Mycoplasma (Eaton Agent)	7 to 21 days	Unknown	Insidious and variable onset; frequent absence of respiratory symptoms; fatigue, muscle pains, chilliness, feverishness, sometimes cough	Symptomatic; antibiotics
Poliomyelitis[a] (Infantile Paralysis) Virus	1 to 5 weeks	Greatest during late incubation and early days of infection; virus remains in feces for weeks	Acute illness, fever, malaise; variable, but usually include headache and stiffness of neck and spine	Symptomatic
Rabies (Hydrophobia) Virus	From 10 days to 2 years; average 50 to 60 days	In dogs and other animals, for 3 to 5 days before onset of symptoms through clinical course of disease; rarely from man to man	Fulminating encephalitis, inevitably fatal; depression, fever, headache, anorexia, nausea, sore throat, malaise, restlessness, hyperesthesia of skin, hypersensitivity to light and sound; convulsions, paralysis	Rabies vaccine and/or rabies immune globulin when bitten by rabid animal; symptomatic once symptoms occur
Ringworm of the Body Several species of fungi	Unknown	During presence of infection	Circinate scaly patches with miliary vesicles in the active border	Fungicides
Ringworm of the Scalp (Tinea Capitis) Microsporum audouini, M. canis, other fungi	Unknown	During presence of infection	Vary from noninflammatory patches with short, brittle, lusterless, broken hairs to deep dusky-red, baggy, swollen areas of infection	Fungicides or x-ray depilation
Rocky Mountain Spotted Fever Rickettsia rickettsii	3 to 10 days	Not communicable from man to man	Sudden onset with fever, headache, photophobia, muscle and joint pains, and chills; characteristic maculopapular rash, usually first on extremities, rapidly spreads over body	Antibiotics

	Incubation Period	Communicability Period	Symptoms	Treatment
Scabies *Sarcoptes scabiei*	Variable	Until itch mites and ova are destroyed	Characteristic burrows of itch mite, not inflammatory unless scratched; severe itching, especially when warm	Miticides
Scarlet Fever (Scarlatina) Hemolytic streptococci, Group A strains	3 to 5 days	From onset until recovery	Sudden onset, sore throat, fever, headache, nausea, vomiting, rapid pulse. Bright-red uniform rash begins on upper chest 1 to 3 days after onset, spreads rapidly over neck, arms, trunk, and legs; velvety skin	Antibiotics
Smallpox[a] (Variola) Virus	7 to 16 days	From 1 to 2 days before first symptoms until crusts drop off. Crusts are infectious	Abrupt onset, with fever, prostration, chills, headache, myalgia, nausea, vomiting; eruption on thighs and lower abdomen on second or third day followed by true exanthema beginning on face and involving head and extremities more than trunk; duration 3 to 6 weeks	Thiosemicarbazone derivatives shorten clinical course of disease; antibiotics for secondary infections
Syphilis *Treponema pallidum* (*Spirochaeta pallida*)	10 to 90 days	During primary and secondary stages and during mucocutaneous relapses	In acquired infection (usually venereal), ulcer occurs at site of inoculation. Constitutional symptoms and generalized lesions of skin and mucous membranes follow. May recur over several years. Late manifestations (tertiary stage) involve circulatory and central nervous systems	Antibiotics
Tetanus *Clostridium tetani*	2 to 50 days; usually between 5 and 10 days	Not communicable from man to man	Acute infectious disease characterized by stiffness of jaw and fever followed by restlessness, irritability, stiff neck, and difficulty in swallowing; rigidity and convulsions as disease progresses	Antitoxin, sedatives, antibiotics

Disease	Incubation period	Period of communicability	Symptoms	Treatment
Trichinosis *Trichinella spiralis*	1 to 28 days	Not communicable from man to man	Variable. Many infections asymptomatic. About 24 hours after infection, nausea, vomiting, abdominal pain, fever, and severe dysentery sometimes develop. Later, during migration of larvae, malaise, weakness, remittent or intermittent fever, myalgia, sweating, periorbital and facial edema, laryngitis, painful swallowing, striate hemorrhages beneath fingernails, and sometimes cardiac and respiratory difficulty occur in varying severity	Symptomatic and supportive
Tularemia *Pasteurella tularensis*	1 to 10 days	Not communicable from man to man	Sudden onset, chills, fever, prostration, headache, severe malaise. Ulceroglandular type is characterized by pustuloulcerative lesion with regional lymphadenopathy. Typhoidal form has no external lesion but may cause local lesions of mouth or pharynx. Fever, vomiting, severe abdominal pain, and diarrhea	Antibiotics
Typhoid Fever[a] *Salmonella typhosa*	1 to 3 weeks	Indefinite, as long as typhoid bacilli occur in feces or urine	Chills, fever, headache, backache, anorexia, diarrhea or constipation, epistaxis, generalized aching, frequently bronchitis. Rose-colored elevated rash which appears in crops about the seventh day is most abundant on abdomen but also on chest and back. Crops last 2 to 3 days, leaving brownish stains. Delirium, listlessness, photophobia, muscle twitching, and somnolence usually indicate severe infection	Antibiotics

[a] Disease best controlled by prophylactic use of vaccine.

6. Food Poisoning

DIFFERENTIAL DIAGNOSIS OF BACTERIAL ETIOLOGIES FOR DIARRHEA AND FOOD POISONING

Bacterial Diarrhea	Pathogenesis	Fever	Diarrhea	Symptoms – Dysentery	Symptoms – Abdominal Pain	Symptoms – Vomiting	Incubation Period (hr)	Effect of Heat	Age Group	Transmission Pattern	Extra Intestinal Symptoms	Culture
Clostridium perfringens	Enterotoxin	−	+	+	++	±	8–12	Thermostable organism	Adults	Poultry, heat-processed meats (stews)	Volume depletion	Food, stool, vomitus
Escherichia coli	Enterotoxin	−	±	±	±	0	24–72	Somatic-thermostable toxin, capsular-thermolabile toxin	Children	Contact	Volume depletion	Stool
Salmonellae	Bacteria	+	+	±	±	±	12–36	Thermolabile organism	All	Prepared foods, poultry, egg products, pet turtles and chicks	Headache, bacteremia	Food, stool
Shigellae	Bacteria	±	+	+	+	±	24–72	Thermolabile organism, thermolabile toxin	Children	Institutions	Seizures, meningismus	Food, stool

Organism	Toxin						Incubation (hr)	Toxin characteristics	Ages affected	Prepared food	Clinical	Diagnostic specimen
Staphylococci	Enterotoxin	−	+	0	+	+	1–6	Thermostable toxin	All	Prepared food (salami, salads, chicken salad), fowl, pastry	Volume depletion, prostration	Food, stool
Vibrio cholerae	Enterotoxin	±	+	0	±	±	24–72	Thermolabile toxin	All	Water, food	Hypokalemic nephropathy	Stool
Clostridium botulinum	Neurotoxin	−	−	−	±	±	12–36	Thermostable spore thermolabile toxin	All	Honey, diverse canned foods	Dysphagia, respiratory paralysis	Serum stool, vomitus for toxin
Bacillus cereus Type I	Enterotoxin	−	+	−	+	++	1–6	Thermolabile toxin	All	Fried rice	Limited	Food, stool
Type II	Enterotoxin	−	++	−	+	±	10–12	Thermolabile toxin	All	Meats, vegetables	Volume depletion	Food, stool

(Modified after Grady and Keusch, 1971, as reprinted from Goldfrank, L. R.: Toxicologic Emergencies (2nd ed). New York, Appleton-Century-Crofts, 1980, p. 244.)
+, occurs regularly; ±, may or may not occur; 0, does not occur.

7. Intestinal Obstruction

Type	Assessment Parameters	Management
Gastric volulus	Severe abdominal pain Brochardt's triad 1. Vomiting followed by retching and then inability to vomit 2. Epigastric distention 3. Inability to pass naso-gastric tube	Immediate laporatomy to prevent gastric necrosis
Gallstone ileus	Right upper quadrant tenderness and mass Distended abdomen Radiopaque gallstone on x-ray Gas in the biliary tree	Emergency laporatomy with removal of obstructing stone
Pyloric obstruction	Increasing pain Anorexia, vomiting of undigested food No relief from antacids Abdominal x-ray shows large gastric fluid level $\downarrow Na, K, Cl$ $\uparrow NaHCO_3$ Metabolic alkalosis	Nasogastric suctioning 5–7 days Surgery—vagotomy, gastrectomy
Small intestinal obstruction Nonstrangulating obstruction	High small bowel, profuse vomiting, variable abdominal pain Mid or distal: Cramping pain, abdominal pain Vomiting, feculent material Obstipation Abdominal distention Peristalic rushes, gurgles and high pitched tinkles Laboratory findings: Hemoconcentration Leukocytosis X-ray findings: Dilated small bowel loops with air-fluid levels	Decompression with intestinal tubes Surgical procedure after rehydration and electrolyte stabilization

Strangulation obstruction	Shock
	Severe, continuous abdominal pain
	Vomiting—gross or occult blood
	Abdominal tenderness and rigidity
	Marked leukocytosis
	X-ray findings:
	    Thumbprinting, loss of mucosal pattern
	    Dilated bowel—fluid between adjacent loops of bowel
		Surgical procedure after rehydration and electrolyte stabilization

Colonic obstruction	Continuous abdominal pain Constipation, obstipation Late vomiting (feculent material) Abdominal distention, tympany High pitched, metallic tinkles X-ray findings: Distended colon—"picture frame" outline of the abdominal cavity	Surgical decompression and removal of the obstructed segment

8. Acid–Base Nomogram

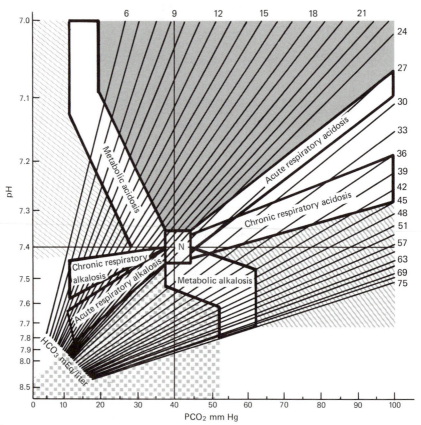

NOTE:

The significance bands for the various simple disorders are labeled on the map. Probable interpretations for points falling in the cross hatched areas between are:

▩ mixed respiratory and metabolic acidosis	▧ mixed metabolic acidosis and respiratory alkalosis
▨ mixed respiratory and metabolic alkalosis	▨ mixed respiratory acidosis and metabolic alkalosis

The lines that fan diagonally from the lower left-hand corner represent serum bicarbonates corresponding to the values given across the bottom and down the left side within the diagram.

A nomogram for the graphical solution of acid–base interrelationships and for converting pH to hydrogen ion concentration. The diagram is based on the Henderson equation $\left[([H^+]) = 24 \dfrac{(Pco_2)}{HCO_3^-} \right]$. Carbon dioxide tension (Pco_2) is shown on the horizontal axis and pH units are shown on the vertical axis. The normal ranges in arterial blood are contained within the shaded square zone near the center of the graph. (*From Flomenbaum, N.: Acid–base disturbances. Emergency Medicine 12(17):27,1980. Adapted from Goldberg, M., Green, S.B., Moss, M.L., et al.: Computer based instruction and diagnosis of acid–base disorders. JAMA 223:269–75, 1973; and Myers, F.J., Pennock, B.E.: The acid–base map—An additional tool for dealing with a difficult problem. Resident Staff Physician 25:49–53, 1979.*)

9. Obstetric Table

Month	1	2	3	4	5	6	7	8	9	10	11	12	13	14	15	16	17	18	19	20	21	22	23	24	25	26	27	28	29	30	31	
Jan.	1	2	3	4	5	6	7	8	9	10	11	12	13	14	15	16	17	18	19	20	21	22	23	24	25	26	27	28	29	30	31	
Oct.	8	9	10	11	12	13	14	15	16	17	18	19	20	21	22	23	24	25	26	27	28	29	30	31	1	2	3	4	5	6	7	Nov.
Feb.	1	2	3	4	5	6	7	8	9	10	11	12	13	14	15	16	17	18	19	20	21	22	23	24	25	26	27	28				
Nov.	8	9	10	11	12	13	14	15	16	17	18	19	20	21	22	23	24	25	26	27	28	29	30	1	2	3	4	5				Dec.
Mar.	1	2	3	4	5	6	7	8	9	10	11	12	13	14	15	16	17	18	19	20	21	22	23	24	25	26	27	28	29	30	31	
Dec.	6	7	8	9	10	11	12	13	14	15	16	17	18	19	20	21	22	23	24	25	26	27	28	29	30	31	1	2	3	4	5	Jan.
April	1	2	3	4	5	6	7	8	9	10	11	12	13	14	15	16	17	18	19	20	21	22	23	24	25	26	27	28	29	30		
Jan.	6	7	8	9	10	11	12	13	14	15	16	17	18	19	20	21	22	23	24	25	26	27	28	29	30	31	1	2	3	4		Feb.
May	1	2	3	4	5	6	7	8	9	10	11	12	13	14	15	16	17	18	19	20	21	22	23	24	25	26	27	28	29	30	31	
Feb.	5	6	7	8	9	10	11	12	13	14	15	16	17	18	19	20	21	22	23	24	25	26	27	28	1	2	3	4	5	6	7	Mar.
June	1	2	3	4	5	6	7	8	9	10	11	12	13	14	15	16	17	18	19	20	21	22	23	24	25	26	27	28	29	30		
Mar.	8	9	10	11	12	13	14	15	16	17	18	19	20	21	22	23	24	25	26	27	28	29	30	31	1	2	3	4	5	6		April
July	1	2	3	4	5	6	7	8	9	10	11	12	13	14	15	16	17	18	19	20	21	22	23	24	25	26	27	28	29	30	31	
April	7	8	9	10	11	12	13	14	15	16	17	18	19	20	21	22	23	24	25	26	27	28	29	30	1	2	3	4	5	6	7	May
Aug.	1	2	3	4	5	6	7	8	9	10	11	12	13	14	15	16	17	18	19	20	21	22	23	24	25	26	27	28	29	30	31	
May	8	9	10	11	12	13	14	15	16	17	18	19	20	21	22	23	24	25	26	27	28	29	30	31	1	2	3	4	5	6	7	June
Sept.	1	2	3	4	5	6	7	8	9	10	11	12	13	14	15	16	17	18	19	20	21	22	23	24	25	26	27	28	29	30		
June	8	9	10	11	12	13	14	15	16	17	18	19	20	21	22	23	24	25	26	27	28	29	30	1	2	3	4	5	6	7		July
Oct.	1	2	3	4	5	6	7	8	9	10	11	12	13	14	15	16	17	18	19	20	21	22	23	24	25	26	27	28	29	30	31	
July	8	9	10	11	12	13	14	15	16	17	18	19	20	21	22	23	24	25	26	27	28	29	30	31	1	2	3	4	5	6	7	Aug.
Nov.	1	2	3	4	5	6	7	8	9	10	11	12	13	14	15	16	17	18	19	20	21	22	23	24	25	26	27	28	29	30		
Aug.	8	9	10	11	12	13	14	15	16	17	18	19	20	21	22	23	24	25	26	27	28	29	30	31	1	2	3	4	5	6		Sept.
Dec.	1	2	3	4	5	6	7	8	9	10	11	12	13	14	15	16	17	18	19	20	21	22	23	24	25	26	27	28	29	30	31	
Sept.	7	8	9	10	11	12	13	14	15	16	17	18	19	20	21	22	23	24	25	26	27	28	29	30	1	2	3	4	5	6	7	Oct.

Numbers shown on the top lines in each section represent the first day of the last menstrual period. Those appearing directly below indicate the probable date of the parturition.

10. Organ Donors

Ideal organ donors are previously healthy individuals who have suffered a total and irreversible cessation of brain function. This may result from:

1. head injury
2. subarachnoid hemorrhage
3. cerebral vascular accident
4. primary brain tumor
5. drug overdose (in some cases)
6. smoke inhalation (in some cases)
7. hepatic coma (the renal failure accompanying this condition is often reversible)
8. anencephalic newborns
9. cardiac arrest

The prospective donor must be free from:

1. sepsis or any active transmissible disease
2. malignant neoplasms (except for primary brain tumor)

DETERMINATION OF BRAIN DEATH

The determination of brain death of a potential organ donor, as with any patient, traditionally remains the clinical judgment of the physician. Strict criteria have been established, however, for determining total and irreversible cessation of brain function when respiration and heart beat are mechanically maintained. The declaration of brain death must be made by two licensed physicians, one of whom will be a Neurology Attending, not affiliated with the transplant team. This provision protects the rights of the potential donor by avoiding conflict of interest by the physicians involved. The primary physician may then pronounce the patient dead.

The following criteria should be met for the determination of brain death:

1. *Deep coma:* The patient must be in deep, unresponsive coma with no movement or response to stimulation (excluding spinal reflexes).
2. *Apnea:* Total lack of spontaneous respirations has to be documented in one of the following ways:
   a. The patient is given room air via respirator for 10 minutes. The respirator is then removed and oxygen is delivered via catheter through the endotracheal or tracheostomy tube at 6 L/minute. Observation must be made for a minimum of 3 minutes off the respirator.
   b. Continuous observation of the patient on the respirator with a nominal arterial P_{CO_2} and no effort to override the machine for 15 minutes.

The material in this section is reprinted courtesy of Downstate Medical Center.

3. *Absence of reflexes:*
   a. The pupils must be fixed and dilated and not respond to a direct source of bright light.
   b. Ocular movements on head turning (oculocephalic reflex) and ice water lavage of the ears (oculovestibular or caloric reflex) are absent.
   c. No corneal reflex.
   d. Swallowing, gagging, yawning, and vocalization are absent.

It must be clearly established that the cessation of brain function is irreversible. This may be obvious in cases of highly evident etiology and extensive discernible brain damage. In such cases, two physicians may be able to determine and pronounce brain death simultaneously.

In less obvious cases an initial stabilization period of 6 hours is suggested from the onset of symptomatology before the initial determination of brain death is made. Furthermore, to establish the irreversibility of total loss of brain function, it is suggested that clinical evaluations be repeated at least 6 hours later.

Every effort must be made to exclude the *reversible* causes of coma. The following categories of patients in coma may have reversible etiology and therefore should not be evaluated for brain death until these conditions are corrected:

1. *CNS depressant drugs:* A toxicology screen may be necessary in strongly suspected cases of drug overdose. In positive cases, 36 to 48 hours are suggested for elimination of the drugs from the body.
2. *Hypothermia:* Less than 90°F.
3. *Metabolic and endocrine disturbances:* Myxedema coma, hypoglycemia coma, diabetic coma, etc. Appropriate diagnostic and therapeutic measures should be taken.

Determination of brain death can be made on clinical criteria alone. However, the following tests may be used for confirmation of the clinical diagnosis:

1. *Electroencephalogram:* The isoelectric EEG is of confirmatory value when drug overdose and hypothermia have been ruled out. Interpretation of the EEG has to be made in conjunction with the totality of the clinical picture.
2. *Cerebral blood flow studies:*
   a. Brain scan
   b. Cerebral arteriography
   Cessation of blood flow to the brian can be safely and expeditiously established by radioisotope studies (brain scan). Cerebral arteriography, on the other hand, is an invasive procedure which carries certain inherent risks.

DONOR MAINTENANCE PROTOCOL

Once brain death has been determined it is imperative to maintain the donor until consents can be obtained and the organs retrieved.

It is important to maintain adequate circulatory volume in order to insure good organ perfusion and urinary output.

SUGGESTED M.D. ORDERS FOR DONOR MAINTENANCE

1. Vital signs q 1 hour
   Notify M.D. If: bp ↓ 100 mmHg
                        pulse ↑ 120/minute
                          or ↓ 70/minute
   (A systolic blood pressure of 100 mmHg or greater is desirable. If necessary, Dopamine is the recommended vasopressor of choice, however, Isuprel, Levophed, or Aramine may be used.)
2. Hourly urine output. Notify M.D. if urine output is less than 50 ml/hour.
   (If hypovolemia has been appropriately corrected as indicated by bp and CVP, and urine output continues to be scanty, a test dose of diuretics, i.e., 25 g Mannitol, IV and 40 mg Lasix IV may be given to induce diuresis.)
3. Record hourly intake and output.
4. Central venous pressure q 1 hour.
   Notify M.D. if CVP: ↓ 10 cm H_2O
                      or ↑ 16 cm H_2O
   (Hypovolemia insidiously develops in patients with brain death, and accounts for nearly 100 percent of all the hemodynamic instability. A central venous catheter should be inserted either by percutaneous technique or by cutdown.)
5. IV fluids for each hour: 5 percent dextrose in Ringer's lactate, to replace previous hour's urinary output plus 40 ml.
   (If patient is becoming hypertensive, 5 percent dextrose in 0.45 saline or 0.33 percent or 0.2 percent saline should be employed. If urine output exceeds 200 ml/hour a diagnosis of diabetes insipidus should be strongly considered and 5–10 units of Pitressin administered subcutaneously.
   Additional fluids may be needed to compensate for pre-existing deficits, particularly in patients where dehydration to reduce cerebral edema has been induced. Test infusions of 250–500 ml of solution in 15 minutes and CVP monitoring is recommended.)
6. CBC, SMA-12 (serum creatinine and blood urea nitrogen), daily.
7. Blood culture × 1 (daily if indicated).
8. Urinalysis daily.
9. Urine culture × 1 (daily if indicated).
10. Sputum culture × 1 (daily if indicated).
11. Blood type, VDRL, and HAA (hepatitis associated antigen) once during hospitalization.
12. Toxicology screen (if indicated).
13. Use hypothermia blanket to maintain temperature ↓100°F and ↑95°F.

Since patients with widespread systemic infections are not considered suitable donors, it is important to take care in avoiding contamination. Rigorous techniques should be employed in catheter, tracheostomy and wound care. However, patients with bacterial infections, such as pneumonia, that can be successfully treated with antibiotics, may be suitable donors if the infection is eliminated prior to the organ retrieval.

MAINTENANCE OF PEDIATRIC DONORS

Pediatric cadaveric kidneys have proven to be at least as good as adult ones for transplantation. Every effort must be made to maintain these potential donors also. Of course the orders for pediatric cases will have to be modified and scaled down. The outstanding problem in the maintenance of pediatric donors as in the adult ones is hypovolemia, therefore the necessity of liberal amounts of IV fluids.

BLOOD SAMPLES

When brain death has been established and it is determined that the patient is a suitable donor, you may be asked to supply the following blood samples for tissue typing and cross-matching procedures prior to the organ procurement:

1. Two (2) 20 ml vials of heparinized blood (total of 40 ml).
2. One (1) 10 ml clotted sample.

CARDIAC ARREST

Even with the most rigorous efforts, the inevitable deterioration of the patient with brain death may lead to cardiac arrest before consent for organ donation may be obtained from the next-of-kin. Recognizing that the grieving family may need some time to make a favorable decision for donation, every reasonable effort to resuscitate the patient and maintain organ perfusion should be employed.

MEDICAL EXAMINER'S CASES

The circumstances of the patient's death may require the medical examiner's permission for removal of organs. Cases falling under the jurisdiction of the medical examiner include:

1. Deaths by homicide or suspicion of homicide
2. Deaths by suicide or suspicion of suicide
3. Deaths due to accidental, traumatic injury
4. All deaths resulting from abortion
5. Deaths from poisoning or suspicion of poisoning
6. Deaths during or immediately following diagnostic, therapeutic, or surgical and/or anesthetic procedures

When in doubt, consult the local medical examiner. In most cases, consent from the medical examiner to remove the donated organs may be obtained over the telephone.

In these cases it is still necessary to obtain the consent from the next-of-kin.

Once death has been pronounced and appropriate consents signed by the next-of-kin, the medical examiner's office should be notified and a case number be obtained. The death certificate and/or medical examiner notification forms should be filled out by the primary physician prior to the organ retrieval, and the hospital admitting office notified as to the time of death.

Once the retrieval has been completed, it is necessary to send copies of the death certificate, next-of-kin consent forms, operative report, and any other information that may be requested to the medical examiner's office. (This may include a microscopic preparation from biopsies of the organs removed.)

ALL OTHER CASES

In all cases death has to be pronounced by two physicians, a death certificate filled out, and the hospital admitting office notified as to the time of death prior to the organ retrieval. An operative report of the organ retrieval should be included in the patient's records.

NEW YORK ANATOMICAL GIFT ACT

Article 43—Anatomical Gifts

4300. Definitions. As used in this section, the following terms shall have the following meanings:

1. "Bank or storage facility" means a hospital, laboratory or other facility licensed or approved under the laws of any state for storage of human bodies or parts thereof, for use in medical education, research, therapy, or transplantation to individuals.

2. "Decedent" means a deceased individual of any age and includes a stillborn infant or fetus.

3. "Donor" means an individual who makes a gift of all or part of his body.

4. "Hospital" means a hospital licensed, accredited, or aproved under the laws of any state and includes a hospital operated by the United States Government, a state, or a subdivision thereof, although not required to be licensed under state laws.

5. "Part" of a body includes organs, tissues, eyes, bones, arteries, blood, other fluids and other portions of a human body, and "part" includes "parts."

6. "Person" means an individual, corporation, government or governmental subdivision or agency, business trust, estate, trust, partnership or association, or any other legal entity.

7. "Physician" or "surgeon" means a physician or surgeon licensed or authorized to practice under the laws of any state.

8. "State" includes any state, district, commonwealth, territory, insular possession, and any other area subject to the legislative authority of the United States of America.

4301. Persons who may execute an anatomical gift.

1. Any individual of sound mind and eighteen years of age or more may give all or any part of his body for any purpose specified in section four thousand three hundred two of this article, the gift to take effect upon death.

2. Any of the following persons, in the order of priority stated, may, when persons in prior classes are not available at the time of death, and in the absence of actual notice of contrary indications by the decedent, or actual notice of opposition by a member of any of the classes specified in paragraphs (a), (b), (c), (d) or (e) give all or any part of the decedent's body for any purpose specified in section four thousand three hundred two of this article:

(a) the spouse,
(b) an adult son or daughter twenty-one years of age or older,
(c) either parent,
(d) an adult brother or sister twenty-one years of age or older,
(e) a guardian of the person of the decedent at the time of his death,
(f) any other person authorized or under the obligation to dispose of the body.

3. If the donee has actual notice of contrary indication by the decedent or that the gift is opposed by a member of any of the classes specified in paragraphs (a), (b), (c), (d) or (e), the donee shall not accept the gift.

4. A gift of all or part of a body authorizes any examination necessary to assure medical acceptability of the gift for the purposes intended.

5. The rights of the donee created by the gift are paramount to the rights of others except as provided by section four thousand three hundred seven of this article.

4302. Persons who may become donees and purposes for which anatomical gifts may be made.
The following persons may become donees of gifts or bodies or parts thereof for the purposes stated:

1. Any hospital, surgeon, or physician, for medical or dental education, research, advancement of medical or dental science, therapy, or transplantation; or

2. Any accredited medical or dental school, college or university for education, research, advancement of medical or dental science, or therapy; or

3. Any bank or storage facility, or medical or dental education, research, advancement of medical or dental science, therapy or transplantation; or

4. Any specific donee, for therapy or transplantation needed by him.

4303. Manner of executing anatomical gifts.

1. A gift of all or part of the body under this article may be made by will. The gift becomes effective upon the death of the testator without waiting for probate. If the will is not probated, or if it is declared invalid for testamentary purposes, the gift, to the extent that it has been acted upon in good faith, is nevertheless valid and effective.

2. A gift of all or part of the body under this article may also be made by document other than a will. The gift becomes effective upon the death of the donor. The

document, which may be a card designed to be carried on the person, must be signed by the donor in the presence of two witnesses who must sign the document in the donor's presence. Delivery of the document of the gift during the donor's lifetime is not necessary to make the gift valid.

3. The gift may be made either to a specified donee or without specifying a donee. If the latter, the gift may be accepted by and utilized under the direction of the attending physician upon or following death. If the gift is made to a specified donee who is not available at the time and place of death, the attending physician upon or following death, in the absence of any expressed indication that the donor desired otherwise, may accept the gift as donee. The physician who becomes a donee under this subdivision shall not participate in the procedures for removing or transplanting a part.

4. Subject to the prohibitions in subdivision two of section four thousand three hundred six the donor may designate in his will, card or other document of gift the surgeon or physician to carry out the appropriate procedures. In the absence of a designation, or if the designee is not available, the donee or other person authorized to accept the gift may employ or authorize any surgeon or physician for the purpose.

5. Any gift by a person designated in subdivision two of section four thousand three hundred one of this article shall be by a document signed by him or made by his telegraphic, recorded telephonic, or other recorded message.

4304. Delivery of document of gift. If the gift is made by the donor to a specified donee, the will, card or other document or an executed copy thereof, may be delivered to him to expedite the appropriate procedures immediately after death delivery is not necessary to validity of the gift. The will, card or other document, or an executed copy thereof, may be deposited in any hospital, bank, storage facility or registry office that accepts it for safekeeping of for facilitation of procedures after death. On request of an interested party upon or after the donor's death, the person in possession shall produce the document for examination.

4305. Revocation of the gift.

1. If the will, card, or other document or executed copy thereof has been delivered to a specified donee, the donor may amend or revoke the gift by:

(a) the execution and delivery to the donee of a signed statement, or
(b) an oral statement of revocation made in the presence of two persons, communicated to the donee, or
(c) a statement during a terminal illness or injury addressed to an attending physician and communicated to the donee, or
(d) a signed card or document, found on his person or in his effects.

2. Any document or gift which has not been delivered to the donee may be revoked in the manner set out in subdivision one of this section or by destruction, cancellation, or mutilation of the document and all executed copies thereof.

3. Any gift made by a will may be revoked or amended in the manner provided

for revocation or amendment of wills or as provided in the subdivision one of this section.

4306. Rights and duties at death.

1. The donee may accept or reject the gift. If the donee accepts a gift of the entire body, he may, subject to the terms of the gift, authorize embalming and the use of the body in funeral services. If the gift is of a part of the body, the donee upon the death of the donor and prior to embalming, may cause the part to be removed without unnecessary mutilation. After removal of the part, custody of the remainder of the body vests in the surviving spouse, next of kin, or other persons under obligation to dispose of the body.

2. The time of death shall be certified by the physician who attends the donor at his death and one other physician, neither of whom shall participate in the procedure for removing or transplanting the part.

3. A person who acts in good faith in accord with the terms of this article or with the anatomical gift laws of another state is not liable for damages in any civil action or subject to prosecution in any criminal proceeding of his act.

4307. Application.
The provisions of this article shall not be deemed to supersede or affect the provisions of the public health law relating to the functions, powers and duties of coroners, coroner's physicians or medical examiners.

11. Bill of Rights for the Emergency Department Client

The emergency department client has the right:

1. To adequate emergency medical care by qualified personnel.
2. To prompt professional assessment and treatment regardless of race, color, creed, sex, national origin, financial resources or political beliefs.
3. To information about diagnosis, prognosis and treatment. These include risks involved and/or alternatives so that he or she and his or her family may give informed consent.
4. To informed participation in all decisions concerning individualized health care. Each patient has the right to determine, without pressure, if he or she will accept the proposed therapy unless the client is medically or mentally unable to make these decisions. In such case the family or legal authorities can be consulted.

Modified from material prepared by Alice W. Deal, R.N., M.S.N., Assistant Professor, Department of Nursing, Old Dominion University, Norfolk, Va., in ETHICON, Point of View, vol. 16, no. 3, 1979, with permission.

5. To be informed of qualifications and identification of the health care team responsible for his or her health care.
6. To refuse observation of those not directly involved in his or her care.
7. To privacy during interview, examination and treatment.
8. To confidential treatment during and concerning emergency care, including communications and records pertaining to care rendered.
9. To refuse treatments, medications or participation in research and experimentation without punitive actions being taken against him or her.
10. To coordination and continuity of health care, including the right to be informed of other health care facilities or educational resources available within the community for correction of the health care problem.
11. To appropriate instruction or education and/or written instruction in reference to his or her illness or injury, to facilitate return to an optimal level of wellness.
12. To select a specialist of the individual's choice as the situation deems necessary. The client also has the right to choose the physician he or she prefers for emergency care.
13. To access to all personal health care records, the right to question the information therein, and a right to have the records corrected for accuracy. Also, the right to have all such records transferred, if necessary, for continuity of care.
14. To be informed prior to the administration of any medication or initiation of any procedure, the name, benefits, the direct and adverse effects involved in such therapy.
15. To receive emotional support and comfort from at least one member of his or her family during treatment and explanations and/or alternatives offered for care. Also the client has the right to expect that his or her family will be informed of the condition, treatment and progress while in the emergency department.
16. To expect a copy of the bill with an explanation or information about charges for services, and the right to challenge these.
17. To be fully informed as to their rights.

12. Pediatric Drug Dosage Calculation

DETERMINATION OF CHILDREN'S DOSES FROM ADULT DOSES ON THE BASIS OF BODY SURFACE AREA

Weight (kg)	Weight (lb)	Approximate Surface Area in Square Meters	Approximate Percentage of Adult Dose[a]
2	4.4	0.15	9
4	8.8	0.25	14
6	13.2	0.33	19
8	17.6	0.4	23
10	22	0.46	27
15	33	0.63	36
20	44	0.83	48
25	55	0.95	55
30	66	1.08	62
35	77	1.2	69
40	88	1.3	75
45	99	1.4	81
50	110	1.51	87
55	121	1.58	91

(*Adapted from Done, A. K.: Drugs for children. In Modell, W. (Ed.): Drugs of Choice, 1970–1971. St. Louis, C. V. Mosby, 1970, p. 48*)
[a] Based on average adult surface area of 1.73 sq M.

13. Radiation Decontamination Procedure

EMERGENCY DEPARTMENT PROCEDURE FOR RADIATION ACCIDENTS

1. *Initial Evaluation.* Although the incidence of injury involving radiation complication is rare, it is possible as a result of nuclear power accidents, transportation, etc. Such patients present special handling problems initially only if they are contaminated (i.e., if they have radioactive material present on the clothing or skin or embedded in wounds. Otherwise they can be initially treated for immediate injury, and radiation injury can be considered later.
2. *Contaminated patients* should be initially treated like isolation patients, the ob-

Reprinted courtesy of Bellevue Hospital Medical Center.

jective being to avoid the spread of contamination while retaining potentially contaminated items for analysis and proper disposal.

a. Restrict patient and personnel movements to avoid spread of contamination.

b. Put on protective clothing such as gloves, gown and mask. Administer urgent first aid if necessary.

c. Keep all clothing and tissue samples removed from the patient in sealed bags or containers.

d. The radiation casualty team will assist in surveying the patient for contamination and decontamination. (If no expert is present and a survey meter is available, check meter operation on battery check scale. Note reading away from any source. Note any significant steady increase in reading as the meter is brought close to the patient or clothing. If a significant increase occurs note whether the contamination is localized by moving the probe slowly over the surface. A small fluctuating reading on the most sensitive scale of the survey meter is normal. Readings on the higher scales indicate that there is significant contamination which should be removed as soon as possible.)

e. If contamination is present set up a controlled area surrounding the area that may be contaminated. Do not permit movement into or out of this area unless essential. Obtain supply of protective clothing (disposable gowns, shoe covers, or operating room clothing as available). Set up changing station at edge of controlled area. Use plastic bags to contain contaminated items.

f. Process to decontaminate using clean soap and water swabs. Discard each swab after use into plastic bag. Avoid the use of instruments that might break the skin.

g. Treat conventional injury as usual with care to avoid spread of contamination. Retain and label all contaminated items for analysis.

PERSONNEL DECONTAMINATION

Method[a]	Surface	Action	Technique	Advantages	Disadvantages
Mixture of 50% Tide and 50% cornmeal	Skin and hands	Emulsifies, dissolves, and erodes	Make into a paste. Use with additional water and a mild scrubbing action. Use care not to erode the skin	Slightly more effective than washing with soap	Will defat and abrade skin and must be used with care
5% water solution of a mixture of 30% Tide, 65% Calgon, 5% Carbose (carboxymethyl cellulose)	Same as above	Same as above	Use with water. Rub for 1 minute and rinse	Same as above	Same as above
A preparation of 8% Carbose, 3% Tide, 1% Versene, and 88% water homogenized into a cream	Same as above	Same as above	Use with additional water. Rub for 1 minute and wipe off. Follow with lanolin or hand cream	Same as above	Same as above
Titanium dioxide paste. Prepare paste by mixing precipitated titanium dioxide (a very thick slurry, never permitted to dry) with a small amount of lanolin. If not successful, go on to next step	Skin, hands, and extremities. Do not use near face or other body openings	Same as above	Work the paste into the affected area for 2 minutes. Rinse and wash with soap and warm water. Monitor	Removes contamination lodged under scaly surface of skin. Good for heavy surface contamination of skin.	If left on too long will remove skin

PERSONNEL DECONTAMINATION

Method[a]	Surface	Action	Technique	Advantages	Disadvantages
Mix equal volumes of a saturated solution of potassium permanganate and 0.2 N sulfuric acid. (Saturated solution of $KMnO_4$ is 6.4)	Skin, hands, and extremities. Do not use near face or other body openings	Dissolves contaminant absorbed in the epidermis	Pour over wet hands, rubbing the surface and using hand brush for not more than 2 minutes. Rinse with water	Superior for skin contamination. May be used in conjunction with titanium oxide	Will remove a layer of skin if in contact with the skin for more than 2 minutes
Apply a freshly prepared 5% solution of sodium acid sulfite. (Solution made by dissolving 5 g of $NaHSO_3$ crystals in 100 ml distilled water.)	Same as above	Removes the permanganate stain	Apply in the same manner as above. Apply for not more than 2 minutes. The above procedure may be repeated. Apply lanolin or hand cream when completed		Same as above
Flushing	Eyes, ears, nose, and mouth	Physical removal by flushing	Roll back the eyelid as far as possible, flush with large amounts of water. If isotonic irrigants are available obtain them without delay. Apply to eye continually and then flush with large amounts of water (Isotonic irrigant [0.9% NaCl solution] 9 g NaCl in beaker, fill to 1000 cc with water). Can be purchased from drug suppliers, etc.	If used immediately will remove contamination. May also be used for ears, nose and throat	When using for nose and mouth, contaminated individual should be warned not to swallow the rinses

	Method	Procedure	Comments	Cautions
Wounds	Physical removal by flushing	Wash wound with large amounts of water and spread edges to stimulate bleeding, if not profuse, stop bleeding first, clean edges of wound, bandage and if any contamination remains, it may be removed by normal cleaning methods, as above	Quick and efficient if wound is not severe	May spread contamination to other areas of body if not done carefully
Sweating	Physical removal by sweating	Place hand or foot in plastic glove or booty. Tape shut. Place near source of heat for 10–15 minutes or until dry	Cleansing action is from inside out. Hand does not dry out	If glove or booty is not removed shortly after profuse sweating starts, the part must be washed with soap and water

Further decontamination should be done under medical supervision

[a] Begin with the first listed method and then proceed step by step to the more severe methods, as necessary.

DECONTAMINATION PROCESS IN CASE OF PATIENT CONTAMINATION

Method[a]	Surface	Action	Technique	Advantages	Disadvantages
Soap and water	Skin and hands	Emulsifies and dissolves contaminate	Wash 2–3 minutes and monitor. Do not wash more than 3–4 times	Readily available and effective for most radioactive contamination	Continued washing will defat the skin. Indiscriminate washing of other than affected parts may spread contamination
Soap and water	Hair	Same as above	Wash several times. If contamination is not lowered to acceptable levels, shave the head and apply skin decontamination methods		
Lava soap, soft brush, and water	Skin and hands	Emulsifies, dissolves, and erodes	Use light pressure with heavy lather. Wash for 2 minutes, 3 times. Rinse and monitor. Use care not to scratch or erode the skin. Apply lanolin or hand cream to prevent chapping	Same as above	Continued washing will abrade the skin
Tide or other detergent (plain)	Same as above	Same as above	Make into a paste. Use with additional water with a mild scrubbing action. Use care not to erode the skin	Slightly more effective than washing with soap	Will defat and abrade skin and must be used with care

[a] Begin with the first listed method and then proceed step by step to the more severe methods, as necessary.

14. Seizure Checklist

Patient's Name _____ I.D. No. _____ Date _____
Time: onset ____ tonic phase ____
    clonic phase ____ completion ____

Pre-Ictal State	Not Observed	Yes	No
1. Was there an aura?	____	__	__
smell?	____	__	__
sound?	____	__	__
sensation?	____	__	__
2. Was there a cry?	____	__	__
3. Did patient fall?	____	__	__

Ictal-State

	Not Observed	Yes	No
1. Eyelids			
Flickering	____	__	__
Open	____	__	__
Closed	____	__	__
2. Pupils			
Dilated	____	__	__
Reactive to light	____	__	__
Nonreactive to light	____	__	__
Staring	____	__	__
3. Head			
Deviated to right	____	__	__
Deviated to left	____	__	__
Facial contorsions	____	__	__
4. Mouth			
Teeth clenched	____	__	__
Jaw clenched	____	__	__
Tongue bitten	____	__	__
Cheek bitten	____	__	__
Lip bitten	____	__	__
Frothing	____	__	__
Drooling	____	__	__
Lip smacking	____	__	__
5. Extremities			
Arms: abducted	____	__	__
adducted	____	__	__
bilateral	____	__	__
unilateral	____	__	__
tonic	____	__	__
clonic	____	__	__
Elbows: flexed	____	__	__
extended	____	__	__
bilateral	____	__	__
unilateral	____	__	__
Hands: suppinated	____	__	__
pronated	____	__	__

	Not Observed	Yes	No
Legs: flexed	____	__	__
extended	____	__	__
bilateral	____	__	__
unilateral	____	__	__
Trunk: rigid	____	__	__
writhing	____	__	__
tremulous	____	__	__
back arched	____	__	__
6. Skin			
Warm	____	__	__
Cool	____	__	__
Moist	____	__	__
Dry	____	__	__
Cyanotic	____	__	__
7. Respirations			
Slow rate	____	__	__
Rapid rate	____	__	__
Apneic	____	__	__
Deep	____	__	__
Shallow	____	__	__
Oral suction required	____	__	__
8. Pulse			
Regular	____	__	__
Irregular	____	__	__
Rapid	____	__	__
Slow	____	__	__
9. LOC			
"Twilight state"	____	__	__
Confused	____	__	__
Excited	____	__	__
Unconscious	____	__	__
Responds to commands	____	__	__
10. Bladder and Bowel			
Loss of urine	____	__	__
Loss of stool	____	__	__
Vomiting	____	__	__
11. Behavior			
Illusions	____	__	__
Hallucinating	____	__	__
Automatisms	____	__	__

(continued)

Post-Ictal State
1. Behavior
   Irritable ⎯⎯ ⎯ ⎯
   Combative ⎯⎯ ⎯ ⎯
   Anxious ⎯⎯ ⎯ ⎯
   Headache ⎯⎯ ⎯ ⎯
   Sleeping ⎯⎯ ⎯ ⎯
   Amnesia ⎯⎯ ⎯ ⎯

Fatigue ⎯⎯ ⎯ ⎯
Muscle soreness ⎯⎯ ⎯ ⎯
2. Vital Signs
   bp ⎯⎯ ⎯ ⎯
   TPR ⎯⎯ ⎯ ⎯

_____
Observer's Signature

(Prepared by Barbara Ann Russo.)

15. Sexual Assault Victim Protocol

TRIAGE NURSE RESPONSIBILITIES

If the patient presents as an alleged sexual assault victim, the triage nurse shall:

1. Escort the patient directly to the GYN room. In cases of severe trauma and/or male victims, escort patient directly to the emergency department examination rooms
2. Assess extent of the patient's injuries and write triage note
3. Notify the crisis counselor
4. Notify emergency department resident and have patient seen as quickly as possible in order to facilitate medical clearance
5. Facilitate the registration process

HEAD NURSE/DESIGNEE RESPONSIBILITIES

Immediately upon notification of the presentation of a rape victim, the head nurse or designee shall:

1. Designate a nursing staff member, to remain with the patient
2. If patient is unescorted by the police, with the patient's consent, notify the police precinct. Please be aware that the patient has the right to refuse police involvement

DESIGNATED NURSE ASSIGNED TO PATIENT

1. Notify GYN of arrival of victim in emergency department
2. Introduce self to patient

_____
Courtesy of Bellevue Hospital Medical Center.

3. Remain with victim until rape counselor is available
4. Note: Do not allow victim to wash or take anything by mouth until the exam is completed
5. Advise patient as to the purpose and procedure for pelvic examination
6. Prepare patient for gynecological examination (take out rape kit, and sexual assault form for physicians)
7. Assist gynecologist
8. Determine with physician the need for other consultations (e.g., social work, psychiatry, or clergy)
9. After the examination:
   a. Arrange for the patient to wash up if he/she wishes
   b. Reinforce instruction given by the physician
   c. Administer, after order is written, prophylactic penicillin (4.8 million units) and Benemid to all victims. In case of allergy to penicillin, have ordered spectinomycin, IM (2 g)
10. Check to see that the sexual assault report form is completed
11. Give to the police officer, if present, all collected evidence. Obtain and record on sexual assault form, the badge number and signature of the receiving officer. *If no police present:* Take collected evidence, with a copy of the assault form, to the administrator, who will notify the appropriate police precinct for pick-up
12. Give to the counselor, before she leaves, one copy of the sexual assault form and the emergency form. The remaining three copies of the sexual assault form are to be distributed as follows:
    a. one to police or administrator with the evidence
    b. one attached to the emergency department record
    c. one to the gynecologist for his/her own records

Note: It is the nurse's responsibility to maintain contact with the patient, counselor, and physician throughout the procedure, to facilitate the process and make it as nontraumatic as possible.

PHYSICIAN RESPONSIBILITIES

1. Refer to guidelines for obtaining the required laboratory data in the GYN room
2. Obtain consent
3. Obtain history from patient
4. Perform a full physical work-up
5. Take VDRL
6. Record examination findings on Sexual Assault Form
7. Obtain vaginal, rectal and oral smears on all female patients. Obtain oral, rectal and urethral smears for male victims
8. Provide necessary treatment to protect patient against V.D. (penicillin, 4.8 million units and Benemid. If allergy to penicillin is suspected, give Spectinomycin 2 g)

9. Complete appropriate lab form, emergency record, sexual assault form, venereal disease reports

RAPE COUNSELOR RESPONSIBILITIES

Primary responsibility is to offer companionship and assurance in response to patient's needs as verbalized by the patient and/or observed by the companion.
    The counselor will:

1. Introduce self to police officer and inquire how police may be contacted re: evidence collection/transportation
2. Proceed to the examination room and introduce self/explain role to the patient
3. *Note:* Do not allow the victim to wash or take anything by mouth prior to the exam
4. Listen to the patient, providing a milieu for ventilation and communication
5. Evaluate patient's needs
6. Offer appropriate crisis intervention to patient/family/friend directly as a consultant
7. Contact male crisis counselor to assist with victim's husband/boyfriend/father when appropriate. The male counselor may wish to contact a female counselor in the reverse situation
8. Assist the patient in making necessary contacts (family, friends, etc.). If someone will be coming to the hospital, instruct them to bring a change of clothing and hygiene items
9. Remain with the patient during the entire hospital period
10. Arrange for transportation home. If family unavailable, taxi fare may be obtained from administration

Prior to Discharge
1. Remain in contact with assigned nurse as to the progress and disposition of the patient
2. Double check assault form for completion and be sure that the patient is given V.D. prophylaxis (including signatures by the doctor and person obtaining evidence), social work appointment in 1 week, and nurse practitioner's appointment in 3 weeks

SPECIMEN COLLECTION FOR SEXUAL ASSAULT VICTIMS

Blood work	VDRL
Nail scrapings	
External exam	Wood's lamp (if available) to look for dried semen. Clip hair and put in labeled jar
	Comb pubic hair. Put specimen in labeled bag
	All samples must be done in duplicate
Internal exam	Swab slide for motile sperm (microscope in PES)
Vaginal	PAP
	Cervical (1)
	Vaginal pool (2)
	GC
Rectal	Swab for motile sperm (2)
	GC
Oral	Swab for motile sperm (2)
	GC
	2 × 2 saturated with saliva to check for secretions

BELLEVUE HOSPITAL CENTER
SUSPECTED SEXUAL ASSAULT REPORTING FORM

Patient's I.D. Number: _____

Instructions:
1. Request immediate consult with the Department of OBS/GYN or other appropriate department.
2. If patient not with a police officer and consents, call police.

I. Identification

Name of Patient: Date: Time Admitted to E.R.:   Sex: Date of Birth:

_____   _____   _____ A.M. _____ P.M.   ____   _____

Address   Telephone   Contact if no phone

_____   Day: _____   Name: _____

_____   Eve: _____   Telephone: _____

_____

II. Consents

I, _____ hereby authorize Dr.(s) _____
   (Print Name)   (Print Name(s))
and the medical staff of Bellevue Hospital Center to perform a physical examination and administer routine treatment to me on the basis thereof.

I do ( ) do not ( ) authorize the hospital to supply laboratory specimens and copies of all medical reports pertinent to this visit to the police department and district attorney's office having jurisdiction. Additionally, the consequences of releasing the aforementioned materials have been fully explained to me in the language I understand.

Patient's Signature:_____   Date:_____

Parent or Guardian Signature: _____   Address: _____

Witness Signature and Title: _____   Address: _____

(continued)

III. Responding Police Officer

Name of Officer: _____   Precinct: _____   Shield No.: _____   Precinct Complaint No.: _____

IV. Physical Examination

Time begun _____ A.M. _____ P.M.   Has the patient bathed, washed, or urinated since the suspected assault. ( ) No   ( ) Yes

Chief complaint (in patient's own words) _____

Is the patient bruised?   Is the patient lacerated?   Has patient any tender areas?
( ) No   ( ) Yes   ( ) No   ( ) Yes   ( ) No   ( ) Yes
Describe: _____   Describe: _____   Describe: _____

Note all other signs of physical trauma not covered by pelvic, rectal, oral examinations.

Pelvic/Rectal/Oral Examination

Instructions: 1. Include all signs of trauma.
2. Note size and development of patient's organs, bleeding, lacerations, and tenderness.
3. Speculum examination: Inspect cervix and vagina with a non lubricated, warm speculum.

		Female	**Male**
Genital	Vulva:	_____	_____
	Vagina:	_____	_____
	Hymen:	_____	_____
	Cervix:	_____	_____
	Fundus:	_____	_____
	Adnexae Left:	_____	_____
	Right:	_____	_____
Rectal		_____	_____
Oral		_____	_____

V. Laboratory Specimens (Evidential)

Take wet mount of material from fornix and cervix. Examine this preparation immediately, note findings:

Instructions:
1. Label all specimens collected for evidence with
    A. Patient's I.D. number and name
    B. Anatomical location taken from
2. Properly protected slides and swabs may be placed in the same evidence envelope along with clothing only.

Take at least three slides of material: two from the vaginal pool and one from the cervix. Allow sufficient streaking to permit analysis. "Fix" slides. Label slides with a diamond pencil, place in protective containers and place in the evidence envelope.

Were specimens taken?   ( ) Yes   ( ) No

Place swabs used for streaking slides in the tubes provided. Label tubes with a diamond pencil, seal the open ends of the tube with tape over the cork. Initial tape with indelible ink. Place in the evidence envelope. Were specimens taken? ( ) Yes   ( ) No

Clothing as Evidence

Instructions:

1. Articles of clothing may only be used as evidence if the patient consents to the release of evidence to the police department and/or the district attorney's office having jurisdiction on part II of this form and if the patient consents to their relinquishment at the time of the visit.
2. Articles of clothing taken in conformance with (1) above must be labeled conspicuously with the patient's I.D. number and name.
3. If more than one article of clothing is taken as evidence, each additional article must be placed in a separate evidence envelope.

Place article(s) of clothing that may be sperm stained and/or used as evidence in the evidence envelope(s) after labelling.

Were such articles obtained ( ) Yes   ( ) No   Number of articles ( )

Instructions:

1. The examining physician must seal the evidence envelope(s) and sign in the space provided over the flap also noting in the space provided the number of slides, swabs, and/or articles of clothing it contains.

VI. Treatment Record

	Yes	No	(Specify drug and dosage)
Was the patient given			
Tetanus toxoid?	( )	( )	
Prophylactic (e.g. for Venereal Disease)	( )	( )	
Other medication?	( )	( )	
Pregnancy prevention drug?	( )	( )	
Was surgical/laceration repair required?	( )	( )	(Describe in detail)
Was the patient given written instructions for victim of sexual assault?	( )	( )	
Was patient admitted to hospital?	( )	( )	

VII. Referral

	Yes	No
Will patient see private physician for follow-up care.	( )	( )

If yes, complete the information required below

Name: _____   Address: _____   Telephone: _____

_____
_____

VIII. Conveyance of Evidence

Instructions:

1. Place signed and sealed evidence envelope(s) in the plain manila envelope with copies 3 and 4 of the hospital report–suspected sexual assault form.
2. Give the plain manila envelope containing the signed and sealed evidence envelope(s) and copies 3 and 4 of the hospital report–suspected sexual assault form to the police or to nursing to be locked away until police pick up.

Specimens given to: _____   Title: _____   Organization: _____

_____
Examining Physician's Signature

16. Shock Syndrome Chart

IDENTIFICATION OF DEGREE OR SEVERITY OF SHOCK

Test or Sign	Normal or Average	Preshock State to Mild Shock	Degree of Shock		
			Moderate	Moderately Severe to Severe	
Sensorium					
Orientation	Well-oriented time/place/person	Oriented	Fairly well oriented	May be confused and dis-oriented	
Enunciation	Distinct	Normal—slurred words	Somewhat slowed and few slurred words	Slow and slurred to mono-syllabic utterances and groans	
Content	Appropriate; structured sentences	Sentences normal	Slow sentences or phrases and words	Often incoherent	
Pupils					
Size	Equal (2–4 mm)	Normal	Normal	Normal to dilatating or dilated	
Constriction with light	Rapid	Rapid	Rapid	Slow or nonreactive	
Pulse					
Rate	60–100/minute	110–120/minute	120–150/minute	Maximal	
Amplitude	Full	Full amplitude to slight de-crease	Variable: mild decrease	Thready	
Blood pressure (mm. of Hg.)					
Systolic	120–145	Normal or slightly low	Decreased—often 40–50 mm. of Hg below usual bp	Less than 80 to unobtain-able	
Diastolic	60–90	Normal or slightly low	Decreased, but less so than systolic	40 to 50 to unobtainable	

	40–70	30–40	20–30	Less than 20
Pulse pressure				
Jugular vein filling Patient flat	Fills to anterior border of sternocleidomastoid muscle	Normal to trace of filling	Trace to no filling	No filling
		May be full in septic shock or grossly distended in cardiogenic shock		
Urinary output via catheter				
ml/minute	0.6–1.5	0.6–0.8	0.4–0.6	0.3 or less
ml/10 minutes	6–15	6–8	4–6	3 or less
Tilt test—Rapid lying to sitting position				
Pulse	Transient increase	Increased	Rapid	Already maximal
Blood pressure	Less than 10 mm decrease	10–25 mm decrease	25–50 mm decrease	Marked decrease to unobtainable
Symptoms	No "lightheadedness"	No lightheadedness	Lightheadedness	Unable to sit up
Therapeutic, if whole blood loss	—	Probably do not transfuse	Transfuse!	Transfuse!
Estimated blood loss	—	To 750 ml	1000 to 1250 ml	1500 to 1750 ml or more
Estimated % blood volume loss	—	15%	20–25%	More than 30–35%
Capillary blanching test Blanching of forehead skin with thumb pressure	Return of circulation in 1.25–1.5 seconds	1.25–1.5 seconds	More than 1.5 seconds	Pallor before and after test
		Note: With hypercapnea, there may be almost instantaneous return		
Central venous pressure	Normal (3–8 cm of saline)	Normal	Low	Extremely low
		May be elevated in cardiogenic shock		

(Reprinted with permission from Flint, T., and Cane, H.D.: Emergency Treatment and Management (4th ed.). Philadelphia, W. B. Saunders, 1970, pp. 546–547.)

17. Tetanus Prophylaxis

A GUIDE TO PROPHYLAXIS AGAINST TETANUS IN WOUND MANAGEMENT (Based on American College of Surgeons Protocol)

General Principles

1. The physician must determine for each patient with a wound, individually, what is required for adequate prophylaxis against tetanus.
2. Regardless of the active immunization status of the patient, meticulous surgical care, including removal of all devitalized tissue and foreign bodies, should be provided immediately for all wounds. Such care is essential as part of the prophylaxis against tetanus.
3. Each patient with a wound should receive absorbed diphtheria tetanus toxoid (dt) intramuscularly at the time of injury, either as an initial immunizing dose, or as a booster for previous immunization, unless he has received a booster or has completed his initial immunization series within the past five (5) years. As the antigen concentration varies in different products, specific information on the volume of a single dose is provided on the label of the package.
4. Whether or not to provide passive immunization with tetanus immune globulin (human) must be decided individually for each patient. The characteristics of the wound, conditions under which it was incurred, its treatment, its age, and the previous active immunization status of the patient must be considered.
5. To every wounded patient, give a written record of the immunization provided, instructing him to carry the record at all times, and, if indicated, to complete active immunization. For precise tetanus prophylaxis, an accurate and immediately available history regarding previous active immunization against tetanus is required.
6. Basic immunization with adsorbed diphtheria tetanus toxoid requires three injections. A booster of absorbed diphtheria tetanus toxoid is indicated 10 years after the third injection or 10 years after an intervening wound booster. All individuals, including pregnant women, should have basic immunization and indicated booster injections.

TETANUS PROPHYLAXIS

A. Uncertain immunization, not previously immunized, or one known dose of tetanus toxoid
   1. Clean, minor wounds—0.5 cc Td as a booster or as initial injection of series.
   2. All other wounds—Give
      a. 0.5 cc Td
      b. 250 units of tetanus immune globulin (TIG)
      c. Deliver with separate syringes at different sites

    d. Consider antibiotics

    e. Debridement.

B. Previously actively immunized with two (two doses of adsorbed, three doses of fluid toxoid) or more doses of tetanus toxoid

    1. Clean, minor wound—No booster necessary

    2. All other wounds—If >5 years since last dose, give 0.5 cc Td.

C. Previously actively immunized with tetanus toxoid more then ten years ago.

    1. Clean, minor wounds—0.5 cc Td.

    2. All other wounds—0.5 cc Td.

    3. Dirty wounds >24 hours old—Add 250 units antitoxin; consider prophylactic antibiotics.

D. Basic immunization (adult) (initiated in the EMS, completed in the OPD)

    1. Give one dose 0.5 cc adsorbed dT toxoid.

    2. 4 to 6 weeks later—0.5 cc adsorbed dT toxoid. If the wound remains unhealed at 4 weeks, a second dose of TIG should be given.

    3. 6 to 12 months later—0.5 cc adsorbed dT toxoid.

    4. Every 10 years give 0.5 cc dT.

E. Basic immunization (children)

    1. 2 months—DPT #1.

    2. 4 months—DPT #2.

    3. 6 months—DPT #3.

    4. 18 months—DPT booster.

    5. 4 to 6 years—DPT booster.

    6. Every 10 years—dT.

F. Consideration of complications

    1. Toxoid

        a. Frequent tetanus toxoid boosters have been associated with urticaria, angioneurotic edema, Arthus-like reactions and excessively high anti-toxin levels.

        b. Local reactions include swelling and erythema, a low grade fever may occur. Both types of symptoms are effectively treated with *aspirin*.

    2. Human antitoxin

    Does not manifest the risks of anaphylaxis or serum sickness noted with horse and bovine anti-toxin.

18. Sexually Transmitted Diseases

TREATMENT OF SEXUALLY TRANSMITTED DISEASES

Type or Stage	Drugs of Choice	Dosage	Alternatives
Gonorrhea			
Urogenital	Tetracycline HCl	500 mg oral qid × 5 days	Doxycycline 100 mg oral bid × 5 days
	or Penicillin G procaine plus probenecid	4.8 million U IM[a] once	Spectinomycin 2 g IM once
		1 g oral once	Cefoxitin 2 g IM once plus probenecid 1 g oral once
	or Amoxicillin plus probenecid	3 g oral once	Cefotaxime 1 g IM once
		1 g oral once	
Anal			
Women	As for urogenital	As for urogenital	
Men	Penicillin G procaine plus probenecid		Spectinomycin 2 g IM once
Pharyngeal	Tetracycline HCl[b]	As for urogenital	Amoxicillin 3 g oral plus probenecid 1 g oral followed by amoxicillin 500 mg oral qid × 2 days
	or Penicillin G procaine plus probenecid	As for urogenital	
Pelvic inflammatory disease[c]			
Outpatients	Tetracycline HCl	500 mg oral qid × 10 days	Doxycycline 100 mg oral bid × 10 days
	or Penicillin G procaine plus probenecid followed by amoxicillin	As for urogenital	
		500 mg oral qid × 10 days	
	or Amoxicillin plus probenecid followed by amoxicillin	As for urogenital	
		500 mg oral qid × 10 days	
Hospitalized patients	Penicillin G crystalline	20 million U IV daily until improvement	Tetracycline HCl 250 mg oral qid[b,d] IV until improvement, then 500 mg oral qid[b] to complete 10 days
	followed by amoxicillin	500 mg oral qid to complete 10 days	

Condition	Treatment	Dosage	Alternative
Acute epididymitis	Tetracycline HCl	500 mg oral qid × 10 days	Doxycycline 100 mg oral bid × 10 days
	or Penicillin G procaine plus probenecid followed by amoxicillin	As for urogenital	
	or Amoxicillin plus probenecid followed by amoxicillin	500 mg oral qid × 10 days As for urogenital	
Bacteremia and arthritis	Penicillin G crystalline followed by amoxicillin	10 million U IV daily × 3 days 500 mg oral qid × 4 days	Tetracycline 500 mg oral qid[b] × 7 days Spectinomycin 2 g IM bid × 3 days Erythromycin 500 mg oral qid × 7 days
Meningitis	Penicillin G crystalline	At least 10 million U IV daily for at least 10 days	Chloramphenicol 4–6 g/day for at least 10 days
Endocarditis	Penicillin G crystalline	At least 10 million U IV daily for at least 3 to 4 weeks	
Neonatal Ophthalmia	Penicillin G crystalline plus saline irrigation	50,000 U/kg/day IV in 2 doses × 7 days	
Arthritis and septicemia	Penicillin G crystalline	75,000 to 100,000 U/kg/day IV in 2 or 3 doses × 7 days	
Meningitis	Penicillin G crystalline	100,000 U/kg/day IV in 3 or 4 doses for at least 10 days	
Children (under 45 kg) Urogenital, anal and pharyngeal	Amoxicillin plus probenecid	50 mg/kg oral once 25 mg/kg (max. 1 g) once	Spectinomycin 40 mg/kg IM once Tetracycline (over 8 years old) 10 mg/kg/day oral qid × 5 days
	or Penicillin G procaine plus probenecid	100,000 U/kg IM once 25 mg/kg (max. 1 g) once	
Arthritis	Penicillin G crystalline	100,000 U/kg/day IV × 7 days	Tetracycline (over 8 years old) 10 mg/kg/day oral qid × 7 days Erythromycin 50 mg/kg/day oral in 4 divided doses × 7 days

TREATMENT OF SEXUALLY TRANSMITTED DISEASES

Type or Stage	Drugs of Choice	Dosage	Alternatives
Meningitis	Penicillin G crystalline	250,000 U/kg/day IV in 6 divided doses for at least 10 days	Chloramphenicol 100 mg/kg/day IV for at least 10 days
Syphilis			
Early (primary, secondary, or latent less than 1 year)	Penicillin G benzathine or Penicillin G procaine	2.4 million U IM[a] once 600,000 U IM/day × 8 days	Tetracycline 500 mg oral qid × 15 days Erythromycin 500 mg oral qid × 15 days
Late (more than one year's duration, cardiovascular)	Penicillin G procaine or Penicillin G benzathine	600,000 U IM/day × 15 days 2.4 million U IM[a] weekly × 3 doses	Tetracycline 500 mg oral qid × 30 days Erythromycin 500 mg oral qid × 30 days
Neurosyphilis	Penicillin G crystalline or Penicillin G procaine	2 to 4 million U IV q 4 hours × 10 days 1.2 million U IM/day × 15 days	Tetracycline 500 mg oral qid × 30 days Erythromycin 500 mg oral qid × 30 days
Congenital			
CSF normal	Penicillin G benzathine	50,000 U/kg IM once	
CSF abnormal	Penicillin G crystalline	25,000 U/kg IM or IV bid for at least 10 days	
	or Penicillin G procaine	50,000 U/kg IM daily for at least 10 days	
Chlamydia trachomatis			
Urethritis or Cervicitis	Tetracycline HCl or Erythromycin	500 mg oral qid × 7 days 500 mg oral qid × 7 days	Doxycyline 100 mg oral bid × 7 days Sulfisoxazole 500 mg oral qid for 10 days
Pelvic inflammatory disease[c]			
Outpatients	Tetracycline HCl	500 mg oral qid × 10 days	Doxycycline 100 mg oral bid × 10 days
Hospitalized patients	Tetracycline HCl	250 mg IV qid until improvement, then 500 mg oral qid to complete 10 days	Doxycycline 100 mg IV bid until improved, then 100 mg oral bid to complete 10 days
Epididymitis	Tetracycline HCl	500 mg oral qid × 10–14 days	Doxycycline 100 mg oral bid × 10–14 days

Condition	Drug	Dosage	Alternative
Oculogenital syndrome	As for urethritis		
Proctitis	Tetracycline or erythromycin	500 mg oral qid for 14 days	
Neonatal			
Ophthalmia	Erythromycin	10 mg/kg oral or IV qid × 14 days	Sulfisoxazole 100 mg/kg/day oral or IV in divided doses (for children over 4 weeks old)
Pneumonia	Erythromycin	10 mg/kg oral or IV qid × 14 days	
Lymphogranuloma venereum	Tetracycline HCl	500 mg oral qid^b × 21 days	Sulfisoxazole 1 g oral qid × 21 days; Erythromycin 500 mg oral qid × 21 days
Vaginitis			
Trichomoniasis	Metronidazole	2 g oral once or 250 mg oral tid × 7 days	
In pregnancy	Clotrimazole	2 100-mg vaginal tablets every night at bedtime × 7 days	
Nonspecific vaginitis	Metronidazole	500 mg oral bid × 7 days	Ampicillin 500 mg oral qid × 7 days
Vulvovaginal candidiasis	Clotrimazole	100 mg intravaginally every night at bedtime × 7 days	Nystatin 100,000 units intravaginally qhs × 14 days
	or Miconazole	2% cream, 5 g intravaginally every night at bedtime × 7 days	
Chancroid	Trimethoprim-sulfamethoxazole	Two tablets^e bid × 14 days	Erythromycin 500 mg oral qid × 14 days; Tetracycline 500 mg oral qid^b × 7–14 days

(*Reprinted from The Medical Letter on Drugs and Therapeutics, 24:31–32, March 19, 1984, copyright © 1982, The Medical Letter, Inc. Used with permission.*)

^{a} Divided into two injections at one visit.
^{b} Or doxycycline 100 mg bid.
^{c} Pelvic inflammatory disease may be caused by several different pathogens and may require multiple antibiotics.
^{d} Adjust dosage if renal function is depressed.
^{e} Each tablet contains 80 mg trimethoprim and 400 mg sulfamethoxazole.

19. Mast Trousers

ANTI-SHOCK TROUSERS MAY SUPPORT LIFE—DEFLATE WITH CARE

- Never deflate unless experienced with anti-shock trousers.
- Never allow deflation by untrained personnel.
- Never deflate prematurely. Wait for qualified clinician to take charge.
- Never deflate quickly except for *immediate* surgery.
- Never remove anti-shock trousers before proper deflation.
- Before deflation: Monitor blood pressure every 3 to 5 minutes. If indicated:

    Start IV fluid therapy

    Monitor ECG

    Take x-rays

    Assemble standby surgical and anesthesiology teams.
- How to deflate:

    Obtain approval from attending physician with anti-shock trouser experience

    Continue blood-pressure monitoring

    Deflate slowly, abdomen section first if multi-chambered

    Stop deflation when systolic pressure drops 5 mm Hg. Resume after IV fluids restore blood pressure level

    If blood pressure fails to recover, complete deflation in operating room with surgical attendance.

INDEX

Page numbers followed by f indicate figures; followed by t indicate tables.

Antispasmodic drugs, in croup, 191
Aortic dissection, hypertension in, 256, 258, 259*t*, 260, 277
Aortic rupture, traumatic, 275–278
Aortography, 256, 276
Apomorphine, in poisonings, 459, 461
Apothecary equivalents, 481*t*–482*t*
ARDS. *See* Adult respiratory distress syndrome
Arginine hydrochloride, in metabolic acidosis, 430
Argyle chest catheter
    in hemothorax, 264
    in pneumothorax, 262
    in tension pneumothorax, 266
Arrhythmias. *See also specific type*
    in cardiac tamponade, 273
    drugs for. *See* Antiarrhythmic drugs; *specific name*
    in myocardial contusions, 271, 272
    in myocardial infarction, 250, 251, 252*t*–253*t*
Arsenic ingestion, 458*t*
Arteriography, in gastrointestinal bleeding, 282
Arteriovenous (AV) malformations, 88*t*–89*t*, 94
Ascariasis, 508*t*
Aspirin ingestion, 419, 458*t*
Assault and battery, 471, 474
Assessment. *See also* Triage
    systems, 4–7
Asthma, 198. *See also* Status asthmaticus
Aspiration. *See also* Near drowning
    freshwater, 207, 208, 209, 213
    seawater, 207, 208
Atrial arrhythmias, 252*t*, 253*t*
Atrial fibrillation, 250, 252*t*
Atropine, in myasthenia gravis, 157
Autoimmune process, cell-mediated, in Guillain-Barré syndrome, 141–142
AV malformations, 88*t*–89*t*, 94

B

Bacillus cereus food poisoning, 515*t*
Back pain, clinical algorithm for, 16
Bacteremia, in bacterial meningitis, 130–131

Barbiturate(s)
    in cranicerebral trauma, 115
    in near drowning, 214
    poisoning, 458*t*
Basilar skull fracture, 102*t*, 107
Battery, 471, 474
Beck triad, in cardiac tamponade, 273
Beta-blockers, 248. *See also specific name*
Beta-hydroxybutyrate (BOHB)-acetoacetate (AcAc) ratio, 367, 368, 418
Beta-stimulating drugs, in shock, 83
Bicarbonate
    in diabetic ketoacidosis, 371
    in metabolic acidosis, 422–425
    in near drowning, 213
    in renal failure, acute, 312
    in respiratory acidosis, 433, 434
    in respiratory alkalosis, 439, 440
    in status asthmaticus, 204
    in status epilepticus, 176
Bicarbonate ion
    gain, 425, 426, 427
    loss, 419–420, 421, 424
Bill of rights, patients', 527–528
Bladder
    in spinal shock, 121, 125
    trauma, 295, 296
Bleeding. *See* Hemorrhage
Blood chemistry, normal values of, 486*t*–489*t*
Blood loss, estimating, 281
Blood pressure, in children, average, 61
Blood replacement
    in abdominal trauma, 298
    in abortion, imminent and inevitable, 317
    in adult respiratory distress syndrome, 226
    in aortic rupture, 277
    in cardiac tamponade, 274
    in ectopic pregnancy, 325
    in flail chest, 269
    in gastrointestinal bleeding, 283
    in hemothorax, 264
    in near drowning, 214
    in peritonitis, 288
    in placenta abruptio, 322